Structure and Function of
Plant Genomes

NATO Advanced Science Institutes Series

A series of edited volumes comprising multifaceted studies of contemporary scientific issues by some of the best scientific minds in the world, assembled in cooperation with NATO Scientific Affairs Division.

This series is published by an international board of publishers in conjunction with NATO Scientific Affairs Division

A	**Life Sciences**	Plenum Publishing Corporation
B	**Physics**	New York and London
C	**Mathematical and Physical Sciences**	D. Reidel Publishing Company Dordrecht, Boston, and London
D	**Behavioral and Social Sciences**	Martinus Nijhoff Publishers The Hague, Boston, and London
E	**Applied Sciences**	
F	**Computer and Systems Sciences**	Springer Verlag Heidelberg, Berlin, and New York
G	**Ecological Sciences**	

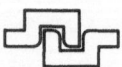

Structure and Function of Plant Genomes

Edited by

Orio Ciferri

Department of Genetics and Microbiology
University of Pavia
Pavia, Italy

and

Leon Dure III

University of Georgia
Athens, Georgia

Plenum Press
New York and London
Published in cooperation with NATO Scientific Affairs Division

Proceedings of a NATO Advanced Study Institute on
Structure and Function of Plant Genomes,
held August 23–September 2, 1982,
at Porto Portese, Italy

Library of Congress Cataloging in Publication Data

NATO Advanced Study Institute on Structure and Function of Plant Genomes (1982:
   Porto Portese, Italy)
   Structure and function of plant genomes.

(NATO advanced science institutes series. Series A, Life sciences; v. 63)
   "Published in cooperation with NATO Scientific Affairs Division."
   "Proceedings of a NATO Advanced Study Institute on Structure and Function of Plant
Genomes, held August 23–September 2, 1982, at Porto Portese, Italy"—Verso t.p.
   Includes bibliographical references and index.
   1. Plant genetics—Congresses. 2. Molecular biology—Congresses. 3. Gene expres-
sion—Congresses. I. Ciferri, Orio. II. Dure, Leon III. Title. IV. Title: Plant genomes. V.
Series.
QK981.N37 1982   581.1′5   83-3955

ISBN 978-1-4684-4540-4
DOI 10.1007/978-1-4684-4538-1   ISBN 978-1-4684-4538-1 (eBook)

© 1983 Plenum Press, New York
Softcover reprint of the hardcover 1st edition 1983

A Division of Plenum Publishing Corporation
233 Spring Street, New York, N.Y. 10013

PREFACE

       This volume contains the presentations of the principal
speakers at the NATO Advanced Study Institute held at Porto
Portese, Italy,23 August - 2 September, 1982. This meeting was the
third in a series devoted to the molecular biology of plants. The
initial meeting was held in Strasbourg, France in 1976 (J. Weil
and L. Bogorad, organizers), and the second in Edinburgh, Scotland
in 1979 (C. Leaver, organizer). As in these previous meetings, we
have attempted to cover the major topics of plant molecular biology
so as to promote the integration of information emerging at an
accelerating rate from the various sub-disciplines of the field.
In addition, we have introduced several topics, unique to higher
plants, that have not yet been approached with the tools of molecular biology, but that should present new and important aspects
of plants amenable to study in terms of DNA $\rightarrow$ RNA $\rightarrow$ Protein.

       This meeting also served to inaugerate the new International
Society for Plant Molecular Biology. The need for this society is,
like the NATO meetings themselves, an indication of the growth,
vitality and momentum of this field of research.

       In our opinion the Italy meeting maintained the tradition of
exciting, catalytic science and of camaraderie and goodwill that
characterized the previous two meetings. We are indebted to the
participants for this. We appreciate greatly the financial support
of the following organizations: NATO, FEBS, IUBS, The British
Council, Italian CNR, AGS, Inc., Agrigenetics, Monsanto, ARCO
Plant Cell Research, Cetus Madison, Chevron Chemical, Zoecon,
Dupont, Phytogen, U.S. NSF and DOE, University of Georgia, Istituto
per il Diritto allo Studio di Universitario Pavia, Istituto G.
Donegani S.p.A., Farmitalia Carlo Erba, Ing. G. Terzano & C. S.p.A.,
Beckman Analytical S.p.A., Banca Popolare di Novara, F.I.A.T. Auto
S.p.A., Boehringer Mannheim GmbH and ICI. Without their support
this meeting could not have taken place. Further, we are indebted
to the young faculty and graduate students of the University of
Pavia for their diligent, selfless handling of the administrative

and logistic aspects of the conference. And finally, we all were fortunate that we were able to gather in the magnificent Lake Garda area of northern Italy.

We hope that this volume will prove useful in broadening and sharpening our perspective of how plants manage the information in DNA sequence so as to develop, function and reproduce.

                                        Orio Ciferri
                                        Leon Dure

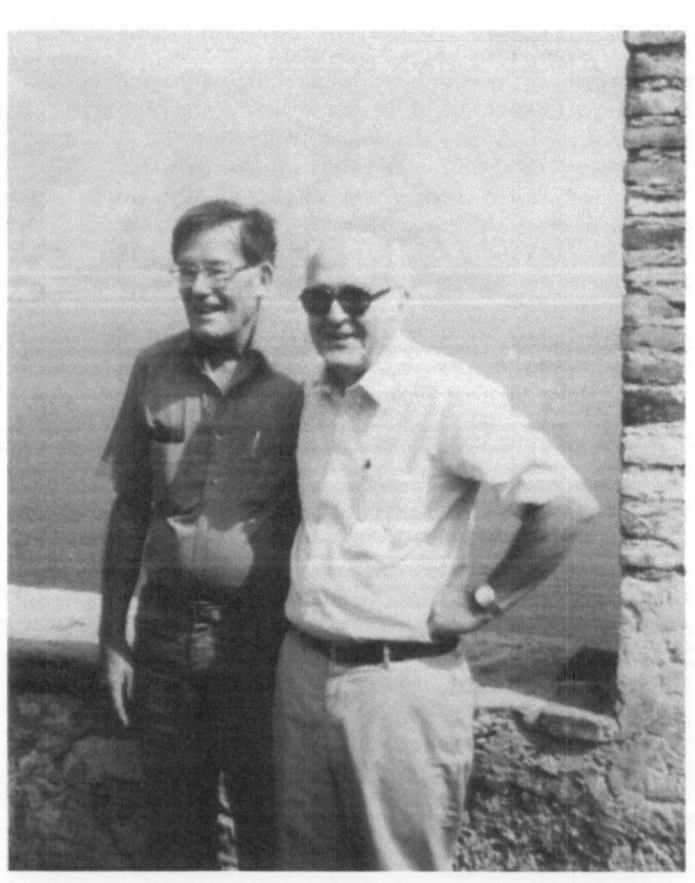

CONTENTS

MOLECULAR BIOLOGY OF PLANT STORAGE PROTEINS

ORGANIZATION AND EXPRESSION OF THE CHLOROPLAST GENOME

SPECIAL TOPICS

REPEATED SEQUENCES AND GENOME ARCHITECTURE

R. B. Flavell

Plant Breeding Institute
Trumpington
Cambridge CB2 2LQ, England

INTRODUCTION

The nuclear genome can be defined as the complement of all
the DNA sequences found in the chromosomes. How the sequences are
arranged with respect to one another, and how they are organised
into chromosomes determines the architecture of the genome. In
this paper I wish to summarise some general features of plant
genome architecture and its evolution, putting special emphasis
on the role played by repeated nucleotide sequences.

The importance of repeated sequences in plant genomes was
evident from the time when they were first shown to constitute a
large proportion of the DNA, especially in plants with larger
genomes (Britten and Kohne, 1968; Flavell et al., 1974). Fig. 1
shows the mass of DNA fragments renaturing in solution with
kinetics that imply they are present in greater than approximately
50 copies per haploid genome, in selected genomes varying in DNA
content (Flavell, 1980). The results show that (1) in species with
DNA contents above 2 pg, greater than 75% of the DNA behaves as
repeated and (2) most of the excess (secondary, Hinegardner, 1976)
DNA which has accumulated in larger genomes consists of repeats.
Therefore the variation in DNA content between species is predominantly (but not exclusively) due to repeated sequences. These
assays of repeated sequence DNA content are underestimates because
they fail to include sequences which originated by amplification
but have subsequently diverged and so behave as unique sequences
(Thompson and Murray, 1980). Furthermore they do not include
sequences which are reiterated only a few times per haploid genome
or which are reiterated but too short to form stable DNA duplexes.

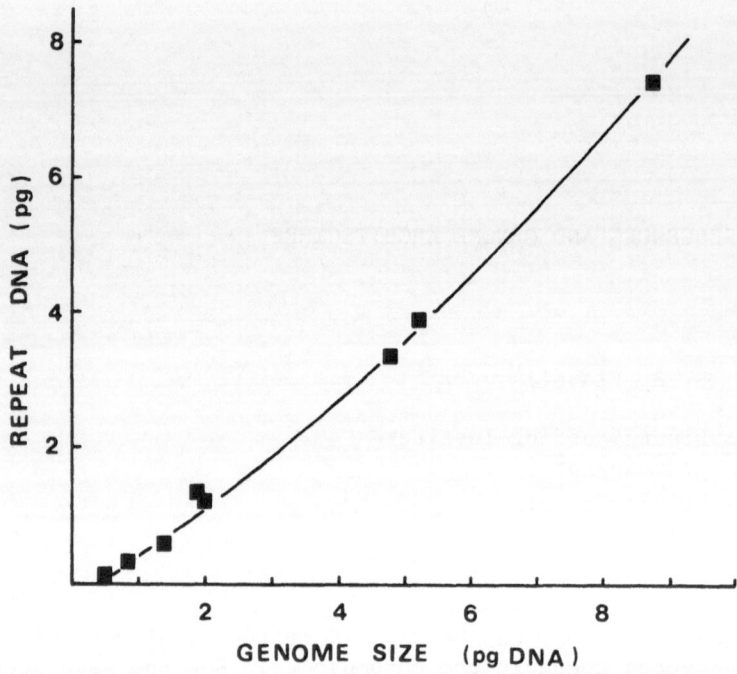

Figure 1. Mass of repeat DNA in plant genomes of different sizes.
The results are replotted from percentage values given in Flavell,
1980. The specific species studies are listed in Flavell, 1980.

Clearly, much of the DNA structure of plant chromosomes is
determined by repeated sequences, especially in species with high
DNA contents.

Classification of repeated sequences

        During the first decade following the discovery of repeated
sequences, it was common to classify them by their copy number in
the genome as calculated from renaturation kinetics (Britten and
Kohne, 1968). This classification has many shortcomings because
it reveals nothing about the structure of the repeats, their
organisation or evolution and is misleading because related DNA
segments are often part of different repeating units (Bedbrook et
al. 1980a,b; Flavell et al., 1979). With the advent of the use of
DNA sequencing, restriction endonucleases and molecular cloning it
became possible to describe the structure and arrangement of repeats
more precisely (e.g. Bedbrook et al., 1980a,b: Appels et al., 1982;
Dennis et al., 1980; Deumling, 1981). As more information of this
kind is gathered a general classification of repeated sequences is
evolving:

(a) <u>Tandem arrays of closely related repeating units</u>.   This
arrangement of repeats is typical of those in highest copy number.
The arrays often lie in chromatin structure recognised as heterochromatic (John and Miklos, 1979), which stains strongly with
Giemsa after denaturation treatments.   The repeating units can be
a few base pairs (Dennis et al., 1980; Deumling, 1981) or
thousands of base pairs (e.g. Bedbrook et al., 1980b).

(b) <u>Multigene families</u>. Many (if not most) genes are present in
multiple copies that are clustered in complex loci (see other
contributions to this volume). Not all of the genes are
necessarily transcribed. Some may be pseudogenes.

(c) <u>Dispersed repeat families</u>. This is the least well defined
and most heterogeneous class. It contains repeat families that
are involved in chromosome pairing and recombination (Stern and
Hotta, 1978) and also probably replication origins (Flavell, 1980).
Hopefully, further research will lead to the recognition of other
defined classes.

     Substantial proportions of plant genomes (>50% in cereals,
Flavell et al., 1981) consist of dispersed families of repeats.
The members of each family occur in a plethora of permutations with
other short repeats and non-repeated sequences. To illustrate
this kind of sequence arrangement the structure of a piece of DNA,
cloned at random from the wheat genome, is shown in figure 2.

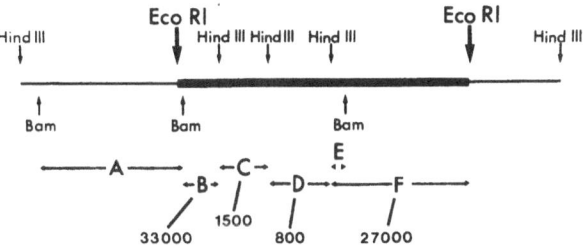

Figure 2. Restriction map of an EcoRI fragment cloned from the
wheat genome. The copy numbers of each subfragment per haploid
<u>Triticum</u> <u>monococcum</u> genome were determined by renaturation
kinetics (see Flavell et al., 1981).

Using Bam HI and Hind III various subfragments (B→F) were cloned separately and used as probes to analyse the fragment further (Flavell et al., 1981). Each of the subfragments shows no homology with any other, yet each belongs to a repeated sequence family within the wheat genome. The approximate copy-number of each type of sequence in a diploid wheat (<u>Triticum</u> <u>monococcum</u>) genome was estimated by renaturation kinetics and is also shown in Figure 2. The different copy number of each sequence within a species and also between several closely related genomes (Flavell et al., 1981) indicates that the sequences in fragments B→F belong to families which have evolved separately in wheat chromosomes.

Many of the sequences homologous to fragment D lie in 1100 base pair Hind III fragments in the wheat genome, just as they do in the cloned example in figure 2. This has been determined by hybridisation of the cloned fragment D to a Hind III digest of total DNA (Flavell et al., 1981; Flavell, 1982). However, the 1100 base pair sequences are dispersed among a large number of different neighbouring sequences in the genome because sequence D hybridises to a wide array of different length fragments when total DNA is cleaved with Eco RI (which does not cut the 1100 base pair sequence).

All of the information we have obtained on the piece of DNA from the wheat genome shown in fig. 2, implies it was constructed by the recombination of several short pieces of DNA. Other examples of similarly complex pieces of repeated DNA have been described by Bedbrook et al. (1980b).

Dispersed repeats appear to be in transposable elements (Burr and Burr, 1982). This may be the means by which complex pieces of DNA, built up from smaller units, have been dispersed around the genome. Clearly DNA complexes that function as transposable elements in certain situtations can be expected to exist in all plant genomes, but many regions of complex DNA permutations may be remnants of transposable elements and no longer capable of being activated to move.

Repeated sequence DNA and the organisation of chromosomes in the nucleus

The mass of nuclear DNA is correlated with many phenotypic characters, for example, minimum mitotic cycle time, meiotic cycle time, cell (Martin, 1966) and pollen volume (Evans et al., 1972; Bennett, 1972; Cavalier Smith, 1978). Therefore it would appear that repeated sequence DNA affects the phenotype by being the major contributor to total DNA mass. It may also affect the spatial organisation of the chromosomes within the nucleus. Recent studies on cereal species by Bennett (1982) have indicated that the

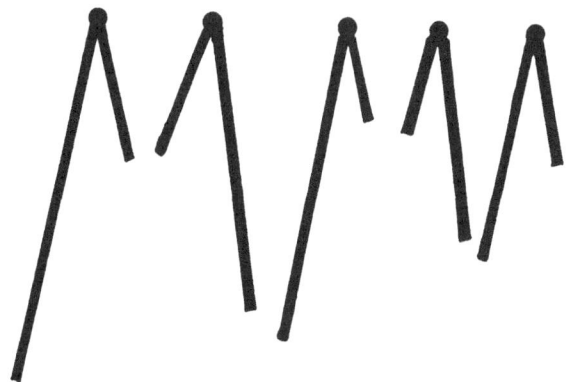

Figure 3. A diagram to illustrate how metaphase chromosomes of a plant (2n=10) are arranged with respect to one another in the nucleus after the model of Bennett (1982). The haploid set of chromosomes are arranged in a chain so that arms of most similar length are adjacent.

chromosomes are arranged in the nucleus in haploid sets, with each chromosome having specific nearest neighbour chromosomes. This chromosome order, detected at somatic metaphase, can be predicted by arranging the chromosomes in a linear array such that chromosome arms of most similar size lie next to one another, as shown in figure 3. If the DNA content of a chromosome arm regulates the position of a metaphase chromosome with respect to other chromosomes in a haploid set, then repeated sequence DNA is a major determinant of chromosome order because it constitutes most of the DNA in many species.

The biological implication of metaphase chromosome order still awaits discovery. Whether an association between similar-sized chromosome arms is maintained during interphase is unknown. If an association of chromosome arms is important for reasons relating to gene function then the relative amount of repeated sequence DNA in each chromosome arm could influence interchromosomal association of genes. If chromosome order is important the relative amounts of repeated DNA in the relevant arms would be expected to be maintained during evolutionary changes in genome size. This is frequently observed in comparisons between related species within a genus.

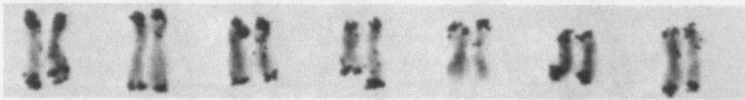

Ae. longissima

Figure 4. Localisation of arrays of a 120 base pair repeat unit
in the chromosomes of <u>Aegilops longissima</u>. The <u>in situ</u> hybridisation was carried out by J. Jones, as described in Jones and
Flavell (1982a,b) using a 120 base pair repeat unit described in
Bedbrook et al. (1980a).

<u>The organisation of arrays of related repeats within the genome</u>

     The localisation of major arrays of closely related repeated
sequences has been determined by <u>in situ</u> hybridisation in several
species (e.g. Bedbrook et al., 1980a; Jones and Flavell, 1982a,b;
Gerlach and Peacock, 1980; Hutchinson and Lonsdale, 1982; Appels
et al., 1982; Deumling, 1981; Deumling and Greilhuber, 1982).
Arrays of the same sequence are frequently found around the centro-
meres, at the telomeres, or interstitially at similar distances away
from the centromere. The localisation of arrays of a 120 bp repeat
unit in <u>Aegilops longissima</u> is shown in fig. 4 as an example. These
results provide proof that members of tandem arrays of repeated
sequences move between chromosomes and provoke the question why are
related repeats often found at similar positions on some or all of
the chromosomes ? Are these sites the only ones where these
particular arrays of sequences are tolerated or where they serve a
specific function ? An alternative explanation is that the distribution reflects how chromosomes physically interact in the
nucleus. If chromosomes do lie in specific positions with respect
to one another and can exchange DNA, say by double crossovers, then
the prediction is that arrays of the same sequence would lie at
similar distances from the centromere on neighbouring arms. To put
it another way, once an array has been formed on one chromosome, a
segment of it has a much higher probability of being transferred to
the equivalent position on its nearest neighbouring arm (this arm
could be the other arm of the same chromosome or of a non-homologous
chromosome) than to any other chromosome arm. To test the hypothesis
it will be necessary to examine where arrays of similar repeats are
localised on chromosomes whose order in the nucleus has been

established. Some support for the hypothesis has already been
gained from analysing the distribution, determined by in situ
hybridisation, of four different arrays or repeats in Secale
cereale (Jones and Flavell, 1982a; Bennett, 1982). Chromosomes
with the most similar hybridisation patterns tend to be adjacent.
However, more data are available from Giemsa banding patterns.
Giemsa bands form at the location of arrays of repeated sequences
(John and Miklos, 1979; Jones and Flavell, 1982a,b) so it is
permissible to use such data. However, because all Giemsa bands
within a species do not contain the same repeats it will be
necessary to learn which bands contain the same repeats before the
Giemsa banding patterns can be unequivocally interpreted.

     Schweizer and Ehrendorfer (1982) have recently discussed the
position of Giemsa bands in several higher plant species, which
provide support for the hypothesis. Some supporting molecular
data are described later. Cytological evidence for the association
of regions of chromosomes carrying the same repeats is available
for many species, including rye (Thomas and Kaltsikes, 1976; Appels
et al., 1982). A new framework for interpreting the distribution
of arrays of repeats in plant genomes is therefore beginning to
emerge which includes the physical association of non-homologous
chromosomes, non-homologous being defined by behaviour at meiosis.

Concerted Evolution of Repeats

     Separate regions of the genome do not evolve independently
of all other regions. The architectural features of different
regions sometimes evolve together if they carry related repeated
DNA sequences. This is because families of repeated sequences
often evolve 'in concert' (Zimmer et al., 1980).

     The phenomenon in plants is best illustrated, with currently
available data, by the repeating units coding for the 18S, 5.8S
and 25S ribosomal RNAs which are organised in tandem arrays at
the nucleolus organisers. From surveys of the structure of the
repeating units present in nucleolus organisers within and between
different wheat plants, it is clear that many different lengths of
repeating unit are present within the species (Fig. 5). The
variation is conveniently recognised by studying BamHI and EcoRI
double digests of total DNA and detecting the rDNA fragments by
hybridisation with ^{32}P labelled rDNA. As shown in figure 5 the
BamHI and EcoRI sites lie within the coding regions. The 3.6 Kb
BamHI-BamHI fragments include parts of the 18S and 25S genes and
the internal transcribed spacer. These fragments are the same
length in all genes in all strains examined. The BamHI-EcoRI
fragments, which include the nontranscribed spacer, are however of
very different lengths in different varieties. The variation in
length of the nontranscribed spacer is due principally to different

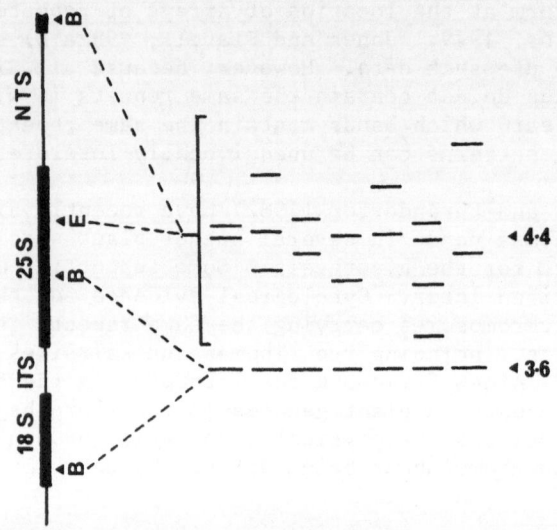

Figure 5. Variation in ribosomal DNA repeat unit length in wheat.
The principal rDNA restriction fragments for BamHI (B) and EcoRI
(E) are shown for 7 different varieties of wheat. NTS = nontranscribed spacer. ITS = internal transcribed spacer. The
fragment sizes shown are in kilobase pairs.

numbers of copies of a small subrepeat localised within the
spacer. Variation in the copy number of this subrepeat probably
results from unequal crossing over between units within the array
of subrepeats.

The presence of many length variants within the species
implies that such variation does not reduce viability and is not

eliminated by selection. However, when individual nucleolus
organisers are examined, a wide array of length variants is not
found. Instead most of the repeating units are of one or a
small number of lengths. This is implied by the similar stoichiometry of the 3.6 Kb BamHI fragments and the BamHI-EcoRI rDNA
fragments (figure 5). Thus most of the repeat units within an
array are much more homogeneous than between arrays.

The homogenisation of repeating units within an array
(concerted evolution) can result from unequal crossing over
between whole repeat units (Smith, 1976; Szostak and Wu, 1980;
Petes, 1980) and by gene conversion (Baltimore, 1981; Klein and
Petes, 1981). The rate of homogenisation of the arrays in wheat
is clearly considerably higher than the production of new length
variants by unequal crossing over within arrays of subrepeats.

Unequal crossing over not only results in the homogenisation
of repeats in an array. It also creates variation in the number
of repeats in the array (Smith, 1976). The number of ribosomal
DNA repeat units at homologous nucleolus organisers in different
plants is very variable (Flavell and Smith, 1974) which suggests
that unequal crossing over is at least partly responsible for the
homogenisation.

Other regions of chromosomes which consist of tandem arrays
of a repeat unit are also usually maintained relatively homogeneous
and differ in DNA content between individuals. This variation in
DNA content can often be observed after staining chromosomes with
Giemsa which highlights regions of tandem arrays of repeats
(Schweizer and Ehrendorfer, 1982).

Separate arrays containing the same sequence also evolve in
concert. This has been concluded from finding, for example, that
ribosomal RNA genes on separate chromosomes are more homogeneous
than would be expected if they evolved independently. Arrays of
a 480 bp repeat unit on different rye chromosomes have also been
shown to possess mutations in a similar frequency, implying homogenisation between chromosomes (Bedbrook et al., 1980a; Appels et
al., 1982). The homogenisation of unlinked sequences is probably
via conversion. Scherer and Davis (1980) and Mikus and Petes
(1982) have provided direct evidence for interchromosomal conversion of genes in yeast.

These examples imply that interactions of related repeated
DNA sequences throughout the genome may be commonplace during
evolution and thus lend further weight to the notion that
different chromosomes interact as suggested above to explain the
movement of sequences from one chromosome to another. The examples
also emphasize that separate regions of the genome do not evolve
independently.

Table 1.   Percentage Homologies between the Repeated
            DNAs of Related Cereal Species

	Wheat	Rye	Barley	Oats
Wheat	100	78	43	20
Rye	70	100	51	26
Barley	59	62	100	28
Oats	19	23	27	100

The percentages are calculated from data in Flavell et al.,
(1977). The % homologies were determined by DNA/DNA
hybridisation between short fragments at 60°C in 0.18 M Na^+.
The data include sequences in >50 copies per haploid genome.

The Repeated Sequence Complement of a Species Evolves Rapidly during Evolution

Comparisons between the repeated sequences of related species
which have diverged from a common ancestor, show that the repeated
sequence complement of a genome changes rapidly during evolution.
The proportions of related repeated sequences in wheat, rye,
barley and oats which diverged from a common ancestor are shown in
Table 1.   The estimates are considerable overestimates of genome
homology because many of the repeats found in more than one species
are present in different copy numbers and are organised differently
in the different species.   Furthermore the sequences are only
related, not identical between species (Flavell, 1982; Rimpau
et al., 1978).   The changes are brought about by the amplification
of sequences to form new tandem arrays, by the dispersal of repeats
around the genome, by deletion of DNA and by the concerted
evolution of repeated DNA families.   These processes result in a
"turnover" of chromosomal DNA during evolution (Flavell, 1979, 1980;
Thompson and Murray, 1980;   Dover et al., 1982).

We are still ignorant of the mechanisms by which sequences are
amplified, deleted and dispersed in the genome. Many of the
mechanisms may act because of the presence of repeated sequences.
Not only is it important to establish how each of these kinds of
mutations occurs in an individual but also how the DNA products are
subsequently fixed in populations of individuals. Selection and
drift are likely to have played major roles in the fixation process
but other processes can be considered where repeats are involved.
Certain repeated sequences, like transposable elements, can become

fixed in a population because of their ability to be duplicated and transferred to other chromosomes. Unequal crossing over between repeats in arrays can also result in the fixation of new variants (see above). Directed gene conversion can homogenise unlinked as well as linked sequences and could therefore be another means of fixing new variants in a population (Nagylaki and Petes, 1980). These sorts of mechanisms, all of which work by stochastic processes to modify the frequency of specific repeated sequences in a population in the absence of selection, have been discussed by Dover (1982) under the heading of "molecular drive". The possibility of fixation of variants of repeats in a population by molecular drive is a particularly intriguing aspect of repeated sequence biology because it suggests that specific chromosomal changes can be established in species without selection or drift.

Thus repeated sequences not only create much of the architecture of the plant genome but also may predispose it to instability and change during evolution. The role of this instability and change in generating phenotypic variation is likely to be a major topic of plant genome research in the coming decades.

REFERENCES

Appels, R., Dennis, E. S., Smyth, D. R., and Peacock, W. J., 1981, Two repeated DNA sequences from the heterochromatic regions of rye (Secale cereale) chromosomes, Chromosoma (Berl.), 84:265-277.
Baltimore, D., 1981, Gene conversion: some implications for immunoglobulin genes, Cell 24:592-594.
Bedbrook, J. R., Jones, J., O'Dell, M., Thompson, R. D. and Flavell, R. B., 1980a, Molecular characterisation of telomeric heterochromatin in Secale species, Cell 19: 545-560.
Bedbrook, J. R., O'Dell, M. and Flavell, R. B., 1980b, Amplification of rearranged sequences in cereal plants, Nature 288: 133-137.
Bennett, M. D., 1972, Nuclear DNA content and minimum generation time in herbaceous plants, Proc. R. Soc. Lond. B 181: 109-135.
Bennett, M. D., 1982, Nucleotypic basis of the spatial ordering of chromosomes in eukaryotes and the implications of the order for genome evolution and phenotypic variation, in: "Genome Evolution", G. A. Dover and R. B. Flavell, eds., Academic Press, London.
Britten, R. J. and Kohne, D. E., 1968, Repeated sequences in DNA, Science 161:529-540.
Burr, B. and Burr, F. A., 1982, Ds controlling elements of maize at the shrunken locus are large and dissimilar insertions, Cell 29:977-986.

Cavalier-Smith, T., 1978, Nuclear volume control by nucleoskeletal
        DNA, selection for cell volume and cell growth rate and
        the solution of the DNA C-value paradox, J. Cell Science
        34:247-278.
Dennis, E. S., Gerlach, W. L. and Peacock, W. J., 1980, Identical
        polypyrimidine polypurine satellite DNA in wheat and
        barley, Heredity 44:345-366.
Deumling, B., 1981, Sequence arrangement of a highly methylated
        satellite DNA of a plant, Scilla : a tandemly repeated
        inverted repeat. Proc. Nat. Acad. Sci. 78:338-342.
Deumling, B. and Greilhuber, J., 1982, Characterisation of
        heterochromatin in different species of the Scilla siberica
        group (Liliaceae) by in situ hybridisation of satellite
        DNAs and fluorochrome banding, Chromosoma 84:535-555.
Dover, G. A., 1982, Molecular drive: a cohesive mode of species
        evolution, Nature 299:111-117.
Dover, G. A., Brown, S., Coen, E., Dallas, J., Strachan, T. and
        Trick, M., 1982, The dynamics of genome evolution and
        species differentiation, in "Genome Evolution", G. A. Dover
        and R. B. Flavell, eds., Academic Press, London.
Evans, G. M., Rees, H., Snell, C. L. and Sun, S., 1972, The
        relationship between nuclear DNA amount and the character-
        isation of the mitotic cycle, in "Chromosomes Today"
        Longman, London 3:24-31.
Flavell, R. B., 1980, The molecular characterisation and organisa-
        tion of plant chromosomal DNA sequences. Ann. Rev. Plant
        Physiol. 31:569-596.
Flavell, R. B., 1982, Amplification, deletion and rearrangement;
        major sources of variation during species divergence,
        in "Genome Evolution", G. A. Dover and R. B. Flavell, eds.
        Academic Press, London, pp 301-324.
Flavell, R. B., Bennett, M. D., Smith, J. B. and Smith, D. B.,
        1974, Genome size and the proportion of repeated nucleotide
        sequence DNA in plants. Biochemical Genetics 12:257-269.
Flavell, R. B., O'Dell, M. and Hutchinson, J., 1981, Nucleotide
        sequence organisation in plant chromosomes and evidence for
        sequence translocation during evolution, Cold Spring Harbor
        Symp'm Quant. Biol. 45:501-508.
Flavell, R. B., Rimpau, J. and Smith, D. B., 1977, Repeated sequence
        DNA relationships in four cereal genomes, Chromosoma (Berl.)
        63:205-222.
Flavell, R. B., Rimpau, J., Smith, D. B., O'Dell, M. and Bedbrook,
        J. R., 1979, The evolution of plant genome structure, in
        "Plant Genome Organisation and Expression", C. J. Leaver,
        ed., Plenum Press, pp 35-47.
Flavell, R. B. and Smith, D. B., 1974, Variation in nucleolus
        organiser rRNA gene multiplicity in wheat and rye,
        Chromosoma (Berl.) 47:327-334.
Gerlach, W. L. and Peacock, W. J., 1980, Chromosomal locations of
        highly repeated DNA sequences in wheat, Heredity 44:269-276.

Hinegardner, R., 1976, Evolution of genome size, in "Molecular
    Evolution", F. J. Ayala, ed., Sinaver Associates Inc. Mass.
    pp 179-199.
Hutchinson, J. and Lonsdale, D., 1982, The chromosomal distribution
    of cloned highly repetitive sequences from hexaploid wheat,
    Heredity 48, 371-376.
John, B. and Miklos, G. L. G., 1979, Functional aspects of hetero-
    chromatin and satellite DNA, Int. Rev. Cytol. 58:1-114.
Jones, J. D. G. and Flavell, R. B., 1982a, The organizing of
    highly repeated DNA families and their relationship to C
    bands in chromosomes of Secale cereale, Chromosoma, in press.
Jones, J. D. G. and Flavell, R. B., 1982b, The structure, amount
    and chromosomal localisation of defined repeated DNA
    sequences in species of the genus Secale, Chromosoma, in
    press.
Klein, H. L. and Petes, T. D., 1981, Intrachromosomal gene
    conversion in yeast, Nature 289:144-148.
Martin, P. G., 1966, Variation in the amounts of nucleic acids in
    the cells of different species, Exp'l Cell. Res. 44:84-90.
Mikus, M. D. and Petes, T. D., 1982, Recombination between genes
    located on non-homologous chromosomes in Saccharymyces
    cerevisiae, Genetics 101:369-404.
Nagylaki, T. and Petes, T. D., 1982, Intrachromosomal gene
    conversion and the maintenance of sequence homogeneity
    among repeated genes, Genetics 100:315-337.
Petes, T. D., 1980, Unequal meiotic recombination within tandem
    arrays of yeast ribosomal DNA genes, Cell 19:765-774.
Rimpau, J., Smith, D. B. and Flavell, R. B., 1978, Sequence
    organisation analysis of the wheat and rye genomes by
    interspecies DNA/DNA hybridisation, J. Molec. Biol. 123:
    327-359.
Scherer, S. and Davis, R. W., 1980, Recombination of dispersed
    repeated DNA sequences in yeast, Science 209:1380-1384.
Schweizer, D. and Ehrendorfer, F., 1982, Evolution of C band
    patterns in Asteraceae-Anthemideae, Biol. Zbl., in press.
Smith, G. P., 1976, Evolution of repeated DNA sequences by unequal
    crossover, Science 191:528-535.
Stern, H. and Hotta, Y., 1978, Regulatory mechanism in meiotic
    crossing over, Ann. Rev. Plant. Physiol. 29:415-436.
Szostak, J. W. and Wu, R., 1980, Unequal crossing over in the
    ribosomal DNA of Saccharomyces cerevisiae, Nature 284:
    426-430.
Thomas, J. B. and Kaltsikes, P. J., 1976, A bouquet-like attachment
    plate for telomeres in leptotene of rye revealed by
    heterochromatin staining, Heredity 36:155-162.
Thompson, W. F. and Murray, M. G., 1980, Sequence organisation in
    pea and mung bean DNA and a model for genome evolution,
    in "Fourth John Innes Symposium", D. R. Davies and D. A.
    Hopwood, eds., John Innes Institute, Norwich, U.K.,
    pp 31-45.

Zimmer, E. A., Martin, S. L., Beverley, S. M., Kan, Y. W. and
    Wilson, A. C., 1980, Rapid duplication and loss of genes
    coding for the α chains of hemoglobin, Proc. Nat. Acad. Sci.
    USA, 77:2158-2162.

DIFFERENTIAL INDUCTION OF mRNAs BY LIGHT AND ELICITOR

IN CULTURED PLANT CELLS

Klaus Hahlbrock, Alain M. Boudet, Joe Chappell,
Fritz Kreuzaler, David N. Kuhn and H. Ragg

Biologisches Institut II der Universität
Schänzlestraße 1, D-7800 Freiburg, FRG

INTRODUCTION

UV irradiation and invasion by microbial pathogens are two potential dangers to which plants must respond by the rapid induction of appropriate defense reactions. A large body of evidence indicates that more than one biochemical pathway is activated in the process of active defense, particularly in the case of microbial attack. At present, however, we are far from understanding - even from being able to enumerate - all of the individual reactions which participate in the complex entirety of the various defense mechanisms against phytopathogens. On the other hand, it is possible, though not known with certainty, that the response to UV irradiation involves fewer biochemical reactions than the response to pathogenic organisms. At least in some cases, partially identical reactions take place in the two responses. One such example is the subject of our present studies.

We are using cultured parsley cells (Petroselinum hortense) to investigate some of the major defense reactions triggered by UV irradiation or treatment with a phytopathogen. For studies of basic induction mechanisms, cell cultures offer very valuable advantages in comparison with intact plants. However, it is important that one is always aware of the limitations of such artificial systems. For example, it is of great value that large amounts of comparatively homogeneous cell populations can be propagated in culture within a few days. Growth conditions can be precisely controlled and easily

15

manipulated for regulatory studies of biosynthetic pathways. In the ideal case, a cell culture is a system
where the high complexity of the biochemical responses
triggered by a certain treatment is reduced to a single
pathway. One such example, where light induces flavonoid biosynthesis, is discussed below.

The second example, the induction of phytoalexins
with a so-called "elicitor" fraction from a phytopathogen, is a typical demonstration of both the value and
the limitations of the use of cell-culture systems.
Here, all cells and cell aggregates of the culture are
treated with the elicitor and can exhibit a response
which, in the intact plant, is limited to a relatively
small number of cells surrounding the area of infection.
Thus, although basic studies of phytoalexin induction
are greatly facilitated by the use of cell cultures, it
is doubtful whether cultured cells show all of the various responses occurring in cells from infected tissue
in intact organisms.

INDUCTION OF PHENYLPROPANOID PATHWAYS

Flavonoids are among the most characteristic and
widely occurring classes of phenylpropanoid derivatives
in higher plants. They serve a variety of functions, including the protection of sensitive tissue against damage by UV irradiation (1,2).

Phytoalexins are antimicrobial substances produced
by plants in response to microbial infection or treatment with an elicitor (3,4). Some phytoalexins, including the furanocoumarins in parsley, are phenylpropanoid
derivatives bearing structural similarities with flavonoids, although the occurrence of furanocoumarins in
higher plants is much less universal (5). Figure 1 depicts the common biosynthetic origin of flavonoids and
furanocoumarins. 4-Coumaroyl-CoA, a product of general
phenylpropanoid metabolism (the 'cinnamate pathway'),
is the central intermediate in both biosynthetic routes.

Two groups of enzymes (designated as Group I and
Group II) catalyze the over-all conversion of phenylalanine to flavone and flavonol glycosides (Fig. 1).
The two groups are induced concomitantly in irradiated
parsley cells, and the enzymes within each group are
coordinately regulated (1,6). When an elicitor, in the
form of an autoclaved mycelial cell-wall preparation
from the fungal pathogen, Phytophthora megasperma f.
sp. glycinea, is given to a cell suspension culture

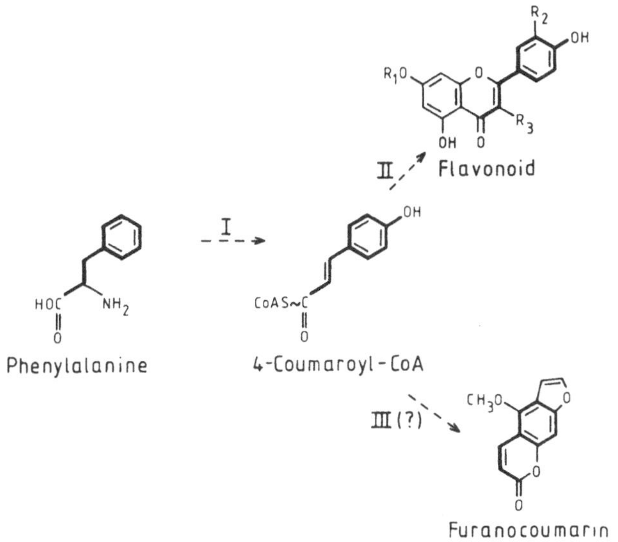

Fig. 1   Common biosynthetic origin of flavonoids and fu-
          ranocoumarins from phenylalanine. Thick lines
          indicate the mode of incorporation of the phenyl-
          propanoid unit. The two groups of inducible en-
          zymes (I and II) leading to the formation of
          flavonoid glycosides have been studied extensive-
          ly in cultured parsley cells (1,6). R_1, R_2 and
          R_3 indicate the positions where substitution
          patterns differ among the various flavones and
          flavonol glycosides isolated from irradiated
          cells (1). The third group (III) is so far hy-
          pothetical and is assumed to catalyze the con-
          version of 4-coumaroyl-CoA to various furano-
          coumarins, including the one shown here, ber-
          gaptene (K. Tietjen and U. Matern, unpublished
          results).

of parsley, the enzymes of Group I, but not those of
Group II are induced. The induction of these enzymes is
much more rapid with elicitor than with light (7) and
is followed by the formation of several furanocoumarins.
The chemical structures of the furanocoumarins have recently been elucidated (K. Tietjen and U. Matern, unpublished results). However, none of the enzymes involved in the conversion of 4-coumaroyl-CoA to these

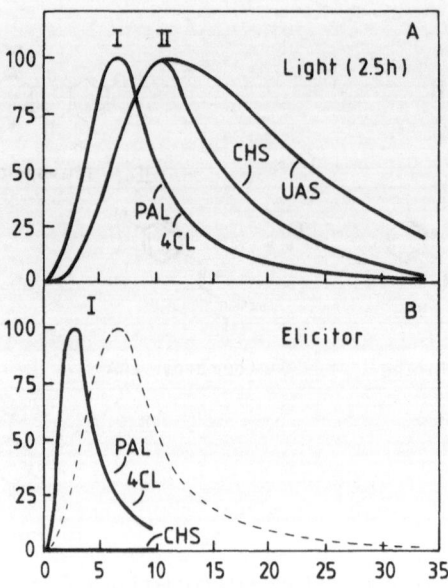

Fig. 2   Kinetics of mRNA induction by 2.5-h irradiation
         (A) or treatment with elicitor (B) of cultured
         parsley cells. PAL, phenylalanine ammonia-lyase;
         4CL, 4-coumarate:CoA ligase; CHS, chalcone syn-
         thase; UAS, UDP-apiose synthase. The broken cur-
         ve in panel B was taken from panel A for compa-
         rison of elicitor light effects on mRNAs of
         Group I. All curves were normalized. Data were
         taken from references (7-10).

products has been identified, and the role of 4-couma-
royl-CoA as an intermediate is only indirectly deduced
from the two observations that (a) its biosynthetic enzyme, 4-coumarate:CoA ligase, is induced by the elicitor and (b) the structural element of 4-coumarate is
found in all furanocoumarins isolated from elicitor-
-treated parsley cells. Accordingly, the proposed existence of a third group of enzymes (Fig. 1) and its
possible induction by the elicitor, though very likely
in view of the existing data, are so far purely hypothetical. The expected small number of enzymic steps
leading to the formation of furanocoumarins from 4-cou-
maroyl-CoA suggests that the proposed Group III com-

prises considerably fewer enzymes than Group II.

mRNA INDUCTION

    Specific antisera have been prepared for four of the
inducible enzymes from parsley cells, two antisera each
for enzymes of Group I (phenylalanine ammonia-lyase and
4-coumarate:CoA ligase) and Group II (chalcone synthase
and UDP-apiose synthase). These antisera were used to
determine the rates of enzyme synthesis, or mRNA activity, by selective immunoprecipitation of the enzyme proteins after synthesis either in vivo or in vitro. The
results obtained with both irradiated and elicitor-
treated cell cultures (7-10) are summarized in Fig. 2
(A and B, respectively). The high degree of coordination
in the induction within each group is even more pronounced at the level of the mRNA activities than at the level
of the enzyme activities. Moreover, the extremely rapid
induction of the Group I mRNAs and the lack of induction
of the Group II mRNAs by the elicitor are clearly demonstrated in Fig. 2B. In all cases shown, essentially the
same results were obtained, regardless of whether the
rates of enzyme synthesis were measured in vivo or in
vitro. This suggests that the rate of synthesis in vivo
is regulated mainly, or exclusively, by the availability
of translatable mRNA.

    We have recently demonstrated that the changes in
mRNA activity are paralleled by changes in mRNA amount.
We have cloned cDNA copies of poly(A)$^+$ mRNAs from irradiated or elicitor-treated parsley cells and isolated
clones with plasmids containing cDNA inserts homologous
to the mRNAs encoding phenylalanine ammonia-lyase, 4-
-coumarate:CoA ligase and chalcone synthase. The insert
from one of these plasmids, pLF56, has been characterized by DNA sequencing and is a cDNA copy comprising
most of the coding sequence, the 3'-untranslated region
and a portion of the poly(A) segment of chalcone synthase mRNA (U. Reimold, M. Kröger and K. Hahlbrock, unpublished results). This cDNA insert was used for the
'Northern' blotting experiment (11) shown inFig. 3A. Hybridization of labeled cDNA with chalcone synthase mRNA
was strongest around 10-11 h after induction. Much less
hybridization occurred at a later stage, and no hybridization was detected prior to induction. This result is
in good agreement with the pattern of changes in mRNA
activity, as shown in Fig. 3B. Similar results were obtained with phenylalanine ammonia-lyase and 4-coumarate:
:CoA ligase mRNAs, again demonstrating that changes in
amount coincided with changes in activity.

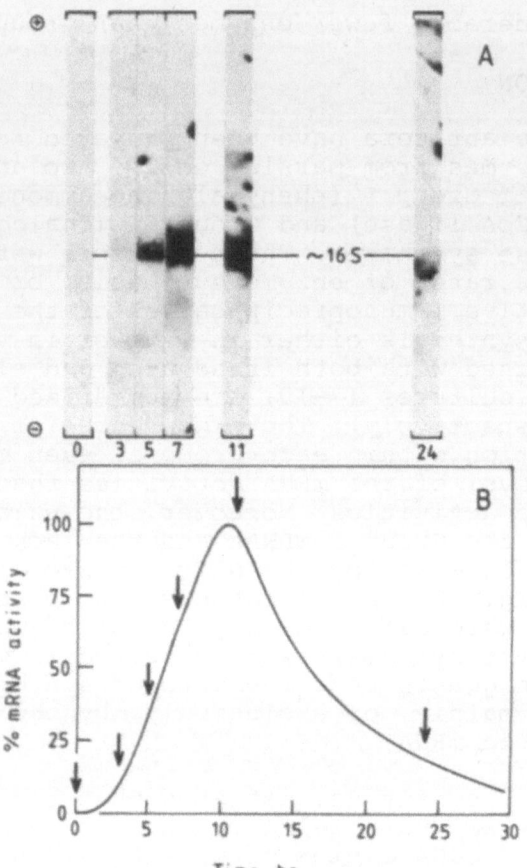

Fig. 3   Comparison of light-induced changes in hybridi-
         zable amount (A) and translatable activity (B) of
         chalcone synthase mRNA. The results shown in pa-
         nel A are described in detail elsewhere (11).
         The data for panel B were taken from Fig. 2A.
         Irradiation of the cells was for 2.5 h.

MATHEMATICAL CALCULATIONS

        A clear-cut relationship between mRNA and enzyme
activities has been observed in all cases studied so far,
independent of whether light or elicitor was the inducing agent (7-10). This relationship can be expressed
by the equation

$$dE(t)/dt = {}^{o}k_{s}(t) - {}^{1}k_{d} \cdot E(t), \qquad \text{(Eqn.1)}$$

where changes in enzyme activity (E) with time (t) are
determined by the zero-order rate constant of enzyme
synthesis (or mRNA activity) ($^{O}k_{s}$), which also changes
with time, and the first-order rate constant of enzyme
degradation ($^{1}k_{d}$). The rate constant, $^{1}k_{d}$, which is assumed
to remain unaltered upon induction, can be calculated from
the apparent half-life of the enzyme activity ($T_{1/2}$) with
the equation

$$^{1}k_{d} = \ln 2/T_{1/2}. \qquad\qquad \text{(Eqn. 2)}$$

The agreement between calculated and experimentally determined data suggests that both light and elicitor act
solely, or at least primarily, through mRNA induction
(7-10).

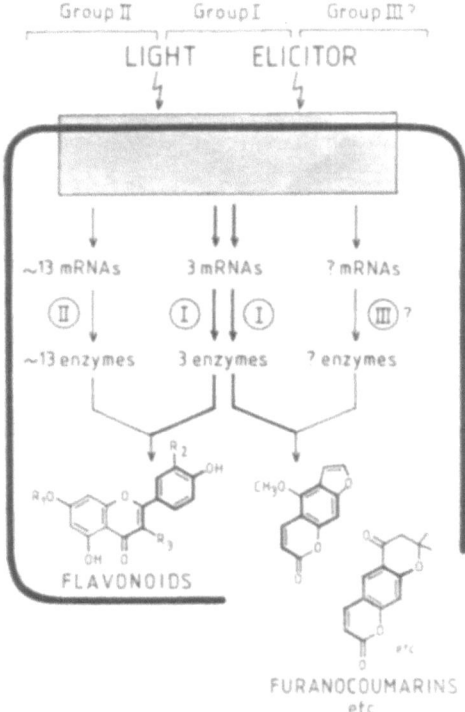

Fig. 4   Scheme summarizing the results presented in this
         article.

CONCLUSIONS

Evidence has been obtained for the coordinated induction of metabolically related enzymes and their mRNAs in
cultured plant cells. Each of the two inducing agents
used in these studies (UV light or elicitor from a phytopathogen) triggers the formation of one class of compounds (UV-protective flavonoids or antimicrobial phytoalexins). The potential function of these compounds is
to protect the challenged plant against possible damage
by the inducing agent. One sequence of biosynthetic
reactions, catalyzed by the enzymes of general phenylpropanoid metabolism (Group I), is the same for both
classes of compounds. The subsequent, more specific reactions are carried out by the enzymes of the flavonoid
glycoside pathway (Group II) and a hypothetical third
group (Group III) comprising the enzymes of furanocoumarin synthesis. A schematic representation of the results obtained so far with cultured parsley cells is
given in Fig. 4.

ACKNOWLEDGEMENTS

Work in our own laboratory was supported by Deutsche
Forschungsgemeinschaft (SFB 46) and Fonds der Chemischen
Industrie. We thank K. Tietjen and U. Matern for making
their data on the structural identification of furanocoumarins from parsley cells available to us prior to publication.

REFERENCES

1. Hahlbrock, K., 1981, In:"The Biochemistry of Plants",
   eds. Stumpf, P. K. and Conn, E. E., Vol. 7, pp. 425-
   456. Academic Press, New York.
2. Wellmann, E. In:"Encyclopedia of Plant Physiology.
   New Series: Photomorphogenesis", eds. Shropshire, Jr.
   W. and Mohr, H. Springer Verlag, Heidelberg. In press.
3. Grisebach, H. and Ebel, J., 1978, Angew. Chem. 90,
   668-681.
4. West, C. A., 1981, Naturwissenschaften 68, 447-457.
5. Brown, S. A., 1981, In:"The Biochemistry of Plants",
   eds. Stumpf, P. K. and Conn, E. E., Vol. 7, pp. 269-
   300. Academic Press, New York.
6. Ebel, J. and Hahlbrock, K. In:"Recent Advances in
   Flavonoid Research 1975-1980", eds. Harborne, J. B.
   and Mabry, J. Chapman and Hall, London. In press.
7. Hahlbrock, K., Lamb, C. J., Purwin, C., Ebel, J.,

Fautz, E. and Schäfer, E., 1981, Plant Physiol. 67, 768-773.

8. Schröder, J., Kreuzaler, F., Schäfer, E. and Hahlbrock, K., 1979, J. Biol. Chem. 254, 57-65.

9. Gardiner, S. E., Schröder, J., Matern, U., Hammer, D. and Hahlbrock, K., 1980, J. Biol. Chem. 225, 10752-10757.

10. Ragg, H., Kuhn, D. N. and Hahlbrock, K., 1981, J. Biol. Chem. 256, 10061-10065.

11. Kreuzaler, F., Ragg, H., Fautz, E., Kuhn, D. N. and Hahlbrock, K., 1982, Proc. Natl. Acad. Sci. USA, in press.

12. Hahlbrock, K., Knobloch, K. H., Kreuzaler, F., Potts, J. R. M. and Wellmann, E., 1976, Eur. J. Biochem. 61, 199-206.

THE HEAT SHOCK RESPONSE IN SOYBEAN SEEDLINGS

Joe L. Key, C. Y. Lin, E. Ceglarz, and F. Schöffl

Botany Department
University of Georgia
Athens, GA 30602

INTRODUCTION

The response of a wide array of organisms to heat shock (hs) has been studied (e.g. Ritossa, 1962; Kelley and Schlesinger, 1978; McAlister and Finkelstein, 1980; Barnett et al., 1980; Guttman et al., 1980; Neidhardt and Van Bogelen, 1981; Key et al., 1981, 1982; Baszczynski et al., 1982; Scharf and Nover, 1982; Altschuler and Mascarenhas, 1982), with Drosophila serving as a model for this work (see Ashburner and Bonner, 1979). In general when the growth temperature is elevated a few degrees ($\pm$ 10°) above "normal", there is a marked decrease in most normal protein synthesis and turn on of synthesis of a new set of proteins (heat shock proteins or hsp's). This dramatic switch in pattern of protein synthesis results from changes in both mRNA production and mRNA utilization in Drosophila (e.g. Ashburner and Bonner, 1979) and in plants (Key, et al., 1981 and Schöffl and Key, 1982). While there is no definitive information on the role or functions of the hsp's, the available evidence generally supports the view that hsp's afford some protection or "thermal tolerance" to the organism (e.g. Mitchell et al., 1979; Loomis and Wheeler, 1980, 1982; McAlister and Finkelstein, 1980; Key et al., 1982; Li and Werb, 1982).

In this report, we shall briefly describe the hs response of etiolated soybean seedlings and present some evidence in support of hsp's (or some other response to hs) providing "thermal protection" to otherwise non-permissive temperature.

25

J. L. KEY ET AL.

RESULTS AND DISCUSSION

Induction of hsp's

When the growth temperature of soybean seedlings, or parts
excised from them, is shifted from 28° to 40° there is a dramatic
change in the pattern of protein synthesis (Fig. 1, lanes a and
b). The synthesis of most normal proteins is decreased and a new
set of proteins (hsp's) is synthesized. This shift in pattern
of protein synthesis is highly temperature-dependent, with low
levels of hsp's being synthesized at 32.5° to 37.5° and essentially
only hsp's being synthesized at 42.5° (Key et al., 1981). The
"induction" of hsp synthesis is rapid with hsp's being detected
during the initial 15 min of hs (unpublished data). The capacity
to synthesize hsp's decreases markedly upon return of seedlings
from a 40° hs to 28° (Fig. 1, lanes c-g); within 4 hr the pattern
of protein synthesis (lane f) is essentially that of normal 28°
tissue (lane a). However, those hsp's which accumulate during
the 40° hs period are stable for at least 12 hr (Fig. 2, lanes e,
f) with only a 15% or so loss of radioactivity from protein during
the 12 hr chase.

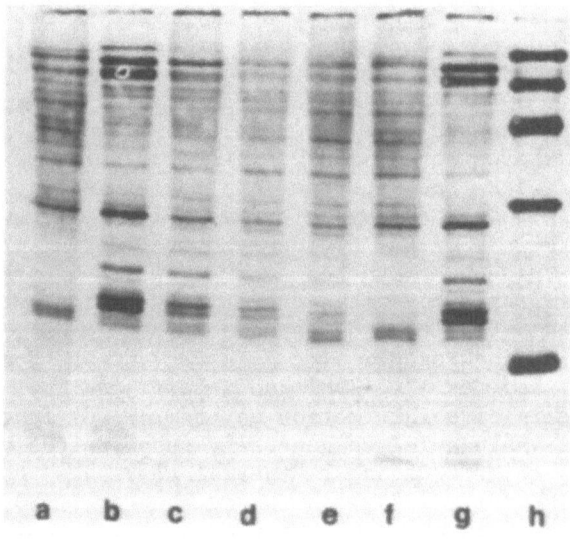

Fig. 1.   Synthesis of Heat Shock Proteins During a 40° Incubation
          and Subsequent 28° Incubation. ^{3}H-leucine-labeled proteins
          were fractionated on a SDS/polyacrylamide gel (Key et
          al., 1981). Lanes: a, normal 28° pattern; b, 4 hr label
          at 40°; c, label during first hour at 28° after 4 hr at
          40°; d, label during second hour as in c; e, label
          during third hour as in c; f, label during fourth hour
          as in c; g, 40° pattern as in b; h, molecular weight
          standards, 92,500; 69,000; 46,000; 30,000, and 12,300.

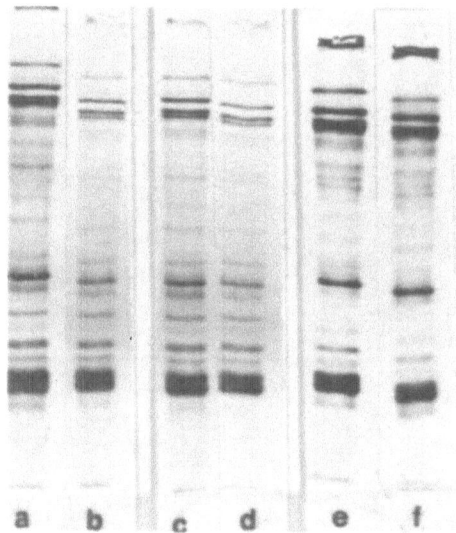

Fig. 2.   Patterns of Heat Shock Proteins Under Different Labeling
          and Chase Regimes. Proteins fractionated as in Fig. 1.
          Lanes: a, 40°, 1-2 hr label; b, 45°, 1-2 hr label; c, 45°,
          1-2 hr label following a 2 hr incubation at 40°; d, 45°,
          1-2 hr label following a 2-hr incubation at 40° and 4 hr
          at 28°; e, patterns of hsp's following a 3 hr label at 40°
          and a 4 hr chase at 28° (1 mM leucine); f, pattern of hsp's
          following a 3 hr label at 40° and a 12 hr chase at 28°
          (1 mM leucine). Individual lanes from different gel runs.

     The rather simple 1D gel pattern of hsp's noted in Fig. 1
is much more complex when viewed on 2D O'Farrell gels (Fig. 3).
There are at least 30 to 40 major proteins synthesized during
hs of the soybean seedlings, and others are likely synthesized
which do not focus in the O'Farrell system. There is a complex
pattern of hsp's in the 15-18 Kd range accounting for a high
proportion of hsp synthesis in the soybean seedling. Of the
8 to 10 different plant species studied to date, all synthesize
a complex, but somewhat different, pattern of 15 to 20 Kd hsp's
(unpublished data). There is considerable homology among several
members of the 15-27 Kd hsp's of soybean based on sequence homologies of their mRNAs (Schöffl and Key, 1982 and unpublished data).

Induction of hs-specific mRNAs

     cDNA cloning and mRNA hybridization analyses (Schöffl and
Key, 1982) were used to ascertain if the changing patterns of
protein synthesis in response to hs related to altered mRNA
patterns. In general, many normal mRNAs persist for several hr
at 40° even though they are poorly translated (Schöffl and Key,

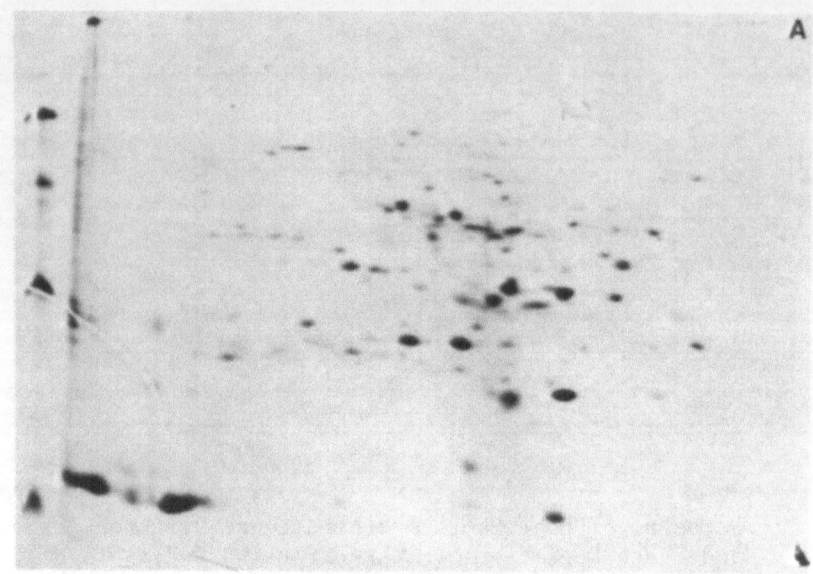

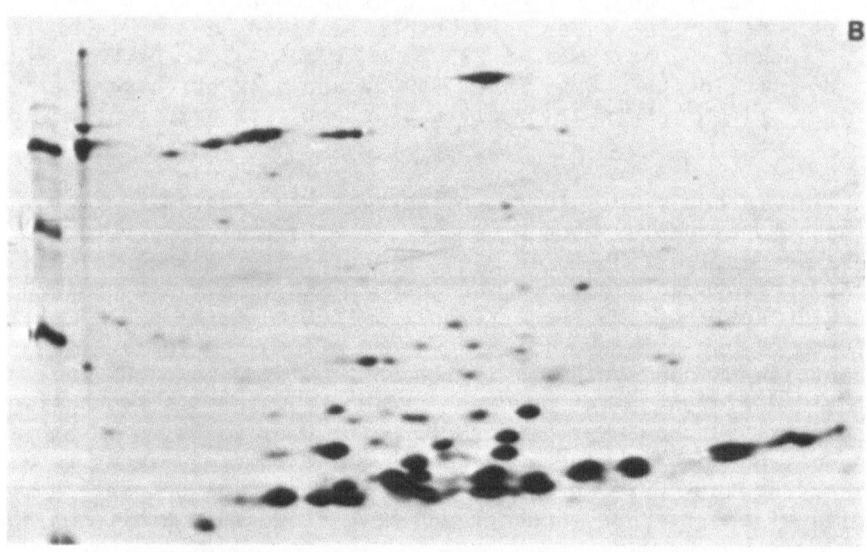

Fig. 3.   Two Dimensional O'Farrell Polyacrylamide Gel Analysis of
          Heat Shock Proteins. A, Tissue was incubated for 4 hr at
          28° followed by a 2 hr incubation in ³H-leucine at 28°;
          B, Tissue was incubated 4 hr at 40° followed by a 2 hr
          incubation in ³H-leucine at 45°. (Total SDS/buffer
          extracted proteins, as used in all reported experiments).

1982 and unpublished data) consistent with the results of studies
in Drosophila (see Ashburner and Bonner, 1979). Additionally,
there is a marked accumulation of mRNAs for the hsp's during hs,
from undetectable levels (or very low levels in some cases) in
control tissue up to 20,000 copies or more per cell for about 20
of the different abundant hs-specific mRNAs studied to date. The
data presented in Fig. 4 demonstrate both the temperature-
dependence and kinetics of hs-specific mRNA accumulation during
hs and recovery from hs. As with hsp accumulation (Key et al.,
1981), hs mRNA for the particular cloned sequence used in Fig. 4
is detected at 32.5°, increases gradually up to 37.5°, then
increases dramatically at 40° and decreases slightly at 42° (Fig.
4C). As the temperature is increased above 40° - 42°, the
accumulation of hs mRNA is significantly reduced and is just
detectable at 47.5° (Fig. 4B, lanes a to e). This mRNA is detected
within 7.5 min at 40° and increases in concentration for 2 hr or
more (Fig. 4A, lanes a to i). Following transfer of the seedlings
from 40° back to 28°, the concentration of the hs mRNA decreases
with a ½ time of about 1 hr (Fig. 4A, lanes j to m, and 4B, lanes
f to i; see also Schöffl and Key, 1982). This loss in hs mRNA
upon return to 28°, coupled with persistence of many normal mRNAs
at 40°, appears sufficient to account for the loss of hsp synthesis and an essentially normal pattern of protein synthesis
within 4 hr (Fig. 1).

"Thermal Protection" to Non-Permissive Temperatures

     The influence of increasing temperatures on amino acid incor-
poration into protein is shown in Fig. 5. When the hs temperature
is increased above some "break point" (40°-41° in the case of
soybean seedlings), there is a precipitous drop in amino acid
incorporation into protein, including into hsp's (Fig. 5). There
also is a marked decrease in accumulation of hs-specific mRNAs
above this "break point" T° (Fig. 4B, lanes a to e). A prior
treatment of soybean seedlings for 2 hr at 40°-41° permits high
levels of protein synthesis (Fig. 5) at these otherwise non-
permissive high temperatures. Those proteins synthesized at the
high (e.g. 45°) hs temperatures are predominantly hsp's (Fig. 2,
lanes b to d); this is true whether the seedlings are shifted
directly from 28° to 45° (lane b), receive a pretreatment at 40°
(lane c), or receive a 4 hr 28° treatment between the 40° and 45°
incubations (lane d). Very different levels of hsp synthesis are
achieved however (Fig. 5, Table 2). Also the hs mRNAs accumulate
to high levels at these high temperatures following a pretreatment
at 40° (Fig. 4B, lanes j to m) and a subsequent 28° incubation to
deplete the hs mRNA (Fig. 4B, lanes f to i). The level of protection afforded amino acid incorporation into protein at the
elevated temperature is dependent upon the time of preincubation
at 40° (Table 1); essentially full protection is achieved within
1 to 2 hr. Also the protection of amino acid incorporation at

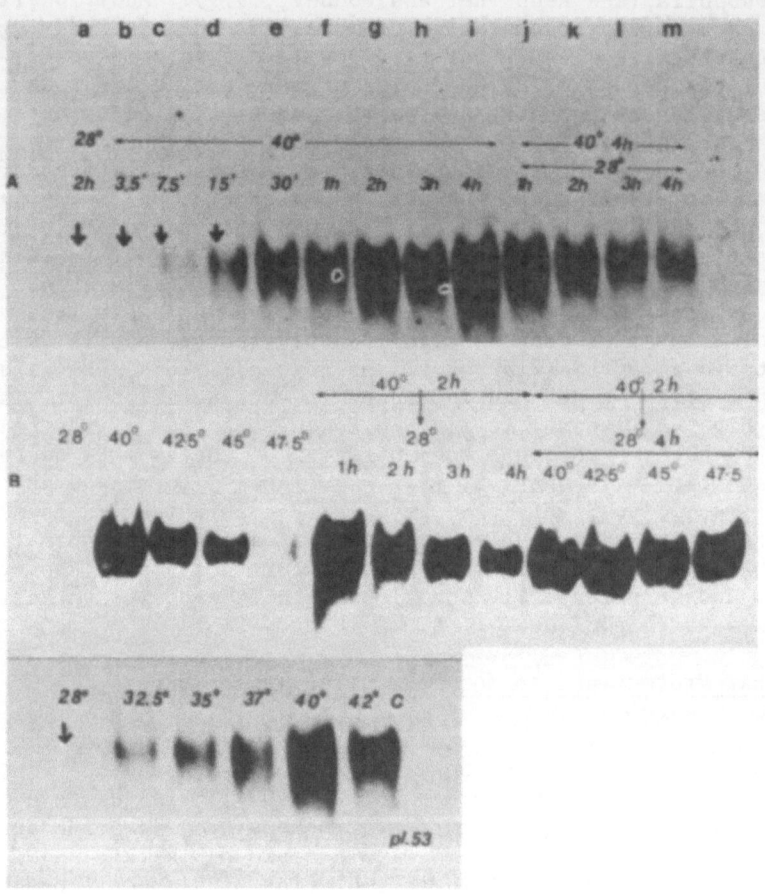

Fig. 4. Northern Hybridization Analyses of the Accumulation and
         Depletion of Heat Shock mRNA. Plasmid 53 (group VII of
         heat shock cDNA clones, Key et al., 1982) was used in
         hybridization analyses to poly(A)RNAs (Schöffl and Key,
         1982) isolated from seedlings treated as follows. A,
         lanes: a, 28° tissue; b to i, tissue incubated at 40°
         for the indicated times; j to m, tissue incubated at
         40° for 4 hr and transferred to 28° for the indicated
         times. B, lanes: a to e, tissue incubated for 2 hr at
         the indicated temperature; f to i tissue incubated for
         2 hr at 40° followed by the indicated times at 28°; j-m,
         tissue incubated as in i prior to 2 hr at the indicated
         temperature. C, tissue was incubated for 2 hr at the
         indicated temperature.

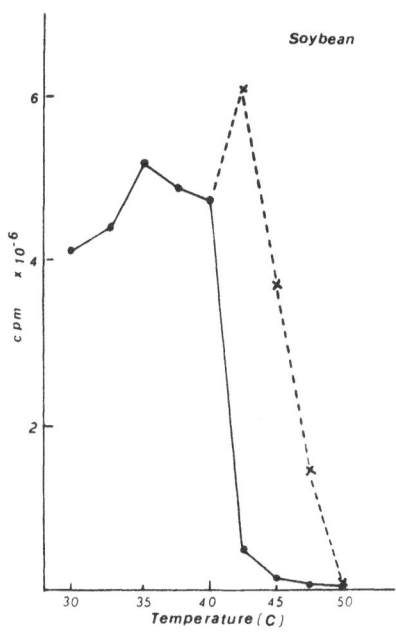

Fig. 5. ^{3}H-Leucine Incorporation
into Protein. Seedlings
were incubated at the
indicated temperature (2 hr,
●——●——●) or after pre-
incubation at 40° (2 hr)
followed by incubation at
the indicated temperature
(2 hr, x---x---x).

Table 1.   Protection of ^{3}H-Leucine Incorporation
at 42.5° by a Preincubation at 40°

Time at 40°[*]	cpm in Protein
(40° - for 2 hr)[**]	12,900
(42.5° - for 2 hr)[**]	1,400
15 min	2,350
30 min	4,150
60 min	12,500
120 min	14,500
180 min	16,600

[*]Tissue was incubated at the indicated times
at 40° prior to a shift to 42.5°; ^{3}H-leucine
incorporation was measured over a 1-2 hr
period at 42.5°.

[**]Tissue was incubated directly for 2 hr at
either 40° or 42.5°; ^{3}H-leucine incorporation was measured over the 1-2 hr period
at the noted temperature.

Table 2. Protective Influence of a 40° Pretreatment
          on Heat Shock Protein Synthesis at Higher
          Temperatures

Temperature Regime	cpm in Protein
28° → 42.5°[1]	68,250
28° → 45°	10,025
28° → 47.5°	725
40° → 28° → 42.5°[2]	147,750
40° → 28° → 45°	70,750
40° → 28° → 47.5°	10,700
40° → 40°[1]	108,500
40° → 45°	79,250

[1]Seedlings incubated for 2 hr at first temperature
followed by 2 hr at the second temperature with
[3]H-leucine added during the final 2 hr.

[2]Seedlings incubated and labeled as in 1 except
that a 4-hr intervening incubation at 28° was
included.

the higher hs temperature provided by a 2 hr incubation at 40° is
achieved even when the tissue is incubated for an intervening 4
hr-period at 28° (Table 2). Thus whatever condition(s) that is
caused by hs at 40° and which permits or generates "thermal
tolerance" to the otherwise non-permissive high temperatures is
stable for at least 4 hr at 28° and "accumulates" in a time- (Table
1) and temperature- (unpublished data) dependent manner. This
occurs even though the hs response (i.e. synthesis of hsp's and
accumulation of hs-specific mRNAs) decays rapidly during the 4-hr
incubation at 28° with the resumption of essentially normal patterns
of protein synthesis (Fig. 1) and depletion of hs mRNAs (Fig. 4A
and B). As noted above those hsp's synthesized during the initial
40° incubation, however, are very stable during a 12-hr incubation
at 28° (Fig. 2) even though their continued synthesis is not (Fig.
1). Thus, the accumulation of hsp's is likely the "condition"
generated during hs at a permissive temperature (e.g. 40°) which
provides protection or "thermal tolerance" to the otherwise non-
permissive hs temperatures (e.g. 45°).

Growth of Soybean Seedlings Following Heat Shock

     Growth (germination) of soybean seedlings is also protected
by hs at 40° during subsequent incubation at otherwise lethal
temperatures (e.g. 45°) (Fig. 6 and unpublished data). This

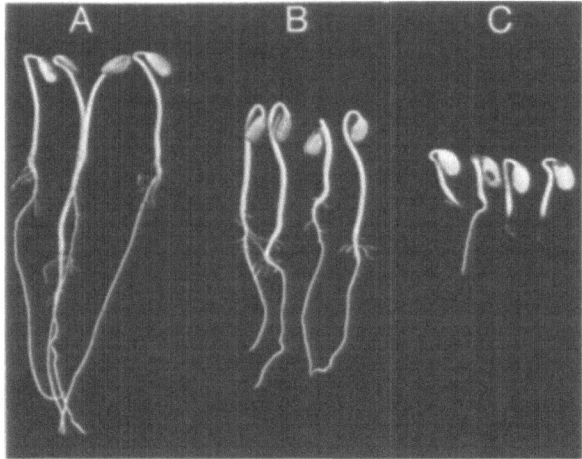

Fig. 6.   Growth of Seedlings Following Heat Shock.   Thirty seeds
          in each treatment were germinated at 28° for 22 hr.   They
          were then incubated for 2 hr at 28° followed by 72 hr at
          28° (A); incubated for 2 hr at 40°, followed by 2 hr at
          45°, then 70 hr at 28° (B); incubated for 2 hr at 45°
          followed by 72 hr at 28° (C).   The average seedling size
          was: A, 15.2 ± 4.3 cm; B, 14.1 ± 3.0 cm; C, 2.1 ± .7 cm.

physiological tolerance to the non-permissive temperatures
develops in a manner consistent again with the accumulation of
hsp's at the permissive hs temperature being of prime importance
to generation of "thermal tolerance" relative to subsequent growth
of the soybean seedlings.   While the appearance and localization
of hsp's has been followed by using ^{3}H-leucine during the initial
hs treatment to label the hsp's, significant levels of hsp's accumulate based on staining of 2D gels (unpublished data); such accumulation of hsp's to high levels would be expected based on the
significant (about 20,000 copies per cell) accumulation of hs
mRNAs, their efficient translation, and the stability of the newly
synthesized hsp's.

SUMMARY AND CONCLUSIONS

     Soybean seedlings (and a wide range of other plants studied
to date) respond to a high temperature by synthesizing a new set

of proteins (hsp's) and slowing the synthesis of most normal (28°)
proteins. Both transcriptional and translational control mechanisms seem to be operative in this hs response. The hs "induces"
the synthesis of mRNAs for the hsp's which accumulate to very high
levels (e.g. 20,000 copies per cell) and become the most abundant
mRNAs after a 2-4 hr hs at about 40°. Many of the 28° mRNAs
persist during the hs and are recruited into protein synthesis
following return of seedlings to the normal growing temperature.
Following hs, the normal pattern of protein synthesis resumes in
a few hr upon return to 28°. However, those hsp's synthesized
during the hs treatment are stable for many hr.

While the specific function of hsp's is not understood, the
evidence presented above indicates that hsp's synthesized at
permissive hs temperatures do provide protection to soybean seedlings to otherwise non-permissive temperatures. There is emerging
a general consensus from studies with a wide range of organisms
that hsp's provide "thermal tolerance" to otherwise non-permissive
temperatures (e.g. Mitchell et al., 1979; Loomis and Wheeler, 1980,
1982; McAlister and Finkelstein, 1980; Li and Werb, 1982; Key et
al., 1982; Yamamori and Yura, 1982). There is suggestive evidence
(e.g. Arrigo et al., 1980; Velasquez et al., 1980; Loomis and
Wheeler, 1982; and Key et al., 1982) that hs-directed localization
of the hsp's plays an important role in the protection provided by
permissive hs temperatures. In the case of soybean seedlings,
some of the hsp's become organelle-associated during hs. This
"association" correlates with preservation of organelle function
during high temperature hs (e.g. synthesis of hs mRNAs and hsp's).
A subsequent chase at 28° results in loss of a majority of the
hsp's from the organelle fractions with their accumulation in the
"soluble" or supernatant phase of the cytoplasm while they remain
localized during a chase at 40°. Furthermore, a second hs treatment at 40° or 45° after the 28° chase results in relocalization
of several of the hsp's in the organelle fractions. Additional
evidence in support of a role of hsp's in "thermal protection"
comes from experiments where hsp-like proteins are induced by
arsenite treatment (unpublished data); some of these proteins
become localized upon hs treatment and appear to confer some
"thermal tolerance" to high (e.g. 45°) hs temperatures. The
nature of the association of hsp's with organelles is not understood.

ACKNOWLEDGEMENT

Research supported by DOE Contract DE-AS09-80ER10678.

REFERENCES

Altschuler, M., and Mascarenhas, J. P., 1982, Heat shock proteins
        and effects of heat shock in plants, Plant Mol. Biol., 1:103.

Arrigo, A., Fakan, S., and Tissieres, A., 1980, Localization of the heat shock-induced proteins in Drosophila melanogaster tissue culture cells, Dev. Biol., 78:86.

Ashburner, M., and Bonner, J. J., 1979, The induction of gene activity in Drosophila by heat shock, Cell, 17:241.

Barnett, T., Altschuler, M., McDaniel, C. N., Mascarenhas, J. P., 1980, Heat shock induced proteins in plant cells, Dev. Gen., 1:331.

Baszczynski, C. L., Walden, D. B., and Atkinson, B. G., 1982, Regulation of gene expression in corn (Zea mays L.) by heat shock, Can. J. Biochem., 60:569.

Guttman, S. D., Glover, C. V. C., Allis, C. D., and Gorovsky, M. A., 1980, Heat shock, deciliation and release from anoxia induce the synthesis of the same set of polypeptides in starved T. pyriformis, Cell, 22:299.

Kelley, P., and Schlesinger, M., 1978, The effect of amino acid analogues and heat shock on gene expression in chick embryo fibroblasts, Cell, 15:1277.

Key, J. L., Lin, C. Y., and Chen, Y. M., 1981, Heat shock proteins of higher plants, Proc. Natl. Acad. Sci., 78:3526.

Key, J. L., Lin, C. Y., Ceglarz, E., and Schöffl, F., 1982, The heat shock response in plants, in "Heat Shock: From Bacteria to Man." M. Schlesinger, M. Ashburner and A. Tissières, eds., Cold Spring Harbor Laboratory. In press.

Li, G. C., and Werb, Z., 1982, Correlation between synthesis of heat shock proteins and development of thermotolerance in Chinese hamster fibroblasts, Proc. Natl. Acad. Sci., 79:3218.

Loomis, W. F., and Wheeler, S., 1980, Heat shock response of Dictyostelium, Dev. Biol., 79:399.

Loomis, W. F., and Wheeler, S. A., 1982, Chromatin-associated heat shock proteins of Dictyostelium, Dev. Biol., 90:412.

McAlister, L., and Finkelstein, D., 1980, Heat shock proteins and thermal resistance in yeast, Biochem. Biophys. Res. Commun., 93:819.

Mitchell, H., Moller, G., Petersen, N., and Lipps-Sarmiento, L., 1979, Specific protection from phenocopy induction by heat shock, Dev. Genet., 1:181.

Neidhardt, F. C. and Van Bogelen, R. A., 1981, Positive Regulatory Gene for Temperature-Controlled Proteins in Escherichia coli. Biochem. Biophys. Res. Commun., 100:894.

O'Farrell, P. H., 1975, High resolution two-dimensional electro-phoresis of proteins, J. Biol. Chem., 250:4007.

Ritossa, F., 1962, A new puffing pattern induced by heat shock and DNP in Drosophila, Experientia, 18:571.

Scharf, K.-D., and Nover, L., 1982, Heat-shock-induced alterations of ribosomal protein phosphorylation in plant cell cultures, Cell, 30:427.

Schöffl, F., and Key, J. L., 1982, An analysis of mRNAs for a group of heat shock proteins of soybean using cloned cDNAs, J. Mol. Appl. Genet., 1:301.

Velasquez, J., DiDomenico, B., and Linquist, S., 1980, Intra-
    cellular localization of heat shock proteins in Drosophila,
    Cell, 20:679.
Yamamori, T., and Yura, T., 1982, Genetic control of heat-shock
    protein synthesis and its bearing on growth and thermal
    resistance in Escherichia coli K-12, Proc. Natl. Acad. Sci.,
    79:860.

ORGANIZATION OF SOYBEAN SEED PROTEIN GENES

AND THEIR FLANKING REGIONS

Robert B. Goldberg, Robert L. Fischer, John J. Harada, Diane Jofuku, and Jack K. Okamuro

Department of Biology, University of California
Los Angeles, California 90024

INTRODUCTION

In this paper we review briefly the research which has been carried out in our lab on the organization of soybean seed protein genes. The genes which we have concentrated our efforts on encode the storage proteins glycinin and β-conglycinin, the Kunitz trypsin inhibitor, seed lectin, and an unidentified 15,500 dalton protein. We are investigating these genes in order to understand the molecular events which regulate gene expression during plant development. Our long term objective is to utilize this information to improve crop plants by molecular genetic engineering procedures.

SOYBEAN SEED PROTEIN GENE EXPRESSION IS DEVELOPMENTALLY REGULATED

Soybean seed protein gene expression is under strict developmental control (Goldberg et al., 1981a, 1981b). This is demonstrated by the mRNA gel blot experiments shown in Figure 1. Seed protein mRNAs accumulate during early maturation, and then decay during late maturation when seed dehydration occurs. In addition, seed protein mRNAs are absent from the nucleus and cytoplasm of cells of the mature plant (Goldberg et al., 1981a; J.K. Okamuro and R.B. Goldberg, unpublished data). These findings suggest that seed protein genes are switched "off" during late development, and that their expression is controlled primarily at the transcriptional level. Recent experiments with "runoff" nuclear RNAs synthesized in vitro by isolated nuclei support this proposition (L. Walling and R.B. Goldberg, unpublished data).

37

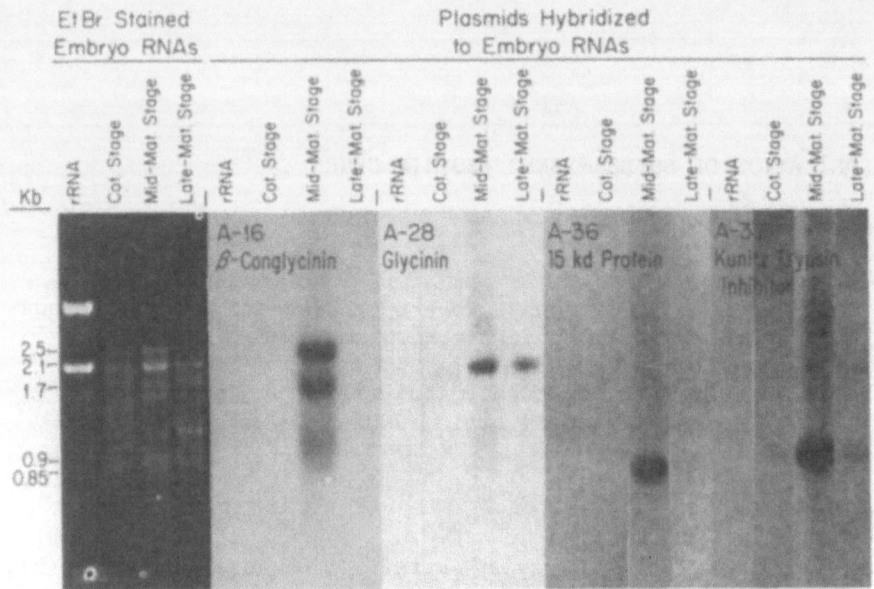

Fig. 1. Hybridization of Seed Protein cDNA Plasmids
with Embryo mRNAs from Various Developmental
Stages. Adapted from Goldberg et al. (1981a).

SOYBEAN SEED PROTEINS ARE ENCODED BY SMALL GENE FAMILIES

Two strategies were used to estimate the copy number of
seed protein genes in soybean chromosomes. First, labeled
single-stranded probes representing specific seed protein
messages were reacted with excess genomic DNA, and their
hybridization rates were measured (Goldberg et al., 1981a).
Secondly, labeled seed protein plasmids were hybridized with
DNA gel blots containing restriction-endonuclease digested
genomic DNA (Fischer and Goldberg, 1982). Representative
examples of both strategies, shown in Figures 2 and 3, indicate
that each seed protein gene is represented a small number of
times in soybean chromosomes. Copy numbers vary between two
and ten depending upon the gene and/or the hybridization conditions employed. In addition, it can be seen that similar
results were obtained with both embryo and leaf DNAs using each
procedure. Together, these findings indicate that glycinin,
β-conglycinin, seed lectin, Kunitz trypsin inhibitor, and 15 Kd
protein genes are organized into small, discrete gene families,
and that these families are not selectively altered or
amplified during development.

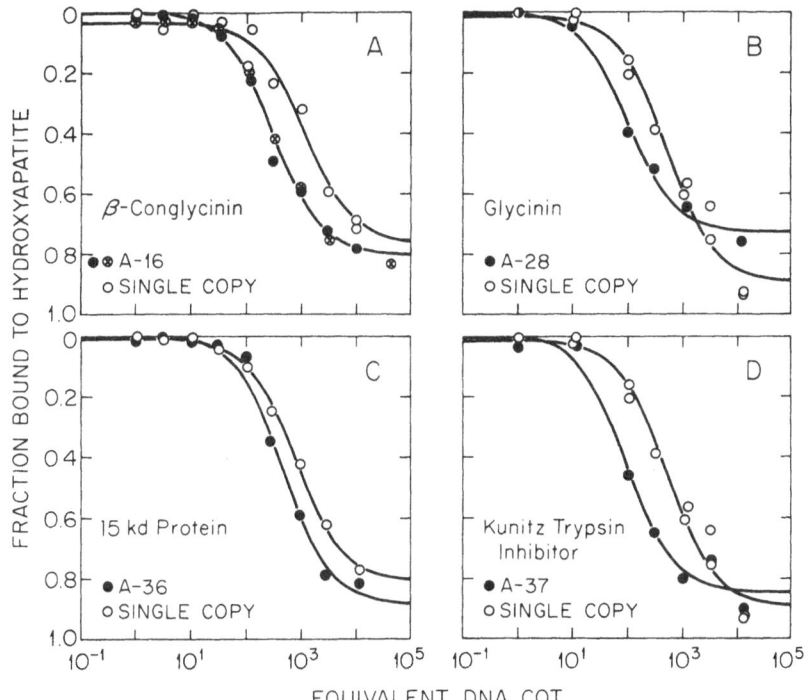

Fig. 2.   Hybridization   of   Single-Stranded   Plasmid
Probes   with   Soybean   DNA.   Closed   circles
represent   plasmid   DNAs   while   open   circles
represent   the   internal   single-copy   DNA
kinetic   standard.   Leaf   DNA   was   used   as   the
"driver"   DNA   in   the   glycinin,   Kunitz   trypsin
inhibitor,   and   15   Kd   protein   plasmid   reactions.   In   the   case   of   the   β-conglycinin
probe,   both   leaf   (closed   circles)   and   embryo
(open   circles   with   x)   DNAs   were   used   as
"drivers".   Adapted   from   Goldberg   et   al.
(1981a).

SEED PROTEIN GENES HAVE RELATIVELY "SIMPLE" STRUCTURES

Seed Protein gene structures were visualized in the
electron microscope by R-loop analysis (Fischer and Goldberg,
1982). Figure 4 presents a collage of different seed protein
genes. No introns are visible in the Kunitz trypsin inhibitor,
seed lectin, and 15 Kd protein genes. S-1 nuclease mapping
studies with the 15 Kd protein and seed lectin genes confirmed
these observations, indicating that if introns are present they

must be short (<0.05 kb) and located near the gene ends. The
top panel of Figure 4 shows that three different glycinin
genes, G_1, G_2, and G_3 (see Figure 3), each have at least
one intron. These introns vary from 0.5 to 0.7 kb in length
depending upon the family member (Fischer and Goldberg, 1982;
N.C. Nielsen, personal communication).

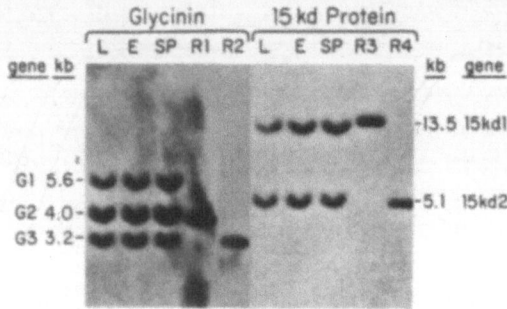

Fig. 3.   Hybridization of Glycinin and 15 Kd Protein
           cDNA Plasmids with Soybean DNA Gel Blots.
           L, E, and SP refer to leaf, embryo, and
           single-plant leaf DNA lanes. R lanes contain
           a single-copy equivalent of each restriction
           endonuclease fragment. Adapted from Fischer
           and Goldberg (1982).

In contrast to the relative structural uniformity of
glycinin genes, β-conglycinin storage protein genes differ from
each other in size and structural organization (J.J. Harada and
R.B. Goldberg, unpublished results). The α-type β-conglycinin
gene displayed in Figure 4 shows strong homology with the 2.5
kb β-conglycinin mRNA size class (see Figure 1). This gene is
approximately 3 kb in length and has no visible introns;
however, the presence of short intervening sequences (<0.1 kb)
has been inferred from restriction endonuclease mapping
studies. The β-type gene shown in Figure 4 is most closely
related to the 1.7 kb β-conglycinin mRNA size class (see Figure
1). This gene is approximately 2 kb in length and has a few,
very small introns. These data show that β-conglycinin gene
structures vary, and that the 2.5 kb and 1.7 kb β-conglycinin
mRNAs are synthesized from different family members, rather
than from the differential processing of a common pre-mRNA.

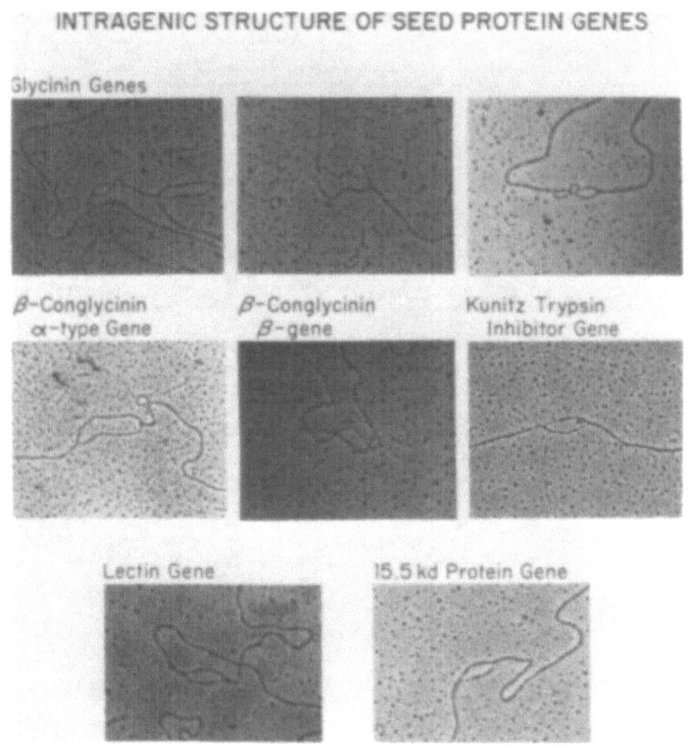

Fig. 4. Visualization of Seed Protein Gene Structures.

SOME SEED PROTEIN GENES ARE LINKED

To describe the arrangement of seed protein gene families in soybean chromosomes, a series of "walks" are currently being carried out. Figure 5 shows a genomic clone which contains two linked glycinin genes (G_1 and G_2), indicating that at least two glycinin gene family members are clustered (R.L. Fischer and R.B. Goldberg, unpublished data). Similarly, three different genomic clones have been isolated which contain two β-conglycinin genes each (J.J. Harada and R.B. Goldberg, unpublished results), and one genomic clone has been characterized which contains two Kunitz trypsin inhibitor genes separated by about 1 kb (D. Jofuku and R.B. Goldberg, unpublished data). These data indicate that intrafamily linkage of some glycinin, β-conglycinin, and Kunitz trypsin inhibitor genes does occur.

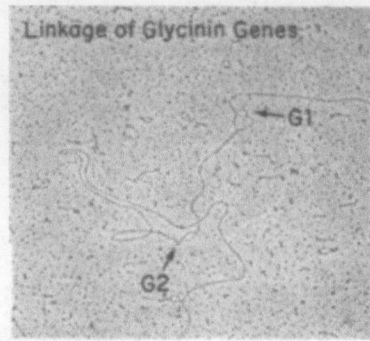

Fig. 5.   Linkage of Two Glycinin Genes.

Whether all members of each family are clustered remains to be
determined.

DISPERSED REPEATED SEQUENCES FLANK SOME SEED PROTEIN GENES

        Repetitive and single-copy DNA sequences are organized in
soybean chromosomes in the short period interspersion pattern
typical of most plants and animals (Goldberg, 1978; Gurley,
Hepburn, and Key, 1979).   To determine whether dispersed
repeats flank different seed protein genes, labeled seed
protein genomic clones were hybridized with DNA gel blots
containing restriction endonuclease digested nuclear DNA.
Representative results, shown in Figure 6, indicate that some
seed protein gene regions have one or more repetitive elements
which are present at many other locations (e.g., 15 Kdl protein
gene region, λA36-2 phage).   Others, however, either have no
dispersed repeats, or repeats restricted to only a few locations (<5) in the genome (e.g., G_2 glycinin gene, λA28-5
phage).   Cross-hybridization experiments between seed protein
genomic clones with dispersed repeats showed that they contained representatives of different repeat families.   Taken
together, these data indicate that dispersed repeats are
contiguous to some seed protein genes, and that common
repetitive sequences are not present within different seed
protein gene regions.

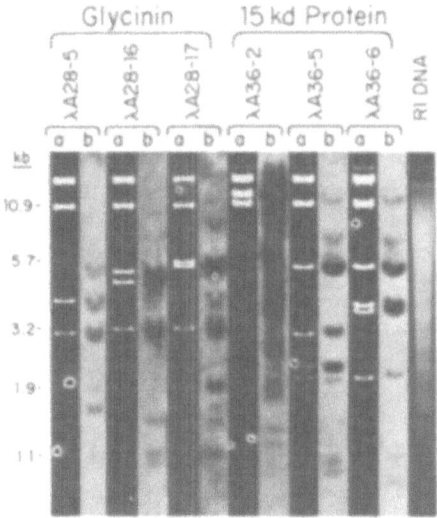

Fig. 6. Hybridization of Seed Protein Genomic Clones
with Soybean DNA Gel Blots. Soybean DNA was
digested with EcoRI, electrophoresed on
agarose gels, blotted, and hybridized with
labeled genomic clones. The washing and
hybridization criteria were 1 M Na$^+$/50%
formamide/32°C. Lanes labeled a represent
EtBr-stained, electrophoresed phage DNAs.
Lanes labeled b are autoradiograms of the
blotted leaf DNA shown in the Rl DNA lane.

DIFFERENTIALLY REGULATED NONSEED PROTEIN GENES ARE CONTIGUOUS
TO SEED PROTEIN GENE REGIONS

     To determine whether nonseed protein genes flank
developmentally regulated seed protein gene regions, labeled
leaf, root, and stem cDNAs were hybridized with DNA gel blots
containing seed protein genomic clones (Fischer and Goldberg,
1982; J.K. Okamuro and R.B. Goldberg, unpublished results).
Relevant findings, portrayed in Figure 7, show that genes
expressed at the mRNA level in the mature plant flank several
different seed protein gene regions. Gel blot studies were
carried out to measure the sizes and prevalences of the nonseed
protein mRNAs (Fischer and Goldberg, 1982; J.K. Okamuro and
R.B. Goldberg, unpublished data). The findings indicated that
each nonseed protein mRNA has a unique size, and that it is

represented only a few times per cell. Since seed protein
genes are not expressed in the mature plant (Goldberg et al.,
1981a; R.B. Goldberg et al., unpublished data), these data show
that there is a short range clustering of genes that are
expressed at distinct periods, and at quantitatively different
levels within the soybean life cycle.

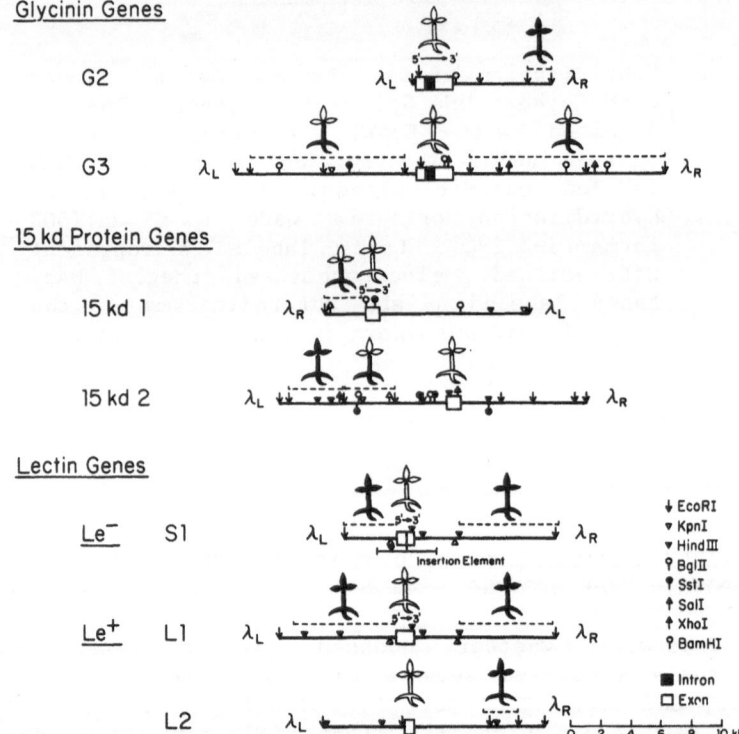

Fig. 7.   Nonseed Protein Genes Linked to Seed Pro-
           tein Gene Regions.   Cartoon-like plants
           summarize the expression pattern for each
           gene region.   Dark areas indicate that the
           gene is expressed in that organ system,
           while light areas indicate that the gene is
           inactive at the mRNA level.

CONCLUSIONS

Soybean seed protein genes represent an excellent model for the study of plant gene regulation. These genes are under strict developmental control, possess relatively "simple" structures, and are organized into discrete gene families. Common repetitive elements, as defined by standard hybridization criteria, do not flank different seed protein genes. This implies that dispersed repetitive elements are unlikely to play a significant role in the regulation of seed protein gene expression. Clusters of uncoordinately expressed genes have been identified within seed protein gene regions. This finding strongly suggests that each plant gene possesses a cryptic, tightly-linked sequence which is responsible for regulating its expression during development. What these sequences are, and how they interact with physiological processes inside the cell, remain to be determined.

ACKNOWLEDGMENTS

We express our gratitude to Gisela Hoschek for expert and dedicated technical assistance. This work was supported by research grants from the National Science Foundation and the U.S. Department of Agriculture.

REFERENCES

Fischer, R. L. and Goldberg, R. B., 1982, Cell 29:651-660.
Goldberg, R. B., 1978, Biochem. Genet. 16:45-68.
Goldberg, R. B., Hoschek, G., Ditta, G. S., and Briedenbach,
    R. W., 1981a, Dev. Biol. 83:218-231.
Goldberg, R. B. Hoschek, G., Tam, S. H., Ditta, G. S., and
    Briedenbach, R. W., 1981b, Dev. Biol. 83:201-217.
Gurley, W.B., Hepburn, A.G., and Key, J. L., 1979, Biochim.
    Biophys. Acta   561:167-193.

EXPRESSION OF NUCLEAR GENES ENCODING THE SMALL

SUBUNIT OF RIBULOSE-1,5-BISPHOSPHATE CARBOXYLASE

Gloria Coruzzi, Richard Broglie,
Gayle Lamppa and Nam-Hai Chua

Laboratory of Plant Molecular Biology
The Rockefeller University
1230 York Avenue
New York, N.Y. 10021

INTRODUCTION

Chloroplast biogenesis requires the coordinate expression of both nuclear and chloroplast genomes. While the chloroplast genome has been shown to encode several polypeptides, structural genes for the majority of the chloroplast proteins are localized in the nucleus (see Ellis, 1981, for a review). In higher plants, the two most prominant nuclear gene products destined for the chloroplasts are the small subunit (S) of ribulose-1,5-bisphosphate carboxylase (RUBISCO) (Chua and Schmidt, 1978b; Highfield and Ellis, 1978; Cashmore et al., 1978) and thylakoid polypeptide 15, the major subunit of the light-harvesting complex (LHC) (Apel and Kloppstech, 1978; Schmidt et al., 1981). In addition to their regulation by light (Apel, 1979; Tobin and Suttie, 1980; Highfield and Ellis, 1981; Sasaki et al., 1981), nuclear genes for these polypeptides are expressed differentially in the mesophyll and bundle-sheath leaf cells of C4 plants (Broglie et al., 1982). The mechanisms for the developmental and tissue-specific regulation of these genes are unknown, although transcriptional control is likely to be a major factor.

The intracellular biosynthetic pathways of S and polypeptide 15 have been investigated. Both polypeptides are synthesized on free cytoplasmic polysomes as soluble precursors (pS and p15), approximately 5,000 daltons larger than the mature forms (see Chua et al., 1980, for a review). After synthesis, the precursors are imported into the chloroplasts by a post-translational mechanism

dependent on ATP (Grossman et al., 1980). During or shortly after
passage through the chloroplast envelope, the precursors are
converted to the mature polypeptides which are assembled into the
RUBISCO holoenzyme (Chua and Schmidt, 1978a,b) or the LHC (Schmidt
et al., 1981).

Although the sequence of events surrounding the synthesis,
transport, and assembly of S and polypeptide 15 have been defined,
molecular details of these processes remain largely unresolved.
Synthesis of these polypeptides as precursors prompted us to
suggest that the precursor extra sequence (transit sequence) may
be important for interaction with the chloroplast envelope during
transport (Chua and Schmidt, 1979). Thus, information regarding
the amino acid sequence of the transit peptides may shed light on
the process.

To study the regulation of the nuclear genes encoding S and
to elucidate the amino acid sequence of the pS transit peptides,
we have isolated cDNA clones for pea (dicot) and wheat (monocot)
small subunits. We have determined the complete nucleotide
sequences of these cDNA clones and deduced the corresponding amino
acid sequences for the mature S and the precursor transit peptides. These cDNA clones were also used as hybridization probes
to isolate the corresponding genomic sequences. The results of
these experiments are summarized here.

Isolation and Characterization of cDNA Clones for the Small Subunit of RUBISCO

We have reported recently the isolation and characterization
of three pea cDNA clones encoding major chloroplast proteins
(Broglie et al., 1981). By hybrid-selection and in vitro transport assays, one of the clones was shown to code for S. Clone
pSS15 contains a cDNA insert of 691 bp, which is slightly less
than the expected full-length (~850 bp), as estimated from Northern blots of mRNA (data not shown). From its complete nucleotide
sequence (Coruzzi et al., 1982) we determined that it encodes 156
amino acid residues of pS. To identify the NH_2 terminus of the
mature S we compared the deduced amino acid sequence of pSS15 to
that determined chemically for the purified S from pea (Takruri
et al., 1981). This comparison allowed us to conclude that pSS15
codes for the entire mature S (123 amino acid residues; M_r =
14,595) and a partial transit peptide (33 amino acid residues) at
the NH_2 terminus of pS (Figs. 1 & 2). Bedbrook et al., (1981)
have reported previously the nucleotide sequence of a cDNA clone
(pSSU1) for the S of pea. There are six nucleotide differences
between pSSU1 and pSS15, which occur in the third base of the
codon. Ten nucleotide differences between the two clones result
in the change of eight amino acid codons at residues 47, 53, 80,
81, 84, 96, 101, and 105 without altering the net charge of the

polypeptide. In addition, the two clones differ in residues
-5, -11 and -13 of the transit peptide. Extensive sequence differences are also detected in the 3' non-coding region. Since
Bedbrook et al., (1980) used the Feltham First Variety and we
used the Progress #9 variety, the differences may reflect either
the use of different strains of peas or the presence of several
RUBISCO small subunit mRNAs in leaf cells.

In an attempt to develop a homologous in vitro transcription
system for plant genes, using wheat-germ extracts or wheat RNA
polymerase II, we have also isolated and characterized a RUBISCO
small subunit cDNA clone from hexaploid wheat (Tritium aestivum

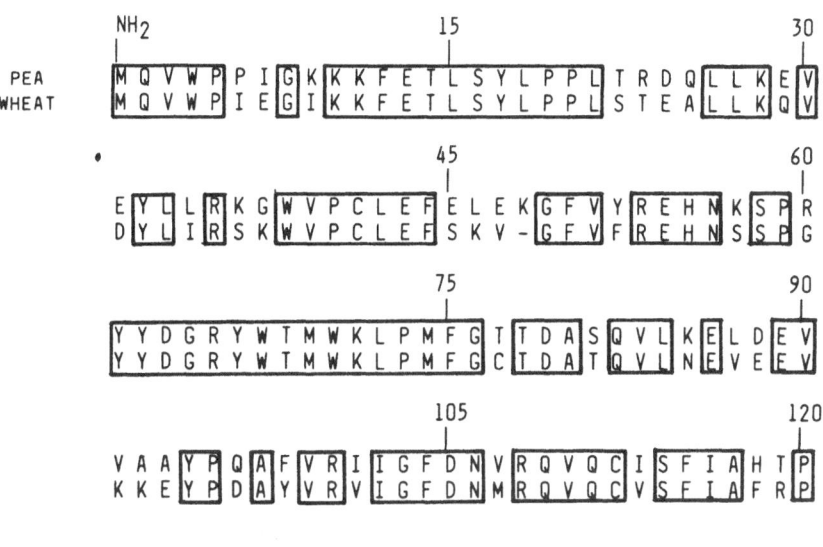

Fig. 1. Comparison of the amino acid sequences of pea and wheat
mature small subunit polypeptides. The amino acid
sequences were deduced from the nucleotide sequences of
cDNA clones pSS15 (Coruzzi et al., 1982) and pW9 (Broglie
et al., in preparation). A single amino acid deletion
at residue 48 of the wheat small subunit polypeptide was
allowed in order to maximize sequence homology. Homologous amino acid sequences are boxed. The RUBISCO small
subunit of pea contains 123 amino acids (M_r = 14,595)
whereas that of wheat contains 128 amino acids (M_r =
14,871). Each amino acid is represented by the standard
single letter code.

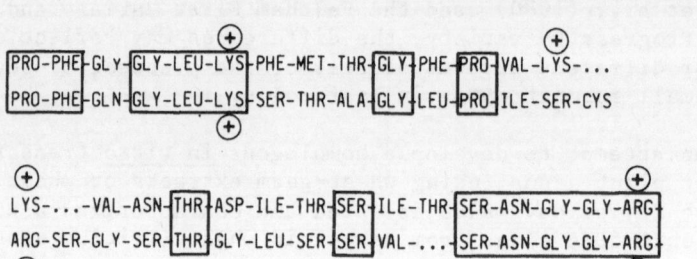

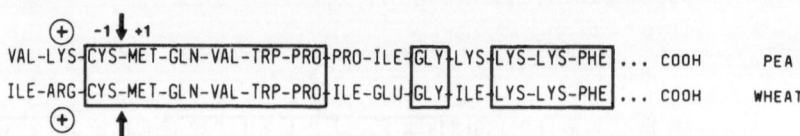

Fig. 2.   Comparison of the transit sequences of pea and wheat
          small subunit precursors. The amino acid sequences of
          the transit peptides were predicted from the nucleotide
          sequences of cDNA clones pSS15 (Coruzzi et al., 1982)
          and pW9 (Broglie et al., in preparation). Deletions
          in both sequences were allowed for maximal homology.
          Homologous amino acid sequences are boxed. Arrows
          indicate the position of cleavage site. Note that the
          transit sequence of pea pS is incomplete.

var. ERA). This clone, designated pW9, has a cDNA insert of
779 bp, which encodes the full length pS (175 amino acids; M_r =
19,450) (Broglie et al., in preparation). By sequence homology
to S of pea and of other higher plants (von Wettstein et al.,
1979) we have localized the NH_2 terminus of mature wheat S to
the 48th residue of pS. Thus, the wheat pS contains an NH_2
terminal transit sequence of 47 amino acid residues (M_r = 4,579)
(Fig. 2) in addition to the mature S (128 amino acids; M_r =
14,871) (Fig. 1).

    The amino acid composition of the small subunit of wheat
RUBISCO has been determined by Yeoh et al., (1979). Table I shows
that their values are quite similar to those predicted from our
cDNA clone, pW9. The complete amino acid sequence of the wheat
small subunit polypeptide deduced from pW9 is the first reported

for any monocot. Poulsen et al., (1976) has obtained partial
amino acid sequence for S of barley. It is remarkable that the
sequence of the first 25 amino acid residues of S is identical
between wheat and barley, although differences are found in other
regions, particularly the COOH terminus. For example, Poulsen et
al., (1976) characterized a tryptic peptide from barley S, which
has the following amino acid sequence: Y-W-T-L-W-K-L-P-M-F-G-I-P-
D-A. Examination of our wheat sequence shows that this tryptic
peptide is most likely homologous to residue 66 to 80 of the wheat
polypeptide. Figure 1 compares the complete amino acid sequence
of the RUBISCO small subunit of pea (dicot) and wheat (monocot)
as predicted from the nucleotide sequences of the cDNA clones,
pSS15 and pW9. The degree of sequence homology between the two
polypeptides is approximately 70%.

Table I. Comparison of Amino Acid Composition of Wheat RUBISCO
Small Subunit Obtained by Chemical Analysis and Deduced
from cDNA Sequence Analysis

Amino Acid	Chemical Analysis[a]	cDNA (pW9) Sequence Analysis[b]
Ala	7	5
Arg	6	6
Asn]	9	3
Asp		5
Cys	2	4
Gln]	14	5
Glu		11
Gly	9	8
His	2	1
Ile	4	5
Leu	9	9
Lys	8	9
Met	3	4
Phe	7	8
Pro	8	9
Ser	7	8
Thr	5	5
Trp	3	4
Tyr	6	7
Val	8	12
Total	117	128

[a] Yeoh et al., 1979
[b] Broglie et al., in preparation

In addition to the mature S, pSS15 also encodes an incomplete
transit peptide of 33 amino acids, and pW9, a full length transit
peptide of 47 amino acids. Comparison of the two transit peptides
(Fig. 2) reveals that the amino acid sequence in this part of the
precursor molecule is less homologous than that in the mature S
(Fig. 1). The wheat transit peptide is characterized by a prepon-
derance of basic amino acids and absence of Asp, Glu, His, Try,
and Tyr. We have suggested previously (Chua et al., 1980) that
the basic property of the transit peptide may be an important
feature in its interaction with the chloroplast envelope, which
is highly acidic at physiological pH (Douce and Joyard, 1980).
In this connection, it is interesting to note that in spite of
the weak sequence homology between the transit peptides of wheat
and pea pS, the number and positions of the positively-charged
amino acids are strongly conserved. Furthermore, there is a conservation of residues (-1 to -8) surrounding the cleavage site
(Cys-Met) which is identical in both plants.

Import of pS by Homologous and Heterologous Chloroplasts and Assembly of Newly-Imported S

Wheat and pea are members of monocots and dicots, respectively. These two major plant groups diverged approximately 150
million years ago; yet, transit peptides of their small subunit
precursors have retained certain structural similarities suggesting that these conserved molecular features may have functional
relevance. To see if polypeptide import is evolutionarily conserved between pea and wheat, poly A RNA translation products
were incubated in pair-wise combination with intact chloroplasts
from the two plants. Figure 3 shows that pS from either plant
is imported into homologous or heterologous chloroplasts and
processed correctly to yield mature S of authentic size. Thus,
transport and processing of pS are interchangeable between pea and
wheat. This finding is not surprising in view of the structural
similarities of the transit peptide and the conservation of the
cleavage site (Cys-Met).

The marked sequence homology between pea and wheat small
subunit polypeptide (Fig. 1) raises the question of whether newly-
imported S shown in Fig. 3 would assemble with heterologous large
subunits to form hybrid holoenzymes. The RUBISCO holoenzyme has
a M_r of about 500,000 and can be clearly resolved from the rest
of the stromal proteins by electrophoresis in a 4-15% native gel.
Since the large subunit of RUBISCO is not labeled under our uptake
conditions, a simple test for small subunit assembly is to deter
mine whether the holoenzyme band is radioactive after precursor
import. Figure 4 shows that the newly-imported S of pea and wheat
can assemble with homologous (lanes 5 & 7) or heterologous large
subunits (lanes 6 & 8). As demonstrated previously for pea and
spinach (Chua and Schmidt, 1978a), the hybrid holoenzyme has iden-

tical electrophoretic mobility as the holoenzyme of the recipient
chloroplast (Fig. 4, lanes 2 & 6; 4 & 8). This observation indicates that the electrophoretic mobility of RUBISCO holoenzyme is
determined solely by the large subunit.

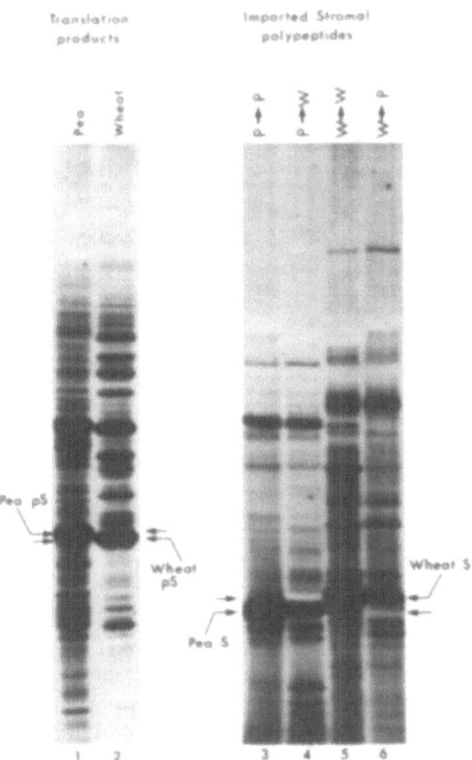

Fig. 3.   Import of stromal polypeptides by homologus and heter-
          ologous chloroplasts in vitro. Pea and wheat poly A
          RNAs were translated in a wheat germ cell-free system
          (Grossman et al., 1982). Uptake of newly-synthesized
          polypeptides into isolated chloroplasts was performed
          in the light as detailed elsewhere (Grossman et al.,
          1982). (1) & (2) Poly A RNA translation products of pea
          and wheat, respectively. Precursors (pS) to the small
          subunits of pea and wheat were identified by immunopre-
          cipitation of cell-free translation products (not shown);
          (3) & (4) Uptake of pea polypeptides into pea and wheat
          chloroplasts, respectively; (5) & (6) Uptake of wheat
          polypeptides into wheat and pea chloroplasts, respect-
          ively. Polypeptides were separated in a 8M urea-SDS
          12-18% gradient gel which was processed for fluorography.
          S, the small subunit of RUBISCO; pS, precursor to the
          small subunit; P, pea; W, wheat.

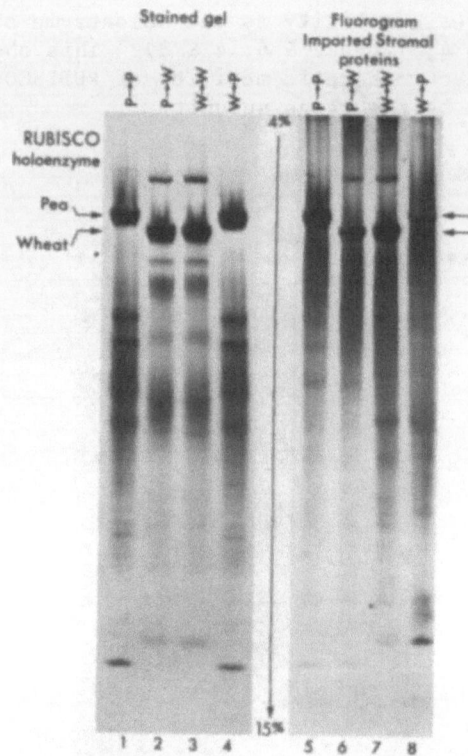

Fig. 4.   Assembly of newly-imported small subunits of pea and
          wheat with homologous and heterologous large subunits
          to form RUBISCO holoenzyme. After uptake (see legend
          to Fig. 3), stromal proteins were resolved in a non-
          denaturing polyacrylamide gel (4-15%) at 4° (Chua &
          Schmidt, 1978a). (1) & (2) Uptake of pea polypeptides
          by pea and wheat chloroplasts, respectively; (3) & (4)
          Uptake of wheat polypeptides by wheat and pea chloro-
          plasts, respectively. Lanes (1) to (4) show the stained
          protein profiles and lanes (5) to (8) the corresponding
          fluorograms. Arrows indicate the position of RUBISCO
          holoenzymes of pea and wheat. P, pea; W, wheat.

Analysis of Small Subunit Genes by Southern Blots and Isolation of Nuclear Genomic Clones Containing the Genes

     cDNA clones from pea (pSS15) and wheat (pW9) were used as
molecular hybridization probes to explore the organization of the
small subunit gene in genomic DNA. Nuclear DNAs from the two
plants were digested to completion with Eco RI, Bam HI, Hind III,
and Bgl II. Eco RI, Bam HI and Bgl II do not cut pSS15 or pW9,
whereas Hind III cuts pSS15 but not pW9. Southern blots of the

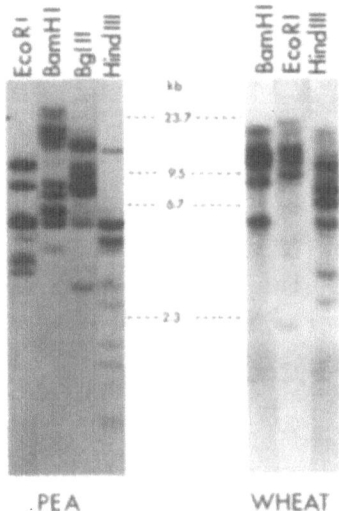

Fig. 5.   Genomic Southern blots of pea and wheat DNA probed with
          cDNA clones pSS15 and pW9. Total nuclear DNA from pea
          and wheat was digested to completion with Eco RI, Bam HI,
          Hind III and Bgl II.   DNA fragments, sized on a 0.8%
          agarose gel were transferred to nitrocellulose paper
          (Southern, 1975) and hybridized to nick translated cDNA
          insert from pSS15 (pea) and pW9 (wheat).   Hind III
          fragments of lambda DNA were used as size standards.

restriction digests were then probed with the respective small
subunit cDNA clones. In both plants, several hybridizing bands
were detected (Fig. 5), indicating that the small subunit is
encoded by a small multigene family.

Genomic clones for the small subunit were constructed from
pea and wheat nuclear DNA using lambda 1059 (Karn et al., 1980)
or Charon 30 (Rimm et al., 1980) as a vehicle. One wheat clone,
chwss 1, has a Bam HI subfragment of 4.3 kb, which was shown by
Southern hybridization to include the entire small subunit gene.
A partial restriction map of the Bam HI fragment is shown in Fig.
6. The small subunit gene was localized on this fragment by
Southern blot analysis, using the 5' and 3' fragments of pW9 as
probes. These hybridization data, in conjunction with results
obtained from R-looping experiments, are summarized in Fig. 6.

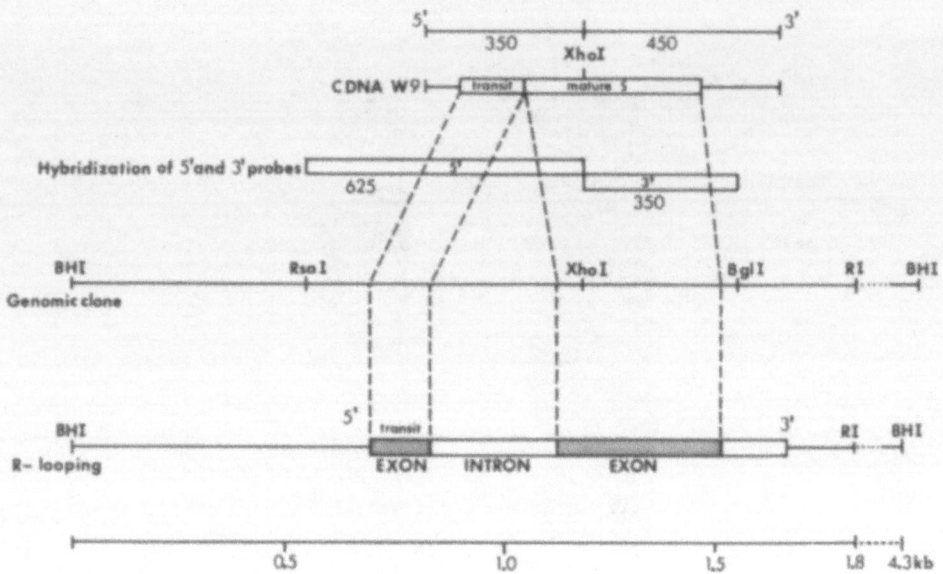

Fig. 6.   Localization of the small subunit gene on the 4.3 kb
          wheat genomic subclone. Partial restriction maps of
          pW9 and the 4.3 kb, Bam HI subfragment from chwss 1 are
          shown. 5' and 3' probes refer to the 5' and 3' fragments
          of pW9 generated by Xho I digestion. Nick-translated
          probes were hybridized to Southern blots of restriction
          fragments generated from the 4.3 fragment. chwss 1
          was hybridized to wheat mRNA under conditions favoring
          DNA:RNA hybrid formation, and visualized by electron
          microscopy. R-looping data is schematically repre-
          sented.

The small subunit gene of wheat is interrupted by an intron of
approximately 300 nucleotides, which separates the transit
sequence from the mature protein. In addition, the 4.3 kb fragment contains 700 nucleotides of 5' upstream sequences. Since
the 3' non-coding region of pW9 does not hybridize to sequences
at the 3' end of the genomic clone, we conclude that pW9 is not
encoded by chwss 1. These results have been confirmed by DNA
sequence analysis of chwss 1 (unpublished results).

     In pea, seven different genomic clones have been isolated.
Southern analysis of these clones reveals that the small subunit
gene is localized within Eco RI fragments ranging in size from
3-15 kb. Detailed analysis of one clone (PG14-3D) shows that it
has a 4 kb Eco RI fragment which contains the entire small subunit
gene. Dot blot hybridization experiments reveal that PG14-3D

hybridizes specifically to a 3' non-coding probe from pSS15 under high stringency (data not shown). Although these results strongly suggest that pSS15 is encoded by PG14-3D, definitive proof must await sequence determination of the genomic clone.

CONCLUSION

In this paper we have summarized our recent results on the isolation and characterization of cDNA and genomic clones for the RUBISCO small subunit of pea and wheat. The complete nucleotide sequences of the cDNA clones pSS15 and pW9, have permitted the deduction of the amino acid sequences of the mature S and the precursor transit peptides. Our *in vitro* reconstitution experiments demonstrated clearly that the wheat and pea small subunit precursors are imported interchangeably into either chloroplast types. Moreover, the precursors are processed correctly in heterologous chloroplasts and the mature forms assembled into hybrid RUBISCO holoenzymes. These experiments suggest that transport, processing, and assembly of the small subunits are conserved between monocots and dicots. As more sequence information for precursor transit peptide accumulates, it may be possible in the future to define structural domains of this extra sequence, which is important for envelope interaction and traversal. Southern hybridization experiments revealed that the small subunit in both pea and wheat is encoded by a small multigene family. This finding is corroborated by the isolation and preliminary characterization of seven different small subunit genomic clones from pea. Characterization of the pea and wheat small subunit genomic clones may help us understand the regulation of different members of the multigene family during plant development.

ACKNOWLEDGEMENTS

We thank Nadera Ahmed, Susan Fiteni and Sara Trillo for skilled technical assistance. This work was supported in part by NIH GM-25114 and by Monsanto Corporation. G.C. and R.B. are recipients of NIH Postdoctoral Fellowships, 5F32 GM-07776 and 5F32 GM-07446, respectively. G.L. is a postdoctoral fellow of the Damon-Runyon Walter-Winchell Fund.

REFERENCES

Apel, K. and Kloppstech, K., 1978, The plastid membranes of barley. Light-induced apearance of mRNA coding for the apoprotein of the light harvesting chlorophyll a/b binding protein, Eur. J. Biochem., 85:581.

Apel, K., 1979, Phytochrome-induced appearance of mRNA activity for the apoprotein of the light-harvesting chlorophyll a/b protein of barley (Hordeum vulgare), Eur. J. Biochem., 97:183.

Bedbrook, J. R., Smith, S. M., and Ellis, R. J., 1980, Molecular cloning and sequencing of cDNA encoding the precursor to the small subunit of the chloroplast enzyme ribulose-1,5 bisphosphate carboxylase, Nature, 287:692.

Broglie, R., Bellemare, G., Bartlett, S. G., Chua, N.-H., and Cashmore, A. R., 1981, Cloned DNA sequences complementary to mRNAs encoding precursors to the small subunit of ribulose-1,5-bisphosphate carboxylase and a chlorophyll a/b binding polypeptide, Proc. Nat. Acad. Sci. USA, 78:7304.

Broglie, R., Coruzzi, G. and Chua, N.-H., 1982, Differential expression of genes encoding polypeptides involved in C4 photosynthesis, in: "Chloroplast Biogenesis," Cambridge University Press, London, in press.

Cashmore, A. R., Broadhurst, M. K., and Gray, R. E., 1978, Cell-free synthesis of leaf proteins: identification of an apparent precursor of the small subunit of ribulose-1,5-bisphosphate carboxylase, Proc. Natl. Acad. Sci. USA, 75:655.

Chua, N.-H. and Schmidt, G. W. 1978a, In vitro synthesis, transport and assembly of ribulose bisphosphate carboxylase subunits, in: "Photosynthetic Carbon Assimilation," H. W. Siegelman and G. Hind, eds., Plenum Press, New York.

Chua, N.-H. and Schmidt, G. W., 1978b, Post-translational transport into intact chloroplasts of a precursor to the small subunit of ribulose-1,5-bisphosphate carboxylase, Proc. Natl. Acad. Sci. USA, 75:6110.

Chua, N.-H. and Schmidt, G. W., 1979, Transport of proteins into mitochondria and chloroplasts, J. Cell Biol. 81:461.

Chua, N.-H., Grossman, A. R., Bartlett, S. G., and Schmidt, G. W., 1980, Synthesis, transport and assembly of chloroplast proteins, in: "Biological Chemistry of Organelle Formation," Th. Bucher, W. Sebald, and H. Weiss, eds., Springer-Verlag Press, New York.

Coruzzi, G., Broglie, R., Cashmore, A. R., and Chua, N.-H., 1982, Nucleotide sequences of two pea cDNA clones encoding the small subunit of ribulose bisphosphate carboxylase and the major chlorophyll a/b-binding thylakoid polypeptide. J. Biol. Chem., in press.

Douce, R. and Joyard, J., 1979, Structure and function of the plastid envelope, Adv. Bot. Res., 7:1.

Ellis, R. J., 1981, Chloroplase proteins: synthesis, transport and assembly, Ann. Rev. Plant Physiol., 32:111.

Grossman, A., Bartlett, S. and Chua, N.-H., 1980, Energy-dependent uptake of cytoplasmically synthesized polypeptides by chloroplasts, Nature, 285:625.

Grossman, A. R., Bartlett, S. G., Schmidt, G. W., Mullet, J. E., and Chua, N.-H., 1982, Optimal conditions for post-translational uptake of proteins by isolated chloroplasts. In vitro synthesis and transport of plastocyanin, ferredoxin-NaDp$^+$ oxidoreductase, and fructose-1,6-bisphosphatase, J. Biol. Chem., 257:1558.

Highfield, P. E. and Ellis, R. J., 1978, Synthesis and transport of the small subunit of chloroplast ribulose bisphosphate carboxylase, Nature, 271:420.

Karn, J., Brenner, S., Barnett, L., and Cesareni, G., 1980, Novel bacteriophage lambda cloning vector, Proc. Nat. Acad. Sci. USA, 77:5172.

Poulsen, C., Strobek, S., and Haslett, B., 1976, Studies on the primary structure of the small subunit of ribulose-1,5-bisphosphate carboxylase, in: "Genetics and Biogenesis of Chloroplast and Mitochondria," Th. Bucher, et al., eds., Elsevier/North Holland Biomedical Press, Amsterdam, The Netherlands.

Rimm, D. L., Horness, D., Kucera, J., and Blattner, P. R., 1980, Construction of coliphage lambda charon vectors with Bam HI cloning sites, Gene, 12:301.

Sasaki, Y., Ishiye, M., Sakihama, T., and Kamikubo, T., 1981, Light-induced increase of mRNA activity coding for the small subunit of ribulose-1,5-bisphosphate carboxylase, J. Biol. Chem., 256:2315.

Schmidt, G. W., Bartlett, S. G., Grossman, A. R., Cashmore, A. R., and Chua, N.-H., 1981, Biosynthetic pathways of two polypeptide subunits of the light-harvesting chlorophyll a/b protein complex, J. Cell Biol., 91:468.

Smith, S. M. and Ellis, R. J., 1981, Light-stimulated accumulation of transcripts of nuclear and chloroplast genes for ribulose bisphosphate carboxylase, J. Mol. Appl. Gen., 1:127.

Southern, E. M., 1975, Detection of specific sequences among DNA fragments separated by gel electrophoresis, J. Mol. Biol., 98:503.

Takruri, I. A. H., Boulter, D., and Ellis, R. J., 1981, Amino acid sequence of the small subunit of ribulose-1,5-bisphosphate carboxylase of Pisum sativum, Phytochem., 20:413.

Tobin, E. M. and Suttie, J. L., 1980, Light effects on the synthesis of ribulose-1,5-bisphosphate carboxylase in Lemma gibba L G-3, Plant Physiol., 65:641.

von Wettstein, D., Poulsen, C. and Holder, A. A., 1978, Ribulose 1,5-bisphosphate carboxylase as a nuclear and chloroplast marker, Theor. Appl. Genet., 53:193.

Yeoh, H. H., Stone, N. E., Creaser, E. H., and Watson, L., 1979, Isolation and characterization of wheat ribulose-1,5-bisphosphate carboxylase, Phytochem., 8:561.

MUTATIONS AT THE <u>SHRUNKEN</u> LOCUS IN MAIZE CAUSED BY THE CONTROLLING

ELEMENT <u>DS</u>

N. Fedoroff[1], D. Chaleff[1], U. Courage-Tebbe[2],
H.-P. Döring[2], M. Geiser[2]*, P. Starlinger[2],
E. Tillmann[2], E. Weck[2], and W. Werr[2]

[1]Carnegie Institute of Washington
Department of Embryology
115 West University Parkway
Baltimore, Maryland 21210
[2]Institut für Genetik
Universität zu Köln
Weyertal 121, D-5000 Köln 41
Federal Republic of Germany
*present address: Friedrich Miescher Institut
P.O. Box 273, CH-4002 Basel, Switzerland

INTRODUCTION

    Controlling elements in maize are transposable elements that
cause insertion mutations, mediate chromosomal rearrangements and
provide sites of chromosome breakage. Several distinct families
of controlling elements have been identified, three of which have
been studied in substantial detail genetically (for reviews, see
McClintock, 1951, 1956b, 1965; Fincham and Sastry, 1974; Nevers and
Saedler, 1977; Starlinger, 1980 and Fedoroff, 1982). Among the best
characterized is the <u>Activator-Dissociation</u> family of elements that
is responsible for the mutations at the <u>Shrunken</u> (<u>Sh</u>) locus described
here (McClintock, 1951). <u>Activator</u> (<u>Ac</u>) is an element capable of
autonomous transposition, while the <u>Dissociation</u> (<u>Ds</u>) element trans-
poses only in the presence of the autonomously-transposing <u>Ac</u>
element (McClintock, 1951). <u>Ds</u> was first identified and named for
its ability to provide a specific site of chromosome breakage and

acentric-dicentric chromosome formation, a property that is also
manifested only in the presence of the Ac element (McClintock, 1946,
1947). Transposition of Ds to a locus affecting plant or kernel
morphology can result in a recessive mutant phenotype (McClintock,
1951, 1956b). Ds insertion mutations are stable in the absence of
Ac, but in its presence revert or further mutate both somatically
and germinally. Somatic mutation can give rise to phenotypically
altered sectors of cells within the organism (for illustrations, see
McClintock, 1965, and Fedoroff, 1982). Both the somatic and germinal
reversion of Ds mutations is commonly, but not invariably, associated
with the loss of the element from the locus. McClintock also
identified strains with Ds elements, which she designated as "non-
transposing", that behave as local mutagens (McClintock, 1952, 1953,
1954, 1955, 1956a). In these strains, the Ds element is characterized
by its ability to provide a site of chromosome breakage during
somatic development and by its ability to give rise to mutations
affecting nearby loci on one side or the other of the original site
of insertion, but not on both sides simultaneously (McClintock, 1952,
1953, 1954, 1955, 1956a). It is the non-transposing Ds elements that
are responsible for the mutations at the Sh locus whose molecular
characterization is described in the present communication.

The Sh locus in maize encodes the enzyme sucrose synthase, which
catalyzes the reversible conversion of sucrose to fructose and UDP-
glucose (Chourey and Nelson, 1976). The Sh-encoded enzyme is the
major, but not the only sucrose synthase activity in immature endosperm tissue (Chourey and Nelson, 1976; Chourey, 1981). There is a
second minor sucrose synthase that is enzymatically indistinguishable
from, and immunologically related to, the Sh-encoded enzyme (Chourey,
1981). The minor sucrose synthase is encoded by a gene that is
distantly related to the coding sequence at the Sh locus (McCormick
et al., 1982). Mutations at the Sh locus substantially reduce, but
do not altogether abolish, endosperm starch biosynthesis. Several
mutant alleles of the Sh locus have been described whose origin is
associated with non-transposing Ds elements (McClintock, 1952, 1953,
1954, 1955, 1956a). The original unstable alleles are designated
sh-m5933, sh-m6233, and sh-m6258. There is also a derivative of
the sh-m6258 strain, designated sh-m6795, which represents a
recessive mutation derived from an unstable Sh revertant of the sh-
m6258 strain. The unstable alleles of the Sh locus arose in strains
containing a non-transposing Ds element just distal to the Sh locus
on the short arm of chromosome 9 (McClintock, 1952, 1953). All four
mutant alleles of the Sh locus are stable in the absence of the Ac
element, but revert to Sh alleles both somatically and germinally
in the presence of Ac. As judged by the location of the Ds-
associated site of chromosome breakage, neither the initial mutations
nor the reversion events are accompanied by transposition of the
element to a genetically distinguishable position (McClintock, 1953).
Revertants remain unstable, mutating to recessive alleles in the
presence of the Ac element (McClintock, 1955). The behavior of the

sh-m alleles is therefore quite different from that of many other Ds insertion mutations and suggests that they arise and revert by local chromosomal rearrangements, although the involvement of extremely short-range transpositions cannot be excluded.

We have examined the structure and expression of the Sh locus in the mutant strains sh-m5933, sh-m6233, and sh-m6258 and sh-m6795 and in a strain carrying the progenitor Sh allele (Fedoroff et al., 1980; Chaleff et al., 1981; Fedoroff et al., 1982; Wöstemeyer et al., 1980; Geiser et al., 1980; Courage-Tebbe et al., 1982), as have Burr and Burr (1980, 1981, 1982). The mutant locus has been characterized in greatest detail in strain sh-m5933, from which a portion of the mutant locus has been isolated (Courage-Tebbe et al., 1982). In addition, preliminary structural studies have been carried out on a number of newly-isolated Sh revertant strains derived from sh-m5933. The results of the structural studies will be described, followed by a summary of experiments on expression of the locus in immature endosperm tissue of mutant strains lacking the Ac element and preliminary molecular studies on several revertants.

STRUCTURAL STUDIES ON THE Sh LOCUS IN sh-m STRAINS.

Studies on the structure of the Sh locus in mutant strains sh-m6233, sh-m5933, sh-m6258 and sh-m6795 have been carried out using cDNA probes representing a portion of the mRNA sequence encoded by the locus (Döring et al., 1981; Burr and Burr, 1980, 1981, 1982; Chaleff et al., 1981; Fedoroff et al., 1982; Fedoroff, Mauvais and Chaleff, 1982), as well as cloned fragments of the Sh locus isolated from a strain carrying the progenitor Sh allele from which the sh-m alleles were derived and two of the sh-m strains (Courage-Tebbe et al., 1982; Fedoroff, unpublished). The presence of extensive restriction endonuclease cleavage site polymorphism in the immediate vicinity of the Sh locus necessitated considerable care in the identification of the correct progenitor locus (Chaleff et al., 1981). A restriction endonuclease cleavage site map of the locus that has been identified as the progenitor appears in Figure 1a. Its identity as the progenitor locus was deduced from the coincidence between its structure and the structure of the unaltered portion of the locus in the mutant strains studied and by its resemblance to the structure of the locus in revertant strains.

Each of the four mutant strains studied had a different structural alteration at the Sh locus. In two of the mutant strains, sh-m5933 and sh-m6233, sequence changes were detected near the 5' end of the transcription unit (Fig. 1b and c). As described in more detail below, the strains differ from each other in the location of the rearrangement breakpoint, as well as the nature of foreign sequence immediately adjacent to the Sh locus sequences. In the

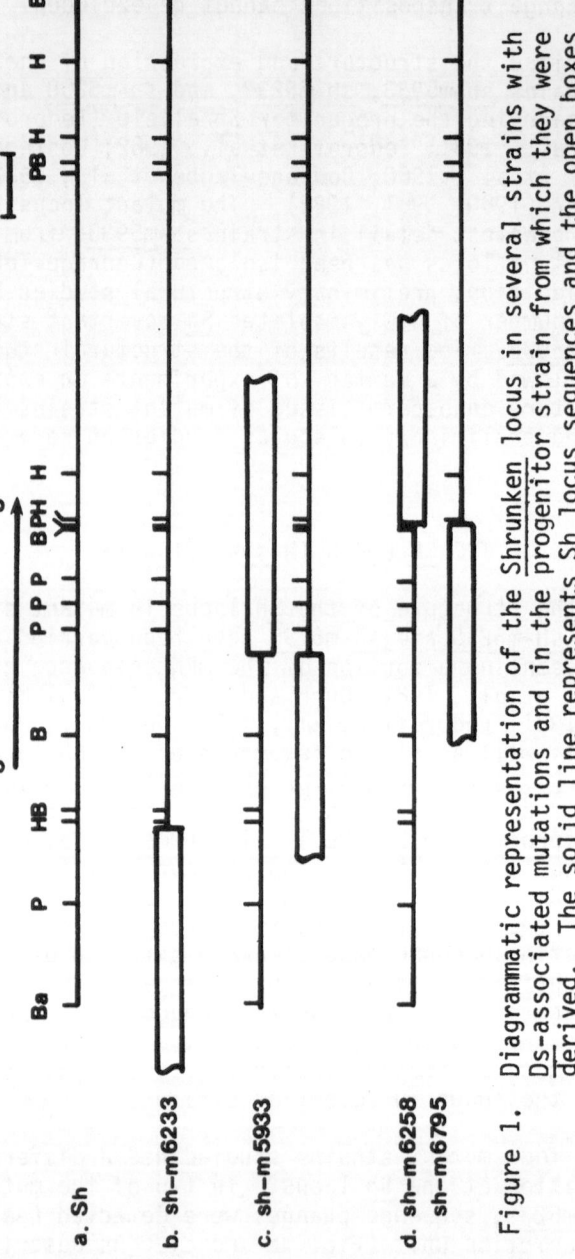

Figure 1.   Diagrammatic representation of the Shrunken locus in several strains with Ds-associated mutations and in the progenitor strain from which they were derived. The solid line represents Sh locus sequences and the open boxes represent foreign sequences adjacent to Sh locus sequences in various mutant strains. The restriction endonuclease cleavage sites are: B = Bgl II, Ba = Bam HI, H = Hind III and P = Pst I. The arrow indicates the direction of transcription and approximately locates the mRNA coding sequence.

related strains sh-m6258 and sh-m6795, the transcription unit is
interrupted within a short intervening sequence near the 3' end of
the mRNA coding sequence (Fig. 1d). The rearrangement breakpoint
maps to the same location in both strains, although the strains
are distinguishable on the basis of the location of restriction
enzyme cleavage sites within the foreign sequence interrupting the
gene (Federoff et el., 1982). There is evidence for the
strains sh-m5933, sh-m6258 and sh-m6795 that sequences originally
present on both sides of the rearrangement breakpoint persist in
the genome. However, as discussed in greater detail below, it is
not yet clear whether the structure of the Sh locus in the Ds
mutant strains is altered due to an insertion or some other type
of chromosomal rearrangement.

The rearrangement breakpoint adjacent to the portion of the Sh
locus containing the transcription unit has been cloned from DNA of
the sh-m6233 and sh-m5933 strains (Courage-Tebbe et al., 1982).
The isolation of a cDNA clone carrying about 500 bp homologous to
the mRNA of the sucrose synthase gene has been reported (Geiser
et al., 1980). Hybridization of this cDNA to recombinant λ1059
phages made possible the isolation of a phage containing an insert
of 16.3 kb. This insert contains the complete sucrose synthase
gene that is the progenitor allele of the Ds-induced sh mutants
described above. The direction of transcription of the gene was
determined by hybridization of mRNA to labeled subfragments,
followed by S1 nuclease digestion. Preliminary studies indicate
that there are several intervening sequences in the sucrose synthase
gene.

Two other recombinant phages were isolated carrying DNA fragments from two different mutable alleles of the Sh locus (sh-m5933
and sh-m6233). A 21-kb Bcl II fragment derived from sh-m5933 DNA
and a 17.6-kb fragment obtained by partial Sau 3A digestion of sh-
m6233 DNA were cloned in λ1059. The cloned fragments of DNA from
the mutant strains contain sequences of several kilobase pairs that
are homologous to the cloned fragment of the progenitor Sh allele.
This common region contains part or all of the sucrose synthase gene.
Both fragments derived from the sh-m strains contain foreign sequences
adjacent to the Sh locus sequences. These sequences are not present
in the cloned fragment containing the progenitor Sh allele. The
foreign DNA may contain part or all of the Ds element; alternatively
it may represent DNA which has been introduced as a result of a Ds-
associated rearrangement. The point at which the sequence of the
fragment derived from the mutant DNA diverges from the Sh locus
sequence differs in the two mutants (Fig. 1b and c). These points
of divergence represent either the insertion site or the rearrangement breakpoint. In the mutant sh-m5933, the point of divergence
is within the transcription unit. The point of divergence in the

mutant sh-m6233 is at a distance of approximately 2.5 kb from the point of divergence in mutant sh-m5933 and on the 5' side of it relative to the direction at transcription. It is not known whether it lies within or outside of the transcription unit.

The segments of foreign DNA sequence in the fragments cloned from sh-m5933 (15 kb) and sh-m6233 (11 kb) DNA contain a limited region of partial homology. In both cases, the region of partial homology is adjacent to the point of divergence of the sequence from that of the Sh locus sequence. This region is approximately 3 kb in length. That these regions are only partially homologous has been deduced from differences in the location of several restriction endonuclease cleavage sites. The region of partial homology was further analyzed in the cloned fragment of sh-m5933 DNA. Two inverted repeats of several hundred nucleotides each were found in this region. One member of the first pair of inverted repeats is characterized by a Bam HI site. There is a distance of approximately 1.3 kb between the two sequences repeated in inverted order. One member of the second inverted repeat is located in this DNA segment. The second member of this repeat is found to the left of the first pair of inverted repeats. In sh-m5933 DNA, one member of the first pair of repeats terminates at the point of divergence. By contrast, in sh-m6233 DNA, one member of the other pair of repeats is found near this point. Although we have no direct evidence that the regions of partial homology adjacent to the rearrangement breakpoints in the mutant strains sh-m5933 and sh-m6233 correspond to Ds element sequences, we have taken this as a working hypothesis, designating these regions "putative Ds DNA" in the following sections. If the regions of sequence homology do indeed comprise Ds element sequences, the absence of complete homology suggests that the elements either differ in their orienta- tion in the two mutant strains or that there are sequence differences among Ds elements.

Cloned subfragments from the region of partial homology (putative Ds DNA) were used as probes in Southern blot hybridization experiments. Up to 40 distinct bands were detected by the probes. Such a pattern is characteristic of neither unique nor highly repetitive DNA. If the DNA is derived from the Ds element, the element must be present in multiple copies in genomic DNA. Because a large number of bands is detected when fragments internal to the putative Ds DNA from the sh-m5933 clone are used as probes, the different copies of the corresponding genomic sequence must be heterogeneous in their restriction endonuclease cleavage patterns.

The results of genomic blot hybridization experiments involving the use of probes from cloned fragments of the progenitor Sh locus indicate that none of the sequences adjacent to the rearrangement breakpoint in the sh-m5933 strain are deleted from the mutant strain. Mapping studies with a variety of enzymes have

invariably identified two separate junction fragments with homology
to the 5' and 3' sides of the rearrangement breakpoint within the
mutant locus. We have deduced from these studies that the distance
between the left and right rearrangement breakpoints must be at
least 20-25 kb in the sh-m5933 strain. Similar studies on mutant
strains sh-m6258 and sh-m6795 indicate that the minimal distance
between the rearrangement breakpoints is 33-38 kb (Fedoroff et al.,
1982). In view of these results, as well as differences between
the restriction maps of the Sh alleles identified by us (Chaleff
et al., 1981; Courage-Tebbe et al., 1982; Federoff et al., 1982)
and by Burr and Burr (1982) as the progenitor allele from which
the mutant strains were originally derived, we cannot support
their conclusion that the mutations are attributable to insertions of 20-22 kb. Our present results are compatible with the
presence either of a large insertion or of another type of
chromosomal rearrangement, such as an inversion.

EXPRESSION OF THE Sh LOCUS IN sh-m STRAINS.

    The sucrose synthase encoded by the Sh locus has been reported
to be a homotetramer (Su and Preiss, 1978). The apparent monomeric
molecular weight of the protein is 92 kD and it is encoded by a
relatively abundant 3-kb mRNA (Su and Preiss, 1978; Burr and Burr,
1980; Chourey, 1981; Fedoroff et al., 1980; Wöstemeyer et al., 1981;
Federoff et al., 1982). The enzyme is expressed only in immature endosperm tissue (Chourey and Nelson, 1976; Chourey
personal communication). Studies on expression of the Sh locus in
sh-m strains were carried out using immature kernels of mutant
strains lacking an active Ac element and therefore measure
expression of the mutant gene under conditions in which Ac-activated
somatic reversion is not occurring. None of the strains contained
detectable amounts of the native sucrose synthase encoded by the Sh
locus in immature endosperm tissue (Table 1; Fedoroff et al.,
1982). Immature endosperm tissue of all of the strains contained only the minor sucrose synthase encoded by the second,
distantly-related sucrose synthase gene (Chourey, 1981; McCormick
et al., 1982). High levels of inactive polypeptides immunoprecipitable with sucrose synthase antiserum were not detected in immature
endosperm of any of the strains (Table 1). However, endosperm
tissue of strains sh-m6258 and sh-m6795 did contain small amounts
of two polypeptides immunologically related to sucrose synthase,
but having apparent molecular weights of 82 kD and 85 kD. The
immunologically cross-reacting 82- and 85-kD proteins were detected
among in vitro translation products of immature kernal poly A[+] mRNAs
of these strains as well (Federoff et al., 1982). The aberrant
sucrose synthase-like polypeptides were more abundant amongst
in vitro translation products than in immature endosperm tissue,
suggesting that the polypeptides are unstable in vivo, despite the
abundance and stability of the mRNA.

Table 1. Expression of the Sh locus in immature kernels of mutant strains whose origin is associated with the controlling element Ds.

	Native Sh-encoded sucrose synthase	Sh-encoded mutant polypeptides	Sucrose synthase mRNA
sh-m5933	-*	-	0.5-1%
sh-m6233	-	-	0.5-1%
sh-m6258 and sh-m6795	-	82 and 85 kD	10-25%, structure aberrant

*-indicates that such proteins were not detectable within the limits of sensitivity of the assays employed.

     Poly A+ mRNA in immature kernels of the sh-m6233 and sh-m5933 contain low levels (0.5-1%) of an mRNA that is homologous to and has the same electrophoretic mobility as the 3-kb sucrose synthase mRNA (Table 1; Federoff et al., 1982). By contrast, strains sh-m6258 and sh-m6795 contain 10-25% of the normal amount of an Sh locus transcript that is approximately 2.8 kb in length and lacks homology with the sucrose synthase locus beyond the rearrangement breakpoint within the coding sequence (Figure 1). The transcripts appear to be the same in both strains and encode the 82- and 85-kD polypeptides immunoprecipitable from immature endosperm tissue with sucrose synthase antiserum (Fedoroff et al., 1982). Transcripts of the portion of the Sh coding sequence 3' to the rearrangement breakpoint are below the level of detection. Thus transcription of the rearranged (Sh) locus in strains sh-m6258 and sh-m6795 is relatively unaffected. The mutant phenotype of these strains is therefore consequent on synthesis of a structurally altered sucrose synthase. Whether the altered sucrose synthase polypeptides are enzymatically inactive or whether they are active, but highly unstable, is not known. The presence of two sucrose synthase-like polypeptides differing slightly in size (82- and 85-kD) is also unexplained.

STRUCTURE OF Sh REVERTANTS DERIVED FROM THE sh-m5933 STRAIN.

     Preliminary studies have been carried out on six different Sh revertants derived from the sh-m5933 strain (Fedoroff, unpublished). In agreement with observations originally reported by McClintock (1953), all of the newly-derived revertants continue to show chromosome breakage at the Sh locus in the presence of the Ac

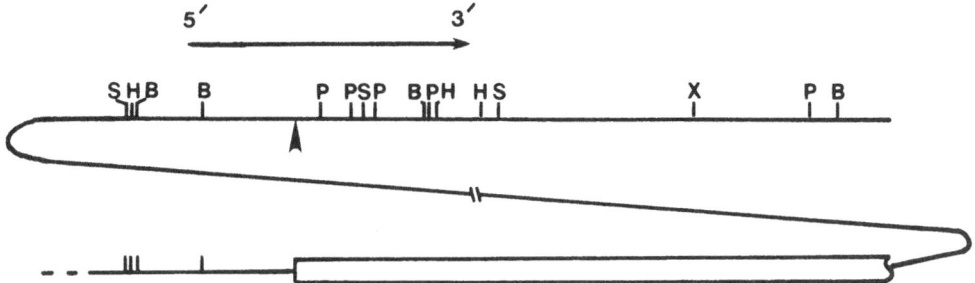

Figure 2. Diagrammatic representation of the structure of several
Sh revertant chromosomes.

        Chromosomes carrying a revertant Sh allele derived from the
sh-m5933 strain contain both a normal Sh locus and a portion of the
rearranged locus present in the sh-m5933 strain on the same
chromosome, although the distance separating them is not known.
The restriction endonuclease cleavage sites are: B = Bgl II, H =
Hind III, P = Pst I, S = Sst I, X = Xba I. The arrow approximately locates and indicates the polarity of the mRNA coding
sequence. The arrowhead below the diagram of the revertant Sh
locus designates the original rearrangement breakpoint in the sh-
m5933 strain. Sh locus sequences 5' to the rearrangement breakpoint are duplicated in the revertant strains, as indicated in the
lower portion of the diagram.

element, indicating the persistance of the Ds element. The results
of Southern blot hybridization experiments on the revertants are
represented diagramatically in Fig. 2. The various revertant
strains are similar or identical structurally. In all of them, the
single restriction endonuclease fragment containing the rearrangement breakpoint in the sh-m5933 strain is detectable and has the
same mobility as the fragment present in the progenitor Sh locus.
However, all of the strains contain an additional fragment that
shows homology to sequences originally present on the 5' side of

the rearrangement breakpoint, but not to sequences initially present
on the 3' side of the rearrangement breakpoint. It is not yet clear
whether the duplication of Sh sequences 5' to the rearrangement
breakpoint occurred during the initial mutation or during the
reversion event. Presently available data are most consistent with
the occurrence of duplication event during reversion. The length
of the duplication is not yet known, although it extends at least
2-2.5 kb to the 5' side of the rearrangement breakpoint.

DISCUSSION

       There is both genetic and molecular evidence that the structural
alteration observed in the sh-m strains whose molecular analysis has
been described here are associated with the Ds element. As is
characteristic of other mutations caused by the Ds element, the
mutations in the sh-m strains are stable in the absence of Ac, but
revert in its presence (McClintock, 1953). The mutations in the
sh-m strains are caused by what McClintock (1956a) termed a "non-
transposing" Ds element. Reversion of the mutations is not accompanied by a genetically detectable change in the location of the
Ds element (McClintock, 1953; Fedoroff, unpublished). The present
studies reveal that the structure of several revertant strains
independently derived from the sh-m5933 strain is very similar and
that the strains contain both a copy of the intact locus and a
duplication of the portion of the locus on the 5' side of the
original rearrangement breakpoint. It is not yet clear whether the
duplication pre-exists in the original mutant strain or is
generated during the reversion event. The existence of the
duplication, however, indicates the involvement of chromosomal
rearrangements in the Ds-mediated mutations at this locus.

       McClintock (1953, 1955) reported that revertant strains
continue to be unstable in the presence of Ac, giving rise to
further unstable derivatives, such as the sh-m6795 derivative of
the sh-m6258 strain. Although the revertant intervening in the
genetic lineage between the two strains has been lost (McClintock,
personal communication), molecular studies on the strains sh-m6258
and sh-m6795 have revealed the presence of very similar genetic
lesions. The mutations in both strains are rearrangements with
one breakpoint at the same site within the transcription unit. The
strains further resemble each other in the location of restriction
endonuclease cleavage sites in the foreign DNA adjacent to the 3'
end of the gene, although they differ in the location of some sites
near the 5' end of the gene (Fedoroff et al., 1982). These
observations are also compatible with the involvement of reversible
rearrangements in the origin and reversion of the Ds-mediated
mutations in the sh-m strains. However, the nature of the
original structural change at the locus in the sh-m strains cannot
be deduced unequivocally from the information presently available.

Although our data do not support the inference drawn by Burr and Burr (1982) that the mutations are caused by 20-22 kb insertions, we cannot rule out the possibility that the sh-m alleles contain extremely large insertions. Nonetheless, the genetic history of the strains, as well as the structure of the revertants, suggest that the mutations are attributable to Ds-mediated local rearrangements rather than to transposition of the element.

ACKNOWLEDGEMENTS

This work was supported by Landesamt für Forschung NRW, the Commission of the European Communities, the National Science Foundation, the USDA Competitive Research Grant Program and the Damon Runyan-Walter Winchell Fund.

REFERENCES

Burr, B., and Burr, F., 1980, Detection of changes in maize DNA at the Shrunken locus due to the intervention of Ds elements, Cold Spring Harbor Symp. Quant. Biol. 45:463.

Burr, B., and Burr, F., 1981, Controlling-element events at the Shrunken locus in maize, Genetics 98:143.

Burr, B., and Burr, F., 1982, Ds controlling elements of maize at the Shrunken locus are large and dissimilar insertions, Cell 29:977.

Chaleff, D., Mauvais, J., McCormick, S., Shure, M., Wessler, S. and Fedoroff, N., 1981, Controlling elements in maize, Carnegie Inst. Wash. Year Book 80:158.

Chourey, P.S., 1981, Genetic control of sucrose synthetase in maize endosperm, Mol. Gen. Genet. 184:373.

Chourey, P.S. and Nelson, O.E., 1976, The enzymatic deficiency conditioned by the shrunken-1 mutations in maize, Biochem. Gen. 14:1041.

Courage-Tebbe, U., Döring, H.-P., Geiser, M., Starlinger, P., Tillmann, E., Weck, E., Werr, W., 1982, Two Partial copies of Heterogeneous Transposable Element Ds Cloned from the Shrunken Locus in Zea mays L., in "Manipulation and Expression of Genes in Eukaryotes", P. Nagley, A.W. Ninnane, W.J. Peacock, and J.A. Pateman, eds., Academic Press, Sydney, in press.

Döring, H.-P., Geiser, M. and Starlinger, P., 1981, Transposable element Ds at the shrunken locus in Zea mays, Mol. Gen. Genet. 184:377.

Fedoroff, N., 1982, Transposable elements in maize, in "Mobile Genetic Elements", J. Shapiro, ed., in press.

Fedoroff, N., McCormick, S., and Mauvais, J., 1980, Molecular studies on the controlling elements of maize, Carnegie Inst. Wash. Year Book 79:51.

Fedoroff, N., Mauvais, J., and Chaleff, D., 1982, Molecular studies

on mutations at the Shrunken locus in maize caused by the
controlling elements Ds, J. Mol. Appl. Gen., in press.

Fedoroff, N., Chaleff, D., Mauvais, J., Shure, M. and Wessler, S.,
1982, Molecular studies on maize genes with controlling
element mutations, Carnegie Inst. Wash. Year Book 81: in press.

Fincham, J.R.S., and Sastry, G.R.K., 1974, Controlling elements in
maize, Ann. Rev. Genet. 8:15.

Geiser, M., Döring, H.-P., Wöstemeyer, Behrens, U., Tillmann, and
Starlinger, P., 1980, A cDNA clone from Zea mays endosperm
sucrose synthetase mRNA, Nucl. Acids Res., 8:6175.

McClintock, B., 1946, Maize genetics, Carnegie Inst. Wash. Year
Book 45:176.

McClintock, B., 1947, Cytogenetic studies of maize and Neurospora.
Carnegie Inst. Wash. Year Book 46:146.

McClintock, B., 1951, Chromosome organization and genic expression,
Cold Spring Harbor Symp. Quant. Biol. 16:13.

McClintock, B., 1952, Mutable loci in maize, Carnegie Inst. Wash.
Year Book 51:212.

McClintock, B., 1953, Mutation in maize, Carnegie Inst. Wash. Year
Book 52:227.

McClintock, B., 1954, Mutations in maize and chromosomal aberrations
in Neurospora, Carnegie Inst. Wash. Year Book 53:254.

McClintock, B., 1955, Controlled mutation in maize, Carnegie Inst.
Wash. Year Book 54:245.

McClintock, B., 1956a, Mutation in maize, Carnegie Inst. Wash.
Year Book 55:323.

McClintock, B., 1956b, Controlling elements and the gene, Cold
Spring Harbor Symp. Quant. Biol. 21:197.

McClintock, B., 1965, The control of gene action in maize,
Brookhaven Symp. Biol. 18:162.

McCormick, S., Mauvais, J., and Fedoroff, N., 1982, Evidence that
the two sucrose synthetase genes in maize are related, Mol.
Gen. Genet., in press.

Nevers, P., and Saedler, H., 1977, Transposable genetic elements
as agents of gene instability and chromosome rearrangement,
Nature 268:109.

Su, J.-C., and Preiss, J., 1978, Purification and properties of
sucrose synthetase from maize kernels, Plant Physiol. 61:389.

Starlinger, P., 1980, A reexamination of McClintock's "Controlling
Elements" in maize in view of recent advances in molecular
biology, in "Genome Organization and Expression in Plants",
C.J. Leaver, ed., Plenum Publishing Corp. New York.

Wöstemeyer, J., Behrens, U., Merckelbach, A., Muller, M., and
Starlinger, P., 1981, Translation of Zea mays endosperm sucrose
synthetase mRNA in vitro, Eur. J. Biochem. 114:39.

STRUCTURE AND EXPRESSION OF ZEIN GENES IN MAIZE ENDOSPERM

B.A. Larkins*, K. Pedersen*, M.D. Marks*, D.R. Wilson*, and P. Argos[+]

*Department of Botany and Plant Pathology, and
[+]Department of Biology
Purdue University, West Lafayette, IN   47907

INTRODUCTION

The storage proteins of maize seed are a group of alcohol-soluble proteins called zeins. These proteins can be separated by SDS polyacrylamide gel electrophoresis into four major groups that have apparent mol wts of 22,000, 19,000, 15,000 and 10,000 (Lee et al., 1976; Gianazza et al., 1977). The M_r 22,000 and M_r 19,000 components are made up of several polypeptides. Their NH_2-terminal sequences are heterogeneous (Larkins et al., 1980) and on 2-dimensional polyacrylamide gels they show substantial charge heterogeneity (Hagen and Rubenstein, 1981). The M_r 15,000 and M_r 10,000 polypeptides are less heterogeneous, and appear to consist of only one or two proteins (Hurkman et al., 1981). Charge heterogeneity among different zeins is genotype specific (Righetti et al., 1977) and has been shown in several instances to be inherited in a simple Mendelian fashion (Soave et al., 1978). These studies suggest that the zeins are a highly homologous group of proteins encoded by multiple and closely related genes.

Mutants of maize have been identified which substantially reduce the synthesis of the different mol wt zein components. The opaque-2 mutation reduces total zein synthesis by about 50% and almost completely eliminates synthesis of the M_r 22,000 zeins (Jones et al., 1977). The opaque-7 mutation also reduces total zein synthesis, but it preferentially inhibits synthesis of the M_r 19,000 zeins (DiFonzo et al., 1980). Both opaque-2 and opaque-7 are recessive mutations, but in floury-2, which causes an equal reduction in both M_r 22,000 and M_r 19,000 zeins, the zein content is dependent upon the number of mutant alleles (Jones, 1978). Preliminary investigations have shown that the reduced level of M_r 22,000

zeins in the opaque-2 mutant results from more than a 100-fold reduction of their mRNAs in the membrane-bound polyribosomes (Pedersen et
al., 1980). This suggests that the opaque-2 mutation causes a significant
reduction in zein mRNA transcription. However, the mechanisms by
which these mutations act are largely unknown (Soave et al., 1981).

To better understand the structural relationships between
different zein proteins we have synthesized and characterized cDNA
clones made from zein mRNAs. These clones have been used to investigate the structure of zein proteins and the sequence homology of
zein mRNAs. They have also been used to study the structure and
organization of zein genes in the maize genome and to investigate
changes in levels of specific zein mRNAs during development of
normal and opaque-2 endosperms.

Characterization of Zein cDNA clones

We analyzed a group of size selected zein cDNA clones to
identify those containing potentially full-length coding sequences
(Marks and Larkins, 1982). Clones corresponding to Mr 22,000, Mr
19,000, and Mr 15,000 zeins were identified based on homology with
zein mRNAs, and several representatives from each of these groups
were characterized by DNA sequence analysis (Pedersen et al., 1982;
Marks and Larkins, 1982). Comparison of the DNA and corresponding
protein sequences showed the presence of signal peptides on both
Mr 22,000 and Mr 19,000 zeins (Larkins et al., 1979). It also revealed a conserved sequence of approximately 60 nucleotides that
was tandemly repeated and present in nine copies in the cDNA clones
of both Mr 22,000 and Mr 19,000 zeins. At the amino acid level this
conserved repeat corresponded to a short peptide of approximately
20 amino acids which occurred near the center of the protein (Fig.
1). The first repeat was 35 or 36 amino acids after the amino
terminus, while the last was either 29 or 10 amino acids before
the COOH-terminus, depending on the zein protein.

Structural analysis of the repeats suggested the potential for
forming α-helices. Fig. 2A shows that when the consensus sequence of
the repeated amino acids is placed on an α-helical wheel polar amino
acids are distributed at three symetrical sites. If the tandem repeats fold back on one another in an antiparallel arrangement, two
polar groups in each repeat can form hydrogen bonds with adjacent
repeats (Fig. 2B). The nine helices would then interact to form a
roughly cylindrical rod shaped molecule. The cylinder would collapse
in the center to accomodate the non-polar side chains of the amino
acids (Fig. 2B). As the zein molecules associate within the endoplasmic reticulum, the third polar group on the surface of the
molecule would hydrogen bond to a different zein molecule. The
glutamine residues at the ends of the helices would also hydrogen
bond with neighboring zein molecules (Fig. 2C). This hypothetical
model for zein protein structure would explain why these proteins

Zein protein	Signal Sequence	Sequence positions
Z22	M A T K I L S L L A L L A L F A S A T N A	1-21
Z19	M A A K I F C L I M L L G L S A S A A T A	1-21

N-Terminal Turn

Z22	S I I P Q C S L A P . S S I I P Q F L P P V T S M A F E H P A V Q A Y R	22-56
Z19	S I F P Q C S Q A P I A S L L P P Y L S P A M S S V C E N P I L L P Y R	22-57

Repeat Sequences

Z22 & Z19 9 repeats	Q Q $^{F}_{L}$ L P $^{A}_{F}$ N Q L $^{A A}_{L V}$ A N S P A Y L Q Q	57-237 58-225

C-Terminal Turn

Z22	Q Q Q L L P Y N R F S L M N P V L S R Q Q P I V G G A I F	238-266
Z19	. . . . Q Q P I I G G A L F	226-235

Fig. 1.   Comparison of structural regions in Mr 22,000 and Mr
          19,000 zein proteins. The amino acid sequences of the
          zein polypeptides were derived from the DNA sequences
          of zein clones as reported by Pedersen et al., (1982) and
          Marks and Larkins (1982). The protein is divided into
          different structural regions as described by Argos et
          el., (1982).

self associate into protein bodies within the rough endoplasmic
reticulum (Hurkman et al., 1981).

Although there is a striking similarity in the structure of
the Mr 22,000 and Mr 19,000 zeins, the mRNAs encoding these proteins
are sufficiently diverged that they do not cross-hybridize at a
moderate (Tm-25° C) hybridization criterion. We isolated the cDNA
inserts from zein clones corresponding to different Mr 22,000, Mr
19,000, and Mr 15,000 mRNAs. These were labeled by nick translation
and hybridized at varying criteria to a set of zein cDNA clones.
The results shown in Fig. 3 demonstrate that lines of sequence
homology can be clearly distinguished between mRNAs corresponding
to different zein mol wt groups. Some very faint cross-hybridization
is detectable under the least stringent condition (Tm-49° C), but at
Tm-35° C there is no apparent cross-hybridization between the Mr
22,000, Mr 19,000, or Mr 15,000 zein sequences. Indeed, at Tm-20° C
differences within the Mr 22,000 and Mr 19,000 classes can be seen.
The two Mr 15,000 clones behave identically, but these have been
found to be derived from the same mRNA sequence. It is therefore
possible to distinguish between different zein DNA sequences by
controlling the criterion of hybridization.

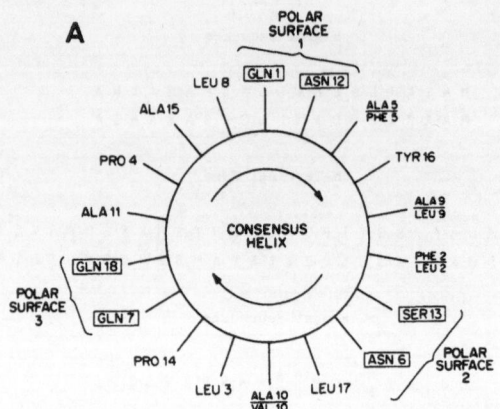

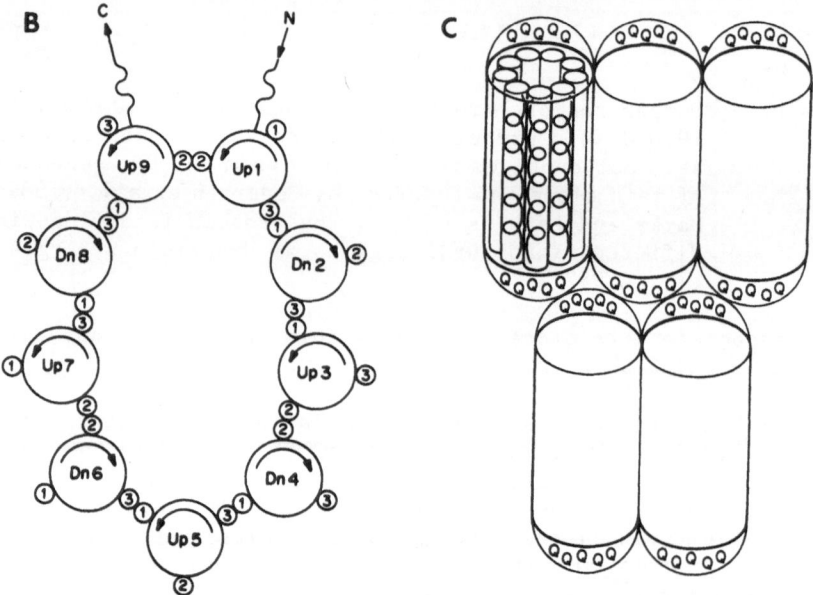

Fig. 2.   A structural model for maize zein proteins. (A) Analysis
           of the consensus repeated peptide on an α-helical wheel.
           (B) Structural arrangement of the nine repeated α-helices.
           Up and Down show the antiparallel arrangement of the
           helices. The positions labeled 1, 2, 3 correspond to the
           polar groups on the helix. (C) Organization of zein poly-
           peptides within the protein body. Q's correspond to gluta-
           mine residues at the end of the helices. (From Argos et
           al., 1982).

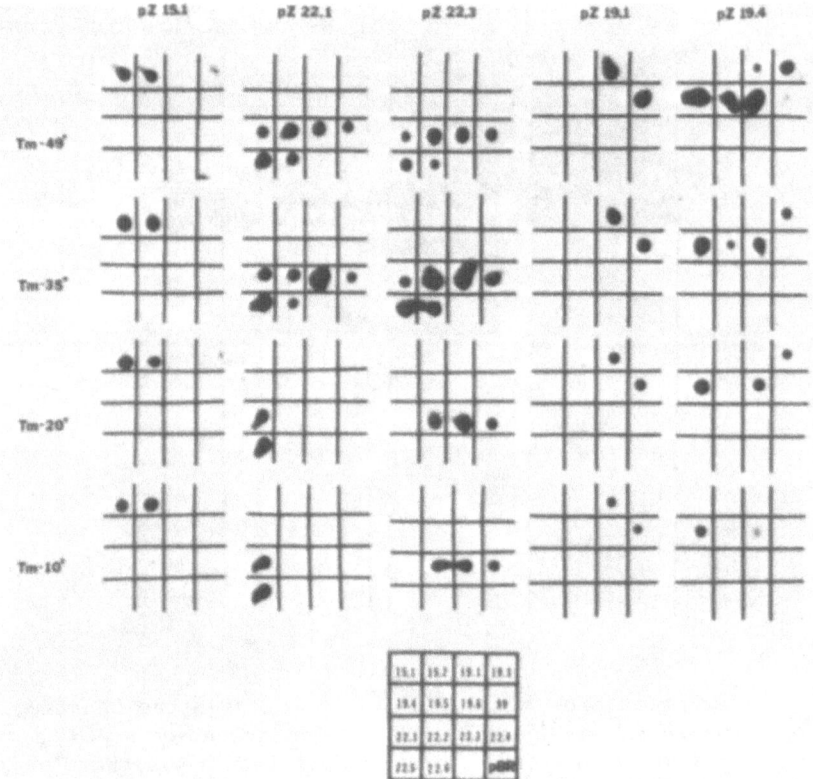

Fig. 3. Analysis of sequence homology among zein clones. Replicate filters were spotted with independently isolated cloned zein sequences and pBR 322. The filters were hybridized to nick translated inserts from the cDNA clones indicated at the top of the figure. The filters were hybridized and washed at the criteria indicated on the left, based on the formula $Tm=(\% \ G+C)/_2 + 81.6 + 16.6 \ \log \ [salt]-0.6(\% \ formamide)$. The cDNA inserts have a G+C content of 46-48% based on their DNA sequence analysis. (From Marks and Larkins, 1982).

Organization and structure of zein genes

Zein genes occur in the maize genome in small multigene families. Figure 4 shows a Southern blot analysis with the insert from one of the M_r 22,000 zein cDNA clones. At Tm-30° C, a criterion where most of the M_r 22,000 sequences cross-hybridize, multiple DNA fragments are detected with varying hybridization intensities. Based on the reconstruction analysis these bands are equivalent to 25-30 gene copies. When this analysis is repeated at a criterion where there is little cross-hybridization (Tm-20° C) the number and intensity of these bands is significantly decreased. At Tm-20° C only

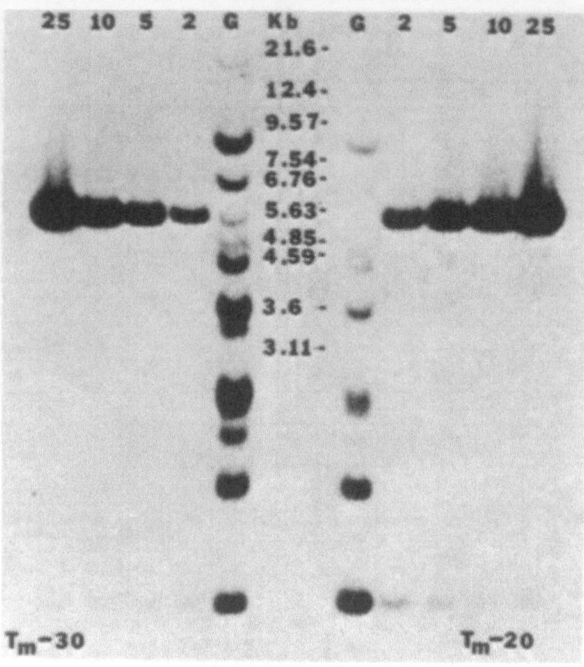

Fig. 4.   Hybridization of pZ 22.1 to Eco RI digested DNA from the
           maize inbred W64A. The DNA was separated on a 0.8% agarose
           gel and transferred to nitrocellulose by Southern blotting.
           The filters were hybridized to the nick translated cDNA
           insert from pZ 22.1 at the criteria indicated, nad then
           washed at the criterion of the hybridization. The recon-
           struction lanes show the image intensity of 25, 10, 5,
           and 2 gene copies.

7-8 gene copies can be detected. Since the results obtained at
Tm-40° C are the same as those at Tm-30° C the simplest interpretation of this data is that there is a maximum of 25-30 genes
encoding Mr 22,000 zeins in this inbred, and there are 7-8 genes
highly homologous to this particular Mr 22,000 cDNA clone.

       Southern hybridization with the Mr 19,000 zein clones give
results similar to the Mr 22,000 zein sequences, although the gene
families are more divergent. The Mr 15,000 zein is also significantly diverged from the Mr 22,000 and Mr 19,000 zeins. Interestingly,
this gene appears to be present in only two to three copies so it is
not repeated to the extent of the Mr 22,000 and Mr 19,000 zeins.

       As an initial step towards characterizing the structure of the
zein genes we isolated a genomic clone corresponding to one of the Mr
19,000 zein sequences (Pedersen et al., 1982). R-loop analysis of
this clone demonstrated the presence of only a single zein gene and

suggested the absence of intervening sequences (Fig. 5). A more
detailed analysis based on DNA sequencing confirmed that there were
no introns in the gene. By comparing the gene sequence with that
of a highly homologous cDNA clone we were able to identify several
putative transcriptional regulatory sequences. Beginning 56 nucleotides 5' of the first base in the cDNA clone is a "TATA" or Hogness
box, and 84 nucleotides 5' of this sequence is a "CCAT" box (Fig.
5). Interestingly, there is a second "TATA" box that precedes this
"CCAT" sequence by 52 nucleotides and a second "CCAT" sequence preceding that "TATA" box by 82 nucleotides (Pedersen, et al., 1982).
The protein coding region of the gene includes a "signal peptide"
of 21 amino acids followed by codons for the mature protein which
contains 214 amino acids.

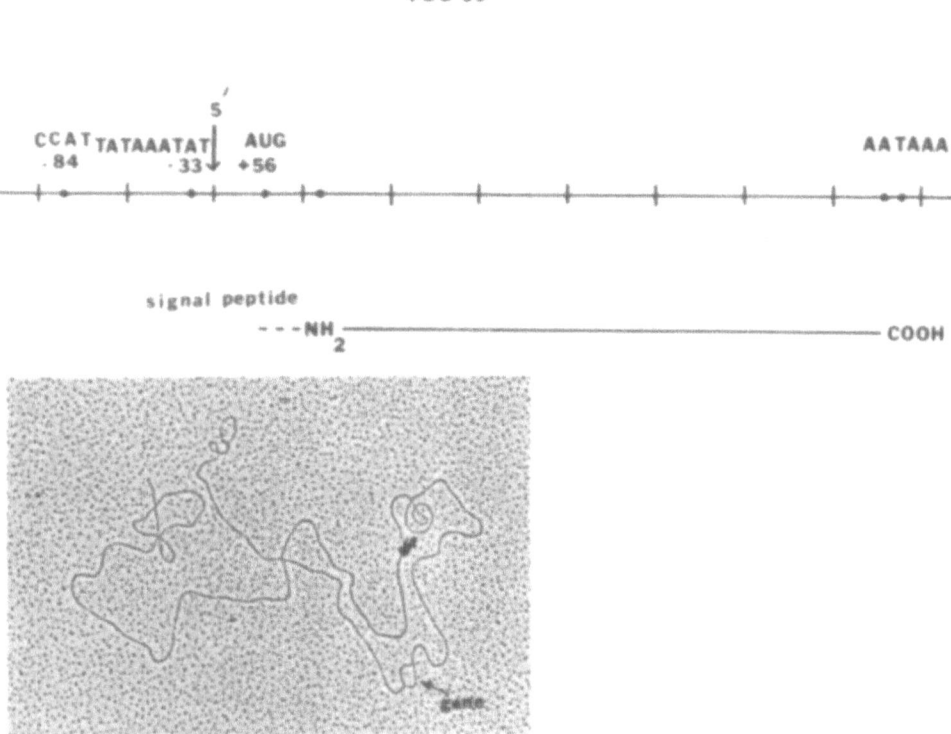

Fig. 5.   Structure of a maize zein gene. The R-loop analysis in
           the lower left shows the presence of a single zein gene in
           the 13 Kb lambda genomic clone and indicates the absence
           of intervening sequences in the gene. This was confirmed
           by the DNA sequence analysis (Pedersen et al., 1982) which
           also demonstrated typical spacing of eukaryotic-type
           promoter sequences flanking the gene (upper part of figure).

There is an "AATAAA" or polyadenylation sequence that follows 23
nucleotides after the amber codon for terminating translation. Thus,
at the DNA level the zein gene is structurally similar to many
other eukaryotic genes. The 1000 nucleotides flanking the 5' and 3'
ends of the gene are very AT-rich and contain little repetitive
DNA (Pedersen et al., 1982).

Zein gene expression during endosperm development

     In normal maize genotypes zein proteins are first detectable
in the endosperm around 12 days after pollination, and they accumulate until maturity which is 45-50 days after pollination (Jones et
al., 1976). In opaque-2 mutants zein synthesis is reduced by about
50%, and the Mr 22,000 zeins are nearly absent (Jones et al., 1977).
To study expression of representative zein genes during this period
we isolated total polysomal poly(A)-containing mRNA from developing
seeds. An analysis of this mRNA on a denaturing methylmercury hy-
droxide gel is shown in Fig 6. In addition to the 18S ribosomal RNA,
which is approximately 2120 nucleotides in length, two prominent RNAs
of 1000 and 1100 nucleotides are resolved in both the normal and
opaque-2 mRNA populations. From Northern blot hybridization analysis
we determined that the 1100 nucleotide mRNA encodes Mr 22,000 zeins,
while the 1000 nucleotide mRNA encodes both Mr 19,000 and Mr 15,000
zein proteins. Both groups of mRNAs are detectable in the normal
genotype at 12 days after pollination, and they become the most abundant mRNAs in the endosperm. In the opaque-2 mutant these mRNAs

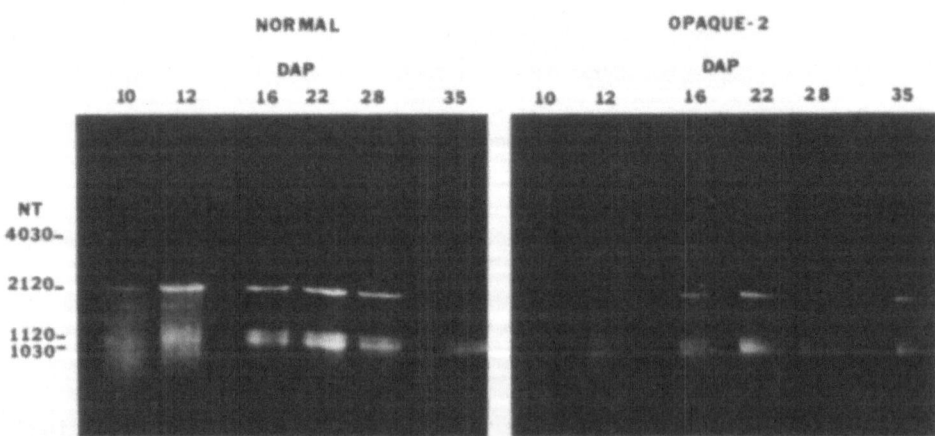

Fig. 6.   Analysis of poly(A) mRNAs from developing kernels of
           normal and opaque-2 maize on denaturing 1.2% agarose gels.
           Total polyribosomes were isolated at the indicated days
           after pollination (DAP) and poly(A)-containing mRNAs were
           isolated by oligo d(T) cellulose chromatography.

are not apparent until 16 days after pollination. They are detectable throughout the remainder of endosperm development, but the 1100 nucleotide mRNA is significantly reduced in abundance.

A developmental Northern dot hybridization analysis of these mRNAs is shown in Fig. 7. The cDNA clones pZ 15.2, pZ 19.1, and pZ 22.3 correspond to mRNAs encoding the Mr 15,000, Mr 19,000, and Mr 22,000 zein proteins, respectively. For comparative purposes we also analyzed these mRNAs with a cDNA clone for the sucrose synthetase mRNA. In the normal genotype trace amounts of each of the different zein mRNAs can be detected as early as 10 days after pollination. Messenger RNAs for all three zein groups are abundant throughout the remainder of development. Although it is present at much lower levels, sucrose synthetase mRNA shows a similar pattern of transcriptional modulation throughout development of the normal endosperm.

The analysis of the opaque-2 mutant indicates a slower accumulation of zein mRNAs. Significant levels of Mr 15,000 and Mr 19,000 zein mRNAs are not detectable until the endosperm is 16 days old. There is a much lower level of Mr 22,000 zein mRNAs until 18 days after pollination, and all the zein sequences decline precipitously after 22 days. On the other hand, sucrose synthetase mRNA is present throughout development, perhaps even in greater abundance in the opaque-2 mutant than in the normal genotype. Thus, it appears that the different zein gene families are coordinately expressed

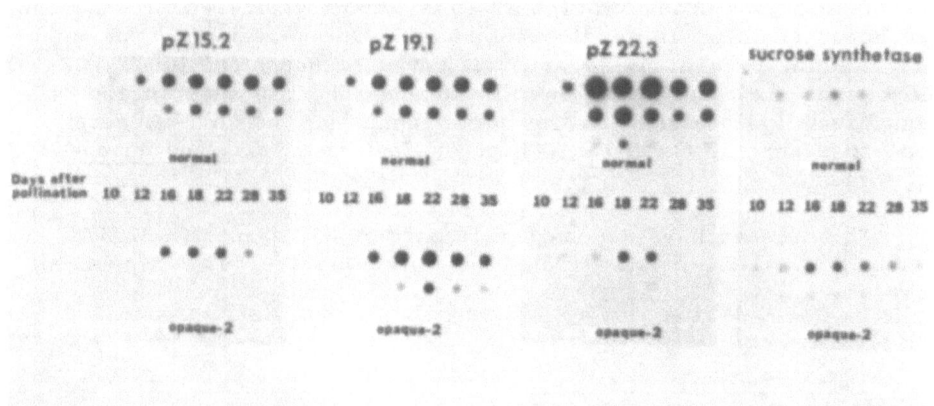

Fig. 7.   Analysis of zein mRNA's in polyribosomes of developing normal and opaque-2 genotypes. Samples of 1.0, 0.5, and 0.1 ug of poly(A)-containing mRNAs from total polysomes isolated between 10 and 35 days after pollination were spotted on nitrocellulose paper and hybridized to cDNA clones corresponding to Mr 15,000, Mr 19,000, and Mr 22,000 zein sequences. An analysis is also shown of a cDNA clone corresponding to the sucrose synthetase mRNA.

throughout normal endosperm development; however, their quantitative and temporal expression is greatly affected by the opaque-2 mutation.

SUMMARY

By characterizing the structure of zein clones we have deter-mined the relationships between zein proteins as well as the homology among related zein mRNAs. The Mr 22,000 and Mr 19,000 zein proteins are translated as precursor polypeptides containing signal peptides. Both of these proteins contain a conserved and tandemly repeated peptide of 20 amino acids. The repeated peptides are present in nine copies and they occur in the central region of the protein toward the COOH-terminus. The peptides appear to be α-helical and cause the molecule to fold into a rod shaped structure. Although there is structural similarity among the different zeins, at the nucleotide level several distinct families of Mr 22,000 and Mr 19,000 sequences can be distinguished. At Tm-35° clones corresponding to Mr 22,000, Mr 19,000, and Mr 15,000 zeins do not cross-hybridize; at Tm-20° subsets of Mr 22,000 and Mr 19,000 zeins can be distinguished. At the nucleotide level zein genes appear to be structurally similar to other eukaryotic genes in that they contain recognized transcriptional regulatory sequences. However, unlike many other eukaryotic genes they contain no intervening sequences. Genes encoding the different mol wt zein proteins are coordinately expressed during normal endosperm development. Translationally active mRNAs can be detected as early as 10 days after pollination, and are present throughout endosperm development. In the opaque-2 mutant zein gene transcription is significantly altered. Transcripts are detected later in development than in the normal genotype, and they decline precipitously after 22 days. Although the Mr 22,000 zein genes are transcribed in this mutant, their transcription is significantly less than in the normal genotype, as well as being less than that of the Mr 19,000 genes in both normal and opaque-2 genotypes.

This research was supported in part by NSF grant PCM-8003757 to B.A.L. Journal Paper No. 9156 of the Purdue Agricultural Experiment Station.

REFERENCES

Agros, P., Pedersen, K., Marks, M.D., and Larkins, B.A. 1982, A structural model for maize zein proteins, J. Biol. Chem. (in press).

DiFonzo, N., Fornasari, E., Salamini, F., Reggianai, R., and Soave, C. 1980, Interaction of maize mutants floury-2 and opaque-7 with opaque-2 in the synthesis of endosperm proteins. J. Heredity, 71, 397.

Gianazza, E., Viglienghi, V., Righetti, P.C., Salamini, F., and Soave, C. 1977., Amino acid composition of zein molecular components, Phytochemistry, 16, 315.

Hagen, G. and Rubenstein, I, 1980, Two-dimensional gel analysis of the zein proteins in maize, Plant Science Lett. 19, 217.

Hurkman, W.J., Smith, L.D., Richter, J., and Larkins, B.A., 1981, Subcellular compartmentalization of maize storage proteins in Xenopus oocytes injected with zein messenger RNAs, J. Cell Biol. 89, 292.

Jones, R.A., Larkins, B.A., and Tsai, C.Y., 1977, Reduced synthesis of a major zein component by the opaque-2 mutant of maize, Plant Physiol. 59, 525.

Jones, R.A., 1978, Effects of floury-2 locus on zein accumulation and RNA metabolism during maize endosperm development, Biochem. Genet. 16, 27.

Larkins, B.A., Pedersen, K., Hurkman, W.J., Handa, A.K., Mason, A.C., Tsai, C.Y., and Hermodson, M.A., 1980, Maize storage proteins: Characterization and biosynthesis in Genome Organization and Expression in Plants, (C.J. Leaver, ed.) Plenum Press, N.Y. pp. 203.

Lee, K.H., Jones, R.A., Dalby, A., and Tsai, C.Y., 1976, Genetic regulation of storage protein synthesis in maize endosperm, Biochem. Genet. 14, 641.

Marks, M.D. and Larkins, B.A., 1982, Analysis of sequence microheterogeneity among zein messenger RNAs, J. Biol. Chem. (in press).

Pedersen, L., Bloom, K.S., Anderson, J.N., Glover, D.V., and Larkins, B.A., 1980, Analysis of the complexity and frequency of zein genes in the maize genome, Biochemistry 19, 1644.

Pedersen, K., Devereux, J., Wilson, D.R., Sheldon, E., and Larkins, B.A., 1982, Cloning and sequence analysis reveals structural variation among related zein genes, Cell 29, 1015.

Righetti, P.G., Gianazza, E., Viotti, A., and Soave, C., 1977, Heterogeneity of storage proteins in maize, Planta, 136, 115.

Soave, C., Suman, N., Viotti, A., and Salamini, F., 1978, Linkage relationships between regulatory and structural gene loci involved in zein synthesis in maize, Theoret. Appl. Genetics. 52, 263.

Soave, C., Tardani, L., DiFonzo, N., and Salamini, F., 1981, Zein level in maize endosperm depends on a protein under control of the opaque-2 and opaque-6 loci, Cell 27, 403.

THE HORDEINS OF BARLEY: DEVELOPMENTALLY AND NUTRITIONALLY

REGULATED MULTIGENE FAMILIES OF STORAGE PROTEINS

B. J. Miflin, S. Rahman, M. Kreis, B. G. Forde,
L. Blanco, and P. R. Shewry

Biochemistry Department
Rothamsted Experimental Station
Harpenden, Herts. AL5 2JQ, U.K.

INTRODUCTION

The endosperm of the grain plays an important role in the life cycle of a cereal plant. It develops over a period of some 40-50 days, finally containing about 70% of the total dry matter and nitrogen of the plant. About 50% of the N in the barley endosperm is in the form of prolamin storage proteins (termed hordeins). At the end of development the grain dries out and the bulk of the endosperm tissue (all except the outer aleurone layer which does not contain hordeins) dies. The endosperm therefore provides an example of a highly specialised tissue which has differentiated to carry out an important and unique function over a limited period of time (see[1] for a further review). The hordeins have been studied because of their influence on nutritional quality[2] and because they are the products of tissue-specific genes. This report summarizes our studies on the nature of the proteins, the genes specifying them and factors controlling the expression of these genes. We have pursued this work using the classical techniques of protein chemistry[3,4,5] and genetics[6,7] and also by constructing a cDNA library made from poly A[+] RNA isolated from developing endosperms.[8]

DEFINITION OF HORDEIN GROUPS

We define hordeins as endosperm-specific proteins which are deposited in protein bodies, have high contents of glutamine and proline, are preferentially synthesized in response to an increased supply of N and are soluble in alcohol-based solvents (e.g. 55% propan-2-ol plus 1% mercaptoethanol). Hordein polypeptides have been classified into three groups: B, C and D[9],[10] (the group originally classified as A hordein is not now considered to be true hordein[5],[11]). The characteristics of the different groups are shown in Figure 1.

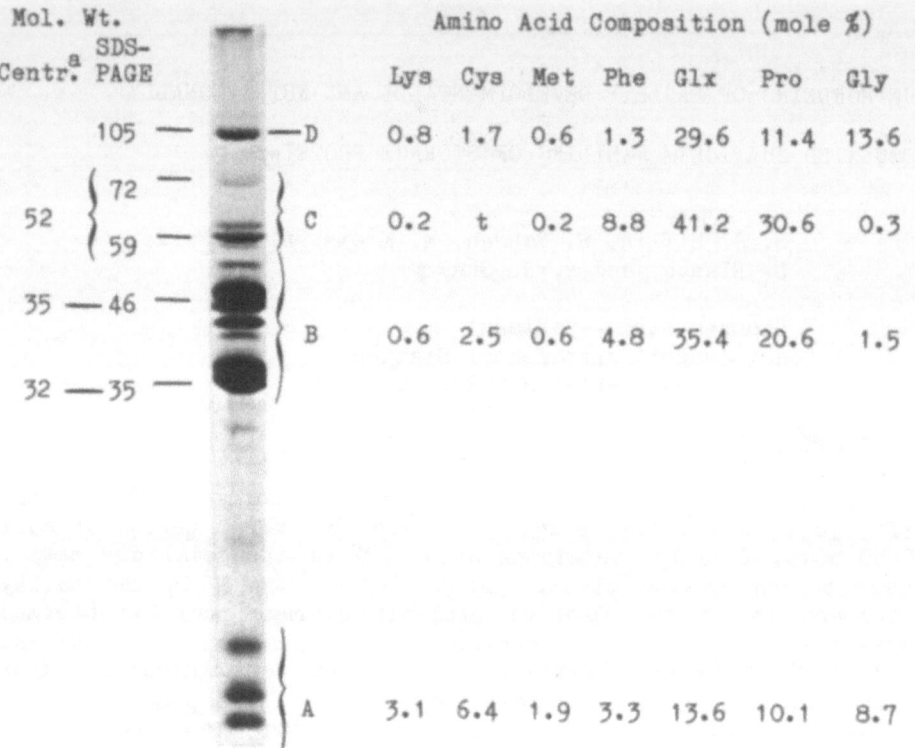

Mol. Wt.			Amino Acid Composition (mole %)						
Centr.[a]	SDS-PAGE		Lys	Cys	Met	Phe	Glx	Pro	Gly
105 —	—D	D	0.8	1.7	0.6	1.3	29.6	11.4	13.6
72 —									
52 {		C	0.2	t	0.2	8.8	41.2	30.6	0.3
59 —									
35 —	46 —								
		B	0.6	2.5	0.6	4.8	35.4	20.6	1.5
32 —	35 —								
		A	3.1	6.4	1.9	3.3	13.6	10.1	8.7

Fig. 1. Characteristics of the groups of hordein polypeptides. The SDS-PAGE separation shows hordein from cv. Sundance, which has the alleles Hor1Pr and Hor2Ze.[6]   [a] Sedimentation equilibrium ultracentrifugation. Data from refs. 3, 5, 9, 10, 11, 24.

Each group appears to consist of a polymorphic series of proteins which differ in number and electrophoretic mobility between varieties.[12] However there are strong similarities between the components in different varieties[3] and homologies extend to similar protein groups in wheat and rye.[9] Genetic analyses of crosses between varieties[6],[7],[13] have shown that there are three loci Hor1, Hor2 and Hor3 on chromosome 5 which code for C, B and D hordein respectively; Hor1 and Hor2 are located on the short arm and are linked (about 10-17% recombination) while Hor3 is located on the long arm.[14] Our working hypothesis is that the Hor loci consist of multigene families which probably arose from ancestral prolamin genes by cycles of gene duplication and mutation. Evidence for this includes the study of CNBr cleavage patterns of different B polypeptides;[3] on the basis of these we have grouped the B hordeins into 3 classes: I, II and III. The barley cultivar Sundance contains both class I and class III polypeptides (Figure 2): the B1 hordein consists largely of class I and B3 of class III.

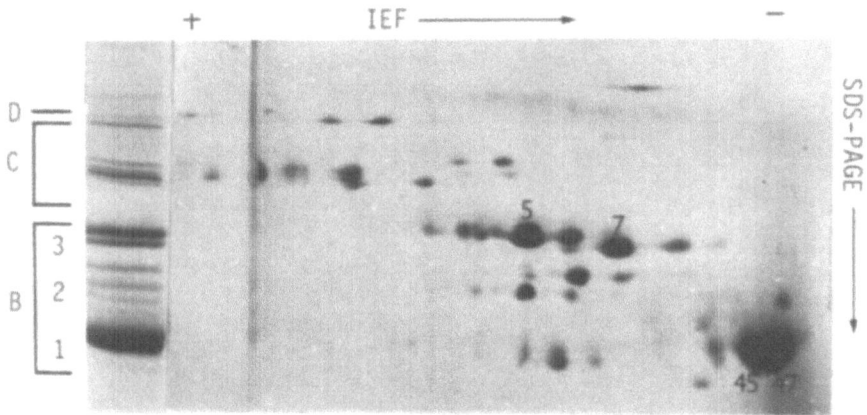

Fig. 2. 2-D analysis of hordein from mature seed of cv. Sundance.[16] B hordein polypeptides are numbered according to ref.3. 5 and 7 are CNBr cleavage class III, 45 and 47 are class I.

By means of hybrid-selection translation[8,15] we have classified our cDNA clones into those which hybridise to Sundance mRNA that directs the synthesis of B1, B3, C and possibly D hordein polypeptides (Figure 3). When mRNA from different cultivars are used, the hybrid-selected translation products correlate with the polypeptide patterns and with the classification based on studies of the proteins.[3,12]

DEVELOPMENTAL CONTROL OF HORDEIN FORMATION

Hordein accumulation begins at about 18 days post-anthesis when the caryopsis is entering its major phase of growth. This is relatively late compared to the initiation of accumulation of the other protein solubility groups and is about the time that the majority of cell division ceases. Hordein accumulates throughout the remainder of endosperm growth until the grain dries out. The different groups of hordeins are not accumulated at the same rate; C and B3 hordeins form a greater proportion of the total early in development, B1 at the later stages.[16] Because hordein does not appear to turn over[17], accumulation is presumed to reflect synthesis. To investigate further the developmental expression of the Hor loci we have isolated and translated membrane-bound polysomes, poly A[+] RNA derived from these and total RNA. After

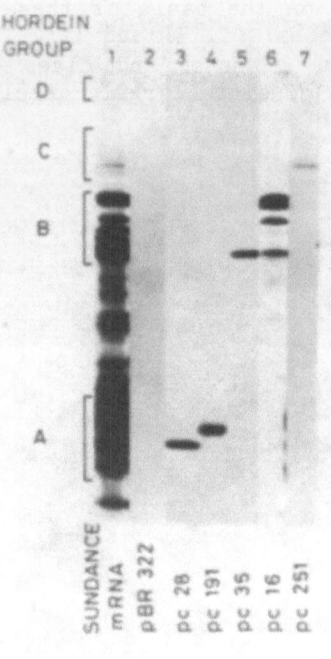

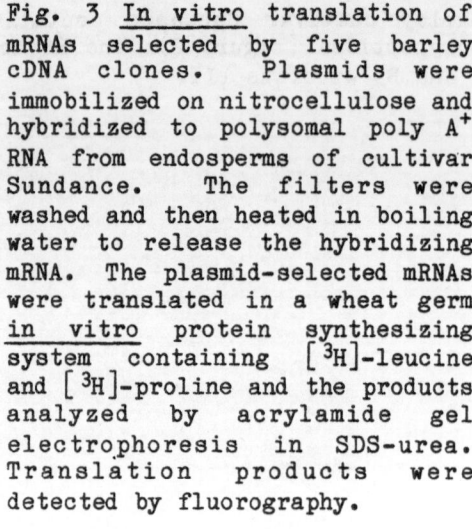

Fig. 3 <u>In vitro</u> translation of mRNAs selected by five barley cDNA clones. Plasmids were immobilized on nitrocellulose and hybridized to polysomal poly A$^+$ RNA from endosperms of cultivar Sundance. The filters were washed and then heated in boiling water to release the hybridizing mRNA. The plasmid-selected mRNAs were translated in a wheat germ <u>in vitro</u> protein synthesizing system containing [^{3}H]-leucine and [^{3}H]-proline and the products analyzed by acrylamide gel electrophoresis in SDS-urea. Translation products were detected by fluorography.

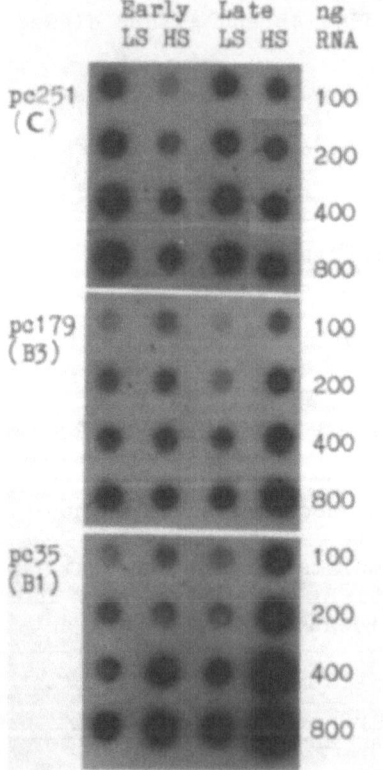

Fig. 4 'Dot' hybridization of three ^{32}P-labelled cDNA clones to different amounts of polysomal poly A$^+$ RNA. RNA was isolated from endosperms of plants grown with high (HS) and low (LS) amounts of S, at 14d (early) and 30d (late) after anthesis and spotted onto nitrocellulose. The plasmids pc251, pc179 and pc35 are related to C, B3 and B1 hordein mRNAs respectively. pc179 cross-hybridizes with and selects the same translatable mRNA as does pc16 (shown in Fig.3).

separation of the translation products by gel electrophoresis and
detection by fluorography the amounts of the different products
have been estimated. The results show that in vitro, as in
vivo, the synthesis of B1 polypeptides relative to that of B3 and
C polypeptides increases during the course of endosperm
development. Finally, some of the RNA fractions have been dotted
on to nitrocellulose and hybridized with ^{32}P-labelled DNA from
various of the cDNA clones. The results show that the amounts of
B1 mRNAs increase relative to C and B3 mRNAs during endosperm
development.

NUTRITIONAL CONTROL OF HORDEIN SYNTHESIS

We have proposed previously[18] that plants have evolved groups
of storage proteins which contain different amounts of
S-containing amino acids so that they can store N independently of
S (e.g. see Fig. 1). We have grown plants on widely different
amounts of N and S and measured the amounts of C (S-poor) and
B (S-rich) hordeins accumulated.[19] The S-starved grain contained
11 µg B1, 13 µg B3 and 134 µg C hordein N/seed whereas the
corresponding values for high-S seed were 233, 123 and 146 µg.
S starvation has therefore prevented the accumulation of B
hordeins without affecting that of C hordein. To test if this was
due to changes in mRNA population, RNA fractions were isolated and
the relative proportions of B and C hordein mRNAs assessed by
translation and dot hybridization (Figure 4). The results were
all consistent with there being a drastic reduction in the amount
of B hordein mRNA relative to C hordein mRNA in the S-starved
seed.

HIGH-LYSINE MUTANTS

Lines of barley have been selected from mutagenized
populations by virtue of their enhanced content of basic amino
acids. These lines contain larger than normal proportions of
lysine in the grain. Risø 1508, derived from cultivar Bomi,
contains a mutant gene lys3a on chromosome 7[20] which has a
number of pleiotropic effects, amongst which is a large decrease
in the amount of hordein per endosperm.[21] The amounts of C and B1
hordein are decreased more than that of B3; D hordein is
unaffected.[22] Risø 56, derived from cultivar Carlsberg II,
contains the mutant allele Hor2ca located at or near the Hor2
locus[23] and has normal or slightly enhanced amounts of C and D
hordein but much reduced amounts of B hordein.[22] The amounts of
the different mRNAs in the mutants and wild types have been
assayed by in vitro translations, "dot" hybridization and colony
hybridization. The effect of the lys3a gene is to decrease the
amount of translatable mRNA for B and C hordeins; that for B1 is
reduced more than that for B3. The Hor2ca gene also leads to
the loss of translatable mRNA for B hordeins but not for C hordein

(Fig. 5A).   DNA isolated from mutants and wild type plants was digested with HindIII, electrophoresed, 'Southern' blotted and hybridized to ^{32}P-DNA from the cloned cDNA. The results show that the Hor2 locus is indeed complex, consisting of multiple copies of B hordein genes. They also confirm the genetic evidence that lys3a has no effect on the Hor2 locus but show that Hor2ca has suffered a deletion of >100 kilobases relative to the wild type allele Hor2Ca (Fig. 5B).

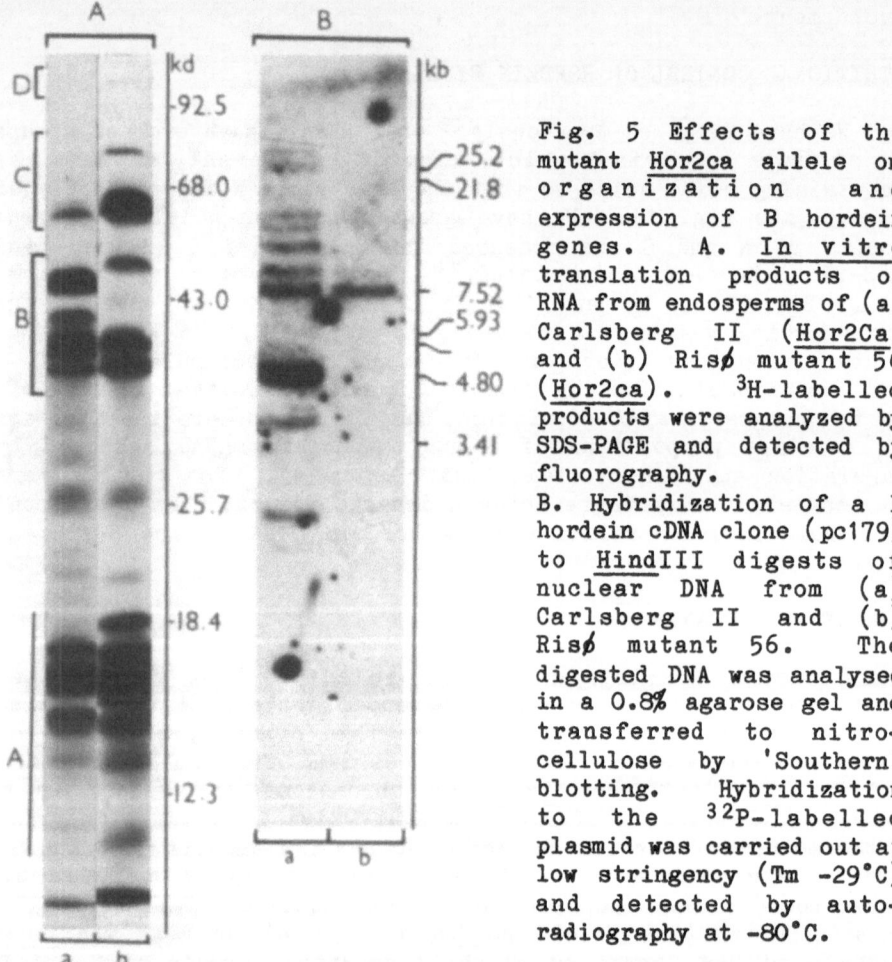

Fig. 5 Effects of the mutant Hor2ca allele on organization and expression of B hordein genes. A. In vitro translation products of RNA from endosperms of (a) Carlsberg II (Hor2Ca) and (b) Risø mutant 56 (Hor2ca). ^{3}H-labelled products were analyzed by SDS-PAGE and detected by fluorography.
B. Hybridization of a B hordein cDNA clone (pc179) to HindIII digests of nuclear DNA from (a) Carlsberg II and (b) Risø mutant 56. The digested DNA was analysed in a 0.8% agarose gel and transferred to nitro-cellulose by 'Southern' blotting. Hybridization to the ^{32}P-labelled plasmid was carried out at low stringency (Tm -29°C) and detected by auto-radiography at -80°C.

CONCLUSIONS

Evidence is accumulating to support the hypothesis that Hor1, Hor2 and Hor3 are multigenic loci. Detailed analyses of B hordein polypeptides and their mRNAs suggest that at least two clearly defined subfamilies of genes are present within the Hor2 locus. The relative rates of expression of the various groups of hordein genes change during development and are also modulated by plant nutrition and by factors controlled by the lys3a gene. These differential controls operate even between the two sub-families at the Hor2 locus. In each case the relative amounts of the proteins are correlated with the relative amounts of their respective mRNAs. This suggests that control is at the level of transcription, although no evidence is available to show that the various mRNAs are equally stable.

ACKNOWLEDGEMENTS

We gratefully acknowledge help from J. Pywell, J. Wallace, J. Franklin and S. Parmar in the experiments reported here.

REFERENCES

1. B. M. Johri, P. S. Srivastava, and A. P. Raste, Endosperm Culture, in "International Review of Cytology, Supplement 11B," G. H. Bourne, J. F. Danielli, eds., Academic Press, New York (1980).

2. P. R. Shewry, B. J. Miflin, B. G. Forde, S. W. J. Bright, Conventional and novel approaches to the improvement of the nutritional quality of cereal and legume seeds, Sci. Prog. 67:571 (1981).

3. A. J. Faulks, P. R. Shewry and B. J. Miflin, The polymorphism and structural homology of storage polypeptides (hordein) coded by the Hor 2 locus in barley (Hordeum vulgare L.), Biochem. Genet. 19:841 (1981).

4. P. R. Shewry, E. J-L. Lew, D. D. Kasarda, Structural homology of storage proteins coded by the Hor 1 locus of barley (Hordeum vulgare L.), Planta 153:246 (1981).

5. P. R. Shewry and B. J. Miflin, Characterization and synthesis of barley seed proteins, in "The Genetics of Seed Proteins of Cereals and Legumes". W. Gottschalk, H. P. Muller, eds. Martinus Nijhoff, The Hague (in press).

6. P. R. Shewry, A. J. Faulks, R. A. Pickering, I. T. Jones, R. A. Finch and B. J. Miflin, The genetic analysis of barley storage proteins, Heredity 44:383 (1980).

7. P. R. Shewry and B. J. Miflin, Genes for the storage proteins of barley. Qual. Plant. (Pl. Foods for Human Nutrition), (in press).

8. B. G. Forde, M. Kreis, M. B. Bahramian, J. Matthews, B. J. Miflin, R. D. Thompson, R. D. Bartels and R. B. Flavell, Molecular cloning and analysis of cDNA sequences derived from poly A$^+$ RNA from barley endosperm: identification of B hordein-related clones, Nucleic Acids Research 9:6689 (1981).

9. B. J. Miflin, J. M. Field, and P. R. Shewry, Cereal storage proteins and their effects on technological properties in "Seed Proteins" J. Daussant, J. Mossé eds., Academic Press, London (in press).

10. J. M. Field, P. R. Shewry, B. J. Miflin and J. F. March, The
     purification and characterization of homologous high
     molecular weight storage proteins from grain of wheat, rye
     and barley, Theor. Appl. Genet. 62:329 (1982).
11. G. Salcedo, R. Sanchez-Monge, A. Aragamentaria and C.
     Aragoncillo, The A hordeins as a group of salt-soluble
     hydrophobic proteins, Plant Sci. Lett. 19:109 (1980).
12. P. R. Shewry, H. M. Pratt, A. J. Faulks, S. Parmar, and B. J.
     Miflin, The storage protein (hordein) pattern of barley in
     relation to varietal identification and disease resistance,
     J. natn. Inst. agric. Bot. 15:34 (1979).
13. J. Jensen, J. H. Jorgensen, H. P. Jensen, H. Giese, and H.
     Doll, Linkage of the hordein loci Hor 1 and Hor 2 with
     the powdery mildew resistance loci Mlk and Mla on
     barley chromosome 5, Theor. Appl. Genet. 58:27 (1980).
14. G. J. Lawrence and K. W. Shepherd, Chromosomal location of
     genes controlling seed proteins in species related to
     wheat, Theor. Appl. Genet. 59:25 (1981).
15. R. P. Ricciardi, J. S. Miller and B. E. Roberts, Purification
     and mapping of specific mRNAs by hybridization-selection
     and cell-free translation, Proc. Natl. Acad. Sci. USA
     76:4927 (1979).
16. S. Rahman, P. R. Shewry and B. J. Miflin, Differential protein
     accumulation during barley grain development. J. exp.
     Bot. 33:717 (1982)
17. P. R. Shewry, H. M. Pratt, M. M. Leggatt and B. J. Miflin,
     Protein metabolism in developing endosperms of high-lysine
     and normal barley, Cereal Chem. 56:110 (1979).
18. B. J. Miflin and P. R. Shewry, Seed storage proteins:
     genetics, synthesis, accumulation and protein quality.
     in: "Nitrogen and Carbon Metabolism", J. D. Bewley ed.,
     Martin Nijhoff, The Hague (1981).
19. P. R. Shewry, J. Franklin, S. Parmar, S. Smith and B. J.
     Miflin, The effects of sulphur starvation on the amino acid
     and protein composition of barley grain, J. Cereal Sci.
     (in press).
20. K-E. Karlsson, Linkage studies in a gene for high lysine
     content in Risø barley mutant 1508, Barley Genet.
     Newslett. 7:40 (1977).
21. J. Ingversen, B. Køie and H. Doll, Induced seed protein
     mutant of barley. Experimentia 29:1151 (1973).
22. B. J. Miflin and P. R. Shewry, The synthesis of proteins in
     normal and high lysine barley seeds, in: "Recent Advances
     in the Biochemistry of Cereals", D. Laidman and R. G. Wyn
     Jones, eds. Academic Press, London (1979).
23. H. Doll, A nearly non-functional mutant allele of the storage
     protein locus Hor 2 in barley, Hereditas 93:217 (1980).
24. P. R. Shewry, J. M. Field, M. A. Kirkman, A. J. Faulks and B.
     J. Miflin, The extraction solubility and characterization
     of two groups of barley storage polypeptides, J. exp.
     Bot. 31:393, (1980)

THE SYNTHESIS, PROCESSING AND PRIMARY STRUCTURE OF PEA SEED LECTIN

T.J.V. Higgins, P.M. Chandler, D. Spencer,
M.J. Chrispeels and G. Zurawski

CSIRO, Division of Plant Industry, P.O. Box 1600
Canberra, A.C.T. 2601, Australia

INTRODUCTION

Pea seed lectin is a protein of Mr approx. 49 000 composed
of two pairs of subunits of Mr 17 000 and 6 000. In mature seeds
it is localized mainly in the protein bodies (1) together with
the storage proteins, legumin and vicilin (2). We became interested in the synthesis and processing of pea seed lectin because
of its association with the storage protein in the protein
bodies. We have found that the biosynthetic pathway which lectin
follows closely parallels that of vicilin and legumin and involves
modifications at different sites in the cell. These modifications fall into two categories, co-translational and post-
translational.

CO-TRANSLATIONAL REMOVAL OF SIGNAL SEQUENCES

When total polysomal RNA from developing pea seeds was
translated in a wheat germ cell-free translation system and the
products fractionated on an immunoaffinity column specific for
pea lectin, the only product which bound to the column was one of
Mr 25 000. When stripped microsomal membranes from dog pancreas
(3) were also present during the translation, two products, Mr
25 000 and Mr 23 000, bound to the affinity gel. The latter
product (Mr 23 000) electrophoresed with the same mobility as the
only lectin-related product detected after pulse-labelling
detached, developing cotyledons with ^{14}C-amino acids. Furthermore,
when membrane-bound pea polysomes, still with their associated
membranes, were translated in a run-off system, the lectin
translation product also co-electrophoresed with the pulse-
labelled product at Mr 23 000.

These results suggested that lectin was synthesized
initially as a precursor molecule (Mr 25 000) with a leader
sequence and that *in vivo*, or in the presence of microsomal
membranes *in vitro*, this leader sequence was removed co-translationally to yield the Mr 23 000 product. To test whether newly-
synthesized lectin (Mr 23 000) was translocated into the
endoplasmic reticulum (ER), cotyledons were pulse-labelled with
[14]C-amino acids and the ER fraction was isolated as described
elsewhere (4). This fraction was then treated with trypsin in
the presence and absence of Triton X-100 and lectin was isolated
by immunochromatography. Analysis by SDS-PAGE showed that only
when Triton X-100 was present together with trypsin was there any
degradation of the lectin. It should be noted that pea seed
lectin is extraordinarily resistant to digestion by any of the
commonly used proteases and the change in mobility after trypsin
treatment is small.

Taken together, these results suggest that, as is the case
with membrane and secreted proteins in animal cells, the primary
lectin translation product contains a signal sequence which
facilitates the binding of the nascent chain to the ER and that
the signal sequence is removed co-translationally during translocation of the nascent chain into the lumen of the ER.

POST-TRANSLATIONAL PROCESSING

The above experiments involving *in vitro* translation and *in
vivo* pulse-labelling showed that the only lectin products were of
Mr 25 000 and 23 000. However, as isolated from mature seed,
lectin is composed of two subunits of Mr 17 000 and 6 000. This
suggested that lectin undergoes a further processing step, in
this case post-translationally. To investigate this further,
pulse-chase labelling experiments were carried out with cotyledons
taken from plants in the mid-phase of seed protein accumulation.
After the pulse and at intervals during the chase period, total
extracts were made of cotyledons and lectin-related products were
then isolated on immunoaffinity gels. SDS-PAGE analysis showed that,
as reported above, only the Mr 23 000 product was present after a
2 h labelling period. After transfer of the cotyledons to a non-
radioactive medium there was a slow reduction in the amount of the
Mr 23 000 product accompanied by the slow appearance of the
subunits of Mr 17 000 and 6 000. At the end of a 22 h chase
period, most, but not all, of the Mr 23 000 product had been
converted to the subunits.

Subcellular fractionation was also carried out on extracts
made during the pulse and chase periods (for methods, see references
4 and 5). These showed that the only lectin product associated
with the ER at any time was the Mr 23 000 form. A trace of
lectin was still detectable in the ER after 22 h of chase, but

this was still in the Mr 23 000 form. At the end of the 2 h
pulse-labelling period the Mr 23 000 product was the only form
detected in the protein bodies where it was slowly converted
to the Mr 17 000 and 6 000 subunits. Cleavage did not go to
completion and small amounts of Mr 23 000 polypeptide were found
even after 22 h of chase. Consistent with this, a trace of Mr
23 000 lectin can also be detected in lectin from mature pea
seeds.

These pulse-chase labelling experiments show that lectin,
which initially appears as a large precursor (pro-lectin) on the
ER, is transported in this form to the protein bodies where it
undergoes a rather slow post-translational cleavage to yield the
two subunits of mature lectin. In all of these features, lectin
resembles the two major storage proteins of pea seeds, legumin
and vicilin. These are also synthesized on the ER as large
precursors and arrive in the protein bodies still in this form
(4,5). Their post-translational cleavage in the protein bodies
also occurs over a period of hours, although this process is not
as slow as in the case of lectin. Processing of the legumin
precursor (Mr 60 000 to 65 000) to form the acidic and basic
subunits (Mr 40 000 and 20 000, respectively) takes about two
hours (4,5,6,7) whereas the processing of some components of the
Mr 50 000 complex to yield the smaller vicilin subunits (Mr 34 000,
30 000, 25 000,18 000,14 000 and 12 000) takes 6 to 20 hours
(4,5,8). In the case of legumin and vicilin, the post-translational processing is known to occur after the oligomeric forms
of these proteins have been assembled and after their arrival in
the protein body (4,5,6).

GLYCOSYLATION

The lectins from a number of legume seeds are known to be
glycosylated as are some of the legume storage proteins. Lectins
from castor bean and broad bean are glycosylated while those from
lentil and jack bean are not (9,10,11). As far as we are aware,
there have been no reports of glycosylation in pea lectin.
We incubated developing pea cotyledons, at a stage when they were
synthesizing lectin, with both ^{14}C-glucosamine and ^{14}C-mannose
but detected no incorporation into lectin. On the other hand,
incorporation of these sugars into some vicilin subunits was
readily detected (12). It thus appears that glycosylation is not
involved at any stage of lectin synthesis and processing.

LECTIN SEQUENCE AND AMINO ACID SEQUENCES AT PROCESSING SITES

The above chain of processing events in the biosynthesis of
lectin was verified by a study of its amino acid sequence. The
entire amino acid sequence of the α-subunits (13) and of the N-
terminal portion of the β-subunit (14) from mature lectin have

previously been determined by protein sequencing. In order to
determine the primary structure of the initial translation
products we made use of recombinant DNA methodology. Cloning of
cDNA complementary to pea polysomal poly(A) RNA, together with
colony hybridization and hybrid release translation, led to the
selection of two putative lectin plasmids. DNA sequencing (15)
and comparison with published amino acid sequences confirmed that
the cloned DNA contained the sequence for pea lectin and the
entire sequence is shown in Figure 1. There was exact agreement
between overlapping sections of the two clones.

From the deduced amino acid sequence (see Figure), it is
clear that there is a sequence, rich in hydrophobic amino acids,
preceding the β-subunit which, in turn, precedes the α-subunit
without any intervening stop codon. This agrees with the predictions of a signal sequence based on the *in vitro* studies and
the formation of an initial pro-lectin of Mr 23 000 indicated by
both *in vitro* and *in vivo* experiments reported above. Very
recent data (not shown), indicates that the leader sequence is in
fact 30 amino acids in length.

The N-terminal amino acid sequence of the β-subunit (14) was
confirmed and the remainder of the β-subunit sequence was deduced
from the cDNA sequence. Comparison with published amino acid
sequences for lentil and broad bean lectins showed that there was
considerable homology between these two lectins and pea lectin.
The sequence of the pea β-subunit extends 30 and 6 amino acids
past the C-terminus of lentil and bean β-subunits, respectively.
The C-terminus of the mature pea β-subunit is not known but, by
analogy with the C-termini of bean and lentil lectins, it is
possible that some further modification occurs after cleavage
between the β and α subunits. The type of enzyme involved in
this cleavage is also unknown but would not appear to involve
trypsin-like proteases because of the absence of the basic
residues lysine and arginine from the sequence on the N-terminal
side of the start of the α-subunit at position 188 in Fig. 1.

It is of interest that the site of glycosylation in broad
bean lectin is the *asn* at the equivalent of postion 167 in Fig. 1
and is associated with the consensus sequence *asn-x-thr*. The
change in the homologous sequence in pea lectin to *asn-x-ala*
(residues 167 to 169) could account for the absence of glycosylation in pea lectin.

The deduced sequence of the α-subunit of pea lectin agrees
completely with the published protein sequence (13). However,
there are four extra C-terminal residues in the deduced amino
acid sequence. Thus, it is possible that in the mature lectin
these amino acids have been removed post-translationally.

```
                                        -10                              1                                 10
TAC GCG ATA TTT CTA TCC ATT CTC TTA ACA ATC CTT TTC TTC AAG GTG AAC TCA ACT GAA ACC ACT TCC TTC TTG ATC ACC AAG TTC
Tyr Ala Ile Phe Leu Ser Ile Leu Leu Thr Ile Leu Phe Phe Lys Val Asn Ser Thr Glu Thr Thr Ser Phe Leu Ile Thr Lys Phe

               20                              30                              40
AGC CCC GAC CAA CAA AAC CTA ATC TTC CAA GGA GAT GGC TAT ACC ACA AAA GAG AAG CTG ACA CTG ACC AAG GCA GTA AAG AAC ACT GTT
Ser Pro Asp Gln Gln Asn Leu Ile Phe Gln Gly Asp Gly Tyr Thr Thr Lys Glu Lys Leu Thr Leu Thr Lys Ala Val Lys Asn Thr Val

               50                              60                              70
GGC AGA GCC CTC TAT TCC TCA CCT ATC CAT ATC TGG GAT AGA GAA ACA GGC AAC GTT GCT AAT TTT GTA ACT TCC TTC ACT TTT GTC ATA
Gly Arg Ala Leu Tyr Ser Ser Pro Ile His Ile Trp Asp Arg Glu Thr Gly Asn Val Ala Asn Phe Val Thr Ser Phe Thr Phe Val Ile

               80                              90                              100
AAT GCA CCC AAC AGT TAC AAC GTT GCC GAC GGG TTT ACG TTC TTC ATC GCA CCT GTA GAT ACT AAG CCG CAG ACC GGC GGT GGA TAT CTC
Asn Ala Pro Asn Ser Tyr Asn Val Ala Asp Gly Phe Thr Phe Phe Ile Ala Pro Val Asp Thr Lys Pro Gln Thr Gly Gly Gly Tyr Leu

               110                             120                             130
GGA GTT TTC AAT AGC GCA GAG TAT GAT AAA ACC ACT CAA ACT GTT GCT GTG ACA GAG TTT GAC ACT TTC TAT AAT GCT TGG GAT CCA AGC
Gly Val Phe Asn Ser Ala Glu Tyr Asp Lys Thr Thr Gln Thr Val Ala Val Thr Glu Phe Asp Thr Phe Tyr Asn Ala Ala Trp Asp Pro Ser

               140                             150                             160
AAC AGA GAT AGA CAT ATT GGA ATC GAT GTG AAC AGT ATC AAA TCC GTA AAC ACT AAG TCG TGG AAG TTG CAG AAT GGT GAA GAG GCT AAT
Asn Arg Asp Arg His Ile Gly Ile Asp Val Asn Ser Ile Lys Ser Val Asn Thr Lys Ser Trp Lys Leu Gln Asn Gly Glu Glu Ala Asn

               170                             180                             190
GTT GTG ATA GCT TTT AAT GCT GCA ACT GTT TTA ACT GTT AGT TTG ACC AAT CCT AAT TCA CTT GAG GAA AAT GTA ACT AGT TAT
Val Val Ile Ala Phe Asn Ala Ala Thr Val Leu Ser Leu Thr Pro Asn Ser Leu Glu Glu Glu Asn Val Thr Ser Tyr

               200                             210                             220
ACT CTT AGC GAC GTT GTG TCT GTG GTT GAT GTT GTT CCT GAG TGG GTA AGG ATT GGT TTC TCA GCT ACC ACA GGA GCA GAA TAT GCA GCA
Thr Leu Ser Asp Val Val Ser Val Lys Asp Val Val Pro Glu Trp Val Arg Ile Gly Phe Ser Ala Thr Thr Gly Ala Glu Tyr Ala Ala

               230                             240
CAT GAA GTT CTT TCA TGG TCT TTT CAT TCT AGT GGA TTG AGT GGA ACT TCA AGT TCT AAG CAA TCA AGT CAA GCT GCA GAT GCA TAG TTTTTTGCTT TTCATCAT
His Glu Val Leu Ser Trp Ser Phe His Ser Ser Lys Gln Ser Gly Thr Ser Lys Gln Ala Ala Asp Ala Ala Stop

CA TGCATGTCAA GTCATGTGTG ACAGATCCAG TTTCTATAAA TAAACTGCGC ATATGCAGTA CTTTTGTAAT GTTGTTATGT ATGCGTTTAT TA15C13
```

Fig. 1. The nucleotide sequence of cloned DNA complementary to pea lectin mRNA and the amino acids derived from this sequence. The N-terminus of the β-subunit is at position 1 and that of the α-subunit at position 188. The position of the β-subunit is not known.

THE FUNCTION OF PROCESSING EVENTS

From the foregoing it is clear that co- and post-translational modifications are common features of the synthesis and deposition of lectin and other protein body proteins. The only processing event with a function which is obvious at this stage is the co-translational removal of the signal sequence during sequestration of the nascent peptide chain into the ER. The presence of a signal sequence seems common to all protein body proteins studied so far. Other modifications are specific to certain classes of protein or to all classes within a species. Their function is unknown. Thus, among the protein body proteins, glycosylation appears to be a more common feature of the 7 to 9S proteins, for example, vicilin in peas, conglycinin in soybean, conglutin β in lupin and phaseolin in beans whereas 12S proteins such as legumin, glycinin and conglutin α are probably not glycosylated. The function of the carbohydrate side-chain is not known. In peas, it is not necessary for any step in polypeptide synthesis, for processing, oligomer assembly or intracellular transport and deposition of vicilin in protein bodies (5,13). Within the one species, post-translational endoproteolytic cleavage may occur in some protein body proteins but not others. For example, in soybean, glycinin is post-translationally cleaved but other protein body proteins such as conglycinin and soybean lectin are not. At the present time it is difficult to decide whether the extensive post-translational cleavage seen in some protein body proteins such as pea vicilin reflect functionally important changes necessary to ensure the protein's survival through desication, dormancy and subsequent re-utilization on germination, or whether they reflect specific, but non-functional changes which can be tolerated without loss of vigour of the developing and germinating seed.

REFERENCES

1.   Van Driessche, E., Smet, G., Dejaegere, R. and Kanarek, L. (1981) Planta 153: 287-296.
2.   Varner, J.E. and Schidlovsky, G. (1963) Plant Physiol. 38: 139-144.
3.   Blobel, G. and Dobberstein, B. (1975) J. Cell Biol. 67: 835-851.
4.   Chrispeels, M.J., Higgins, T.J.V., Craig, S. and Spencer, D. (1982) J. Cell Biol. 93: 5-14.
5.   Chrispeels, M.J., Higgins, T.J.V. and Spencer, D. (1982) J. Cell Biol.
6.   Spencer, D., and Higgins, T.J.V. (1980) Biochem. Internatl. 1: 502-509.
7.   Croy, R.R.D., Gatehouse, J.A., Evans, M.I. and Boulter, D. (1980) Planta 148: 49-56.

8. Gatehouse, J.A., Croy, R.R.D., Morton, H., Tyler, M. and
    Boulter, D. (1981) Eur. J. Biochem. 118: 627-633.

9. Roberts, L.M. and Lord, J.M. (1981) Europ. J. Biochem. 119:
    31-41.

10. Cunningham, B.A., Hemperley, J.J., Hopp, T.P. and Edelman, G.M.
    (1979) Proc. Natl. Acad. Sci. USA 76: 3218-3222.

11. Foriers, A., Lebrun, E., Van Rapenbusch, R., de Neve, R. and
    Strosberg, A.D. (1981) J. Biol. Chem. 256: 5550-5560.

12. Badenoch-Jones, J., Spencer, D., Higgins, T.J.V. and Millerd,
    A. (1981) Planta 153: 201-209.

13. Richardson, C., Behnke, W.D., Freisheim, J.H. and Blumenthal,
    K.M. (1978) Biochim. Biophys. Acta 537:310-319.

14. Van Driessche, E., Foriers, A., Strosberg, A.D. and Kanarek, L.
    (1976) FEBS Letters 71: 220-222.

15. Maxam, A.M. and Gilbert, W. (1980) Methods in Enzymol. 65:
    499-560.

STRUCTURE AND EXPRESSION OF GENES ENCODING THE SOYBEAN 7S SEED STORAGE PROTEINS[1]

R.N. Beachy, J.J. Doyle, B.F. Ladin, and M.A. Schuler

Plant Biology Program, Department of Biology
Washington University, St. Louis, MO 63130, U.S.A.

SUMMARY

The 7S seed storage proteins (vicilins) of soybean (Glycine max) are trimeric holoproteins that accumulate during the cotyledon and maturation stages of seed development. The α', α and β subunits represent the majority of the subunits. To a lesser degree another group of subunits (the γ subunits) are also found in the vicilin proteins. The synthesis of each of these subunits is differentially regulated. Several of the messenger RNAs (mRNAs) encoding these subunits contain identical nucleotide sequences, but also unique sequences specific for the individual subunits.

The nucleotide sequence of a gene encoding an α' subunit of soybean vicilin was compared with the published partial sequence of a gene encoding a subunit of the vicilin protein of Phaseolus vulgaris (Sun et al., 1981). The overall structure of the genes and the predicted secondary structures of the subunits were similar. The differences in the lengths of the mRNAs that encode the two subunits result, at least in part, from a number of nucleotide deletions and duplications that have occurred in their respective genes.

---

[1]This research was supported by research grants to RNB by the National Science Foundation, the U.S. Department of Agriculture, and the U.S. Department of Energy, and by an NIH-NRSA Fellowship to BFL.

The two major storage proteins of soybeans (Glycine max) which
have sedimentation coefficients of 7S and 11S are referred to as the
vicilins and legumins, respectively. The research in our laboratory
deals primarily with the vicilin proteins. In this paper we present
a summary of the information that has accumulated on these proteins.
Our discussion will focus on (1) the biosynthesis of the soybean
vicilins, (2) the differential accumulation of vicilin subunits,
(3) the structure of the messenger RNAs and genes that encode some
of the vicilin subunits, and (4) a comparison of a soybean vicilin
subunit with a subunit of Phaseolus vulgaris vicilin. By a
combination of such research approaches we hope to better understand
the structure and function of the soybean vicilins.

Biosynthesis and structure of the soybean vicilins

The predominating subunits of the vicilin proteins, α' (83,000
d.), α (76,000 d.), and β (53,000 d.) are synthesized as precursor
polypeptides on membrane bound polyribosomes (Sengupta et al., 1981;
Beachy and Jarvis, unpublished). These precursor polypeptides
undergo both the loss of a signal peptide and core glycosylation
concurrent with translation (Sengupta et al., 1981). Additional
glycosylation of the α', α, and β polypeptides takes place one to
three hours post translation (Beachy et al., 1981). It is not known
whether these additional maturation steps occur on rough endoplasmic
reticulum, in transit vesicles or in protein bodies. Subunits of
vicilin or the vicilin holoproteins themselves are transported in
vesicles to the vacuole of the cell and deposited therein.
The proteins are compartmentalized into protein bodies by the
vacuolar membrane.

Soybean vicilin trimeric holoproteins which contain different
combinations of the α', α, and β subunits have been isolated from
mature seeds (Thanh and Shibasaki, 1976). Thus it appears that a 7S
protein can be assembled from mixtures of subunits that are produced
at any given period in seed maturation. This conclusion is
supported by the fact that while α' and α subunits of soybean
vicilin accumulate in the seed six to fourteen days in advance of
the β subunit (Meinke et al., 1981; Gayler and Sykes, 1981), vicilin
holoproteins assemble and accumulate throughout this developmental
period.

In addition to the α', α, and β subunits of soybean vicilins we
have recently identified three polypeptides, designated γ_1, γ_2, and
γ_3, that co-purify with the 7S holoproteins. These subunits are
present only in small amounts throughout seed maturation and in
the mature mature seed (Ladin et al., manuscript in preparation).
The role of these subunits in the structure and assembly of the
vicilins is unknown, and experiments are currently underway to
determine their pattern of synthesis and assembly into vicilin
holoproteins.

Although the majority of the storage proteins are produced in the cotyledons, a small amount of 7S and 11S storage proteins accumulate in the plumule and radicle of the embryonic axis. In contrast to the vicilins in the cotyledon, those in the embryonic axis contain greater amounts of α' subunits relative to α subunits and lack the β subunit (Meinke et al., 1981). Electron microscopic examination of protein bodies in axes and cotyledons has revealed that protein bodies in the axes are smaller and morphologically distinct from those in cotyledons (Ladin et al., manuscript in preparation).

When soybean vicilins were subjected to isoelectric focusing followed by SDS-PAGE (O'Farrell, 1975) α' and α, γ_1, γ_2 and γ_3 subunits are each resolved into multiple isomeric forms. The β subunit remained as a single species. We present data elsewhere to show that each of these isomeric forms represents the product of a different gene (Schuler et al., in press).

Cloned cDNAs of the 7S protein subunit messenger RNAs

In order to study the structure and expression of the genes encoding the soybean vicilins cloned cDNAs were prepared to the vicilin mRNAs.

A. Identification of cloned cDNAs by hybridization to messenger RNAs (mRNAs). Cloned cDNAs prepared from seed mRNAs as previously described (Beachy et al., 1979; Schuler et al., in press) were identified by several criteria. First, the cloned cDNAs were used to hybrid-select homologous mRNAs which were then translated in vitro (Beachy et al., 1981). The results of these experiments indicated that each cloned cDNA contained sequences complementary to several different mRNAs (see Table 1). However, each clone exhibited greater homology to one type of mRNA than to the others. By this method we identified cloned cDNAs which were complementary to mRNAs encoding the pre-α' and pre-α polypeptides. Other cloned cDNAs were identified which were complementary to mRNAs encoding polypeptides of 68 kd, 60 kd, and 53 kd (p68, p60, p53). These cloned cDNAs exhibited a low degree of homology with the mRNAs for the pre-α' and pre-α polypeptides.

Second, the cloned cDNAs were hybridized to mRNAs that were previously transferred to activated paper following electro-phoresis in agarose gels. Cloned cDNAs which were complementary to mRNAs for the pre-α' (76 kd), pre-α (73 kd), p68, p60 and p53 polypeptides hybridized to mRNAs 2400 to 2500 nucleotides in length. This result suggested that since the mRNAs encoding poly-peptides from 76 kd to 53 kd were similar in length, the mRNAs, would contain different amounts of untranslated sequence. This suggestion was substantiated by the DNA sequencing of the cloned cDNAs discussed below. Several of the cloned cDNAs also hybridized to a 1700 nucleotide mRNA that potentially encodes the β subunit (Schuler et al., in press). We have concluded from these data that each of the mRNAs encoding the vicilin subunits contain sequences unique to each mRNA and sequences common to a number of the vicilin subunit mRNAs.

Table 1. Characterization of Soybean Vicilin Cloned cDNAs by Hybrid-select-release of Soybean mRNAs[1]

In vitro translation reaction product[2] as a function of mRNA release temperature[3]

Cloned cDNA	50°	55°	60°	65°	70°	75°	Identity of clone
Gmc 236	-	p60	p60 p68	α' α p60 β	α	α	α (Gmc α•236)
Gmc 32	p68 p60 p53	-	(p68) (p60) (p53)	-	(α') α	α' (α)	α' (Gmc α'•32)
Gmc 232	-	(α') (α) (p60)	α' α (p68) p60	α p68 p60	p68	-	p68 (Gmc p68•232)
Gmc 58	α' α p68	-	p60 p53	-	p60 p53	-	p60 p60 (Gmc p53•58) p53

[1]Hybrid-select-release experiments were done according to the method of McGrogan et al. (1978). Released mRNAs were translated in a wheat germ extract, and the translation products were analyzed by SDS-polyacrylamide gel electrophoresis.

[2]The identity of polypeptide products is detailed in Beachy et al. (1981) and Schuler et al. (in press).

[3]Parentheses are used to indicate that lesser amounts of the mRNAs are released at the temperatures indicated than are released at other temperatures.

B.   Restriction endonuclease mapping of the cloned cDNAs.
Restriction maps of cloned cDNAs encoding the α', α, p68, p60, and
p53 polypeptide mRNAs were compared (Figure 1).   Cloned α' subunit
cDNAs (Gmc α' 16 and Gmc α' 32) and α subunit cDNAs (Gmc α 21 and
Gmc α 236) have similar but not identical restriction maps.   Likewise the p68 polypeptide cDNA (Gmc p68·232) and the cDNA complementary to p60 and p53 polypeptide mRNAs have similar but not
identical maps.   However, there is little relationship between α'
and α cDNA clones and the p68/p60/p53 cDNA clones, either at the
level of endonuclease restriction sites or gross sequence homology.
We determined that the homology between α' and α subunit cDNAs,
and between the p68 and p60/53 cDNAs occurred throughout the
cloned cDNAs, but that the homologies between α'/α cDNAs and the
p68/p60/p53 cDNAs were restricted to the 3' termini of the cloned
cDNAs.   It is this homology that is responsible for the
hybrid-selection of the several mRNAs by the individual cloned
cDNAs.   These nucleotides, termed the 7S subunit 3' conserved
sequence, is one characteristic feature of the members of the 7S
protein multigene family.

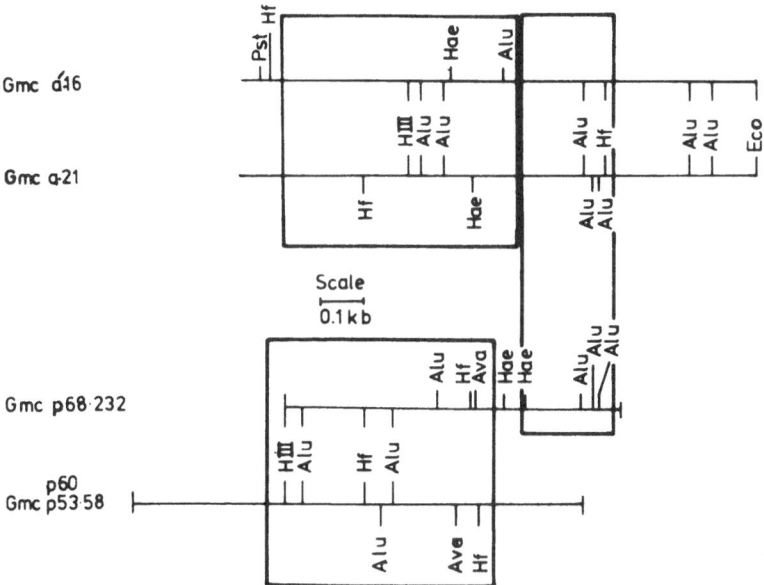

Figure 1. Restriction maps of cloned cDNAs encoding the α', α,
p68, p60, and p53 polypeptide mRNAs. Restriction endonuclease
sites have been diagrammed in a pairwise fashion to reflect
restriction site conservation between various cloned cDNAs. Areas
of sequence homology between clones have been enclosed in boxes.

C. Nucleotide sequencing of the cloned cDNAs. A number of cloned cDNAs were sequenced by the method of Maxam and Gilbert (1980) as modified by Smith and Calvo (1980). These included Gmc '16, Gmc α 21, Gmc p68·232, and Gmc p60/p53·58. The 400 nucleotides closest to the 3' end of the mRNAs are presented in Figure 2. Nucleotide homologies are indicated by vertical bars. Several features of the mRNAs for the various proteins are evident. (1) The α' and α-subunit mRNAs share a high degree of homology within the translated portion of the mRNA and within the 3' untranslated portion of the mRNAs (Schuler et al., in press). From the DNA sequence analysis we estimate that the α' and α subunit mRNAs differ in 7% of their nucleotides. The nucleotide sequences of the individual α' subunit cDNAs differ only by 0.5%. The amino acid differences caused by these nucleotide differences potentially result in the charge heterogeneity that has been observed in the α' subunits. Similar nucleotide variations occur in the α subunit cDNAs. (2) The α' and α subunit mRNAs share no homology with the coding regions of the p68, p60 or p53 polypeptide mRNAs. The 7S subunit 3' conserved sequence is present within the 3' noncoding region of the p68 polypeptide mRNAs, and in the coding of the α' and α subunit mRNAs. (3) Although the p60/p53 polypeptide mRNAs do not contain the 7S subunit conserved sequences, they share a high degree of homology with p68 polypeptide mRNA. This homology extends to a position directly downstream from the AAUAAA sequence characteristic of polyadenylation signals (Brownlee and Proudfoot, 1976). The p68 polypeptide mRNA cloned cDNA Gmc p68·232 contains an additional 155 nucleotides but does not include the 3' end of the mRNA encoding the p68 polypeptide. (4) Both the p68 and p60 mRNAs contain several AAUAAA polyadenylation signals in their long 3' untranslated sequences. The α' and α subunit mRNAs contain only two overlapping polyadenylation signals in their short 3' untranslated sequences. These additional AAUAAA sequences in the p60/p53 mRNAs occur 95 to 100 nucleotides 5' (upstream) of the correct AAUAAA in Gmc p60/p53·58, and more than 300 nucleotides from the correct polyadenylation signal of Gmc p68·232. (5) The 3' untranslated region of the α' and α subunit mRNAs is highly conserved and can be modeled into a stem-loop structure (Schuler et al., in press).

Figure 2. The nucleotide sequences for the cDNAs encoding the α' and α subunits and the p68 and p60/p53-polypeptides. The nucleotide sequence, the cloned cDNAs, Gmc α 16, Gmc α 21. Gmc p68·232 and Gmc p60/p53·58 are shown on lines 2, 3, 6, and 7, respectively. Nucleotides included in the brackets at the center, the Gmc α 16 sequence are derived from the closely related genomic DNA, Gmc α 17 (Schuler et al., in press). The amino acids encoded by Gmc α 16, Gmc α 21, Gmc p68·232, Gmc p60/p53·58 are presented on lines 1, 4, 5, and 8, respectively. Vertical lines (|) between the sequences mark identical nucleotides.

GlyAlaLeuPheLeuProHisPheAsnSerLysAlaIleValLeuValIleAsnGluGlyGlyIleLeuLysGluGluGluArgGluGlnGlu

Gmc α'16 GAGCGCTCTTTTCTACCACACTTCAATTCAAAGGCCATAGTGCTACTAGTGATTAATGAAGGAGAAGCAAACATTGAACTTGTTGGCATTAAAGAACAACAACAGAGGCAGCAACAGGAA

                              Leu   Ile   Asp   Leu   Glu

Gmc α 21 GGAGCTCTCTTCTTCTACCACACTTCAATTCAAAGGCCGATAGTGCTAATTAATGAACGAGATGCAAACATTGAACTTGTGGCCTAAAAGAACAACAACAGGAGCAGCAACAGGAA

Gmc p68·232   .........GTATTAAAGTCGGCATAAATGACAAGCATGGAGGATGAGGCCATCTCATGAAATAATAAC
    p60
Gmc p53·58 || |||||||||||||||||||||||||||||||||||||||||||||||||||
          TATGAAGGAATTGGGGTCCTTTGCTAACCCTGAGTCTCAACAAGGCTCACCCCGTGTTAAAGTCCCATAAATGACAAGCATGGAGGATGAGGCCATCTTATGAAATAATAAC
          TyrGluGlyIleGlyValLeuTrpLeuThrLeuSerLeuAsnLysAlaHisProValLeuProValLeuSerHisLyster

GluGlnProLeuGluValArgLysTyrArgAlaGluLeuSerGluGlnGlnAspIlePheValIleProAlaGlyTyrProValMetValAsnAlaThrSerAspLeuAsnPhePheAla

Gmc α'16 GAGCAACCTTTGGAAGTGCGGAAATATAGAGCTGAATTGTCTGAACAAGATATATTTGTAATCCCAGCAGGTTATCCAGTTATGGTCAACGCTACCTCAGATCTGAATTCTTTGCTTT

                                           Val   Asn   Ile

Gmc α 21 GAGCAACCTTTGGAAGTGCGGAAATATAGAGCTGAATTGTCTGAACAAGATATATTTGTAATCCCAGCAGGTTATCCAGTTATGGTCAACGCTACCTCAAATCTGAATTCTTTGCTATT

Gmc p68·232   AATAATAAATTTGTATGATAATAAAAGTATGGCCCATGTACCATCCAGCGAGCCTATGTTTATATCTGAGTGGCGTTATACCTTCAATCGCCTTAATAAAATTCTTTGCTATT
    p60 || ||||||||||||||||| ||||||||||||||||||||||||||||||||||||||||||||||||||||||||||||||||||||||||||||||
Gmc p53·58   AATAATAAATTTGTATGGTAATAAAAGTATGGCCCATGTACCATCCAGCGAGCCTATGTTTATATCTGAGTGGCGTTACCTTCAATCGCCTTAATAAAATGCAGTCTTCAC

GlyIleAsnAlaGluAsnAsnGlnArgPheLeuLeuAlaGlySerLysAspAsnValIleSerGlnIleProSerGlnLeuValGlnLeuGluAlaPheLeuGlySerAlaLysAspIleGlu

Gmc α'16 GGTATCAATGCCGAGAACAACCAGAGGAACTTCCTTGCAGGTTCGAAAGACAATGTGATAAGCCAGATACCTAGTCAAGTTGCAGGAGCTTGCGTTCCTTGGGTCTGCAAAAGATATTGAG

                                                         Gln   GlnAlaVal

Gmc α 21 GGTATTAATGCCGAGAACAACCAGAGGAACTTCCTCGCAGGTTCGCAAGACAATGTGATAAGCCAGATACCTAGTCAAGTGCAGGAGCTTGCATTCCTTGGGTCTGCAAAGCTGTCGAG

Gmc p68·232   GGTATTAATGCCGAGAACAACCAGAGGAACTTCCTCGCCAGGTTCCCAAGACAATGTGATAAGCCAGATAATGTCAACCAGAGCTTGCAGGAGCTTGCAGGAGTGCCAAGCTGTGTGAG
    p60
Gmc p53·58   GTTTGTCTT·poly A

AsnLeuIleLysSerGlnSerGlnSerTyrPheValAspAlaGlnProGlnGlnLysGluGlyGlnGlnLysGlyLysGlyLysGlyGlyLysLysGlyAsnLysGlyGlyAsnLysGlyGlyAsnLysAsnLeuSerIleLeuArgAlaPheTyrter

Gmc α'16 AATCTAATAAAGAGCCAAAGTGAGTCCTACTTTGTGGATGCTCAGCCTCAGCAGAAAGAGGACGGGCAACAAGCGAAGGGTCCTTGTCTTCAATTTTGAGGGCCTTTACTGAATAA

          Lys   Leu   Asn   Arg   LysLys

Gmc α 21 AAGCTATTAAAGAACCAAAGTGAGTCCTACTTTGTGCATGCTCAGCCTCAGCCTAAGAAGAAAAAGAGGGGAATAAGGGAAGAAAAGGGGTCCTTTGTCTTCAATTTTGAGGGCTTTTACTGAATAA

Gmc p68·232   AAGCTATTAAAGAACCAAAGTGTAACCXCGTGGTCCAGCCACACCATGTGGTCCTAAGGCTGCAGGAGCC

Although the existence of these structures in vivo has not been demonstrated, secondary structures may regulate expression of the α and α' subunit mRNAs by altering the stability of the mRNA or its efficiency of translation.

Structure of the α' subunit gene

Several α'-subunit genes have been isolated from a library of soybean DNA cloned in lambda phage Charon 4A that was prepared by R. Nagao, D. Shah and R. Meagher (University of Georgia, Athens, GA, U.S.A.) as previously described (Schuler et al., in press). The genomic DNAs were identified as α' subunit genes rather than the closely related α subunit genes because the endonuclease restriction map of the genomic clone, Gmg 17.1, was identical to that of the α' subunit cDNA clone Gmc α'16. Furthermore the amino acid sequence derived from the genomic DNA sequence matched the partial amino acid sequence of a cyanogen bromide fragment of the α' subunit (Mederios, Ph.D. Thesis, Purdue University, W. Lafayette, IN, U.S.A.). The α' subunit gene represented in Gmg 17.1 extends 3050 nucleotides from the site of initiation of transcription to the polyadenylation site (Schuler, unpublished). More than 99% of the nucleotides in the α' subunit cDNA Gmc α'16, are identical to the nucleotides in Gmg 17.1. By comparing the sequences of the 1600 nucleotides of Gmc α'16 with the genomic DNA, four short intervening sequences (IVS) 40, 85, 115 and 133 nucleotides in length were located (Schuler et al., in press).

Studies of the structure of the protein subunits of soybean vicilin

An understanding of the function of the soybean vicilins as controlled by the subunit structure can be gained by a variety of research approaches, several of which are presented in this section.

A. The primary and secondary structures of α' and α subunits of the soybean vicilins. Within the 609 nucleotides in the coding region at the 3' end of the α' and α mRNAs, 47 nucleotide (7.5%) mismatches resulted in 30 amino acid differences. Seven of these differences lie within an 11 amino acid sequence (Figure 2) near the carboxyl terminus. Predictions of secondary structures of the subunits were derived from primary amino acid sequences according to the methods of Chou and Fasman (1974, 1977) and Garnier et al. (1978). These analyses indicate that the secondary structures of the α' and α subunits are nearly identical and that the region of high amino acid replacements lies within a region of random coil and do not alter the predicted secondary structure (Schuler and Godette, unpublished data). Similar analyses with the amino acid sequences derived from nucleotide sequences of the β subunit mRNAs and those encoding the p68, p60 and p53 polypeptides are in progress. This research approach may eventually make it possible to predict how these subunits assemble into a 7S holoprotein.

B. Comparison of the soybean vicilins with the vicilins of
other plants within the Leguminosae. Since vicilin-like proteins
are found in a large number of different leguminous species, one
might logically expect that the features essential to the structure and function of the vicilins have been conserved evolutionarily. If such conservation exists, however, it is not detectable
by immunochemical tests. A number of researchers (Derbyshire et
al., 1976; Dudman and Millerd, 1975; Klozova and Kloz, 1972)
reported that the antigenic relatedness of legume seed storage
proteins is confined to a narrow taxanomic range within the
Leguminoseae. Antibodies raised against G. max vicilins do not
cross react with Phaseolus vulgaris proteins, although, despite
wide variation in molecular weights (up to 25,000 d.) these antibodies do cross react with proteins from a number of members of
the subtribes Glycininae and Phaseolinae of the tribe Phaseoleae
(Doyle and Ladin, unpublished). The data suggest that common
structural features have been conserved within the tribe
Phaseoleae and, therefore, a close comparison of vicilin genes and
their proteins may provide a means to identify critical structural
features of these proteins.

We have compared the nucleotide sequence, amino acid sequences
and the predicted secondary structures of a P. vulgaris storage
protein gene (phaseolin, Sun et al., 1981) and the α' subunit gene
of G. max vicilin (Schuler et al., manuscript in preparation). The
phaseolin subunit mRNA has a length of 1800 nucleotides while the
soybean α'-subunit mRNA is 2500 nucleotides. Within the roughly 800
nucleotides of the two genes that were compared, three intervening
sequences interrupted the same amino acid positions in both genes.
Excluding deletions and insertions of nucleotides within the genes,
the overall nucleotide homology between the genes within the coding
and intervening sequences was 73%. The nucleotide sequences
surrounding apparent gaps in the nucleotide sequences were analyzed,
using the models of Efstratiadis et al. (1980) and Shen et al.
(1981), to differentiate between duplications or deletions. Of the
four large gaps occurring in this section of the gene, it appears
that one duplication event and three deletion events have occurred.
Each of the deletions or duplications in the coding region occurred
as a multiple of three nucleotides and introduces or deletes one to
nine amino acids from the sequences. In all, six such events were
identified, accounting for 90 nucleotides or approximately 11% of
the difference in length of the Glycine and Phaseolus vicilin mRNAs.
If the ten deletions and duplications in the intervening sequences
are not considered, the nucleotide homology within the intervening
sequences is 71%, which is similar to the homology within the exons.

The amino acid homology between the two genes is 58%. The
amino acid differences result from nucleotide differences in each
of the three codon positions. The degree of homology varied from

50% to 78% in each of the exons. This variable degree of homology suggests that some regions of the protein, perhaps those that evolved as discrete protein domains, are subject to sequence constraints which are not common to other portions of the proteins. To determine if features of the secondary structure constrained the evolution of the proteins the primary amino acid sequence of these subunits were subjected to secondary structure analyses as described above. The predicted secondary structures of the Glycine and Phaseolus subunits remain remarkably similar when the deletion and duplications in the proteins are excluded from the evaluation. This supports the suggestion that protein structure rather than amino acid sequence has been conserved during the evolution of these two subunits. This is not surprising since the function of the seed storage proteins is as a nutrient reserve for the germinating seedling.

These types of comparisons will be the more valuable when vicilin proteins of other legumes, from subtribes other than the Phaseoleae, can be evaluated in like fashion. In the future we can hope to arrive at a clearer understanding of the structure and function of the legume vicilin proteins by using a number of research approaches including, but not exclusively, those described here.

ACKNOWLEDGEMENTS

We wish to thank V. Zenger and D. Goddette for their help with computer programs for DNA sequence analyses, and Mrs. J. Doyle for assistance in preparing the manuscript. Travel funds to enable RNB to attend the N.A.T.O./EMBO Workshop were provided by the DOE-BER.

REFERENCES

Beachy, R.N., Jarvis, N.P., and Barton, K.A., 1981, Biosynthesis of subunits of the soybean 7S storage protein, J. Mol. Appl. Genet., 1:19.
Beachy, R.N., Thompson, J.F., and Madison, J.T., 1979, Isolation and characterization of messenger mRNAs that code for the subunits of soybean seed protein, in: The Plant Seed: Development, Preservation and Germination," I. Rubenstein, R.L. Phillips, C.E. Green, and B.C. Gengenbach, eds., Academic Press, New York.
Chou, P.Y. and Fasman, G.D., 1974, Conformational parameters for amino acids in helical, β-sheet, and random coil regions calculated from proteins, Biochem., 13:211.

Chou, P.Y. and Fasman, G.D., 1977, β-turns in proteins, J. Mol.
    Biol., 115:135.
Derbyshire, E., Wright, D.J., and Boulter, D., 1976, Legumin and
    vicilin, storage proteins of legume seeds, Phytochem., 15:3.
Dudman, W.F., and Millerd, A., 1975, Immunochemical behavior of
    legumin and vicilin from Vicia faba: a survey of related
    proteins in the leguminosae subfamily faboideae, Biochem.
    System and Eco., 3:25.
Efstratiadis, A., Posakony, J.W., Maniatis, T., Lawn, R.M.,
    O'Connell, C., Spritz, R.A., DeRiel, J.K., Forget, B.G.,
    Weissman, S.M., Slightom, J.L., Blechl, A.E., Smithies, O.,
    Bralle, F.E., Shoulders, C.C., and Proudfoot, N.J., 1980, The
    structure and evolution of the human β-globin gene family,
    Cell, 21:653.
Garnier, J., Osguthorpe, D.J., and Robson, R., 1978, Analysis of
    the accuracy and implications of simple methods for
    predicting the secondary structure of globular proteins, J.
    Mol. Biol., 120:97.
Gayler, K.R., and Sykes, G.E., 1981, β-conglycinin in developing
    soybean seeds, Plant Physiol., 67:958.
Klozova, E., and Kloz, J., 1972, Distribution of the protein
    "phaseolin" in some representatives of Viciaceae, Biol.
    Planta., 14:379.
Maxam, A.M., and Gilbert, W., 1980, Sequencing end-labeled DNA
    with base-specific chemical cleavages, Vol. 65, in: "Methods
    in Enzymology", L. Grossman, and K. Moldare, eds., Academic
    Press, New York.
McGrogan, M., Spector, D.J., Goldenberg, C.J., Halbert, D., and
    Raskas, H.J., 1979, Purification of specific adenovirus 2
    RNAs by preparative hybridization and selective thermal
    electron, Nuc. Acid Res., 6:593.
Meinke, D.W., Chen, J., and Beachy, R.N., 1981, Expression of
    storage protein genes during soybean seed development,
    Planta, 153:130.
O'Farrell, P.H., 1975, High resolution two-dimensional
    electrophoresis of proteins, J. Biol. Chem., 250:4007.
Proudfoot, N.J., and Brownlee, G.G., 1976, 3'Non-coding region
    sequences in eucaryotic messenger RNA, Nature, 263:211.
Schuler, M.A., Ladin, B.F., Polacco, J.C., Freyer, G., and Beachy,
    R.N., 1982. Structural sequences are conserved in the genes
    coding for the α, α' and β-subunits of the soybean 7S seed
    storage protein. Nucl. Acids Res., in press.
Schuler, M.A., Schmitt, E.S., and Beachy, R.N., 1982. Closely
    related families of genes code for the α and α' subunits of the
    soybean 7S storage protein complex, Nucl. Acids Res., in press.
Sengupta, C., Deluca, V., Bailey, D.S., and Verma, D.P.S., 1981,
    Post-translational processing of 7S and 11S components of
    soybean storage proteins, Plant Mol. Biol., 1:19.
Shen, S., Slightom, J.L., and Smithies, O., 1981, A history of the
    human fetal globin gene duplication, Cell , 6:191.

Smith, D.R., and Calvo, J.M., 1980, Nucleotide sequence of the E.
    coli gene coding for dihydrofolate reductase, Nuc. Acid Res.,
    8:2255.
Sun, S.M., Slightom, J.L., and Hall, T.C., 1981, Intervening
    sequences in a plant gene-comparison of the partial sequence of
    cDNA and genomic DNA of French bean phaseolin, Nature, 289:37.
Thanh, V.H., and Shibasaki, K., 1976, Heterogeneity of
    beta-conglycinin, Biochim. et Biophys. Acta., 439:326.

COTTONSEED STORAGE PROTEINS AS A TOOL FOR DEVELOPMENTAL BIOLOGY

Leon Dure III, Caryl Chlan and Glenn A. Galau

Department of Biochemistry, University of Georgia
Athens, Georgia 30602, U.S.A.

INTRODUCTION

Our interest in the storage proteins of the cotton seed stems
from the fact that they represent the products of genes that are
expressed during a specific period during seed development. Thus
their expression is regulated by developmental cues, and it is the
comprehension of the molecular nature of these cues that is the
principle interest of our laboratory. In order to provide a background to searching for these cues, we have attempted to describe
the embryogenesis of this organism in terms of changes in the population of expressed genes by following the changes in the population
of mRNAs and proteins during this phase of ontogeny. We have observed
other sets of gene products (mRNAs) that are expressed before, after
or overlapping with the storage protein genes. Presumably each set
is expressed in response to different cues that arise in the tissue
at specific times in embryogenesis so as to produce the mature seed
capable of successful germination. In order to use the storage protein genes as a tool in the search for the molecular bases of developmental cues, we have examined storage protein properties and
biosynthesis in some detail.

The initial translation products of the storage protein mRNAs
are modified considerably to form the finished proteins of the
mature cotton seed. This processing sequence of events has been
determined in order to equate the finished proteins with the pre-
pro-proteins synthesized in vitro in the wheat germ system from
mRNA isolated at stages during embryogenesis. The identification of
proteins synthesized in vitro and the magnitude of their synthesis
during embryogenesis (both determined by 2D electrophoresis) are the

113

principal bases for identifying the developmentally regulated gene
subsets among which the storage proteins represent a single subset.
The processing pathways uncovered for the cotton storage proteins
have features in common with those reported for both the vicilins
and legumins of many legumes (1,2,3) and may reflect some general
features of storage protein metabolism common to most dicots (4).

BRIEF DESCRIPTION OF THE PROCESSING OF THE COTTONSEED STORAGE PROTEINS

The principal storage proteins of the mature cotton embryo have
the properties outlined in Table I. (For primary data, see 5,6).

Table I

SOME PROPERTIES OF COTTON PRINCIPAL STORAGE PROTEINS

	apparent final size	glycosylated	# Isoelectric variants	% of total protein mature seed	amino terminal	amino acid composition
α globulins	52kD	+	6-8	16	BLOCKED	VERY SIMILAR
						VERY HIGH GLX
β globulins	48kD	−	3-4	11	BLOCKED	VERY LOW TRP, MET

These proteins have been designated α and β globulins because
of the requirement for relatively high salt concentration (> 0.25 M)
for solubility. Both α (52 kD) and β (48 kD) globulins are in reality
sets of isoelectric variants that are partially resolved on 2D gels.
Their mRNAs, however, yield initial translation products in in vitro
synthesis of 60 kD for the 52 kD set and 69 kD for the 48 kD set.
Note that the larger set of products (69 kD) give rise after processing to the smaller set of mature proteins (48 kD). Figure 1
outlines the sequence of events involved in converting the mRNA
products to the finished proteins.

The cotton storage proteins occur cytologically in membrane-
bound protein bodies as do most seed proteins that are considered
storage proteins. This deposition requires a transit through membranes and, in every instance studied, storage protein mRNAs have
been found to associate with membrane-bound ribosomes and their
protein products lose a signal peptide co-translationally (7,8,9)
The wheat germ in vitro translation system does not carry out this
signal peptide cleavage. Hence the 60 and 69 kD initial translation
products seen by electrophoresis probably do not occur in vivo.
Rather protein sets of 58 kD and 67 kD are thought to be the initial

PROCESSING SCHEME OF PRINCIPAL STORAGE PROTEINS
(PROTEIN APPARENT SIZE GIVEN IN kD)

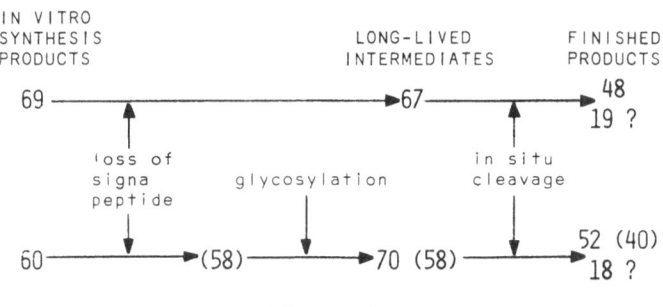

Figure 1.

products of in vivo translation. The 67 kD protein set can be seen
on 2D gels of in vivo synthesized proteins (via labelling of intact
cotton cotyledons) and as stainable protein as well (6,10). The
58 kD protein set is not seen in these instances and its existence
is assumed. What is seen in in vivo synthesis and as stainable protein
is a protein set of 70 kD that is glycosylated. From evidence presented below we believe that the 70 kD protein set is the glycosylated derivative of the 58 kD set. Both the 67 and 70 kD protein
sets are subsequently cleaved to give the 48 and 52 kD finished protein sets plus smaller polypeptide fragments of 15-20 kD that are
abundant in cotton cotyledons, contained in the protein bodies, but
not yet identified as to origin. By the completion of embryogenesis
both the 67 and 70 kD sets of intermediates have disappeared.

Antibodies to the 48 kD set and to the 52 kD set have been
prepared and their cross reactivity with the postulated initial
translation products and intermediates tested. When the antigen-
antibody reactions were allowed to proceed for a long period
(generally overnight) all the initial in vitro products and in vivo
intermediates shown in Figure 1 were found to react with antibodies
to both the 48 and 52 kD protein sets (6). Thus the processing of
the in vitro products to the finished proteins had to be deduced from
other evidence, which is summarized below:
 1. The 70 and 52 kD species are glycosylated (6)
 2. In a short pulse of developing embryos, no radioactivity
    appears in the 52 kD species, whereas the 70, 67 and
    48 kD species are heavily labelled (6)

3. Radioactivity can be "chased" from the 70 kD into the 52 kD species with time (6)
4. On 2D gels, the 70 kD species appear to have the same number of isoelectric variants as do the 52 kD species and to have the same isoelectric points
5. The same relationship as in 4 is observed between the 67 and 48 kD species
6. Antibodies to the 48 kD species show a kinetic selectivity for the 69 kD species seen in in vitro synthesis (15).

The last bit of evidence (#6), obtained more recently, reinforces the processing scheme of Figure 1 which was initially deduced from the data in #1-5.

The sequence of events shown in Figure 1 requires that two assumptions be made: first, that the cleavage of the 67 kD protein set to give the 48 kD set is rather fast, since the 67 kD set does not accumulate to a large extent as stainable or in vivo labelled proteins. Second, that the cleavage of the 70 kD set to give the 52 kD set is very slow. The 70 kD proteins are very abundant as stainable proteins and as in vivo labelled proteins until late embryogenesis. The latter observation causes the accumulation of the 52 kD proteins to appear to lag relative to the accumulation of the 48 kD proteins until late in embryogenesis.

RELATEDNESS OF 52(60) kD AND 48(69) kD PROTEINS

From the foregoing it is apparent that these two protein sets represent a rather large multigene family that contain common antigenic determinants and thus homologies in their gene sequences. It is also apparent that each set represents a subfamily of genes since they differ in molecular weight and since there is a kinetic preference between the 48 kD antibodies and the 69 kD antigens. The degree of homology between these gene subfamilies has been investigated through the use of cloned cDNA probes constructed from mRNAs coding for the 69 and 60 kD proteins. The strategy for obtaining these probes is discussed below and diagrammed in Figure 2.

We knew from in vitro protein synthesis patterns obtained with mRNA from different times in development (10) and from the kinetics of reassociation of cDNA: mRNA, using mRNA and cDNA from the different developmental stages, that the storage protein mRNA concentration drops 50-100 fold during the last few days of embryo growth (12). In the dry seed mRNA it is even lower. Prior to this point, the storage protein mRNAs are the most abundant mRNAs in embryonic cotyledons, comprising about 30% of the total sequences beginning about mid way through embryogenesis. Knowing this, the preparation of cloned cDNA probes to the storage protein mRNAs proved to be straightforward. cDNA was prepared from the mRNA of young embryos

ISOLATION OF STORAGE PROTEIN cDNA CLONES
BY HOMOLOGOUS AND HETEROLOGOUS COLONY HYBRIDIZATION

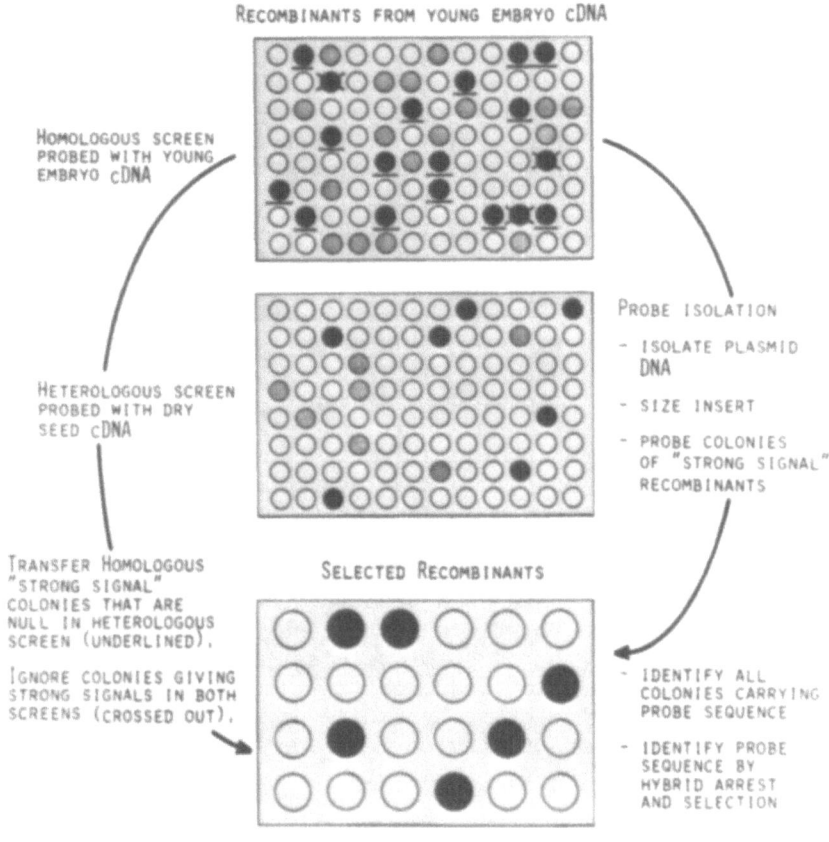

Figure 2

that contained the storage protein mRNA at its maximum level. The cDNA was inserted into the plasmid pBR 325 by conventional techniques and used to transform E. coli. Colonies that contained recombinant plasmid DNA were transferred to colony grids and probed with the same young embryo cDNA (radioactive). It was assumed that the strength of the radioactive signal emanating from recombinant colonies reflected the concentration of homologous sequences in the cDNA probe and that the frequency of recovering recombinants containing the same sequence reflected the concentration of that sequence in the cDNA used to construct the recombinant plasmids.

Thus when the recombinant colonies were probed (via replica filters) with the same young embryo cDNA as was used to produce

recombinants, most of the strong radioactive signals were assumed
to have been produced by the most abundant sequences in the probe,
i.e. the storage protein sequences. Further, many recombinants
carrying the storage protein sequences were anticipated since the
high concentration of storage protein sequences in young embryo mRNA
were manifested in the recombinants as well.

When the replica grid of recombinant colonies was then probed
with radioactive cDNA made to mRNA from cotyledons of the mature
seed, no detectable signals were anticipated from colonies carrying
storage protein sequences since their concentration in the probe
population was so low. Rather, the signals that did appear were
generated from colonies carrying sequences that were moderately
abundant in the cDNA (mRNA) from both developmental stages. These
colonies were ignored and only those colonies that putatively carried
storage protein sequences were transferred to another colony grid.
This grid was then probed with individual cDNA sequences that
carried a putative storage protein sequence.

We had anticipated finding 2 groups of recombinant colonies
on this latter grid - one group that hybridized with all the individual cDNAs carrying sequences for the 69 kD protein set, and the
other carrying sequences for the 60 kD protein set. Surprisingly
we found 3 sets of colonies that hybridized to 3 sets of cDNA
probes. The identity of the cDNA probe sequences were determined
by "hybrid arrest" and "hybrid select" techniques (13,14). These
results revealed that the 60 kD protein set (mature 52 kD set) is
encoded by 2 subfamilies of sequences that do not have enough
homology between them to cross hybridize at moderate stringency
(15). However, cross reactivity could be demonstrated if the criterion for reassociation was lowered.

Thus the genes for the principal storage proteins of the cotton
seed can be considered to be a multigene family that contains 2
distantly related subfamilies (60 and 69 kD genes) that still contain common antigenic sites, but insufficient nucleotide homology
to be detected by routine techniques. Further, the 60 kD genes
appear to be comprised of 2 sub-subfamilies that share homologies
that can only be detected at low hybridization criteria.

STORAGE PROTEIN GENES AS A DEVELOPMENTAL SUBSET IN EMBRYOGENESIS

Coincident with tracing the mature storage proteins back to
their initial translation products, we have followed the rise and
fall in concentration during embryogenesis and germination of
other abundant mRNAs. This was accomplished by the 2D electrophoresis of the radioactive protein products obtained from the in vitro
translation of mRNA isolated from cotyledons of different age
embryos and from in vivo labelled proteins extracted from cotyledons
of corresponding ages. From these "catalogues" a picture has emerged

of sets of mRNAs that are abundant at different periods of development. Very likely there are many changes in mRNA abundancy in
cotyledon tissue in embryogenesis and early germination that involve
mRNA species too sparse to be detected by 2D electrophoresis (12).
We have confined our catalogues to those species whose presence/
absence or rise/fall are clearly discernable.

Seven mRNA subsets are readily identifiable on the gels as
groups that change in abundancy in a roughly coordinate fashion -
perhaps in response to group-specific developmental signals.
Figure 3 presents a temporal view of these subsets. The ordinate
dimensions shown for these groups of mRNAs are not intended to
represent the relative mass of mRNAs comprising each subset, but
are solely for clarity. Subset 1 contains mRNA sequences that are
constitutive to the entire developmental span studied, e.g. from
very small embryo cotyledons of 5 mg wet weight through mature
cotyledons (125 mg wet weight) up to 48 hour germinated cotyledons.
This subset has the largest number of individual numbers, although
individually these sequences never appear to comprise more than
1-2% of the mRNA mass. Subset 2 contains those sequences that are
demonstrable throughout the embryogenesis period study, but
disappear in early germination. This group contains the least
number of members. Subset 3 are mRNA species that are no longer
seen on gels after the embryo cotyledons reach 40 mg in wet weight.

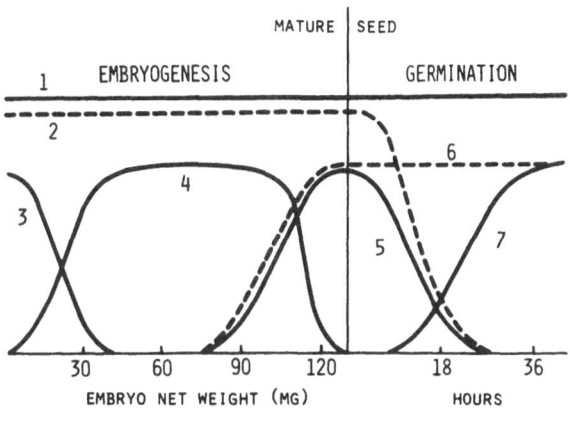

Figure 3

Subset 4 is comprised of the storage protein sequences. They comprise about 2% of the total mRNA mass at the earliest cotyledon stage (5 mg) and increase in abundancy rapidly until they constitute about 30% of the mRNA mass by the 40 mg stage (16). Each of the 3 subfamily mRNAs appear to increase coordinately as shown by dot blot analysis using cloned cDNA probes and stage specific RNA (16). However, when a cloned probe for each of the families was reassociated with the cDNA of 40 mg cotyledons to cDNA saturation, it was found that the 3 mRNA subfamilies are not present to the same extent. The mRNAs for the 69 kD proteins and one of the 60 kD protein mRNA subfamilies each comprise 12-13% of the total mRNA, whereas the other 60 kD protein mRNA subfamily exists in about 1/3 this amount (16).

The storage proteins mRNAs remain in super abundant concentration throughout most of the remainder of embryogenesis until, dramatically, they as a whole decline at least 16 fold between the 110 and 120 mg cotyledon stage (12,16) which is roughly a 3 day period. If this decline is due entirely to the cessation of the transcription of the storage protein genes, the half lives of the storage protein mRNAs would be about 18 hours. These sequences continue to decline as the embryo desiccates to form the mature dry seed to a level 0.01 of its maximum concentration (12,16). Oddly, these sequences do not disappear entirely during early germination, but are demonstrable by reassociation kinetics of 24 hour germinated cotyledon RNAs (12). Perhaps these genes continue to "lead" a low level of mRNA sequences until the cotyledons become senescent (about 2-3 weeks of germination). Since the cotyledon cells do not appear to undergo further cell division after the 60-80 mg stage of embryogenesis, such a leakage would occur from the same genome from which these genes were maximally expressed rather than from replicated genomes.

Two mRNA subsets become abundant late in embryogenesis and constitute the most abundant sequences in the dry seed cotyledon mRNA. One of these subsets (number 5) drops out of the abundant class in the first day of germination whereas the other (number 6) remains abundant. The former of these subsets is of interest in that it appears to be a group of sequences "induced" by the plant growth regulator Abscisic Acid (ABA). They can be caused to appear prematurely when young embryos are dissected and incubated on moist filter paper in ABA. Such embryos so incubated without ABA precociously germinate. This prevention of precocious germination by ABA may reflect the in vivo role of ABA in late embryogenesis when its endogenous level rises in cotton embryos (12).

Storage protein mRNAs, seen in this developmental context, appear to be a subset that rise and fall in abundancy independently from the other abundant subsets that characterize cotton embryogenesis. Thus they may represent a group of genes that are controlled by their own set of regulatory signals.

It should be noted in Figure 3 that by preparing mRNA from cotyledons at specific points in embryogenesis and germination, it is possible to prepare and clone cDNA enriched for specific mRNA subset sequences. By employing the homologous/heterologous screening strategy, illustrated in Figure 2, cDNA clones for each of the seven mRNA subsets can be recognized, specifically identified by hybrid arrest and used to isolate the genes for specific subsets from a genomic library.

REFERENCES

1. J. A. Matthews, J. E. S. Brown and T. C. Hall, Nature 294, 175-176 (1981).
2. D. W. Meinke, J. Chen and R. N. Beachy, Planta 153, 130-139 (1981).
3. R. R. D. Croy, J. A. Gatehouse, I. M. Evans and D. Boulter, Planta 148, 49-56 (1980).
4. C. A. Chlan and L. Dure, Mol. and Cell. Biochem., In Press (1982).
5. L. Dure and C. A. Chlan, Plant Physiol. 68, 180-186 (1981).
6. L. Dure and G. A. Galau, Plant Physiol. 68, 187-194 (1981).
7. B. A. Larkins and W. A. Hurkman, Plant Physiol. 62, 256-263 (1978).
8. T. C. Hall, Y. Ma, B. O. Buchbinder, J. W. Pyne, S. M. Sun and F. A. Bliss, Proc. Natl. Acad. Sci. (U.S.A.) 75, 3196-3200 (1978).
9. T. J. V. Higgins and D. Spencer, in Genome Organization and Expression in Plants, C. J. Leaver, ed., Plenum Press, New York, 245-258 (1980).
10. L. Dure, S. C. Greenway and G. A. Galau, Biochem. 20, 4162-4168 (1981).
11. J. P. Rogers, South African Jour. of Science 76, 471-474 (1980).
12. G. A. Galau and L. Dure, Biochem. 20, 281-292 (1981).
13. B. M. Paterson, B. E. Roberts and E. L. Kuff, Proc. Natl. Acad. Sci. (U.S.A.) 74, 4370-4374 (1977).
14. A. P. Ricciardi, J. S. Miller and B. E. Roberts, Proc. Natl. Acad. Sci. (U.S.A.) 76, 4927-4931 (1979).
15. G. A. Galau, C. A. Chlan and L. Dure, Plant Mol. Biol., In Press.
16. J. B. Pyle, J. A. Baker, C. A. Chlan, G. A. Galau and L. Dure, Plant Mol. Biol., In Press.

PHASEOLIN: NUCLEOTIDE SEQUENCE EXPLAINS MOLECULAR WEIGHT AND CHARGE HETEROGENEITY OF A SMALL MULTIGENE FAMILY AND ALSO ASSISTS VECTOR CONSTRUCTION FOR GENE EXPRESSION IN ALIEN TISSUE

T. C. Hall, J. L. Slightom, D. R. Ersland, M. G. Murray, L. M. Hoffman, M. J. Adang, J. W. S. Brown, Y. Ma, J. A. Matthews, J. H. Cramer, R. F. Barker, D. W. Sutton, J. D. Kemp

Agrigenetics Advanced Research Laboratory
5649 East Buckeye Road
Madison, Wisconsin 53716 USA

INTRODUCTION

It is now well established that the seed storage proteins of major crop species are encoded as families of closely related genes. Similarities and divergencies are being defined at the levels of protein structure, amino acid sequence, and nucleotide sequence, (see Brown, Ersland, and Hall, 1982, and Ersland et al., 1983 for reviews). Phaseolin, the major storage protein of the French bean (Phaseolus vulgaris L.) can be separated into a group of about ten closely related polypeptides by two-dimensional PAGE. Analysis of some 150 cultivars yielded only three different patterns, characterized as T (Tendergreen), S (Sanilac) and C (Contender) types (Brown et al., 1981a). The component polypeptides range in apparent molecular weight from 45 to 51 kd, and in isoelectric point from pH 5.6 - 5.8 (Fig. 1). The T, S and C patterns contained 5, 8 and 8 polypeptides respectively.

The genes controlling the phaseolin polypeptides of the three phenotypes are closely linked, no recombinants having been observed in some 300 F_2 progeny and each group of genes is inherited as a co-dominant allelic alternative (Romero et al., 1975; Brown et al., 1981b). Recently, evidence has been obtained for a regulatory system controlling the expression of these genes (J. Romero and F. A. Bliss, personal communication). The present article discusses the molecular basis for heterogeneity of the phaseolin family, and describes current progress in the expression of cloned phaseolin genes utilizing several different experimental systems.

123

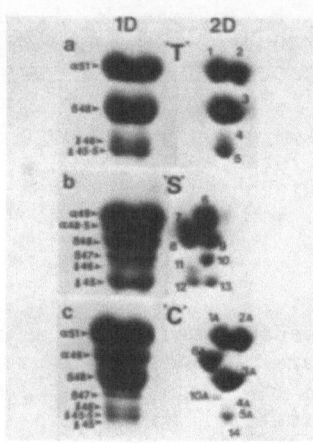

Fig. 1.   Electrophoretic patterns of phaseolin from bean
           cultivars: a, 'Tendergreen' (T) types; b, 'Sanilac' (S)
           types; and c, 'Contender' (C) types. The 2-D separations
           are aligned with the 1-D by M_r values, showing the poly-
           peptide composition of the 1-D bands. The 2-D separations
           are aligned vertically by isoelectric points.   The 14
           polypeptides which make up the three phaseolin types lie
           in the molecular weight range 45 kd to 51 kd and in the pH
           range of 5.6 to 5.8 (reproduced from Brown *et al.*, 1981b).

COMPLEXITY OF THE PHASEOLIN FAMILY

As shown in Fig. 1a, most of the native protein from T-type seeds is found in three molecular weight variants: α of about 51 kd, β of about 48 kd and γ of about 45 kd. Peptide mapping (Ma, Bliss, and Hall, 1980) suggested considerable homologies among the phaseolin polypeptides, but CNBr cleavage suggested that the α forms have an extra methionine residue.   Glycosylation studies (Hall *et al*., 1980 and Y. Ma and T. C. Hall, unpublished) indicated that the γ forms were less glycosylated than the others. Fourteen phaseolin polypeptides have been described if the complete range of variants found in the T, S and C types are combined. If each of the protein spots represents a single gene product, this sets the phaseolin gene family number at about 14, but the possibilities that several identical genes exist, or that differential processing (glycosylation, cleavage) of identical products from a single gene occurs, allows for the presence of more, or fewer, copies of the phaseolin gene per haploid genome.

Experiments to establish the complexity of the phaseolin family at the DNA level have included reassociation kinetics using solution hybridization and Southern (1975) blot analyses (Ersland *et al*., in preparation). C_0t curve determination yields a copy number of about 7 per haploid genome. Digestion of Tendergreen DNA with *Eco* RI, *Bam* HI and *Bgl* II endonucleases followed by Southern (1975) hybridization to phaseolin sequences also yields an estimate of approximately 7 copies per haploid genome (Fig. 2). *Eco* RI digestion gives three classes of phaseolin gene fragments. Class I is represented by a 12.3 kbp fragment (1-2 copies) that is cut to 3.0 kbp in a *Bam* HI–*Eco* RI double digest. Class II is defined as a 7.0 kbp *Eco* RI fragment (~3 copies) that is also cut to 3.0 kbp in a *Bam* HI–*Eco* RI double digest. Class III sequences (~3 copies) are

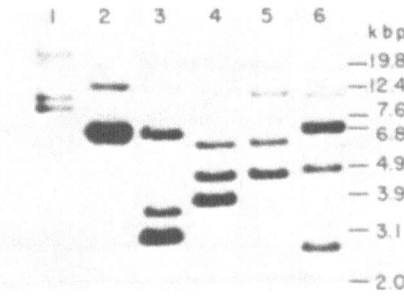

Fig. 2.   Analysis of the phaseolin gene family by digestion with different restriction enzymes followed by Southern (1975) blot hybridization to phaseolin gene sequences. Restriction digests are, lane: (1) *Bam* HI, (2) *Eco* RI, (3) *Bam* HI and *Eco* RI, (4) *Bam* HI and *Bgl* II, (5) *Bgl* II, and (6) *Bgl* II and *Eco* RI.

present on a 6.7 kbp *Eco* RI fragment that is cut into 4.8 and 2.8 kbp fragments in a *Bgl* II-*Eco* RI double digest.

ORGANIZATION OF PHASEOLIN GENES AT THE NUCLEOTIDE LEVEL

A partial sequence of genomic clone λ177.4 has been published (Sun, Slightom and Hall, 1981). Subsequently, we have made additional phaseolin clone selections from the Charon 24A *Eco* RI genomic library, and from a λ1059 (Karn, *et al*., 1980) *Mbo* I library. Comparison of the sequence of long cDNA clones (Slightom, *et al*., Murray *et al*., in preparation) with the genomic sequences present on clone λ177.4 yields the organization shown in Fig. 3. This phaseolin gene includes 1990 bp from a presumptive m⁷G cap site to the poly(A) addition point. It comprises 77 bp of 5' untranslated DNA, 1263 bp of protein-coding DNA which is interrupted by five introns (a total of 515 bp) and 135 bp of untranslated DNA at the 3'-end.

Over 4.5 kbp of λ177.4 have now been sequenced, and the 2 kbp region that includes the phaseolin gene is shown, together with the derived amino acid sequence, in Fig. 4. Several sequences believed to be important in controlling the transcription of eukaryotic genes (Efstradiatis *et al*., 1980) can be identified. Three TATA box (putative promoter) sequences (overlined in Fig. 4) are located at positions -28, -37 and -39, upstream from the mRNA cap site. Two putative distant promoter regions are evident (double overlines), a CCAT sequence at -67 bp and a CCAAAT sequence at -74 bp.

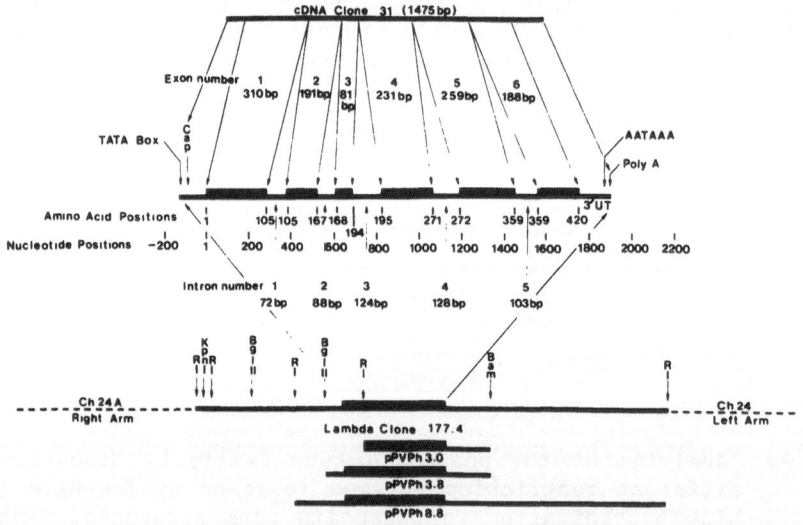

Fig. 3. Diagram of the structure of the phaseolin gene from clone λ177.4. Coding regions (six exons) are shown as raised bars, separated by five introns (IVS).

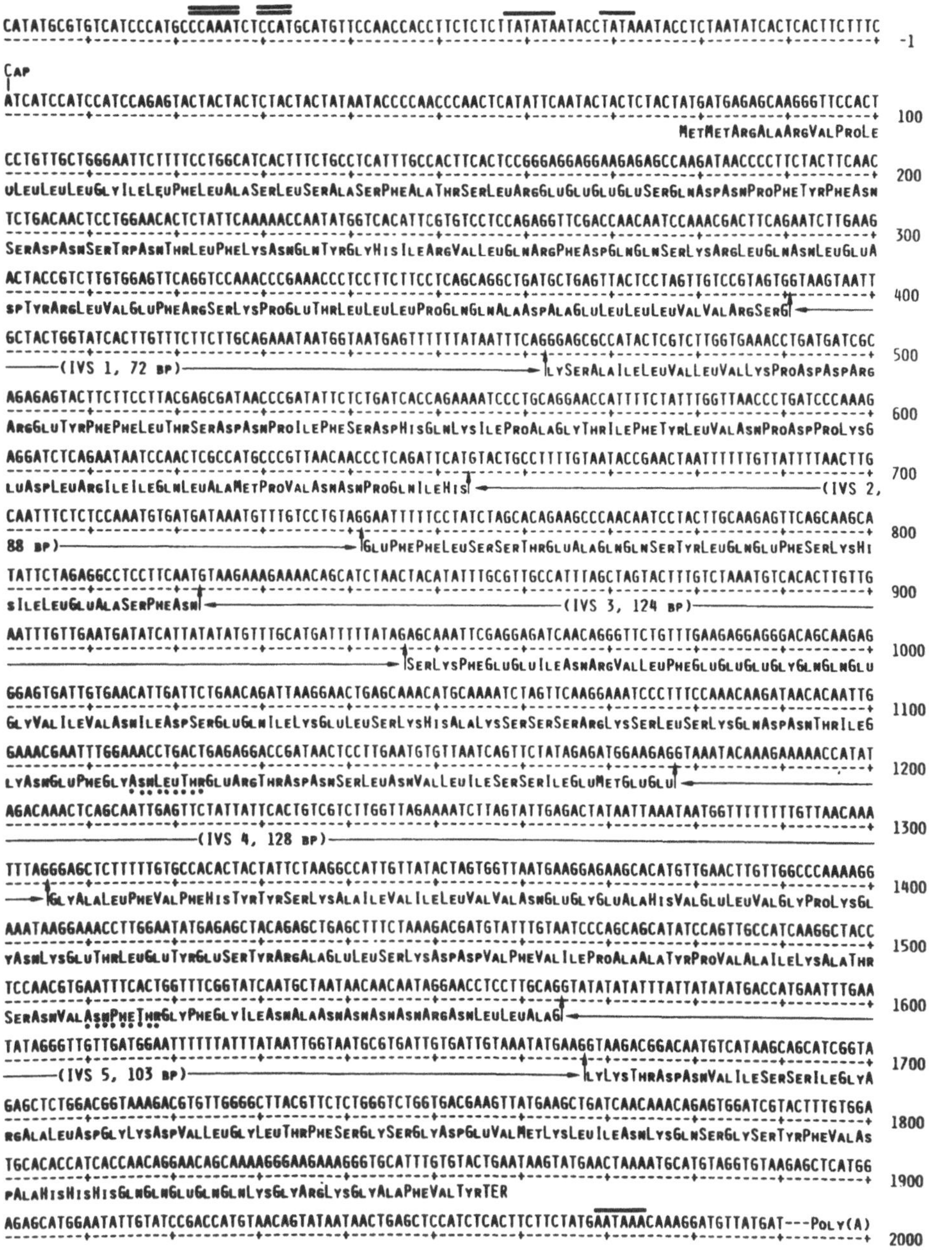

```
CATATGCGTGTCATCCCATGCCCAAATCTCCATGCATGTTCCAACCACCTTCTCTCTTATATAATACCTATAAATACCTCTAATATCACTCACTTCTTTC
----------+---------+---------+---------+---------+---------+---------+---------+---------+---------+  -1

CAP
 |
ATCATCCATCCATCCAGAGTACTACTACTCTACTACTATAATACCCCAACCCAACTCATATTCAATACTACTCTACTATGATGAGAGCAAGGGTTCCACT
----------+---------+---------+---------+---------+---------+---------+---------+---------+---------+  100
                                                                           MetMetArgAlaAlaArgValProLeu

CCTGTTGCTGGGAATTCTTTTCCTGGCATCACTTTCTGCCTCATTTGCCACTTCACTCGGGAGGAGGAAGAGAGCCAAGATAACCCCTTCTACTTCAAC
----------+---------+---------+---------+---------+---------+---------+---------+---------+---------+  200
uLeuLeuLeuGlyIleLeuPheLeuAlaSerLeuSerAlaSerPheAlaThrSerLeuArgGluGluGluGluSerGlnAsnAsnProPheTyrPheAsn

TCTGACAACTCCTGGAACACTCTATTCAAAAACCAATATGGTCACATTCGTGTCCTCCAGAGGTTCGACCAACAATCCAAACGACTTCAGAATCTTGAAG
----------+---------+---------+---------+---------+---------+---------+---------+---------+---------+  300
SerAspAsnSerTrpAsnThrLeuPheLysGlnTyrGlyHisIleArgValLeuGlnArgPheAspGlnAsnSerLysArgLeuGlnAsnLeuGluA

ACTACCGTCTTGTGGAGTTCAGGTCCAAACCCGAAACCCTCCTTCTTCCTCAGCAGGCTGATGCTGAGTTACTCCTAGTTGTCCGTAGTGGTAAGTAATT
----------+---------+---------+---------+---------+---------+---------+---------+---------+---------+  400
spTyrArgLeuValGluPheArgSerLysProGluThrLeuLeuLeuProGlnGlnAlaAspAlaGluLeuLeuLeuLeuValValArgSerG|

GCTACTGGTATCACTTGTTTCTTCTTGCAGAAATAATGGTAATGAGTTTTTTATAATTTCAGGGAGCGCCATACTCGTCTTGGTGAAACCTGATGATCGC
----------+---------+---------+---------+---------+---------+---------+---------+---------+---------+  500
————(IVS 1, 72 bp)————————————————————————————|lySerAlaIleLeuValLeuValLysProAspAspArg

AGAGAGTACTTCTTCCTTACGAGCGATAACCCGATATTCTCTGATCACCAGAAATCCCTGCAGGAACCATTTTCTATTTGGTTAACCCTGATCCCAAAG
----------+---------+---------+---------+---------+---------+---------+---------+---------+---------+  600
ArgGluTyrPhePheLeuThrSerAspAsnProIlePheSerAspHisGlnLysIleProAlaGlyThrIlePheTyrLeuValAsnProAspProLysG

AGGATCTCAGAATAATCCAACTCGCCATGCCCGTTAACAACCCTCAGATTCATGTACTGCCTTTTGTAATACCGAACTAATTTTTTGTTATTTTAACTTG
----------+---------+---------+---------+---------+---------+---------+---------+---------+---------+  700
luAspLeuArgIleIleGlnLeuAlaMetProValAsnAsnProGlnIleHis| ————————————————————————————————(IVS 2,

CAATTTCTCTCCAAATGTGATGATAAATGTTTGTCCTGTAGGAATTTTTCCTATCTAGCACAGAAGCCCAACAATCCTACTTGCAAGAGTTCAGCAAGCA
----------+---------+---------+---------+---------+---------+---------+---------+---------+---------+  800
88 bp)—————————————————————————————|GluPhePheLeuSerSerThrGluAlaGlnGlnAsnSerTyrLeuGlnGluPheSerLysHi

TATTCTAGAGGCCTCCTTCAATGTAAGAAAGAAAACAGCATCTAACTACATATTTGCGTTGCCATTTAGCTAGTACTTTGTCTAAATGTCACACTTGTTG
----------+---------+---------+---------+---------+---------+---------+---------+---------+---------+  900
sIleLeuGluAlaSerPheAsn| ————————————————————————(IVS 3, 124 bp)————————————————————

AATTTGTTGAATGATATCATTATATATGTTTGCATGATTTTTATAGAGCAAATTCGAGGAGATCAACAGGGTTCTGTTTGAAGAGGAGGGACAGCAAGAG
----------+---------+---------+---------+---------+---------+---------+---------+---------+---------+  1000
—————————————————————————|SerLysPheGluGluIleAsnArgValLeuPheGluGluGluGlyGlnGlnGlu

GGAGTGATTGTGAACATTGATTCTGAACGAGATTAAGGAACTGAGCAAACATGCAAAATCTAGTTCAAGGAAATCCCTTTCCAAACAAGATAACACAATTG
----------+---------+---------+---------+---------+---------+---------+---------+---------+---------+  1100
GlyValIleValAsnIleAspSerGluGlnIleLysGluLeuSerLysHisAlaLysSerSerSerArgLysSerLeuSerLysGlnAspAsnThrIleG

GAAACGAATTTGGAAACCTGACTGAGAGGACCGATAACTCCTTGAATGTGTTAATCAGTTCTATAGAGATGGAAGAGGTAAATACAAAGAAAAACCATAT
----------+---------+---------+---------+---------+---------+---------+---------+---------+---------+  1200
lyAsnGluPheGlyAsnLeuThrGluArgThrAspAsnSerLeuAsnValLeuIleSerSerIleGluMetGluGlu|

AGACAAACTCAGCAATTGAGTTCTATTATTCACTGTCGTCTTGGTTAGAAAATCTTAGTATTGAGACTATAATTAAATAATGGTTTTTTTTGTTAACAAA
----------+---------+---------+---------+---------+---------+---------+---------+---------+---------+  1300
————————————————————(IVS 4, 128 bp)————————————————————

TTTAGGGAGCTCTTTTTGTGCCACACTACTATTCTAAGGCCATTGTTATACTAGTGGTTAATGAAGGAGAAGCACATGTTGAACTTGTTGGCCCAAAAGG
----------+---------+---------+---------+---------+---------+---------+---------+---------+---------+  1400
———|GlyAlaLeuLeuPheValPheHisTyrTyrSerLysAlaIleValIleLeuGluValValAsnGluGlyGluAlaHisValGluLeuValGlyProLysGl

AAATAAGGAAACCTTGGAATATGAGAGCTACAGAGCTGAGCTTTCTAAAGACGATGTATTTGTAATCCCAGCAGCATATCCAGTTGCCATCAAGGCTACC
----------+---------+---------+---------+---------+---------+---------+---------+---------+---------+  1500
yAsnLysGluThrLeuGluTyrGluSerTyrArgAlaGluLeuSerLysAspAspValPheValIleProAlaAlaAlaTyrProValAlaIleLysAlaThr

TCCAACGTGAATTTCACTGGTTTCGGTATCAATGCTAATAACAACAATAGGAACCTCCTTGCAGGTATATATATTTATTATATATGACCATGAATTTGAA
----------+---------+---------+---------+---------+---------+---------+---------+---------+---------+  1600
SerAsnValAsnPheThrGlyPheGlyIleAsnAlaAsnAsnAsnAsnArgAsnLeuLeuAlaG|

TATAGGGTTGTTGATGGAATTTTTTATTTATAATTGGTAATGCGTGATTGTGATTGTAAATATGAAGGTAAGACGGACAATGTCATAAGCAGCATCGGTA
----------+---------+---------+---------+---------+---------+---------+---------+---------+---------+  1700
————(IVS 5, 103 bp)—————————————————————|LyLysThrAspAsnValIleSerSerIleGlyA

GAGCTCTGGACGGTAAAGACGTGTTGGGGCTTACGTTCTCTGGGTCTGGTGACGAAGTTATGAAGCTGATCAACAAACAGAGTGGATCGTACTTTGTGGA
----------+---------+---------+---------+---------+---------+---------+---------+---------+---------+  1800
rgAlaLeuAspGlyLysAspValLeuGlyLeuThrPheSerGlySerGlyAspGluValMetLysLeuIleAsnLysGlnSerGlySerTyrPheValAs

TGCACACCATCACCAACAGGAACAGCAAAAGGGAAGAAAGGGTGCATTTGTGTACTGAATAAGTATGAACTAAAATGCATGTAGGTGTAAGAGCTCATGG
----------+---------+---------+---------+---------+---------+---------+---------+---------+---------+  1900
pAlaHisHisHisGlnGlnGluGlnGlnLysGlyArgLysGlyAlaPheValTyrTER

AGAGCATGGAATATTGTATCCGACCATGTAACAGTATAATAACTGAGCTCCATCTCACTTCTTCTATGAATAAACAAAGGATGTTATGAT---PoLy(A)
----------+---------+---------+---------+---------+---------+---------+---------+---------+---------+  2000
```

Fig. 4   The genomic sequence for phaseolin encoded in clone
         λ 177.4.   Comparison with the identical coding sequence
         expressed in mRNA obtained by sequencing of cDNA clone 31
         reveals the mRNA start (nucleotide 1), derived amino acid
         sequence, five introns (IVS 1-5) and termination region.
         Other features are described in the text.

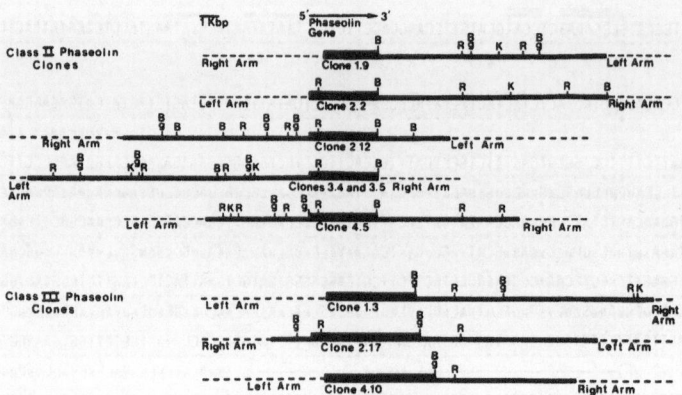

Fig. 5.   Restriction enzyme site mapping of λ1059 phaseolin clones
          shows non-allelic genes from phaseolin gene classes II and
          III.   Restriction enzymes used are: R=*Eco* RI, B=*Bam* HI,
          Bg=*Bgl* II, and K=*Kpn* I.

It will be interesting to determine which of these CCAAT and TATA
sequences is functional in mRNA transcription.   It is tempting to
speculate that if more than one transcription system exists, the
high levels of storage protein expression during cotyledon development may result from the combined efforts of the multiple systems,
each responding to the slightly different promoter signals.
Interestingly, there are several AATAAA (polyadenylation signal)
sequences at the 3' end of the gene (only one is shown, overlined,
in Fig. 4); in connection with the above conjecture, these may be
functional in different transcripts.

     The derived peptide sequence shown for nucleotides 630-653
(Fig. 4) has been confirmed by amino acid sequencing of native
phaseolin (J. Marsh and R. Casey, personal communication).   The N-
terminal region of the derived amino acid sequence is very hydrophobic and may well represent a signal sequence involved in
membrane transport.   It is possible that the N-terminus of
phaseolin polypeptides that accumulate in the protein bodies is at
or close to the four glutamic acid residues coded by nucleotides
162-173.   This would explain the difficulties that have been
encountered in obtaining an N-terminal sequence for phaseolin polypeptides.   Likely positions for N-glycosylation (Sun, 1974; Sharon
and Lis, 1979) are coded by nucleotides 1115-1123 (asn, leu, thr)
and 1510-1518 (asn, phe, thr), see dotted underline in Fig. 4.

     As mentioned above, several cDNA and genomic clones have now
been subjected to restriction endonuclease and nucleotide sequence
analysis.   These include five Class II and three Class III genomic
clones from the λ1059 library (Fig. 5).   To date, no clone repre-

sentative of the 12.3 kbp (Class I) *Eco* RI genomic fragment has been identified. Detailed analysis of the available genomic clones has not yet resulted in linking any of the phaseolin sequences, indicating that they are separated by distances greater than 20 kbp, despite the close linkage observed from sexual crosses.

MOLECULAR BASIS FOR SIZE AND CHARGE HETEROGENEITY

Comparison of the nucleotide sequences of the available cDNA clones (Fig. 6a–c) explains how differences in size and charge of the phaseolin polypeptides arise (Slightom *et al.*, in preparation). Variations in molecular weight can be seen to arise in several ways. The putative α-type polypeptide coding sequences shown in Fig. 6a–c (clones 6, 13, 39, 69, 110, 134 and 169) contain two direct repeats, one of 15 bp (between positions 711 and 740), the other of 27 bp (positions 1322–1375). Although the absence of these sequences from the putative β-type clone 31 can be considered to be a deletion, it appears simpler to assume that the repeats represent insertions into the archetype. Although explanations such as divergence from a common ancestor are available, it is unclear why these two insertions are either both present or both absent; the possibility remains that clones containing only one of the repeats may yet be identified.

Repeated sequences may be a general feature of seed storage proteins. Zeins of corn have been found to have 7–9 tandem repeats of a conserved amino acid sequence about 20 residues long (Geraghty *et al.*, 1981; Pedersen *et al.*, 1982). Short, nontandem internal repeats have been observed in acidic subunits of soybean glycinin (11S) storage proteins (Moreira *et al.*, 1981). Unlike the phaseolin and glycinin repeats, the repeats in zein make up a major proportion of the protein molecule.

Contrary to widely held notions, the vital and complex functions of seed storage protein (membrane transit during synthesis or accumulation, general insolubility to minimize osmotic potential at high concentrations, stability during harsh climatic conditions such as overwintering, resistance to microbial degradation despite susceptibility to rapid yet controlled hydrolysis during germination and suitable amino acid composition—often including a high nitrogen content) almost certainly impose stringent constraints on their amino acid sequence. The phaseolin sequences analyzed thus far support this concept, there being great conservation even at the nucleotide level. Nevertheless, point deletions do account for small molecular size differences. Single or double base deletions would induce frameshifts, and it is noteworthy that almost all observed deletions occur in triplets, restoring the reading frame. Instances are seen between positions 456 and 462 in Fig. 6. An exception to this situation may be clone 72 which has a base deletion at position 179. If this is a

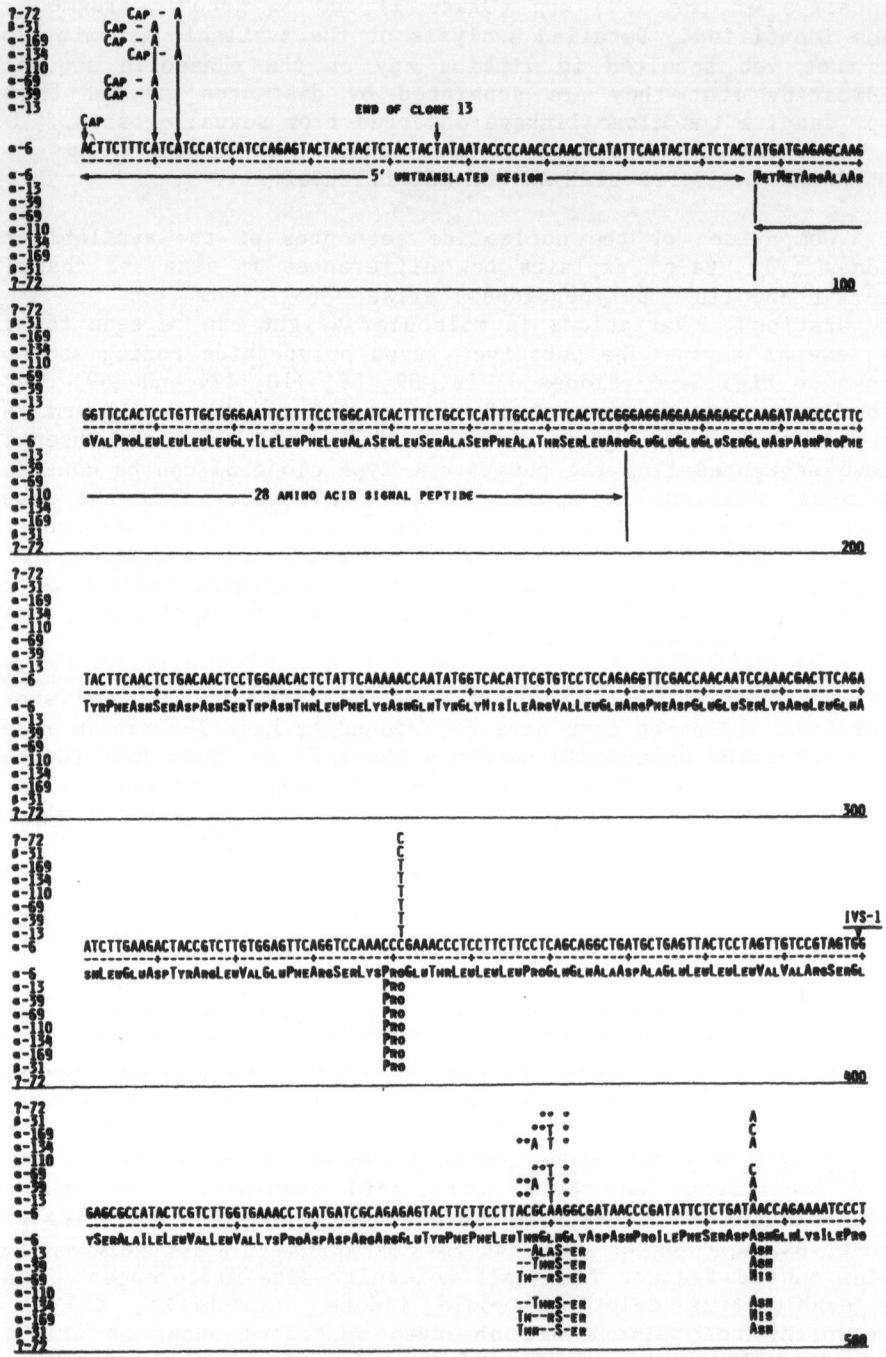

Fig. 6a

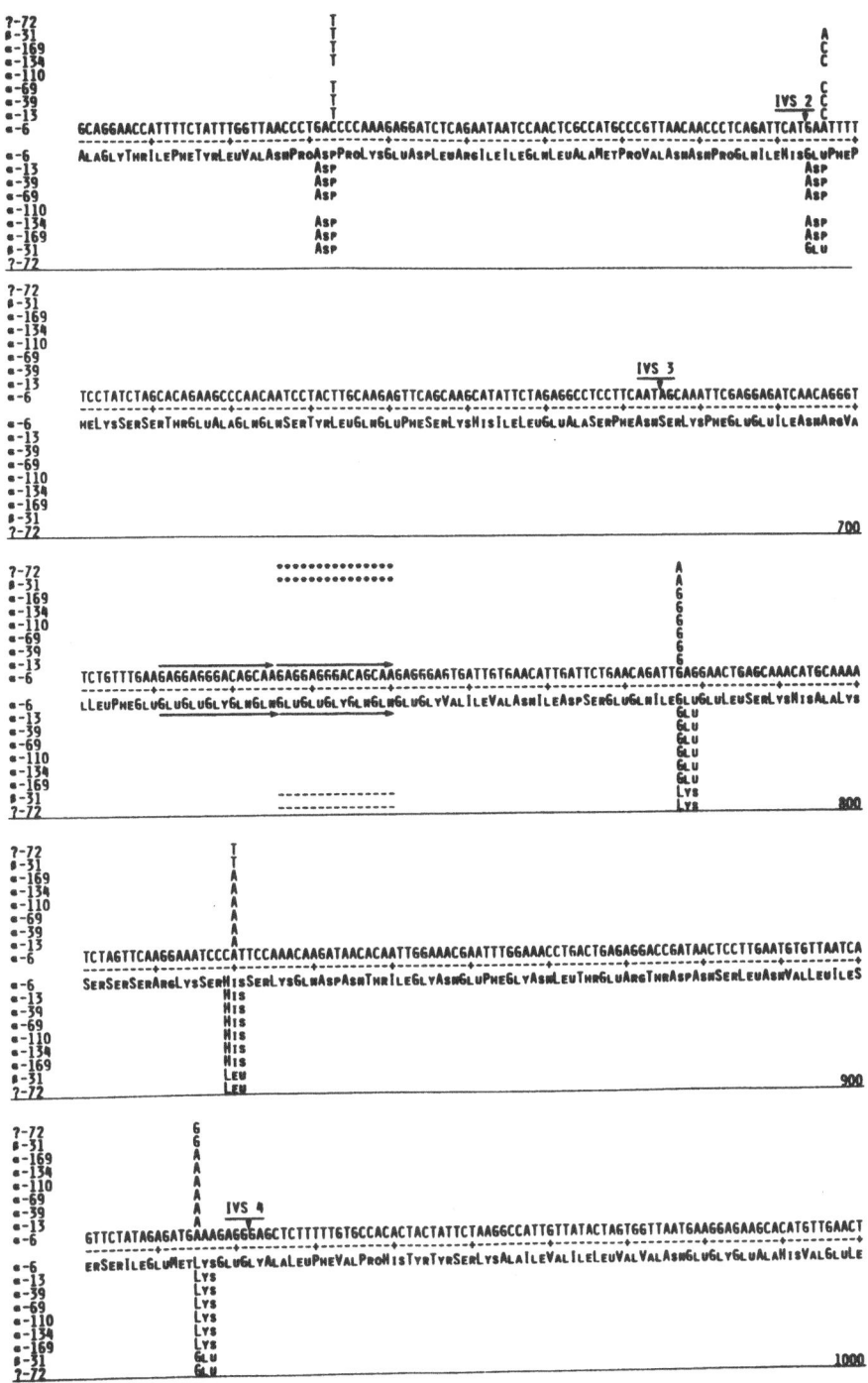

Fig. 6b

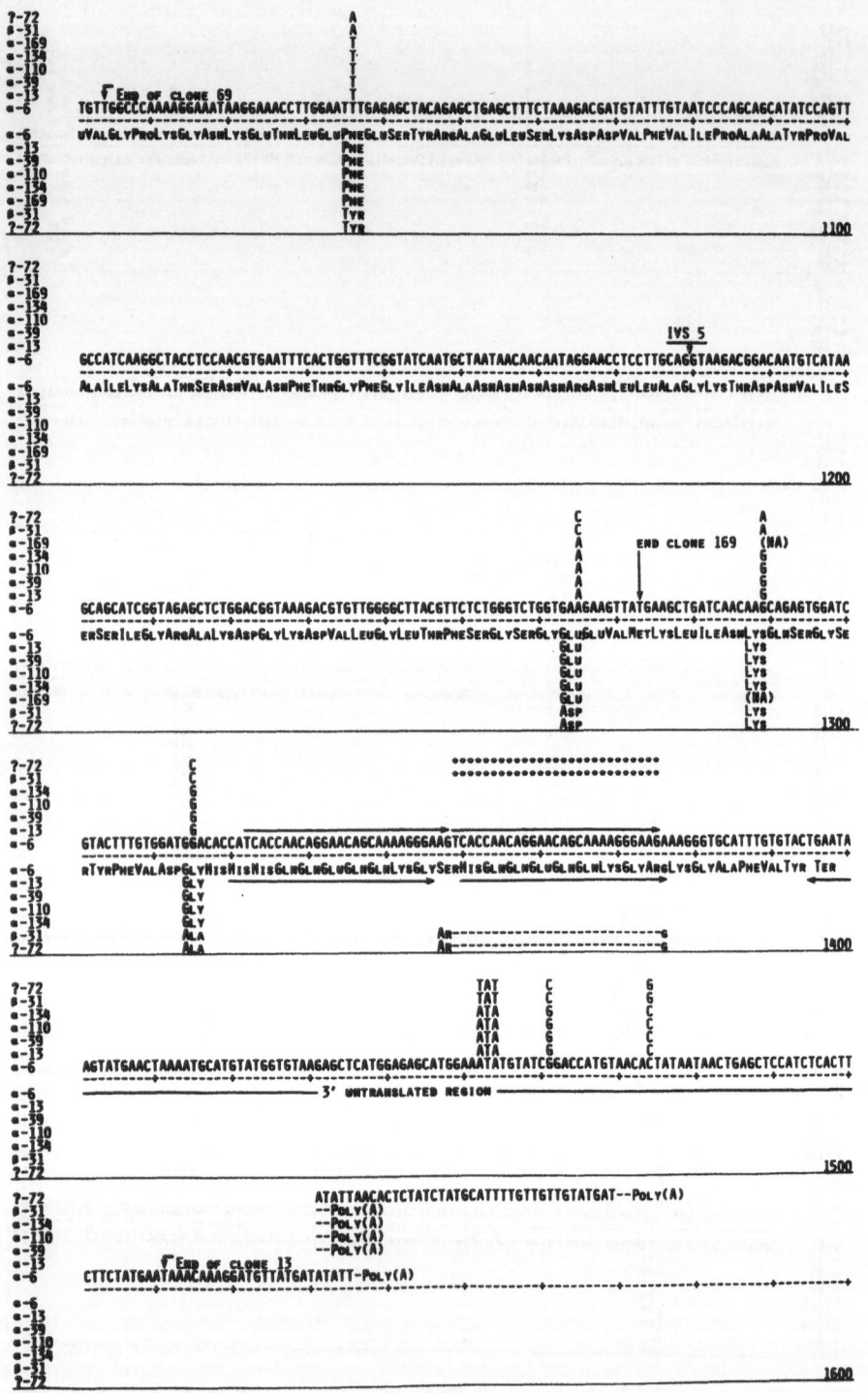

Fig. 6c

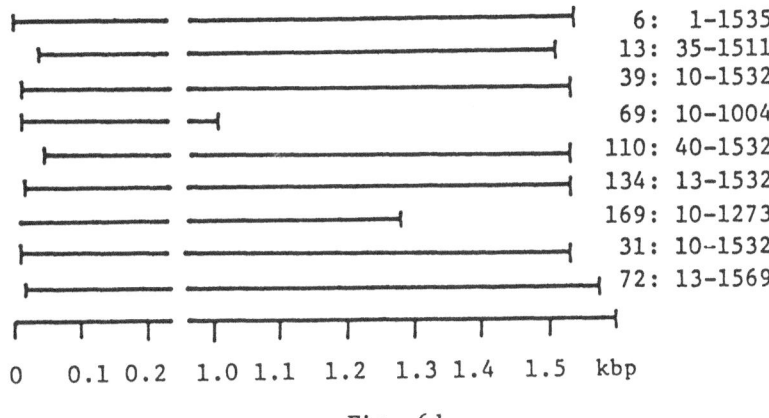

6:	1–1535
13:	35–1511
39:	10–1532
69:	10–1004
110:	40–1532
134:	13–1532
169:	10–1273
31:	10–1532
72:	13–1569

0   0.1 0.2 1.0 1.1 1.2 1.3 1.4 1.5 kbp

Fig. 6d

Fig. 6 a-c Comparison of nine cDNA clones; see Fig. 6d above for
relative coding regions covered by these clones. The
nucleotide sequences and derived amino acid sequences are
displayed as mirror images. Clone 31 is identical in
sequence with genomic clone λ177.4. Only positions
varying from the sequence of clone 6 are indicated;
further details of these locations are given in Table I.

functional gene, the methionine codon at bases 567–569 may be N-
terminal; however, the resulting sequence would be short even for a
γ-type phaseolin. The possibility cannot be excluded at this time
that the deletion at position 179 is an error in the reverse
transcriptase reaction (Hartley *et al*.,1982). Such errors appear
not to be very common as evidenced by the sequence identity of
several cDNA clones shown in Fig. 6. The derived amino acid
changes and molecular weights of unglycosylated forms of putative α
and β phaseolins are shown in Table I. The sugar residues would be
expected to add about 4 kd to these α and β polypeptides, yielding
a M_r of 50–51 kd (assuming cleavage of a 2–3 kd signal polypeptide)
for clone 6, in close agreement with the apparent molecular weight
for T-type α-phaseolins obtained by electrophoretic analysis (Fig.
1). The nucleotide sequences of overlapping regions of clones 39
and 134 were identical, as were those for clones 69 and 169.
Because of sequence similarity of these pairs, only data for clones
39 and 169 are shown in Table I. The sequence obtained for clone
110 (Fig. 6) was identical to that obtained for clones 6, 13, 39
and 169 and was therefore omitted from the analysis.

Table I. Compilation of base substitutions and deletions obtained in a comparison of nine phaseolin cDNA clones (see Figure 6). Deletions (DEL) at positions 726-740 (inclusive) result in the loss of $(Glu)_2$, $(Gln)_2$, and Gly residues in peptides coded by clones 31 and 72. Deletions (√) between positions 1348 and 1375 (inclusive) delete Ser, His, $(Gln)_4$, Glu, Lys, Gly residues and result in the addition of an Arg residue. Clone 31 is identical in sequence with the coding regions of genomic clone λ177.4. A = amino acid coded, C = charge, M = mol. wt.

Position:	341	456-462	486	533	596	726 DEL	777	820	915	1036	1265	1289	1315	1348 DEL	SUMMARY
CLONE SEQUENCE															
α- 6	CCC	ACGCAAG..	AAC	GAC	GAA	—	GAG	CAT	AAA	.TTT	.GAA	.AAG	GGA.	—	
α- 13	CCT	--GCTA-;;	AAC	GAT	GAC	—	GAG	CAT	AAA	.TTT	.GAA	.AAG	GGA.	—	
α- 39	CCT	--ACTA-;;	AAC	GAT	GAC	—	GAG	CAT	AAA	.TTT	.GAA	.AAG	GGA.	—	
α-169	CCT	AC--TA-;;	CAC	GAT	GAC	—	GAG	CAT	AAA	.TTT	.GAC	.AAA	GCA.	√	
β- 31	CCC	ACG--A-;;	AAC	GAT	GAA	√	AAG	CTT	GAA	.TAT	.GAC	.AAA	GCA.	√	
?- 72							AAG	CTT	GAA	.TAT	.GAC	.AAA	GCA.	√	
PEPTIDE DERIVATION															
α- 6	Pro	ThrGlnGly	Asn	Asp	Glu	—	Glu	His	Lys	Phe	Glu	Lys	Gly.	—	49,034.5 Daltons (REFERENCE SEQUENCE)
α- 13A	Pro	--AlaS-er	Asn	Asp	Asp	—	Glu	His	Lys	Phe	Glu	Lys	Gly.	—	-1 RESIDUE POSSIBLE SMALL CHANGE 48,892.4 (-142.1)
C	0	±	0	0	±	0	0	0	0	0	0	0	0	0	
M	0	-128.1	0	0	-14	0	0	0	0	0	0	0	0	0	
α- 39A	Pro	--ThrS-er	Asn	Asp	Asp	—	Glu	His	Lys	Phe	Glu	Lys	Gly.	—	-1 RESIDUE POSSIBLE SMALL CHANGE 48,922.4 (-112.1)
C	0	±	0	0	±	0	0	0	0	0	0	0	0	0	
M	0	-98.1	0	0	-14	0	0	0	0	0	0	0	0	0	
α-169A	Pro	Th--rS-er	His	Asp	Asp	—	Glu	His	Lys	Phe	Glu	Lys	Gly.	(-)	-1 RESIDUE LIKELY +1 48,945.5 (-89)
C	0	±	+1	0	±	0	0	0	0	0	0	{0}	{0}	{0}	
M	0	-98.1	+23.1	0	-14	0	0	0	0	0	0	{0}	{0}	{0}	
β- 31A	Pro	Thr--S-er	Asn	Asp	Glu	-5	Lys	Leu	Glu	Tyr	Asp	Lys	Ala	-9	-15 RESIDUES LIKELY +4 47,462 (-1572.5)
C	0	±	0	0	0	+2	+2	-1	-2	±	±	0	±	+3	
M	0	-98.1	0	0	0	-571.5	-0.9	-24	+0.9	+16	-14	0	+14	-894.9	
?- 72A		(Thr--S-er)	(Asn)	Asp	Glu	-5	Lys	Leu	Glu	Tyr	Asp	Lys	Ala	-9	-15 RESIDUES LIKELY +4 47,462 (-1572.5)
C		(±)	{0}	0	0	+2	+2	-1	-2	±	±	0	±	+3	
M		(-98.1)	{0}	0	0	-571.5	-0.9	-24	+0.9	+16	-14	0	+14	-894.9	

The foregoing provides a clear basis for molecular weight heterogeneity. Derived Mr values for the putative α-phaseolin shown in Table I differ only slightly: -142.1, -112.1 and -89 for clones 13, 39 and 169 compared with clone 6. Amino acid substitutions account for small differences in molecular weight, but the lack of repeats in the vicinity of positions 726 and 1348 result in a loss of nearly 1.6 kd from the putative β-type clones (31 and 72).

Despite extensive sequence conservation, it is evident from the data shown in Fig. 6 that variable regions are present. Some of the base substitutions observed are conservative and make no change in amino acid composition. Others give rise to amino acid replacements that would affect the charge on the polypeptide. Because the environment in which such substitutions occur will affect the overall result, it is difficult to precisely correlate charge changes with the two-dimensional peptide map. However, the substitution of His for Asn resulting from the A→C mutation at position 486 is likely to give a +1 charge difference for the peptide coded by clone 169 when compared with the other putative α-coding clones (6, 13, and 39). Such changes presumably represent the basis for charge heterogeneity in the phaseolin family of peptides.

EXPRESSION OF PHASEOLIN SEQUENCES

Toad (*Xenopus laevis*) oocytes have proven to be useful for investigating coupled transcription and translation of cloned DNA (McKnight and Gavis, 1980; Gurdon and Melton, 1981). Phaseolin mRNA injected into the oocyte cytoplasm is efficiently translated, and the products undergo glycosylation events that yield polypeptides which migrate to positions similar to those of native phaseolin on two-dimensional electrophoresis (Matthews, Brown and Hall, 1981). Preliminary experiments in which the entire λ177.4 clone was injected into the nucleus and oocytes were incubated in [^{3}H]leu resulted in the synthesis of material immunoprecipitable with phaseolin antibody that migrated to a position close to that of authentic β-phaseolin polypeptides (Fig. 7). A 3.8 kbp subclone (pPVPh 3.8, see Fig. 3) has recently been constructed and used for microinjection. Hybridization of ^{32}P-labeled oocyte poly(A) RNA from microinjected oocytes to different digests of phaseolin-containing clones indicated that transcription of the injected DNA occurred (Fig. 8).

Several recombinant plasmids composed of phaseolin sequences inserted into yeast vectors have been constructed and transformed into *Saccharomyces cerevisiae*. Although no positive data with regard to expression of the phaseolin gene have been obtained, we have determined that the clone λ177.4 contains at least one, possibly several sequences which have *ars* (autonomously replicating sequence) activity in yeast. Although yeast integrative plasmids

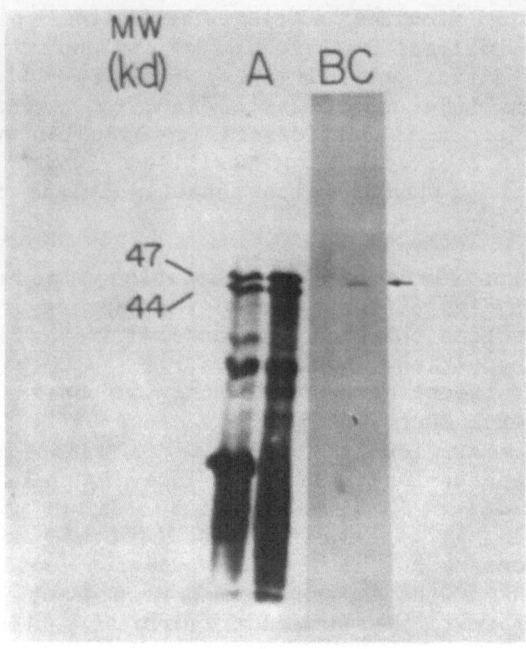

Fig. 7. Analysis of proteins by SDS-PAGE. Wheat germ translation
products of phaseolin mRNA (lane A) (Hall *et al*., 1978)
were separated along with proteins immunoprecipitated with
anti-phaseolin antibodies from oocytes injected with 20 ng
of Charon 24A DNA (lane B) or with 20 ng λ177.4 DNA (lane
C). The samples were all run on the same gel but required
different exposures during printing.

such as the vector YIp5 transform with low frequency, their
transformation efficiency increases by several orders of magnitude
when *ars* elements are incorporated (Struhl *et al*., 1979). When the
3.0 kbp *Eco* RI-*Bam* HI restriction fragment from λ177.4 was cloned
into YIp5, the transformation frequency of the resultant plasmid
increased by a factor of 10^3. We have localized the *ars* activity
in the bean DNA to a region of approximately 1100 bp adjacent to
the 3' end of the phaseolin gene. This segment contains several
sequences with a single base difference from an 11 bp consensus
sequence (5'$_T^A$TTTAT$_G^A$TTT$_T^A$3') found in seven different yeast *ars*
elements (Broach *et al*., 1982). Two of the consensus sequences in
bean DNA are only 11 bp apart and are included in an A+T-rich
region (79%) similar to that for the yeast sequences. Thus it
appears that plant DNA which serves as an *ars* in yeast has features
in common with yeast *ars* elements. A plant sequence capable of
autonomous replication linked to a selectable marker should be
valuable in plant transformation systems.

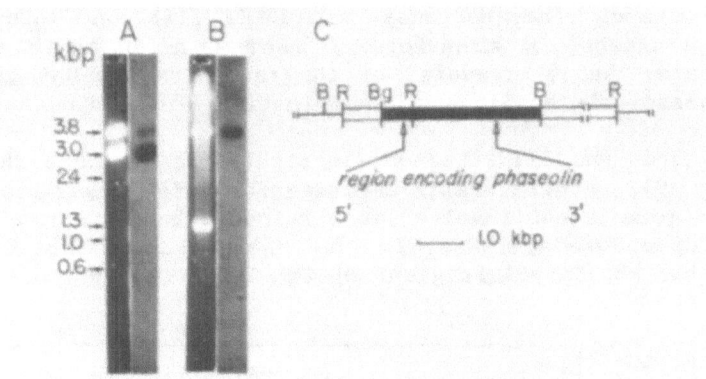

Fig. 8.   Hybridization of ^{32}P-labeled oocyte poly(A) RNA, isolated
from oocytes injected with pPVPh3.8, onto different
digests of phaseolin gene-containing clones.   Panel A,
left lane, *Bam* HI-*Eco* RI digest of pPVPh 3.0 stained with
ethidum bromide; right lane, autoradiogram of the same
digest showing strong hybridization to the 3.0 kbp *Eco* RI-
Bam HI band which contains the phaseolin gene.   Panel B,
left lane, ethidium bromide-stained *Bgl* II-*Bam* HI digest
of pPVPh8.8, right lane, autoradiogram showing strong
hybridization to the 3.8 kbp *Bgl* II-*Bam* HI band.   Panel C
shows the phaseolin gene region in pPVPh8.8 which
hybridized to oocyte poly(A) RNA (solid box).   Solid
lines, pBR322 vector DNA; open boxes, cloned genomic DNA
sequences flanking the phaseolin gene; arrows, the limits
of the phaseolin gene in pPVPh8.8 (Figures 3,4).

VECTOR TRANSFER

     Currently, the most advanced of all the available DNA transfer
systems for engineering plants is the Ti plasmid of *Agrobacterium
tumefaciens*.   A portion of the plasmid DNA, termed T-DNA (Chilton
et al., 1977) integrates into the plant nuclear genome (Yadav *et
al*., 1980).   Recently, plants have been regenerated from Ti-
transformed plant cells and the T-DNA found to be   retained and
active at least through the F$_1$ generation (Wullems *et al*., 1981).
Consequently, T-DNA is an appealing vehicle for the transfer and
stable integration of foreign DNA into plants.

     The use of T-DNA as a transfer vehicle involved: 1) cloning a
fragment of T-DNA in *E. coli* using the broad host range plasmid
pRK290 (Ditta *et al*., 1980); 2) inserting the phaseolin gene and

the neomycin phosphotransferase II (NPTII) gene into the cloned T-
DNA fragment; 3) transforming *A. tumefaciens* with the recombined
plasmid; and 4) transfer of the recombinant T-DNA fragment to the
Ti plasmid by homologous recombination (Ruvkun and Ausubel, 1981).

   The *Hind* III sites on the right side of the T-DNA of pTi-15955
(Fig. 9), were initially selected for foreign DNA insertion because
this area is not involved in virulence, but is actively transcribed
(Murai and Kemp, 1982a,b). The *Hind* III sites are centered within
the 5.3 kbp *Eco* RI fragment of the T-DNA (heavy lines in Fig. 9).

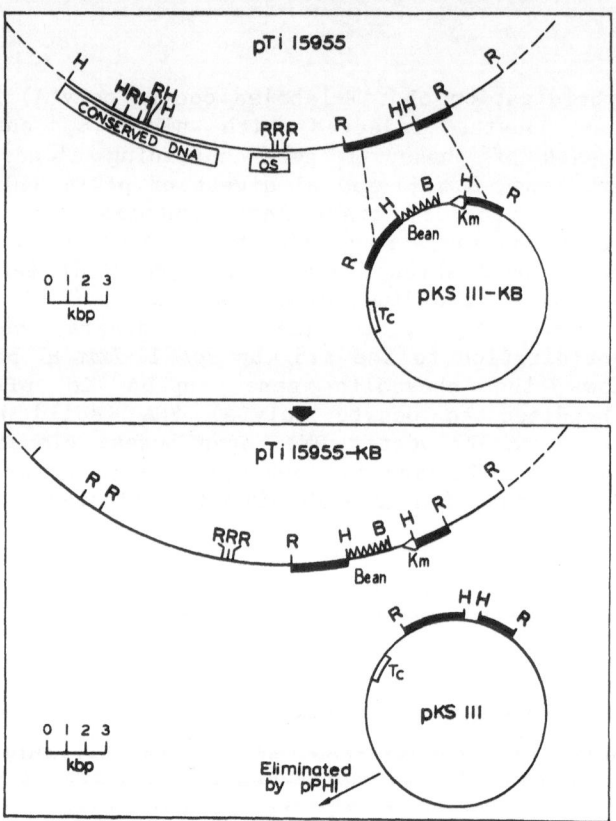

Fig. 9.   Selection of *A. tumefaciens* in which the Km and Bean DNA
          had recombined into pTi. The T-DNA of pTi-15955 is shown
          as a thin solid curved line. Conserved DNA is that
          portion of the T-DNA found in most Ti plasmids. OS is the
          position of the octopine synthase gene. The heavy line is
          that portion of the 5.3 kbp *Eco* RI fragment that is common
          between pTi and pKSIII-KB. Km is the portion of Tn5 DNA
          carrying the NPT-II gene and Bean is the *Eco* Ri-*Bam* HI
          fragment of the phaseolin gene.

This fragment was cloned into pRK290 and the new recombinant designated pKSIII (Fig. 9). The phaseolin gene was tailored to exclude
its promoter region and the first 12 amino acids of the coding
sequence (nucleotides 1-112, Figure 4). It did, however, contain
five introns, the translation termination signal, and the poly(A)
addition site. The insertion of the phaseolin gene and NPT II gene
into the *Hind* III site of pKSIII resulted in a "shuttle" vector
pKSIII-KB that was moved to *A. tumefaciens* by transformation (Kemp
et al., 1982).

Recombinant T-DNA was inserted into the resident Ti plasmid by
homologous recombination. This was accomplished by conjugation
with *E. coli* carrying a plasmid that is incompatible with pRK290
and selecting for the exclusion plasmid, as well as kanamycin
resistance (Ruvkun and Ausubel, 1981). Plasmid DNA was isolated
from one of the exconjugants (*A. tumefaciens* 15955-KB) to demonstrate that both genes had recombined into pTi-15955 by flanking T-

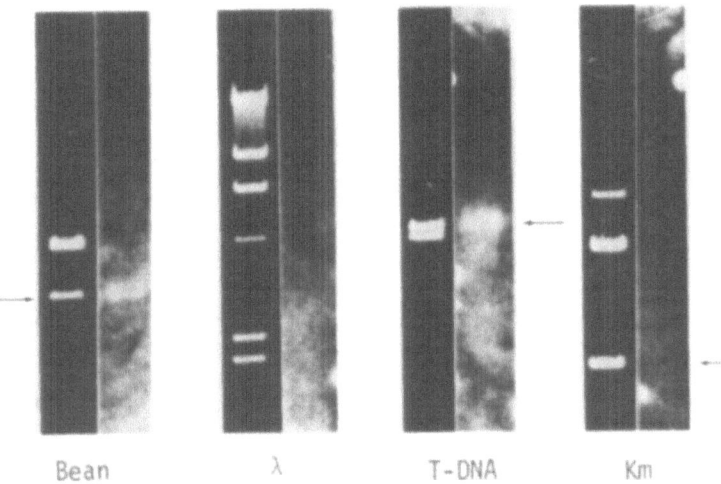

Bean   λ   T-DNA   Km

Fig. 10.   Hybridization of [^{32}P] RNA from PSCG-15955-KB tumor
            tissue with restriction fragments of various DNAs.   DNA
            was fractionated by agarose gel electrophoresis, trans-
            ferred to nitrocellulose filters and hybridized with [^{32}P]
            RNA isolated from *in vivo* labeled tissue. The left-hand
            lane of each pair is an ethidium bromide stain of the gel
            and the right-hand lane is the autoradiograph. DNA bound
            to filters is as follows: (Bean pBR322 clone of the 7.2
            kbp *Eco* RI fragment of the phaseolin DNA restricted with
            Eco RI-*Bam* HI, (λ) *Hind* III restriction of λ bacteriophage
            DNA, (T-DNA) pBR322 clone of the 5.3 kbp *Eco* RI, (Km)
            pBR322 clone of the neomycin phosphotransferase II gene
            from Tn5 restricted with *Bam* HI-*Hind* III.   Arrows
            indicate the position of DNA fragments known to be integ-
            rated into the DNA of PSCG-15955-KB.

DNA sequence homology (pTi-15955-KB is shown in Figure 9). Sunflower plants were infected with the exconjugant and the resulting
crown galls were established in tissue culture. The phaseolin gene
is stably integrated into the tissue culture DNA and no detectable
reorganization has occurred since its insertion one year ago.

The engineered tissue PSCG-15955-KB appears to be synthesizing
an RNA that has sequence homology to the phaseolin DNA (Figure 10),
but antibodies to phaseolin did not detect this protein in the
tissue. A possible reason that the phaseolin gene is only partly
expressed may be that the gene is transcribed as part of the active
T-DNA gene; but it was not translated because its reading frame did
not match that of the T-DNA gene.

Recently, similar procedures were used to insert the nopaline
synthase gene from pTi-C58 into the incompatible plasmid pTi-15955
(Kemp *et al.*, 1982). Normal levels of nopaline and nopaline
synthase activity were detected in sunflower tissues innoculated
with *A. tumefaciens* containing the engineered plasmid. Such
evidence supports the feasibility of full protein expression of
genes transferred by this means.

The sequence definition provided in Fig. 3 shows that the N-
terminus of phaseolin and of the promoter regions lie some 30-100
bp upstream of the *Eco* RI site used in the original 'sunbean' construction. Several clones using the KSIII shuttle vector that
contain the entire phaseolin coding region (from both genomic or
cDNA clones) together with either nopaline synthase promoter or
phaseolin promoter sequences have been constructed.

Acknowledgement. Data shown in Figs. 1,3,4,7,9 and 10 were
obtained in part through grants from NSF, U.S.D.A., and the Herman
Frasch Foundation to T. C. Hall and J. D. Kemp at the University of
Wisconsin. We thank Rod Klassy, Roger Drong and Michael Staver for
expert technical assistance and Barry Buchbinder for discussions.
J. A. Matthews address is: Dept. of Botany, Univ. of Leicester,
England.

REFERENCES

Broach, J. R., Li, Y. Y., Feldman, J., Abraham, J., Nasmyth, K.,
    and Hicks, J. B., 1982, Localization and sequence analysis of
    yeast origins of DNA replication, Cold Spring Harbor Symp.
    Quant. Biol: 47. In press.
Brown, J. W. S., Ma, Y., Bliss, F. A., and Hall, T. C., 1981a,
    Genetic variation in the subunits of globulin-1 storage
    protein of French bean, Theor. Appl. Genet., 59:83.
Brown, J. W. S., Bliss, F. A., and Hall, T. C., 1981b, Linkage
    relationship between genes controlling seed proteins in French
    bean, Theor. Appl. Genet., 60:251.

Brown, J. W. S., Ersland, D. R., and Hall, T. C., 1982, Molecular aspects of storage protein synthesis during seed development, in: "The Physiology and Biochemistry of Seed Development, Dormancy and Germination", A. A. Khan, ed., Elsevier Biomedical Press, Amsterdam. In press.

Chilton, M. D., Drummond, M. H., Merlo, D. J., Sciaky, D., 1978, Highly conserved DNA of Ti plasmids overlaps T-DNA maintained in plant tumours, Nature 275:147.

Ditta, G., Stanfield, S., Corbin, D. and Helinski, D. R., 1980, Broad host range DNA cloning system for gram-negative bacteria: construction of a gene bank of Rhizobium meliloti, Proc. Natl. Acad. Sci. USA 77:7347.

Efstradiatis, A., Posakony, J. W., Maniatis, T., Lawn, R. M., O'Connell, C., Spritz, R. A., DeRiel, J. K., Forget, B. G., Weissman, S. M., Slightom, J. L., Blechl, A. E., Smithies, O., Baralle, F. E., Shoulders, C. C., and Proudfoot, N. J., 1980, The structure and evolution of the human β-globin gene family, Cell 21:653.

Ersland, D. R., Brown, J. W. S., Casey, R., and Hall, T. C., 1983, The storage proteins of Phaseolus vulgaris L., Vicia Faba L., and Pisum sativum L., in: "The Genetics and Biochemistry of Seed Proteins", W. Gottschalk and H. P. Müller, eds., Martinus Nijhoff, The Hague. In press.

Geraghty, D., Peifer, M. A., Rubenstein, I., and Messing, J., 1981, The primary structure of a plant storage protein: zein. Nucl. Acids Res. 9:5163.

Gurdon, J. B., and Melton, D. A., 1981, Gene transfer in amphibian eggs and oocytes, Ann. Rev. Genet. 15:189.

Hall, T. C., Ma, Y., Buchbinder, B. V., Pyne, J. W., Sun, S. M., and Bliss, F. A., 1978, Messenger RNA for G1 protein of French bean seeds: Cell-free translation and product characterization, Proc. Natl. Acad. Sci. USA 75:3196.

Hall, T. C., Sun, S. M., Buchbinder, B. V., Pyne, J. W., Bliss, F. A., and Kemp, J. D., 1980, Bean seed globulin mRNA: Translation, characterization and its use as a probe towards genetic engineering of crop plants, in: "Genome Organization and Expression in Plants", C. J. Leaver, ed., Plenum Publishing Corp., New York. p. 259.

Hartley, J. L., Chen, K. K., and Donelson, J. E., 1982, A mercury-thiol affinity system for rapid generation of overlapping labeled DNA fragments for DNA sequencing, Nucl. Acids Res. 10:4009.

Karn, J., Brenner, S., Barnett, L., and Cesarini, G., 1980, Novel bacteriophage λ cloning vector, Proc. Natl. Acad. Sci. USA 77:5172.

Kemp, J. D., Sutton, D. W., Fink, C., Barker, R. F., and Hall, T. C., 1982, Agrobacterium-mediated transfer of foreign genes into plants, Beltsville Symposium VII, "Genetic Engineering: Applications to Agriculture".

Ma, Y., Bliss, F. A., and Hall, T. C., 1980, Peptide mapping

reveals considerable sequence homology among the three polypeptide subunits of Gl storage protein from French bean seed,
Plant Physiol. 66:897.

Matthews, J. A., Brown, J. W. S., and Hall, T. C., 1981, Phaseolin
mRNA is translated to yield glycosylated polypeptides in
Xenopus oocytes, Nature 294:175.

McKnight, S. L., and Gavis, E. R., 1980, Expression of the herpes
thymidine kinase gene in *Xenopus laevis* oocytes: An assay for
the study of deletion mutants constructed *in vitro*, Nucl.
Acids Res. 8:5931.

Moreira, M. A., Hermodson, M. A., Larkins, B. A., and Nielsen, N.
C., 1981, Comparison of the primary structure of the acidic
polypeptides of glycinin, Arch. Biochem. Biophys. 210:633.

Murai, N., and Kemp, J. D., 1982a, T-DNA of pTi-15955 from *Agrobacterium tumefaciens* is transcribed into a minimum of seven
polyadenylated RNAs in a sunflower crown gall tumor, Nucl.
Acids Res. 10:1679.

Murai, N., and Kemp, J. D., 1982b, Octopine synthase mRNA isolated
from sunflower crown gall callus is homologous to the Ti
plasmid of *Agrobacterium tumefaciens*, Proc. Natl. Acad. Sci.
USA 79:86.

Pedersen, K., Devereux, J., Wilson, D. R., Sheldon, E., and
Larkins, B. A., 1982, Cloning and sequence analysis reveal
structural variation among related zein genes in maize, Cell
29:1015.

Romero, J., Sun, S. M., McLeester, R. C., Bliss, F. A., and .Hall,
T. C., 1975, Heritable varition in a polypeptide subunit of
the major storage protein of the bean (*Phaseolus vulgaris L.*),
Plant Physiol. 56:776.

Ruvkun, G. B., and Ausubel, F. M., 1981, A general method for site-
directed mutagenesis in prokaryotes, Nature 289:85.

Sharon, N., and Lis, H., 1979, Comparative biochemistry of plant
glycoproteins, Biochem. Soc. Trans. 7:783.

Southern, E. M., 1975, Detection of specific sequences among DNA
fragments separated by gel electrophoresis, J. Mol. Biol.
98:503.

Struhl, K., Stinchcomb, D. T., Scherer, S., and Davis, R. W., 1979,
High frequency transformation of yeast: Autonomous replication of hybrid DNA molecules, Proc. Natl. Acad. Sci. USA
76:1035.

Sun, S. M., 1974, Ph.D. Thesis, University of Wisconsin.

Sun, S. M., Slightom, J. L., and Hall, T. C., 1981, Intervening
sequences in a plant gene: comparison of the partial sequence
of cDNA and genomic DNA of French bean phaseolin, Nature
289:37.

Wullems, G. J., Lucy, M., Ooms, G., and Schilperoort, R. A., 1981,
Retention of tumor markers in F_1 progeny plants from *in vitro*-
induced octopine and nopaline tumor tissues, Cell 24:719.

Yadav, N. S., Postle, K., Saiki, R. K., Thomashow, M. F., and
Chilton, M. D., 1980, T-DNA of a crown gall teratoma is covalently joined to host plant DNA, Nature 287:458.

IDENTIFICATION AND CHARACTERIZATION OF GENES FOR POLYPEPTIDES OF

THE THYLAKOID MEMBRANE

R. G. Herrmann[1], P. Westhoff[1], J. Alt[1], P. Winter[1],
J. Tittgen[1], C. Bisanz[1], B. B. Sears[1], N. Nelson[2],
E. Hurt[3], G. Hauska[3], A. Viebrock[4] and W. Sebald[4]

[1]Botanisches Institut der Universitat, Universitsstr.
1.4 Dusseldorf 1, F.R.G.
[2]Department of Biochemistry, Technion, Haifa, Israel
[3]Institut fur Botanik der Universitat, Universitsstr.
31, 84 Regensburg, F.R.G.
[4]Gesellschaft fur Biotechnologische Forschung
Marscheroder Weg 1, 53 Braunschweig, F.R.G.

I. INTRODUCTION

Biosynthesis of the chloroplast depends upon the cooperative expression of both nuclear and plastid genes. Characterization of the integrative mechanisms involved in this interaction will necessarily first require more basic information about the component genomes. Despite its moderate complexity, our knowledge about the informational content of the plastid chromosome is still quite limited: only the genes for two polypeptides and the genes for structural RNAs of the organelle's translation machinery have been identified and physically mapped, collectively covering approximately 10% of the chromosome's coding capacity (reviewed in Herrmann and Possingham 1980).

Thylakoid membranes catalyze light-induced charge separation, electron transport, proton uptake and ATP synthesis in photosynthesis. In higher plants this membrane is composed of roughly 40 major protein species ranging in M_r from 70 to less than 5 kd. Most of these polypeptides are organized into five discrete supramolecular complexes which are characteristically apportioned among appressed and non-appressed membrane regions: photosystem I and photosystem II reaction centres plus associated light-collecting systems, the cytochrome f/b6 complex, and the ATP synthase (Arntzen 1978, Nelson and Hauska 1979). The formation of thylakoids requires protein

143

synthesis in plastids and cytosol suggesting coordinated expression of plastid and nuclear genes (reviewed in Herrmann and Possingham 1980). Thylakoid biogenesis must also have the potential of
physiological adaptation of the membrane to different environments.
Moreover, developmental disturbances frequently observed in thylakoids of interspecific genome/plastome hybrids indicate that the
two genetic compartments have evolved a finely-tuned interplay (see
Herrmann et al. 1980a). Studies on the molecular biology of this
complex structure will, therefore, provide fundamental information
relating to plastome functions, various aspects of structure/func-
tion relationships, as well as the mechanisms involved in genome/
plastome interaction.

We report here on the bipartite organization of genes for polypeptides of the thylakoid membrane among plastome and genome, the
physical localization and transcript analysis of plastome-encoded
genes, as well as our initial cloning of nuclear components. These
investigations have relied upon our previous construction of physical maps of plastid chromosomes from several dicotelydons (*Spinacia
oleracea*, Crouse et al. 1978, Herrmann et al. 1980; five species
of *Oenothera*, Gordon et al. 1981, 1982; *Nicotiana tabacum*, Seyer
et al. 1981), the development of a sensitive procedure for hybrid
selection-mapping (Bünemann et al. 1982, Westhoff et al. 1981) combined with immunology and cell-free translation systems. Our data
provide evidence that the plastome is the principal determinant for
constituent thylakoid polypeptides. The identification of these
genes increases the known functions of the plastid chromosomes to
approximately 20% of its total coding capacity. Results of earlier
work can be found in a previous review dealing with the same topic
(Herrmann et al. 1980a).

II. CLONE BANKS FOR PLASTOMES OF SEVERAL DICOTYLEDONS

We have used cloned restriction fragments as a means for obtaining defined, pure segments of ptDNA in high yield. Overlapping
fragments produced by infrequently cutting enzymes (Sal I, Pst I,
Bam HI, Xho I) have been cloned in *E. coli* C 600 using primarily
the vectors pBR 322 and pWH 300 in shotgun experiments. In order
to increase for low-frequency clones carrying large inserts, and
to reduce the number of colonies to be screened, newly ligated DNA
was fractionated on and recovered from low-gelling-temperature
agarose gels prior to transformation. In particular cases limited
or partial digest fragments for transformation were purified by
electroelution from agarose gels. The three-step procedure employed to identify the cloned fragments has been outlined elsewhere
(Herrmann et al. 1980a). Recombinant DNA was designated by a let-
ter/number code (pWHsp) which specifies organism (*Spinacia*) and
compartment (plastid). The 100 series describes Pst I fragments,
the 200 series those obtained with Sal I, the 300 series with Xho I,

and the 400 series with Bam HI. Clones are numbered consecutively
in decreasing size of fragments.

Fig. 1 illustrates a collection of stably cloned fragments of
spinach ptDNA. Similar clone banks are available for DNA from the
Euoenothera plastomes I and V (not shown; restriction maps in Gordon et al. 1981, 1982). These libraries were utilized for subcloning experiments (Section III, Fig. 4), hybrid selection mapping,
DNA programmed cell-free translation (Fig. 4), nucleotide sequence
analysis and studies in interspecific plastome homology (Section V)
outlined in this paper.

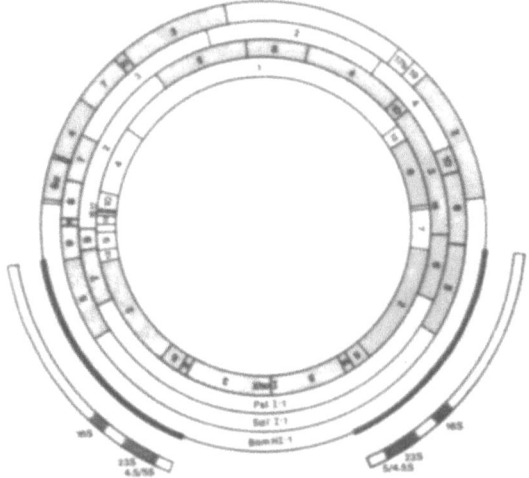

Fig. 1. A map of primary cloned fragments (hatched areas) spanning
the entire spinach plastid chromosome. All recognition sites for
the endonucleases Sal I, Pst I and Xho I are included. Locations
are shown for relevant Bam HI fragments (by courtesy of Dr. P.
Whitfeld) and rRNA genes. The extended parts indicate the inverted
repeat of the chromosome. The fragments are numbered in decreasing
size; for fragment molecular weights see Crouse et al. (1978) and
Herrmann et al. (1980b).

III. IDENTIFICATION AND LOCATION OF PLASTOME-CODED GENES

The identification of transcripts and genes for thylakoid
membrane polypeptides depended upon initial preparation of biochemically active membrane complexes, eliciting antisera against individual constituents of these complexes, and the use of these antisera to identify specific polypeptides among the products of DNA-
or RNA-programmed cell-free translation. The complexes were obtained by differential extraction of the plastid membranes with detergents, ion exchange chromatography and sucrose gradient centrifugation. Octylglucoside/cholate extraction releases the ATP synthase (Nelson et al. 1980, Westhoff et al. 1981) and cytochrome f/b6

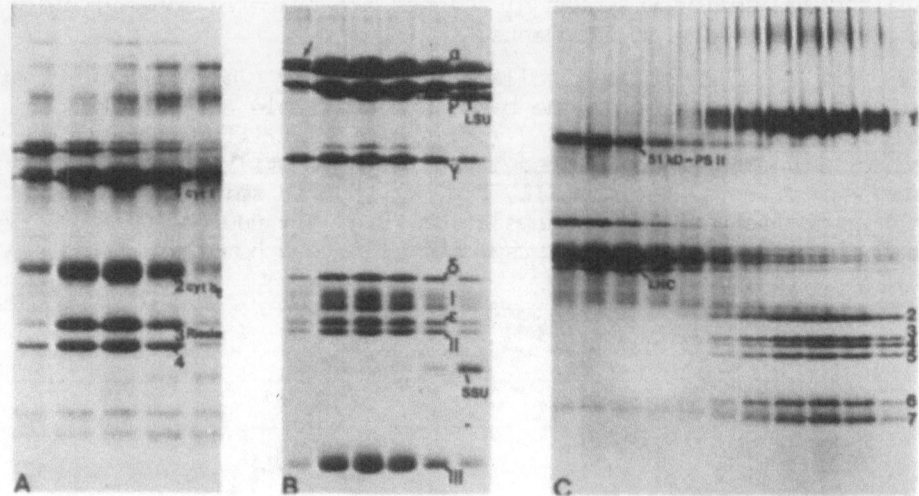

Fig. 2. Purification of thylakoid membrane complexes (spinach) by
zone centrifugation in sucrose gradients. The gravity field is
directed to the right. Individual gradient fractions were analyzed
for their polypeptide composition on SDS polyacrylamide gels and
visualized by Coomassie Blue staining. Panel A: cytochrome f/b6
complex (subunits 1-4); Panel B: ATP-Synthase complex, CF_1 subunits
$\alpha-\epsilon$; CF_O subunits I - III, subunit III: proteolipid ; Panel C:
photosystem I reactin center (subunits PS I 1-7) and light-harvesting chlorophyll a/b complex (LHC).

complex (Hurt and Hauska 1981). Subsequent Triton X-100 treatment
of the insoluble fraction solubilizes photosystem I reaction center (Bengis and Nelson 1975), light-harvesting chlorophyll a/b complex and photosystem II particles (Fig. 2).

    We have previously shown that both ptRNA and total cellular
poly A^+-RNA direct the synthesis in a rabbit reticulocyte ribosomal system of a complex mixture of polypeptides, and that ptRNA
and poly A^--RNA yield similar protein patterns in the in vitro
system (Herrmann et al. 1980a; Westhoff et al. 1981). Immunoprecipitation with antisera specific for individual membrane proteins has allowed identification of about 20 components studied to
date from either the poly A^+- or ptRNA (poly A^--RNA) translation
products. Those components derived from ptRNA represented prime
candidate genes located on the plastid chromosome. They are listed in Section VI. (For products directed by poly A^+-RNA see next
Section).

    The location of genes for these proteins was established u-
sing two complementary procedures. In the hybrid-selection system,
DNA fragments of known map positions (see Fig. 1) spanning the

entire circular ptDNA molecule were immobilized onto macro-
porous Sephacryl S-500 (Bünemann et al. 1982). Then total ptRNA,
poly A^-- or poly A^+-RNA was added under conditions which promote
hybridization, to select for complementary transcripts. After thermal dissociation these transcripts were translated in a rabbit reticulocyte lysate. The ^{35}-S-methionine labelled products were identified immunologically, by peptide mapping and by electrophoresis
in various one- and two-dimensional polyacrylamide gel systems for
comparison with the authentic membrane proteins. One of the first
results of this hybrid selection mapping was the identification of
genes for three CF_1 subunits alpha, beta and epsilon (Westhoff et
al. 1981). In each instance only one region in the chromosome selected a particular component. No poly A^+-transcripts for constituents of the thylakoid membrane were selected by any ptDNA fragment.

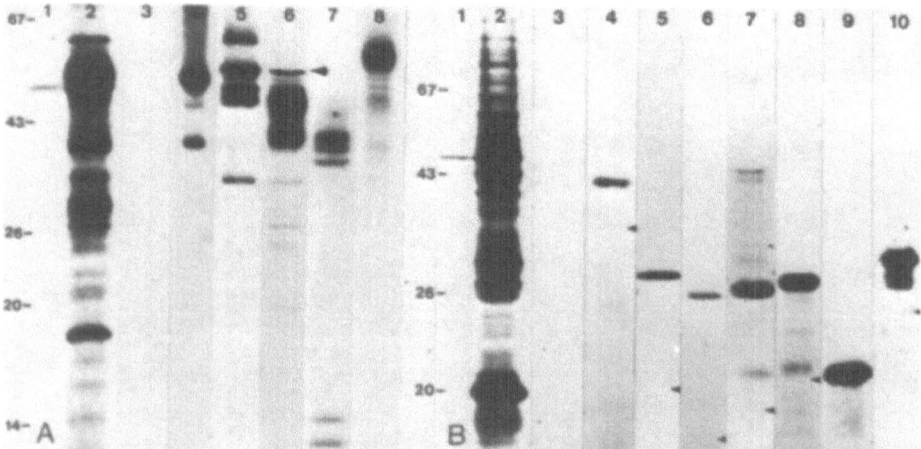

Fig. 3. Cell-free translation of ptRNA and poly A^+-RNA in rabbit
reticulocyte lysates. Fluorography of SDS/urea polyacrylamide gels.
RNA fractions from spinach seedlings illuminated for 14 h after illumination. Panel A: No message control (track 1), ptRNA pattern
(track 2), immunoprecipitates with non-immune serum (track 3),
antisera to LSU (track 4), α plus β (track 5), 51 kd and 44 kd
photosystem II polypeptides (tracks 6 and 7) and the photosystem
I reaction center apoprotein (track 8). Panel B: No message control (track 1), poly A^+-RNA pattern (track 2), tracks 3 - 10 immunoprecipitates with non-immune serum, anti-γ, anti-δ, CF_o-II,
anti-Rieske, anti-PS I/2, antiplstocyanin and anti-LHCP. The
positions of the respective authentic proteins are indicated by
arrow; the plastocyanin standard has migrated off the gel. The
low molecular weight antigenic determinants seen in some tracks
are premature termination products as indicated by Northern blot
and protein fingerprint analysis (cf. also Westhoff et al. 1981).
Arrow in Panel A, track 6: contaminating ATP synthase β-subunit.

The second technique involved DNA-programmed coupled transcription-translation in cell-free lysates derived from *E. coli* (Zubay et al. 1970), as an alternative to hybrid-selection mapping. Such a DNA-directed system has two major advantages. It can refine positions of structural genes (transcript sizes in hybrid-selection!). Moreover, expression of partial gene sequences in which promotors are retained provides information on transcription polarity. The experimental design involved subcloning secondary fragments from

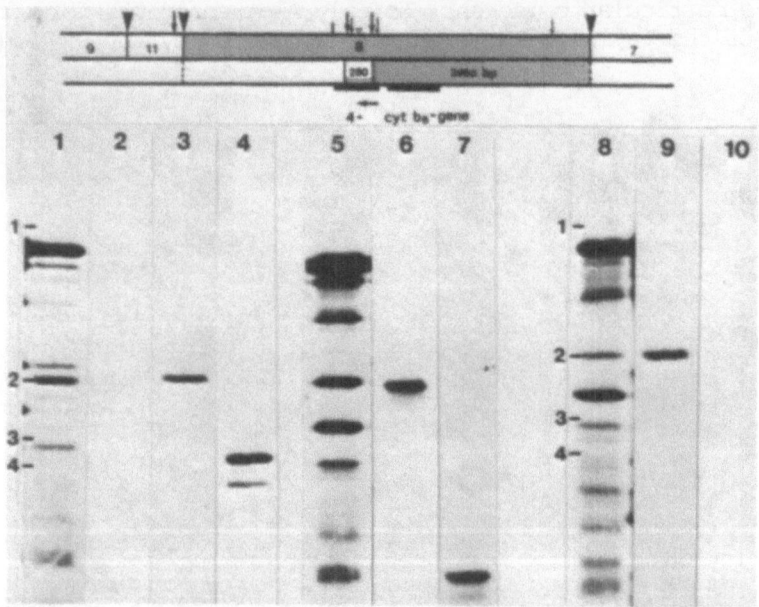

Fig. 4. Fine structure maps of the region of spinach ptDNA bearing the genes for cytochrome b6 and polypeptide 4 of the cytochrome complex (Panel A): Hatched areas indicate cloned sequences (Sal I; Bam HI). Their use in DNA-programmed cell-free translation determined the relative positions of genes for both proteins and the direction of transcription for polypeptide 4. (Panel B): Left: Translation patterns of the cloned DNA fragments (tracks 1, 5, 8). Precipitation with non-immun serum (track 2), with anti-cytochrome b6 (tracks 3, 6, 9) and anti-polypeptide 4 (tracks 4, 7, 10). Note that all clones direct the synthesis of cytochrome b6. Complete polypeptide 4 is precipitated from the products of pWHsp 208 DNA (track 4) and a short polypeptide from the added 1950 + 280 bp DNA clone (track 7). The protein is missing from the 2950 bp clone (track 9-10). Fluorograph of a SDS polyacrylamide gel; 1-4: subunits of the cytochrome f/b6 complex.

limited or partial digests of primary fragment clones (Section II) with restriction enzymes that possess cleavage sites in or near structural genes. Thus the ability of the derivative clones to direct the synthesis of full-length or truncated proteins could be analysed by immunoprecipitation, and compared with the polypeptides derived from the original primary fragment. Expression of fragments cloned in both orientations relative to the plasmid vector was evaluated, to exclude the possibility of read-through from vector sequences. Fig. 4 illustrates an example for these approaches.

IV. TRANSCRIPTS AND CLONING FOR POLYPEPTIDES OF NUCLEAR ORIGIN

The translation products of poly A^+-RNA contained components which are immunologically related to several thylakoid membrane polypeptides (authentic protein/pre-sequence kd): the gamma (37/ 8 kd) and delta (19.5/8 kd) subunits of CF_1 (Westhoff et al. 1981), polypeptide CF_0-II (16/7 kd) of the ATP synthase, the Rieske Fe/S protein (18/7 kd) of the cytochrome complex, the polypeptide PS I/ 2 (22/4 kd), constituent polypeptides of the chlorophyll a/b light harvesting complex (25/4 kd; Apel and Kloppstech 1978) and plastocyanin (10/11 kd; Grossman et al. 1982). All these polypeptides were synthesized in vitro as precursors with pre-sequences differing considerably in size (Fig. 3). These polypeptides can be imported by unbroken chloroplasts (Bartlett and Westhoff, unpublished) indicating that they are accurately translated by wheat germ extracts and that their excess sequences function in postranslational transport (Chua and Schmidt 1979) of polypeptides from the cytosol, their site of synthesis, into the organelle.

In order to gain information about these genes, we have constructed a cDNA library from polyadenylated RNA isolated from spinach seedlings at a mid-greening stage. The RNA was first size-fractionated on sucrose gradients and then converted into double-stranded DNA copies by AMV reverse transcriptase and terminal deoxynucleotidyl transferase 3'-end homopolymer tailing (dCTP, Land et al. 1981). The selfpriming step followed by S1 nuclease digestion was omitted, because it leads to losses of the 5'-terminal mRNA sequence. The double-stranded cDNA was inserted into the G-tailed Pst I site of pBR 322 by G-C annealing and the resulting recombinant DNA molecules were used to transform competent *E. coli* C 600 cells. Tetracycline resistant transformants were screened by insert excision and by their ability to select mRNA species for specific proteins.

To date, cDNA clones for the small subunit of ribulose bisphosphate carboxylase/oxygenase and for three thylakoid proteins, plastocyanine, the 23 kd polypeptide of photosystem I and the constituent polypeptide for the chlorophyll a/b light harvesting complex have been isolated. The insert sizes ranged from 200 to 1600 bp.

V. COMPARATIVE GENE MAPPING

The plastid chromosomes of spinach, tobacco and *Euoenothera* species share remarkable structural similarity in that they are organized into an inverted repeat interspersed by two unique-sequence segments of different size (Herrmann et al. 1980a). The restriction maps for these chromosomes are drawn to scale in Fig. 5. Their alignment with the aid of a 0.6 kbp (0.45 Md) Sal I primary fragment (Herrmann et al. 1980a, Seyer et al. 1981) has now been established by hybridization experiments that demonstrate the sequence homology of this fragment (and others) at corresponding map positions. To locate the positions of genes in heterologous DNA, we

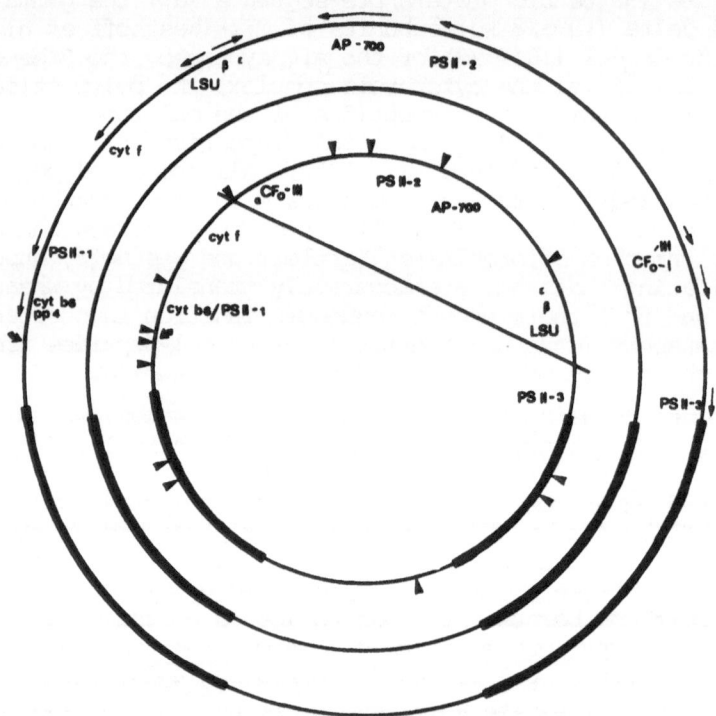

Fig. 5. The positions of genes for thylakoid membrane polypeptides on plastid chromosomes of spinach (outer circle), tobacco (central circle) and *Oenothera* sp. (inner circle). The maps were matched by putting the 0.45 Md Sal I primary fragment left (thick arrow, see text). The bold black line represents the duplicated segments; arrow heads: Sal I cuts. Transcription polarities are indicated by parallel arrows; that of CF$_O$-III (proteo-lipid gene) is tentative. The straight line is the *Oenothera* chromosome designates the inversion.

used cloned spinach probes that contained exclusively structural gene sequences. Cross-reaction of the spinach antisera with corresponding thylakoid proteins from *Oenothera* and tobacco indicated that these genes possess phylogenetically conserved sequences. We have determined the positions of genes on the plastid chromosomes of these other plants by hybridization of nick translated spinach probes to Southern blots of restricted heterologous ptDNAs; specific hybridization was obtained in each instance. Fig. 5 compares the position of genes in these three chromosomes.

VI. CONCLUSIONS

There are several points of interest in this early stage of gene mapping for thylakoid membrane polypeptides: 1) The thylakoid membrane complexes are of dual genetic origin, with the plastome being a principal genetic determinent for polypeptide components. This is in striking contrast to the situation in mitochondria. Of 20 components studied to date, structural genes for 12 are encoded in the plastome, and these include almost all "reaction center" proteins (Fig. 5). 2) Each plastome-coded gene exists as a single copy per chromosome. The structural DNA sequences are uninterrupted with the possible exception of CF_O-1. 3) All genes are located in the large single-copy segment of the plastid chromosome. There is no obvious economy of gene arrangement or organization. Even the genes for polypeptides of a discrete complex are not organized into a typical operon structure, but are scattered over the entire single-copy segment (Fig. 5). 4) Both complementary strands code for genes (Fig. 5). Genes (Krebbers et al. 1982) and transcripts can overlap. 5) In contrast to nuclear-derived thylakoid components, transcripts for plastome-coded components are exclusively found in poly A^--RNA. The latter polypeptides are apparently translated to the correct size. Exceptions are the 32 kd protein (Grebanier et al. 1978) and cytochrome f, which is synthesized as a precursor of substantially greater size (approximately 30 amino acids) irrespective of the cell-free system used. 6) The transcript sizes, determined by hybrid-selection and Northern blotting range from 500 (CF_O-III) to 7000 (P 700 apoprotein) nucleotides. Untranslated regions can vary exceedingly, from ca. 250 (CF_O-III) through ca. 500 (PS II-1; ß) to more then 1000 bp (PS II-2; PS I-1). 7) Transcription can be polycistronic even for overlapping genes (e.g. β, ε, Krebbers et al. 1982). There is no firm evidence that such transcripts are processed, although plastids are known to possess enzymatic equipments for RNA modification (Herrmann et al. 1980a). 8) Overall gene order and relative distance of the genes probed are the same for the tobacco and spinach chromosomes within the accuracy of the maps (Fig. 5) and this will probably apply with minor adjustments to a number of ptDNAs (Palmer and Stein 1982). However, a 44.7 kbp inversion within the large single-copy segment of the *Oenothera* chromosomes shows that phylogenetic divergence of plastomes

can involve major rearrangements of gene order in addition to dele-
tion/insertion (Herrmann et al. 1980a, see also Palmer and Stein
1982). It is probably not mere coincidence that this inversion is
boardered by regions where deletions and insertions have occurred
(Gordon et al. 1982). 9) Deletion/insertion can occur in structural genes. Analysis of thylakoid polypeptides from _Euoenothera_
wildspecies and their interspecific genome/plastome hybrids has uncovered allelic forms of proteins with nuclear and plastid inheritance (Herrmann et al. 1980a). Fine mapping and translation of appropriate cloned DNA segments suggest that the difference seen in
the PS II-1 polypeptide between plastomes I and V has been caused
by a single deletion/insertion event in the gene rather than by secondary modification of the transcript or protein.

        In summary, our data suggest that the functional organiza-
tion of plastid chromosomes as well as genetic fluxes in higher
plant cells must be highly complex. Their use should aid in understanding the control of gene expression in and between compartments
with respect to subunit stoichiometry of thylakoid membrane complexes, developmental differences in membrane composition, and the coordinated expression of genes with highly different cellular copy
numbers in plastids and nucleus (Herrmann and Possingham 1980).

ACKNOWLEDGEMENTS

        The skillful technical assistance of Ms. Monika Streubel,
Ms. Barbara Schiller and Ms. Gabriele Schewe is gratefully acknow-
ledged. This work was supported by the DFG (He 693) and the
Stiftung Volkswagen.

VII. REFERENCES

Apel, K. and Kloppstech, K. (1978) Eur. J. Biochem. 85, 581-588
Arntzen, C.J. (1978) Curr. Topics in Bioenerget. 8, 111-160
Bengis, C. and Nelson, N. (1975) J. Biol. Chem. 250, 2783-2788
Bünemann, H., Westhoff, P. and Herrmann, R.G. (1982) Nucl. Acids
        Res., in press
Chua, N.-H. and Schmidt, G.W. (1979) J. Cell Biol. 81, 461-483
Crouse, E.J., Schmitt, J.M., Bohnert, H.J., Gordon, K., Driesel, A.
        J. and Herrmann, R.G. (1978) in: "Chloroplast Development"
        G. Akoyunoglou, J.H. Argyroudi-Akoyunoglou, eds., Elsevier/
        North Holl., pp. 565-572
Gordon, K.H.J., Crouse, E.J., Bohnert, H.J. and Herrmann, R.G.
        (1981) Theor. Appl. Genet. 59, 281-296
Gordon, K.H.J., Crouse, E.J., Bohnert, H.J. and Herrmann, R.G.
        (1982) Theor. Appl. Genet. 61, 373-384
Grebanier, A.E., Coen, D.M., Rich, A. and Bogorad, L. (1978) J. Cell
        Biol. 78, 734-746
Grossman, A.R., Bartlett, S.G. Schmidt, G.W., Mullet, J.E. and Chua
        N.-H. (1982) J. Biol. Chem. 257, 1558-1563

Herrmann, R.G., Seyer, P., Schedel, R., Gordon, K., Bisanz, C., Winter, P., Hildebrandt, J.W., Wlaschek, M., Alt, J. Driesel, A.J. and Sears, B.B. (1980a) in: "Biological Chemistry of Organelle Formation", Th. Bücher, W. Sebald, H. Weiss, eds., Springer Berlin-Heidelberg-New York, pp. 97-112

Herrmann, R.G., Whitfeld, P.R. and Bottomley, W. (1980b) Gene 8, 179-191

Herrmann, R.G. and Possingham, J.V. (1980) in "Results and Problems in Cell Differentiation", J. Reinert, ed., vol. 10, Springer Berlin-Heidelberg-New York, pp. 45-96

Hurt, E. and Hauska, G. (1981) Eur. J. Biochem. 117, 591-599

Krebbers, E.T., Larrinua, I.M., McIntosh, L. and Bogorad, L. (1982) Nucl. Acids Res. 10, 4985-5001

Land, H., Grez, M., Hauser, H., Lindenmaier, W. and Schütz, G. (1981) Nucl. Acids Res. 9, 2251-2266

Nelson, N. and Hauska, G. (1979) in "Membrane Bioenergetics", C.P. Lee, G. Schatz, L. Ernster, eds., Addison-Wesley Publ. Comp., London-Amsterdam-Don Mills-Sidney-Tokyo, pp. 189-202

Nelson, N., Nelson, H. and Schatz, G. (1980) Proc. Natl. Acad. Sci. USA 77, 1361-1364

Palmer, J.D. and Stein, D.B. (1982) Curr. Genet. 5, 165-170

Seyer, P., Kowallik, K.V. and Herrmann, R.G. (1981) Curr. Genet. 3, 189-204

Westhoff, P., Nelson, N., Bünemann, H. and Herrmann, R.G. (1981) Curr. Genet. 4, 109-120

Zubay, G., Chambers, D.A. and Cheong, L.C. (1970) in "The Lactose Operon", J.R. Beckwith, D.Z. Zipser, eds., Cold Spring Harbor Lab. Press, New York, pp. 375-392

ORGANIZATION AND EXPRESSION OF THE CHLOROPLAST

GENOME OF *Euglena gracilis*

Richard B. Hallick, Bruce M. Greenberg, Wilhelm Gruissem,
Margaret J. Hollingsworth, Gerald D. Karabin, Jonathon O.
Narita, Jac A. Nickoloff, Charles W. Passavant, and Gary
L. Stiegler

University of Colorado
Boulder, Colorado 80309 U.S.A.

INTRODUCTION

We have been involved in a characterization of the chloroplast
(ct) genes of the unicellular photosynthetic eucaryote *Euglena
gracilis*. Previous work from several different laboratories on physical mapping and cloning of this DNA, and on the characterization of
the ribosomal RNA (rRNA) operons has been recently reviewed.[1] In the
present article we describe our recent studies on the organization and
expression of transfer RNA (tRNA) genes. Nucleotide sequence data is
now available for 18 different species. We also describe a new
Euglena chloroplast extract that catalyzes DNA-dependent, selective *in
vitro* transcription of *Euglena* ct tRNA genes.

The second part of this article concerns the identification of ct
protein coding loci for the α and β subunits of the CF_1 coupling factor, a 32 kd thylakoid membrane polypeptide (32 kd), and protein
synthesis elongation factor Tu (EF-Tu). The mRNA transcripts of these
genes, and of the large subunit of ribulose-1,5-bisphosphate carboxylase (LS) were further analyzed in cells at various stages of light
induced chloroplast development.

ORGANIZATION OF *Euglena* CT tRNA GENES

Our work on ct tRNA genes has involved identification of tRNA
coding loci via Southern[2] hybridization experiments, purification of
genes as recombinant plasmid DNAs, and DNA sequence analysis. A long
range goal has been the characterization at the DNA sequence level of

155

the complete set of ct tRNA genes. At present, we do not know how many different tRNAs are necessary for ct protein synthesis. The identification of tRNA coding loci has been reviewed.[1,2,4,5] As shown in Figure 1, these loci are scattered around the ct genome.

The DNA sequence for four of these loci have now been determined. In each case, multiple, clustered tRNA genes have been found. The gene organization for the known tRNA loci is as follows: (1) Thrice repeated tRNA^{Ile}-tRNA^{Ala} of the rRNA operons[6,7] in *Eco* P; (2) tRNA^{Val}-tRNA^{Asn}-tRNA^{Arg}-tRNA^{Leu} of *Eco* G;[8] (3) tRNA^{Tyr}-tRNA^{His}-tRNA^{Met}-tRNA^{Trp}-tRNA^{Glu}-tRNA^{Gly} of *Eco* V-H;[9] and (4) tRNA^{Thr}-tRNA^{Gly}-tRNA$_I^{Met}$, tRNA^{Gln}-tRNA^{Ser} of *Eco* Q.[10] Of the seventeen genes described to date, all have the same polarity as the rRNA genes except tRNA^{Leu} of *Eco* G, the tRNA^{Thr}-tRNA^{Gly}-tRNA^{Met} cluster of *Eco* Q, and tRNA^{Phe} of *Eco* A.

The tRNA^{Phe} coding locus, although not sequenced, was mapped using chemically synthesized tetradecanucleotide probes complementary

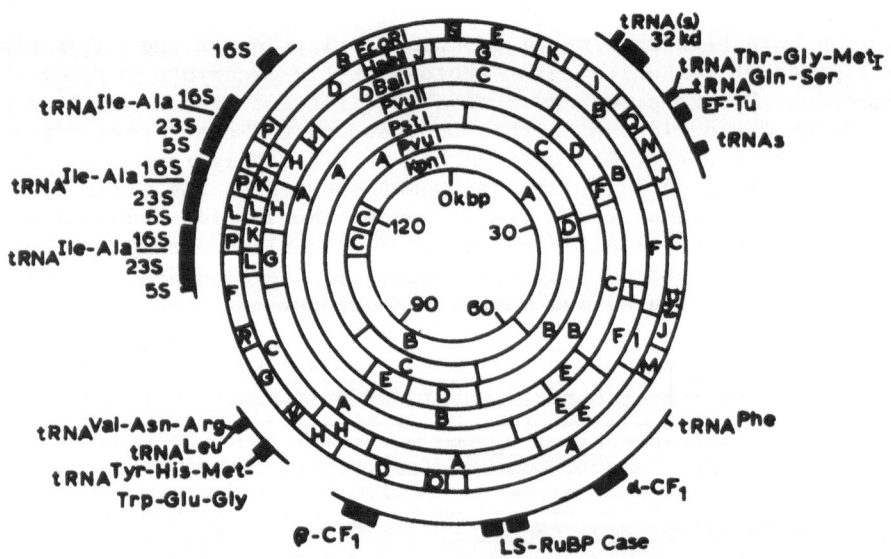

Fig. 1.   Restriction endonuclease cleavage map for the 145 kbp *Euglena gracilis* Z ct genome. The restriction mapping data have been reviewed.[1] In addition to the nine tRNA loci which have been precisely mapped, there is at least one additional locus within *Eco* A.[4,5] There may also be additional tRNA genes at the tRNA^{Phe} locus (see text). The identification of protein coding loci is described in the text.

to either the DHU- of TψC- stem and loop of the tRNA, which had been
sequenced previously.[11] These oligonucleotides are 5'-d(CTACCAACTGA-
GCT) and 5'-d(AGATTTGAACTGGT), respectively. Using ^{32}P-labeled synthetic oligonucleotides as probes, the single tRNA[Phe] locus was mapped
to a 2.5 kilobase pair (kbp) HindIII fragment within Eco A (Fig. 1).
This fragment was isolated as a recombinant plasmid. The tRNA[Phe] gene
locus and polarity (same as tRNA[Leu]) were defined precisely with
respect to a unique Dde I cleavage site internal to the gene, and also
to one of the probes. A similar locus was described by El Gewely et
al.[16] Several different synthetic DNAs have been used for fine mapping other tRNA genes.[9,10,12] This is a novel method of tRNA gene
mapping that is widely applicable to other genomes.

Based on the available data, it is possible to make some gener-
alizations about Euglena ct tRNA genes. First, the genes are tightly
clustered at coding loci, and are separated by short AT-rich spacers.
For example, the genes in Eco Q (Fig. 1) have the organization tRNA[Gln]
-14 bp-tRNA[Ser]-174 bp-tRNA[Met]-12 bp-tRNA[Gly]-5 bp-tRNA[Thr]. Such clustering is consistent with the model that some genes are initially
transcribed into multicistronic precursors. Second, none of the
known genes are interrupted by intervening sequences, nor is the
3'-CCA terminus DNA coded. Third, the normally expected[13] invariant
and semi-invariant bases, and tRNA secondary structure are generally
found. Fourth, the nucleotide sequence homology of Euglena ct tRNAs
is highest with homologous tRNAs from higher plant chloroplasts
(average 76%, n = 14) and E. coli (70%, n = 17). The homology with
cytoplasmic or mitochondrial tRNAs is much lower.[10]

SELECTIVE in vitro TRANSCRIPTION OF CHLOROPLAST tRNA GENES

We have previously described the isolation of a nucleoprotein
complex from Euglena chloroplasts active in selective in vitro rRNA
transcription.[14] The DNA-dependent RNA polymerase responsible for
rRNA synthesis remains tightly DNA-template bound in chloroplast
lysates. By contrast, a crude extract from isolated, intact chloroplasts has been obtained that gives mature chloroplast tRNAs as in
vitro transcription products when appropriate DNA templates are used.
The methods used to prepare an extract from isolated, intact chloroplasts, to carry out in vitro DNA-dependent RNA transcription, and to
characterize tRNA products are essentially the same as previously
described for transcription of ct tRNA genes by a HeLa cell extract.[15]

An illustration of the products of transcription, separated by
electrophoresis through a polyacrylamide gel is shown in Fig. 2. Five
different plasmid DNA templates were used to direct in vitro tRNA synthesis. Three contain previously sequenced tRNA gene clusters. With
reference to Fig. 1, they are from Eco G, Eco V-H, and Eco Q. Two
other plasmid DNA templates contained known tRNA coding loci from Eco
J' and Eco I, respectively, which have not been sequenced.

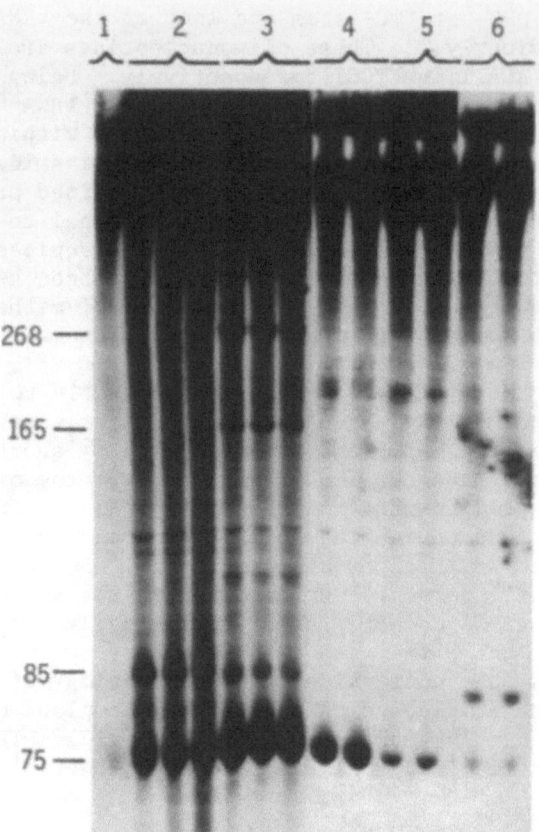

Fig. 2.   Acrylamide gel electrophoresis of *in vitro* transcription
products of chloroplast tRNA genes. For methods, see Gruissem et al.[15] The DNA templates were as follows: Lane 1, no
exogenous DNA. Lane 2, pPG14,[8] a recombinant between *Eco* G
and pMB9. Lane 3, pPG76,[9] a recombinant between *Bam-Sal* 9
containing the *Eco* V-H tRNA locus and pBR322. Lane 4, pPG689,
a recombinant between *Eco* J' and pMB9. Lane 5, pEZC514, a
recombinant between *Eco* I and pBR322. RNA size estimates in
nt, based on the mobility of RNA standards are shown to the
left of the figure.

In each case there are one or two prominent RNA products of the
size of tRNAs with either a short or long variable arm when tRNA genes
are used as templates. No tRNA sized products are obtained in the
absence of plasmid DNA, nor when the following genes (data not shown)
were present on plasmid DNA templates: (1) 16 S rRNA-tRNA^{Ile}-tRNA^{Ala}
of *Euglena* ct DNA *Eco* P (Fig. 1). (2) 23 S rRNA-5 S rRNA of *Eco* F
(Fig. 1). (3) *E. coli* tRNA^{Asp}-tRNA^{Trp}. (4) *Drosophila* tRNA^{Arg}.

Several lines of evidence are consistent with the conclusion that the tRNA sized products (Fig. 2) are tRNAs transcribed *in vitro* in the chloroplast extract. A summary of this work is as follows: (1) The gel purified pPG76 and pPG14 tRNA-sized transcripts hybridized only to restriction fragments from tRNA coding loci when Southern hybridization experiments were employed. (2) When plasmid DNA templates were treated with restriction enzymes prior to transcription, synthesis of tRNA-sized products was abolished when internal sites in tRNA genes were involved, i.e. a *Pvu* I cut in tRNA^{Asn} of pPG14 or an *Ava* I in tRNA^{Tyr} of pPG76. There was no effect when DNA was cleaved outside of the tRNA transcription units. (3) The pPG76 transcripts in the 75 nt fraction could be resolved into at least four discrete RNAs by 2D gel electrophoresis. There are five tRNA genes in this size category coded in pPG76 DNA. (4) The preliminary RNAse T$_1$ fingerprint of the 75 nt RNAs from pPG14 was as expected for a tRNA^{Val}, tRNA^{Asn}, tRNA^{Arg} mixture.[15]

It has been possible to extend this work to higher plant chloroplasts. A soluble extract was prepared from chloroplasts of *Spinacia oleracea*. The extract was active in the synthesis of tRNA-sized transcripts with either cloned *Euglena* or spinach chloroplast tRNA genes as DNA templates.

LOCATION OF *Euglena* CHLOROPLAST PROTEIN GENES

With ^{32}P-labeled DNA restriction fragments from known chloroplast genes as hybridization probes, several *Euglena* ct protein coding loci have been identified via heterologous Southern hybridization experiments. The methods and strategy for these studies have previously been described for mapping of the RuBP carboxylase LS gene.[17] The work has been extended with the following additional gene probes: (1) A 1.1 kbp *Pst* I-*Sal* I fragment containing 804 bp of the spinach ct 32 kd gene.[18,19] (2) A 2.4 kbp spinach ct DNA *Sal* I fragment coding for the α-subunit of CF$_1$-ATPase.[20] (3) A 1.6 kbp *Eco* RI-*Kpn* I fragment from the spinach ct β-subunit gene for CF$_1$-ATPase.[19,20] (4) A 1.2 kbp *Eco* RI fragment of *Chlamydomonas* ct DNA containing the 3'-end of the EF-Tu gene.[21] (5) A 621 bp *Hha* I fragment internal to the EF-Tu gene of *E. coli*.[22,28]

For each gene probe, the locus of hybridization to *Euglena* ct DNA was determined with several different sets of restriction enzyme digestion products. In each case except the α-gene hybridization, the locus was confirmed by hybridization to cloned ct DNAs. An example of the data for the 32 kd gene probe is shown in Fig. 3. Hybridization is shown with the 5.1 kbp *Eco* I (lane A), the 3.2 kbp *Hind*10 which is internal to *Eco* I (lane B), and to the 1.7 kbp *Pvu* II-*Hind*III and 1.1 kbp *Hind*III restriction fragments of the plasmid pEZC514, a recombinant DNA between *Eco* I and pBR322 (lane C).

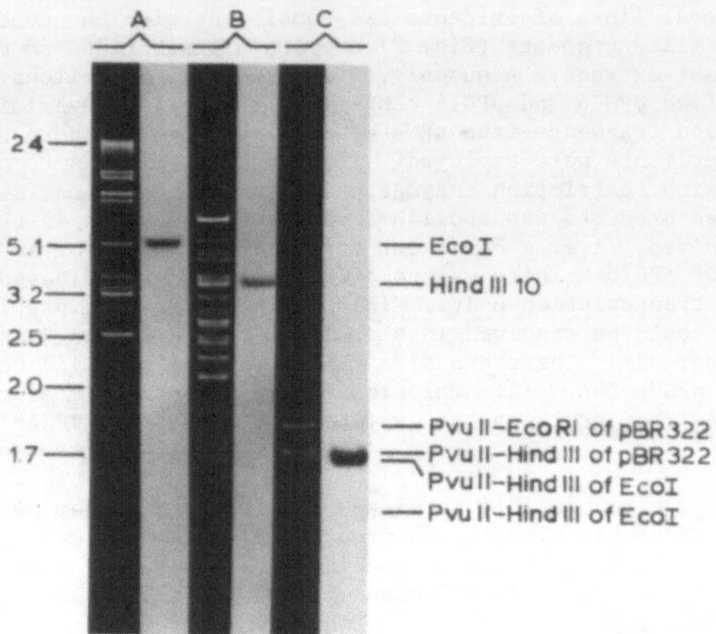

Fig. 3.   Hybridization of ^{32}P-labeled 32 kd gene probe to *Euglena* ct
          DNA.   Shown are gel photos (left) and autoradiograms (right)
          for the following DNA samples: A.   *Eco* RI digested *Euglena*
          ct DNA.   B.   *Hind*III digested *Euglena* ct DNA.   C.   *Pvu* II-
          *Hind*III-*Eco* RI digested plasmid pEZC514 DNA.   DNA fragment
          size in kbp is shown to the left of the figure.   Digestion
          products are also identified.

        A summary of the protein coding loci for all gene probes is
shown in Fig. 1.   The α- and β- subunit genes of CF$_1$-ATPase are in *Eco*
A and *Eco* D respectively, the 32 kd gene is in *Eco* I, and EF-Tu is
coded in *Eco* N.   For each protein gene, the locus within these fragments with respect to various restriction sites is as illustrated.

CHLOROPLAST GENE TRANSCRIPTION DURING LIGHT INDUCED CHLOROPLAST
DEVELOPMENT

        The RNA transcripts of several ct protein genes have been ana-
lyzed by the membrane filter (Northern) blot hybridization method.
RNA was isolated from dark-adapted *Euglena*, and from cells following
12, 24, 36, 48, 60 and 72 hr of light induced ct development.[23]   RNA
samples were fractionated by electrophoresis in formaldehyde-agarose

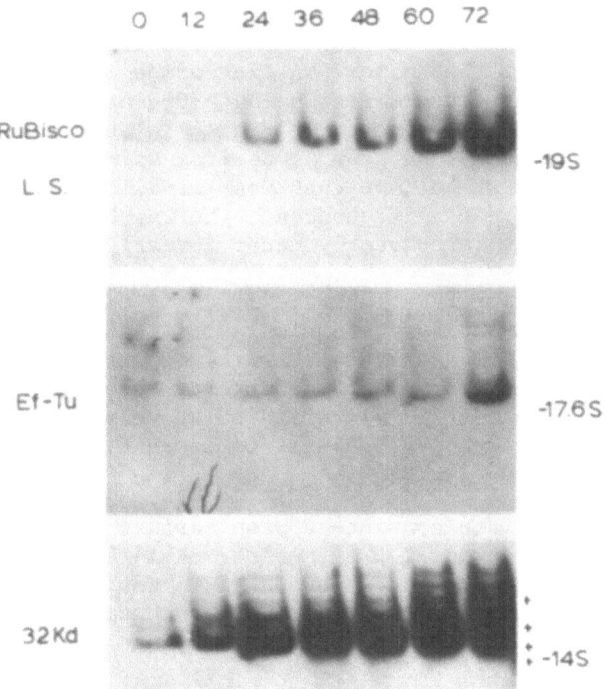

Fig. 4.   Autoradiograms following membrane filter hybridization of
[32]P-labeled DNAs and *Euglena* RNA separated by gel electrophoresis.   RNA was isolated from dark grown cells following
0-72 hr of exposure to light[23] as indicated.   Individual
filters were hybridized with the following ^{32}P-labeled DNAs:
Top, pEZC738 DNA,[17] containing part of the RuBP carboxylase
LS gene.   Middle, gel purified *Eco* N, containing the EF-Tu
gene.   Bottom, pEZC25 DNA, a recombinant between *Hind*10,
which codes for the 32 kd gene, and pBR322.

gels,[24] and transferred to nitrocellulose membrane filters.[25]   Filters
were incubated under hybridization conditions with ^{32}P-labeled
restriction fragments from recombinant plasmids containing the *Euglena*
ct protein genes described above.   Some of the results are shown in
Fig. 4.

The ^{32}P-labeled LS probe hybridizes predominately to an RNA of
approximately 19 S size, as previously reported.[17]   Several larger,
less abundant RNAs are also evident, especially with longer x-ray film
exposure (not shown).   This LS mRNA is developmentally regulated.   The

mRNA is barely detectable in dark adapted cells ("0" hour). Following
the onset of growth in the light, mRNA levels increase throughout the
period of ct development.

A similar induction of 32 kd mRNA transcription during ct development is observed. The major RNA transcript is 14 S in size. At
least 5 larger RNAs, the largest being >3000 nt, are also evident.
Four of these six RNAs (denoted +, Fig. 4) also hybridize with the
1.1 kbp, ^{32}P-labeled 32 kd gene probe from spinach ct DNA (described
above). Therefore we believe that most or all of these higher MW RNAs
contain 32 kd mRNA coding sequences. The reason for this multiplicity
of mRNA transcripts is currently under investigation.

Transcription of the β-subunit locus is also developmentally regulated, with a temporal pattern similar to that of the LS and 32 kd
genes. Transcripts larger than the size expected for the mRNA are
also found (data not shown). By contrast, the levels of mRNA detected
with the EF-Tu probe (Fig. 4) remain relatively constant through the
first 60 h of development. This is followed by a significant RNA
increase between 60-72 h.

These results are consistent with earlier reports[23,26,27] that
several different temporal programs for mRNA regulation occur during
light induced chloroplast development. In addition, there is now
preliminary evidence that multiple RNA processing events may be necessary for the maturation of several chloroplast mRNAs.

THE RIBULOSE-1,5-BISPHOSPHATE CARBOXYLASE GENE IS INTERRUPTED BY MUL-
TIPLE INTERVENING SEQUENCES

A description of the LS coding locus, and evidence that this
gene is a split gene have previously been reported.[17] In order to
know the precise LS gene structure, the number of introns, and the
nature of exon-intron boundaries, a DNA sequence analysis of this
locus has been initiated. This work is not yet complete, but it is
possible to summarize the progress to date, and the conclusions that
are possible based on the preliminary DNA sequence data. A restriction map of the LS coding locus based on the report of Stiegler et
al.[17] is shown in Fig. 5.

The three HindIII fragments Hind 15, 41, and 53, which contain
most of the LS gene were each cloned in the single strand phage vector
M13mp5 in both possible orientations. Primed dideoxy DNA sequence
analysis has been carried out from each HindIII site (Fig. 5B). LS
amino acid coding loci were identified by comparison of the DNA
sequence to that of the LS genes of maize,[29] spinach,[30] pea,[19] and
Chlamydomonas.[31] As shown diagramatically in Fig. 5C, there are at
least 2 coding regions in Hind41-53 separated by non-coding sequences.
A large coding region is centered around the HindIII site between

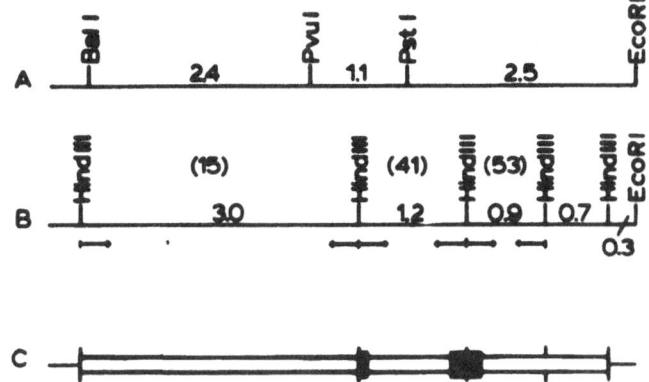

Fig. 5.   Restriction map of *Euglena* ct DNA LS coding locus. DNA fragment sizes are in kbp. A. General map. B. *Hind*III map,
and designation of fragment nomenclature, i.e. *Hin*d 15, *Hin*d
41, and *Hind*III 53. The direction and extent of DNA sequence
is shown with arrows. C. LS protein coding regions (exons)
(see text) are shown as shaded boxes.

*Hin*d 41 and *Hin*d 53. This *Hind*III site is located at codons 129–
131,[31] and is a conserved sequence with respect to the *Chlamydomonas*
LS gene. This entire exon codes for at least 100 amino acids, codons
85–184. These 100 amino acids have 85% amino acid sequence homology
with the *Chlamydomonas* LS gene, and 82–87% homology to the three
higher plant ct LS genes. A second, putative short exon, containing
codons ca. 253–267, is found immediately preceeding the *Hind*III site
between *Hin*d 41 and *Hin*d 15. In these two examples, the precise exon-
intron boundaries cannot yet be determined. Intron sequences are
recognized by the complete loss of homology to the known LS genes, the
high AT-base content, and the appearance of termination codons in the
amino acid reading frame.

Based on the preliminary sequence data and the previously reported[17] hybridization results, the following conclusions can be made:
(1) There are at least three intervening sequences in the gene, one
in each of fragments *Hin*d 15, 41 and 53. This is a minimal estimate.
More than three is a definite possibility. (2) The expected 475
codons,[29,30,31] or 1425 bp of the gene, are dispersed over at least
2.5 kbp of ct DNA, and perhaps as much as 3.5–4 kbp or more. (3) The
gene is transcribed, and processed to yield a major transcript of ca.
19 S (Fig. 4). The appearance of this mRNA is developmentally
regulated.

ACKNOWLEDGEMENTS

    This work was supported by NIH Grants GM21351 and GM28463. W. G.
is supported by a research grant from the Deutsche Forschungsgemeinschaft. We are grateful to Reinhold Herrmann for providing a spinach
ct DNA restriction fragment with β-gene sequences, to Jeffrey Palmer
and William Thompson for cloned spinach ct DNA fragments, to John
Watson, Stefan Surzycki, and Jean-David Rochaix for a *Chlamydomonas*
ct DNA recombinant plasmid, and to Gerard Zurawski and Michel Dron for
the communication of results prior to publication.

REFERENCES

1. R. B. Hallick, Chloroplast DNA, in "The Biology of *Euglena*,
    Vol. IV," D. E. Buetow, ed., Academic Press, New York, in
    press.
2. E. M. Southern, Detection of Specific Sequences Among DNA Frag-
    ments Separated by Gel Electrophoresis, J. Mol. Biol. 98:503
    (1975).
3. R. B. Hallick, K. E. Rushlow, E. M. Orozco, Jr., G. L. Stiegler,
    and P. W. Gray, Chloroplast DNA of *Euglena gracilis* Gene Map-
    ping and Selective in vitro Transcription of the Ribosomal RNA
    Region, ICN-UCLA Symp. Mol. Cell. Biol. 15:127 (1979).
4. E. M. Orozco, Jr., and R. B. Hallick, *Euglena gracilis* Chloro-
    plast Transfer RNA Transcription Units. I. Physical Map of
    the Transfer RNA Gene Loci, J. Biol. Chem. 257:3258 (1982).
5. M. R. El-Gewely, M. I. Lomax, E. T. Lau, R. B. Helling, W.
    Farmerie, and W. E. Barnett, A Map of Specific Cleavage Sites
    and tRNA Genes in the Chloroplast Genome of *Euglena gracilis*
    bacillaris, Mol. Gen. Genet 181:296 (1981).
6. E. M. Orozco, Jr., K. E. Rushlow, J. R. Dodd, and R. B. Hallick,
    Euglena gracilis Chloroplast Ribosomal RNA Transcription Units
    II. Nucleotide Sequence Homology Between the 16 S-23 S Ribo-
    somal RNA Spacer and the 16 S Ribosomal RNA Leader Regions,
    J. Biol. Chem. 255:10997 (1980).
7. L. Graf, H. Kossel, and E. Stutz, Sequencing of 16 S-23 S Spacer
    in a Ribosomal RNA Operon of *Euglena gracilis* Chloroplast DNA
    Reveals Two tRNA Genes, Nature 286:908 (1980).
8. E. M. Orozco, Jr., and R. B. Hallick, *Euglena gracilis* Chloro-
    plast Transfer RNA Transcription Units. II Nucleotide
    Sequence Analysis of a $tRNA^{Val}-tRNA^{Asn}-tRNA^{Arg}-tRNA^{Leu}$ Gene
    Cluster, J. Biol. Chem. 257:3265 (1982).
9. M. J. Hollingsworth, and R. B. Hallick, *Euglena gracilis* Chloro-
    plast Transfer RNA Transcription Units. Nucleotide Sequence
    Analysis of a $tRNA^{Tyr}-tRNA^{His}-tRNA^{Met}-tRNA^{Trp}-tRNA^{Glu}-tRNA^{Gly}$
    Gene Cluster, J. Biol. Chem. in press (1982).

10. G. D. Karabin and R. B. Hallick, *Euglena gracilis* Chloroplast Transfer RNA Transcription Units. Nucleotide Sequence Analysis of a tRNA^{Thr}-tRNA^{Gly}-tRNA^{Met}-tRNA^{Ser}-tRNA^{Gln} Gene Cluster, submitted for publication.

11. S. H. Chang, C. K. Brum, M. Silberklang, U. L. RajBhandary, L. I. Hecker, and W. E. Barnett, The First Nucleotide Sequence of an Organelle Transfer RNA:Chloroplastic tRNA^{Phe}, Cell 9:717 (1976).

12. J. A. Nickoloff and R. B. Hallick, Synthetic Deoxyoligonucleotides as General Probes for Transfer RNA Genes, submitted for publication.

13. R. P. Singhal and P. A. M. Fallis, Structure, Function, and Evolution of Transfer RNAs (with Appendix Giving Complete sequences of 178 tRNAs), Prog. Nucl. Acids Res. and Molec. Biol. 23:227 (1979).

14. K. E. Rushlow, E. M. Orozco, Jr., C. Lipper, and R. B. Hallick, Selective *in Vitro* Transcription of *Euglena* Chloroplast Ribosomal RNA Genes by a Transcriptionally Active Chromosome, J. Biol. Chem. 255:3786 (1980).

15. W. Gruissem, D. M. Prescott, B. M. Greenberg, and R. B. Hallick, Transcription of *E. coli* and *Euglena* Chloroplast tRNA Gene Clusters and Processing of the Polycistronic Transcripts in a HeLa Cell Free System, Cell 30:81 (1982).

16. M. R. El-Gewely, R. B. Helling, W. Farmerie, and W. E. Barnett, Location of a Phenylalanine tRNA Gene on the Physical Map of the *Euglena gracilis* Chloroplast Genome, Gene 17:337 (1982).

17. G. L. Stiegler, H. M. Matthews, S. E. Bingham, and R. B. Hallick, The Gene for the Large Subunit of Ribulose-1,5-bisphosphate Carboxylase in *Euglena gracilis* Chloroplast DNA: Location, Polarity, Cloning, and Evidence for an Intervening Sequence, Nucleic Acids Res. 10:3427 (1982).

18. A. J. Driesel, J. Speirs, and H. J. Bohnert, Spinach Chloroplast mRNA for a 32000 Dalton Polypeptide, Size and Localization on the Physical Map of the Chloroplast DNA, Biochim. Biophys. Acta 610:297 (1980).

19. G. Zurawski, personal communication.

20. P. Westhoff, N. Nelson, H. Bünemann, and R. G. Herrmann, Localization of Genes for Coupling Factor Subunits on the Spinach Plastid Chromosome, Curr. Genetics 4:109 (1981).

21. J. C. Watson and S. J. Surzycki, Extensive Sequence Homology in the DNA Coding for Elongation Factor Tu from *Escherichia coli* and the *Chlamydomonas reinhardtii* Chloroplast, Proc. Natl. Acad. Sci. USA 79:2264 (1982).

22. G. An and J. D. Friesen, The Nucleotide Sequence of *tuf*B and Four Nearby tRNA Structural Genes of *Escherichia coli*, Gene 12:33 (1980).

23. B. K. Chelm and R. B. Hallick, Changes in the Expression of the Chloroplast Genome of *Euglena gracilis* during Chloroplast Development, Biochemistry 15:593 (1976).

24. H. Lehrach, D. Diamond, J. M. Wozney, and H. Boedtker, RNA Molec-
     ular Weight Determinations by Gel Electrophoresis under
     Denaturing Conditions, a Critical Reexamination, Biochemistry
     16:4743 (1977).
25. P. S. Thomas, Hybridization of Denatured RNA and Small DNA Frag-
     ments Transferred to Nitrocellulose, Proc. Natl. Acad. Sci.
     USA 77:5201 (1980).
26. B. K. Chelm, R. B. Hallick, and P. W. Gray, Transcription Pro-
     gram of the Chloroplast Genome of Euglena gracilis during
     Chloroplast Development, Proc. Natl. Acad. Sci. USA 76:2258
     (1979).
27. J. R. Y. Rawson, C. L. Boerma, W. H. Andrews, and C. G. Wilkerson
     Complexity and Abundance of Ribonucleic Acid Transcribed from
     Restriction Endonuclease Fragments of Euglena Chloroplast
     Deoxyribonucleic Acid during Chloroplast Development,
     Biochemistry 20:2639 (1981).
28. T. Yokota, H. Sugisaki, M. Takanami, and Y. Kaziro, The Nucleo-
     tide Sequence of the Cloned tufA Gene of Escherichia coli,
     Gene 12:25 (1980).
29. L. McIntosh, C. Poulsen, and L. Bogorad, Chloroplast Gene
     Sequence for the Large Subunit of Ribulose Bisphosphatecar-
     boxylase of Maize, Nature 288:556 (1980).
30. G. Zurawski, B. Perrot, W. Bottomley, and P. R. Whitfeld, The
     Structure of the Gene for the Large Subunit of Ribulose-1,5-
     bisphosphate Carboxylase from Spinach Chloroplast DNA,
     Nucleic Acids Res. 9:3251 (1981).
31. M. Dron and J.-D. Rochaix, personal communication.

COMPARATIVE STUDIES ON tRNAs AND AMINOACYL-tRNA SYNTHETASES FROM VARIOUS PHOTOSYNTHETIC ORGANISMS

J. H. Weil[1], M. Mubumbila[1], M. Kuntz[1], M. Keller[1],
E. J. Crouse[1], G. Burkard[1], P. Guillemaut[1], R. Selden[2],
L. McIntosh[2], L. Bogorad[2], W. Löffelhardt[3], H. Mucke[3],
H. J. Bohnert[4], A. Dietrich[1], G. Souciet[1], B. Colas[1],
P. Imbault[1], V. Sarantoglou[1]

[1]IBMC, 15 rue Descartes, Strasbourg, France
[2]Harvard University, 16 Divinity Ave, Cambridge, USA
[3]Institut für Biochemie, Währingerstrasse 38
 Wien, Austria
[4]EMBL, Postfach 1022.09, Heidelberg, Germany

MAPPING OF tRNA GENES ON THE CHLOROPLAST DNA OF VARIOUS PHOTOSYNTHETIC ORGANISMS

Chloroplasts have their own protein synthesizing system, using chloroplast-specific tRNAs which are different from their cytoplasmic counterparts and are coded for by chloroplast DNA (Weil, 1979 ; Weil and Parthier, 1982). Total chloroplast tRNA can be fractionated by two-dimensional polyacrylamide gel electrophoresis (Burkard et al., 1982) into individual tRNAs, which can be recovered from the gel, identified by aminoacylation and labeled with ^{32}P at their 3' end using α-^{32}P-ATP and tRNA nucleotidyl transferase (Mubumbila et al., 1980). Each labeled tRNA can then be hybridized to DNA fragments which have been generated by the action of a restriction endonuclease on chloroplast DNA, fractionated by agarose gel electrophoresis, and transferred to nitrocellulose strips. As the position of these fragments on the circular map of the chloroplast chromosome has been previously determined, this approach allows the localization of the tRNA genes. Such a tRNA gene map was first established in the case of the spinach chloroplast genome (Driesel et al., 1979), which is a circular molecule containing two inverted repeats ; each of these inverted repeats contains a set of ribosomal RNA genes, and the spacer located between the 16S and the 23S

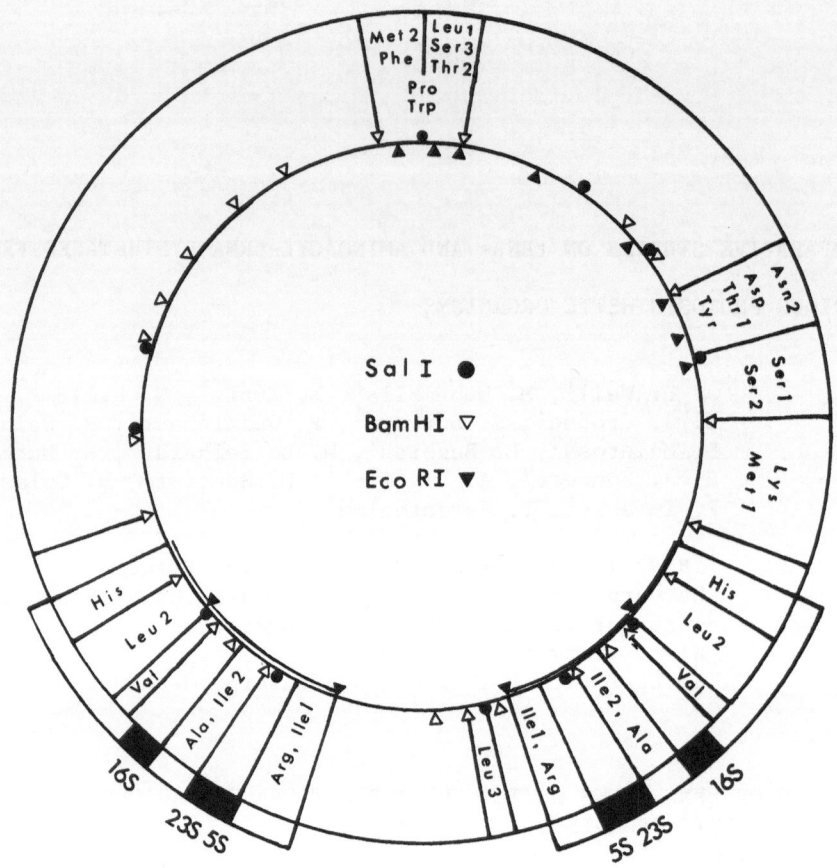

Fig. 1   Localization of tRNA genes on the restriction endonuclease
         cleavage site map of *Zea mays* chloroplast DNA. The smallest
         DNA segment to which hybridization was observed is indicated
         for each chloroplast tRNA tested.

rRNA gene was shown to contain a tRNA^{Ile} gene (Bohnert et al.,
1979). Such tRNA gene mapping studies have now been extended to the
chloroplast genomes of other photosynthetic organisms.

Localization of tRNA Genes on the Chloroplast Genome of *Zea mays*

A collaboration between Harvard University and Strasbourg,
using maize chloroplast DNA fragments obtained by action of Sal I,
Bam H I or Eco R I restriction endonucleases has allowed the localization of 25 tRNA genes. As shown on fig. 1, 15 tRNA genes are

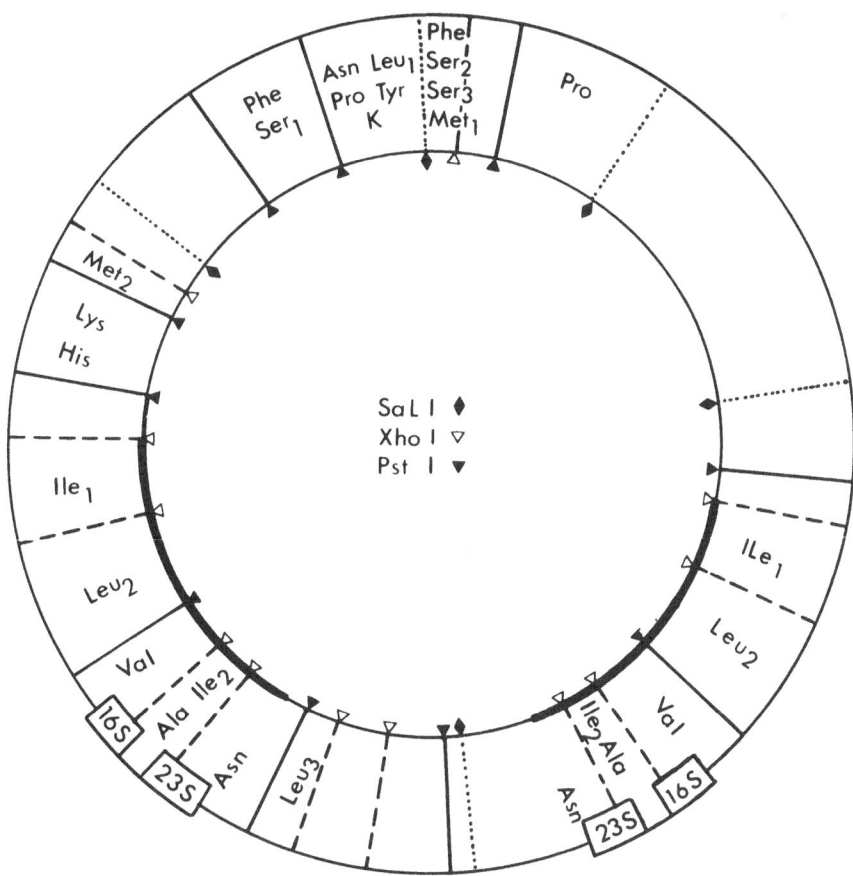

Fig. 2   Localization of rRNA genes on the restriction endonuclease
cleavage site map of *Phaseolus vulgaris* chloroplast DNA.
The thick line corresponds to the two copies of the inverted
repeat region.

located in the large single copy region, 1 gene (that of tRNA$_3^{Leu}$)
in the small single copy region, while 9 genes are found on each
copy of the two inverted repeats and among them 2 genes (those for
tRNA^{Ala} and tRNA$_2^{Ile}$) are located in the spacer between the 16S and
23S rRNA genes.

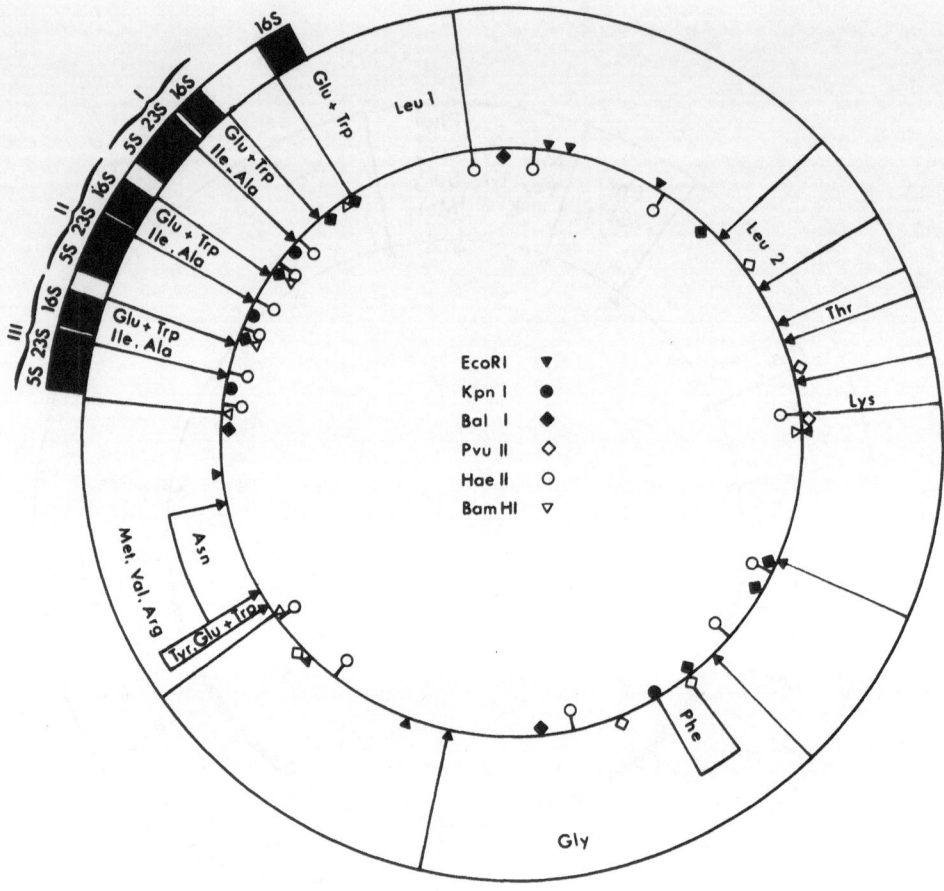

Fig. 3 Localization of tRNA genes on the restriction endonuclease
cleavage site map of *Euglena gracilis* Z chloroplast DNA.

Localization of tRNA Genes on the Chloroplast Genome of *Phaseolus vulgaris*

In the case of *Phaseolus vulgaris* no map of the chloroplast
genome was available, so that chloroplast tRNAs were used as markers,
to localize the respective position of the restriction fragments
obtained with Sal I, Xho I and Pst I endonucleases and to obtain a
physical map of this genome. As shown on fig. 2, about 20 tRNA genes
have been located on this map. As in maize, most of them are found
in the large single copy region, one gene is found in the small
single copy region (that of $tRNA_3^{Leu}$), 7 gnees are found on each copy
of the two inverted repeats ; again the genes for $tRNA^{Ala}$ and

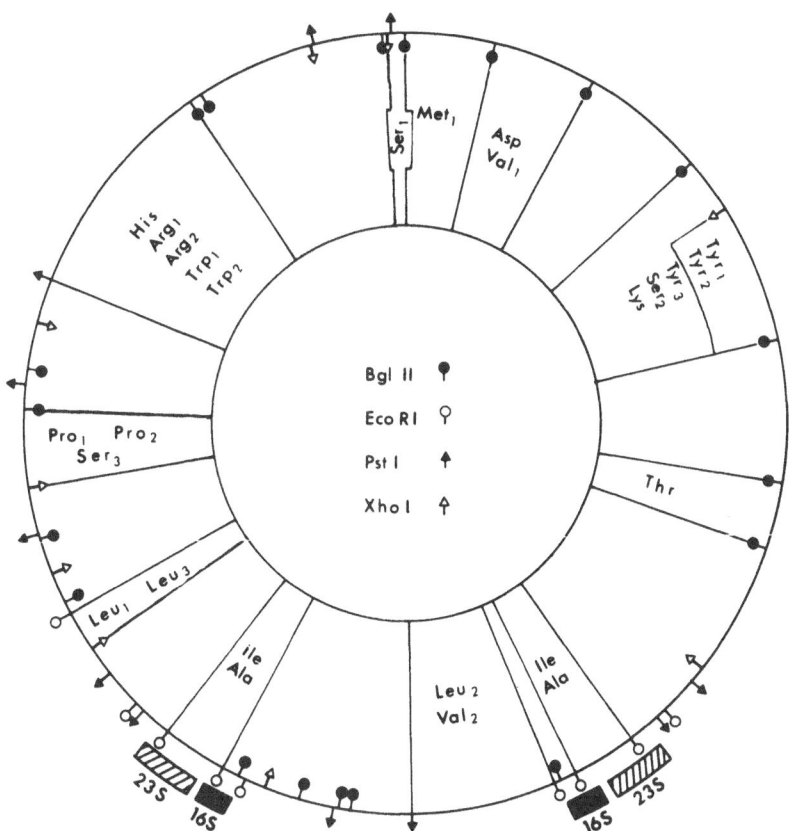

Fig. 4 Localization of tRNA genes on the restriction endonuclease cleavage site map of *Cyanophora paradoxa* cyanelle DNA.

$tRNA_2^{Ile}$ are located in the ribosomal spacer.

Localization of tRNA Genes on the Chloroplast Genome of *Euglena gracilis*

The presence of a rDNA unit on two inverted repeats is not a feature common to all chloroplast DNAs. In at least two *Euglena gracilis* strains (Z and *Bacillaris*), the chloroplast genome contains

three tandemly repeated rDNA units, and part of a fourth one
(Rawson et al., 1978 ; Gray and Hallick, 1978 ; Jenni and Stutz,
1978 ; El Gewely et al., 1981). About 15 tRNA genes have been
localized on this genome (see fig. 3) and again two genes, coding
for a tRNA^{Ala} and a tRNA^{Ile}, are present in the ribosomal spacer
in at least two (and possibly all three) rDNA units (Keller et al.,
1980).

Localization of tRNA Genes on the Cyanelle Genome of *Cyanophora paradoxa*

Cyanelles are photosynthetic organelles which can be considered as intermediates between procaryotic organisms (they have a
peptidoglycan cell wall similar to that of cyanobacteria) and
chloroplasts (the size of their DNA is similar to that of
chloroplast DNA). A collaboration was established between Wien,
Heidelberg and Strasbourg, to study the localization of tRNA genes
on the cyanelle genome. As shown on fig. 4, two tRNA genes, coding
for a tRNA^{Ala} and a tRNA^{Ile}, are again found in the ribosomal spacer
of the rDNA unit present on each of the two inverted repeats.

SEQUENCE OF THE MAIZE CHLOROPLAST ISOLEUCINE tRNA ENCODED IN THE RIBOSOMAL SPACER

It is interesting to note that genes for tRNA^{Ala} and tRNA^{Ile}
are located in the ribosomal spacer not only in chloroplast and
cyanelle genomes (see fig. 1-4), but also in bacterial (*E. coli* and
B. subtilis) genomes (Morgan et al., 1977 ; Loughney et al., 1982).
Hybridization of total chloroplast 4S RNA had suggested the presence of tRNA genes in the ribosomal spacer of chloroplast DNA in
Euglena gracilis (Hallick et al., 1978) and *Chlamydomonas reinhardi*
(Malnoe and Rochaix, 1978). Hybridization studies performed with
purified individual tRNA species have revealed that a tRNA^{Ile} gene
is present in the spacer in spinach chloroplast DNA (Bohnert et al.,
1979) and that a tRNA^{Ile} and a tRNA^{Ala} genes are present in the
spacer in the chloroplast genome of Euglena (Keller et al., 1980)
and of *Zea mays* (Weil et al., 1981). More recently the sequence of
the genes coding for tRNA^{Ala} and tRNA^{Ile}, located in the spacers of
Euglena (Orozco et al., 1980 ; Graf et al., 1980) and maize (Koch
et al., 1981) chloroplast DNA, has been determined. In the case of
maize it was shown that the tRNA^{Ala} gene and the tRNA^{Ile} gene
contain a long intron consisting of 806 and 949 base-pairs
respectively.

The positions, where the excision of such an intron takes
place, could only be postulated (Koch et al., 1981) and in fact
there was no evidence that such a large gene (over 1000 base-pair
long) is transcribed and processed into a mature functional tRNA.
In order to answer these questions, the sequence of maize chloroplast
tRNA$_2^{Ile}$, which had been shown to hybridize to the spacer (Weil et

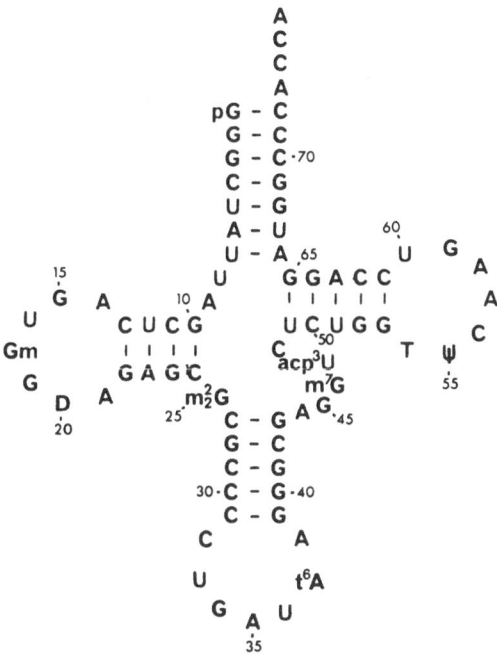

Fig. 5 Nucleotide sequence of *Zea mays* chloroplast $tRNA_2^{Ile}$

al., 1981), was determined (Guillemaut and Weil, 1982) and is shown in fig. 5. This sequence is identical to that predicted from the corresponding gene sequence by Koch et al., 1981, but it shows the post-transcriptional modifications of this tRNA. Three putative splicing points had been postulated, namely i) immediately after the GAU anticodon (on its 3' side), ii) after the first base following the anticodon, iii) after the second base following the anticodon (Koch et al., 1981). Depending upon where the splicing occurs the anticodon loop of the mature tRNA should have the following sequence : i) GAUAC, ii) GAUAC, iii) GAUAA, respectively. As shown on fig. 5, the third hypothesis is correct, as the anticodon is followed by two A residues (the first of which is modified into t^6A).

It therefore appears that the intron of maize chloroplast tRNA$_2^{Ile}$ is located at a position different from that found for the split yeast tRNA gene (Knapp et al., 1979), which is found after the first base following the anticodon. There seems to be no general rule for the position of introns even among maize chloroplast split tRNA genes, as Steinmetz et al. (1982) have located an intron after the first base of the anticodon in maize chloroplast tRNA^{Leu} gene.

The fact that the tRNA$_2^{Ile}$ which has been sequenced is the only tRNA^{Ile} which hybridizes to the chloroplast DNA of the spacer region and the fact that it does not hybridize to any other chloroplast DNA restriction fragment, show that its gene, which is over 1000 base-pair long, must be transcribed and processed *in vivo* to yield a mature functional tRNA.

The sequence of spinach chloroplast tRNA$_2^{Ile}$ has also been determined (Guillemaut and Weil, 1982). It is identical to that of maize chloroplast tRNA$_2^{Ile}$ shown on fig. 5, except for a lower percentage of methylation of the G residue at position 46. Spinach chloroplast tRNA$_2^{Ile}$ has been shown to hybridize to the ribosomal spacer (Bohnert et al., 1979), but in this case, no DNA sequence information is available and it is not known whether this tRNA^{Ile} gene contains any intron.

COMPARATIVE STUDIES ON CYTOPLASMIC AND CHLOROPLASTIC LEUCYL-AND VALYL-tRNA SYNTHETASES

In contrast to chloroplastic-specific tRNAs, which are coded for by the chloroplast genome, chloroplast-specific aminoacyl-tRNA synthetases are coded for by the nuclear genome (Weil and Parthier, 1982). As such is also the case for the cytoplasmic enzymes, one may wonder what are the differences between a cytoplasmic amino-acyl-tRNA synthetase and the chloroplastic enzyme specific for the same amino-acid. In order to approach this problem, two pairs of *Euglena gracilis* aminoacyl-tRNA synthetases, namely the cyto-plasmic and chloroplastic valyl- (Imbault et al., 1979 ; Sarantoglou et al., 1980) and leucyl-tRNA synthetases (Imbault et al., 1981 ; Sarantoglou et al., 1981) and the chloroplastic and cytoplasmic leucyl -tRNA synthetases from *Phaseolus vulgaris* (Souciet et al., 1982) have been purified, allowing a comparison of their catalytic, structural and immunological properties.

Whereas *Euglena* and *Phaseolus* chloroplastic leucyl-tRNA synthetases and *Euglena* chloroplastic valyl-tRNA synthetase have a high substrate specificity and only aminoacylate chloroplastic or procaryotic tRNAs, cytoplasmic leucyl-tRNA synthetases (from *Euglena* and *Phaseolus*) are less specific, as they aminoacylate not only cytoplasmic tRNAs, but also some *E.coli* isoacceptors (Imbault et al., 1982 ; Guillemaut et al., 1975).

Euglena cytoplasmic and chloroplastic valyl-tRNA synthetases have both a monomeric structure and a molecular weight of 126,000 (Colas et al., 1982a). Leucyl-tRNA synthetases are also monomeric (Colas et al., 1982a ; Souciet et al., 1982), but the molecular weight of the chloroplastic enzyme is somewhat smaller (100,000 in *Euglena*, 122,000 in *Phaseolus*) than that of its cytoplasmic conterpart (116,000 in *Euglena*, 132,000 in *Phaseolus*).

Examination of the trypic peptide maps shows that the structure of chloroplastic valyl- and leucyl-tRNA synthetases differs from that of their cytoplasmic conterpart, in *Euglena* as well as in *Phaseolus*. Comparison of the amino acid compositions also reveals differences and rules out the possibility that the chloroplastic enzyme derives from its cytoplasmic counterpart, as the former (which has a smaller molecular weight in the case of *Euglena* leucyl-tRNA synthetases) contains some amino acid residues in larger amounts than the latter (Colas et al., 1982a).

Taken together, the results obtained are not in favor of the hypothesis of post-translational modifications to explain the differences between chloroplastic and cytoplasmic valyl- and leucyl-tRNA synthetases. Addition of a subunit is ruled out by the fact that the enzymes studied are all monomeric, and removal of a peptide is unlikely considering the aminoacid compositions and the fact that - at least in the case of the two *Euglena* valyl-tRNA synthetases - the chloroplastic and the cytoplasmic enzymes have the same molecular weight.

Finally, immunological studies (Colas et al., 1982b) have shown that antibodies raised against a cytoplasmic or a chloroplastic enzyme (valyl- or leucyl-tRNA synthetase) are able to inhibit the activity of the corresponding enzyme, but not that of its counterpart from the other cellular compartment (fig. 6). Similarly, immuno-electrophoretic analyses (fig. 7) reveal a precipitate only when the enzymatic extract tested contains the aminoacyl-tRNA synthetase which was used to prepare the antiserum present in the agarose gel (no precipitate occurs in the presence of the homologous enzyme from the other cellular compartment). The results of these comparative

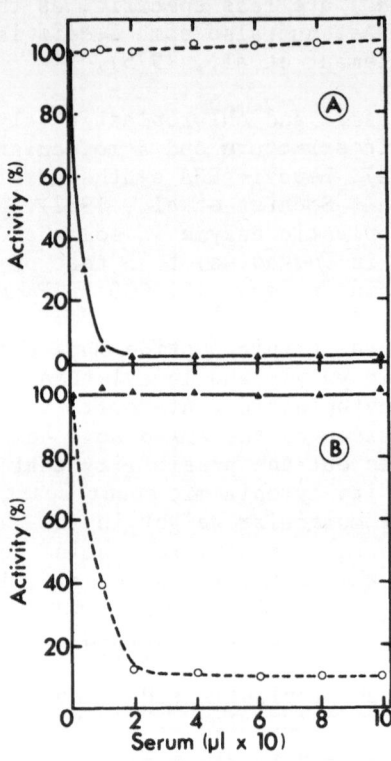

Fig. 6   Immuno-inactivation of chloroplastic (▲——▲) and
          cytoplasmic (o----o) valyl-tRNA synthetases by antibodies
          raised against chloroplastic (A) and cytoplasmic (B) valyl-
          tRNA synthetases respectively. Data are expressed as
          percentages of the activity determined under the same
          conditions but using pre-immune serum only.

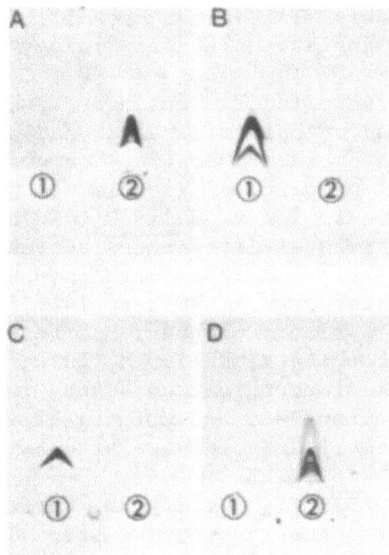

Fig. 7 Rocket immuno-electrophoresis. A) cytoplasmic valyl-tRNA
        synthetase antiserum with chloroplastic (well 1) or
        cytoplasmic (well 2) valyl-tRNA synthetase. B) chloroplastic
        valyl-tRNA synthetase antiserum with chloroplastic (well 1)
        or cytoplasmic (well 2) valyl-tRNA synthetase. C) cytoplasmic
        leucyl-tRNA synthetase antiserum with cytoplasmic (well 1)
        or chloroplastic (well 2) leucyl-tRNA synthetase. D)
        chloroplastic leucyl-tRNA synthetase antiserum with
        cytoplasmic (well 1) or chloroplastic (well 2) leucyl-tRNA
        synthetase.

studies on the structural and immunological properties suggest
that chloroplastic and cytoplasmic valyl-tRNA synthetases (and
leucyl-tRNA synthetases) are coded for by different (nuclear)
genes.

Bohnert HJ, Driesel AJ, Crouse EJ, Gordon K, Herrmann RG,
    Steinmetz A, Mubumbila M, Keller M, Burkard G, Weil JH (1979).
    Presence of a transfer RNA gene in the spacer sequence
    between the 16S and 23S rRNA genes of spinach chloroplast DNA.
    FEBS Lett 103:191.
Burkard G, Steinmetz A, Keller M, Mubumbila M, Crouse EJ, Weil JH
    (1982). Resolution of chloroplast tRNAs by two-dimensional
    gel electrophoresis. In Edelman M, Hallick RB, Chua NH (eds) :
    "Methods in Chloroplast Molecular Biology", Amsterdam,
    Elsevier, in press.
Colas B, Imbault P, Sarantoglou V, Boulanger Y, Weil JH (1982a)
    chloroplastic and cytoplasmic valyl- and leucyl-tRNA
    synthetases from *Euglena gracilis*. Comparative studies of
    their structural properties. Biochim Biophys Acta 697:71.
Colas B, Imbault P, Sarantoglou V, Weil JH (1982b). Immunological
    evidence for structural differences between *Euglena gracilis*
    chloroplastic valyl- and leucyl-tRNA synthetases and their
    cytoplasmic counterparts. FEBS Lett 141:213.
Driesel AJ, Crouse EJ, Gordon K, Bohnert HJ, Herrmann RG,
    Steinmetz A, Mubumbila M, Keller M, Burkard G, Weil JH (1979).
    Fractionation and identification of the individual spinach
    chloroplast transfer RNAs and mapping of their genes on the
    restriction endonuclease cleavage site map of chloroplast DNA.
    Gene 6:285.
El Gewely MR, Lomax MI, Lau ET, Helling RB, Farmerie W, Barnett WE
    (1981). A map of specific cleavage sites and tRNA genes in
    the chloroplast genome of *Euglena gracilis bacillaris*. Mol
    Gen Genet 181:296.
Graf L, Kössel H, Stutz E (1980). Sequencing of 16S-23S spacer in
    a ribosomal RNA operon of *Euglena gracilis* chloroplast DNA
    reveals two tRNA genes. Nature 286:908.
Gray PW, Hallick RB (1978) Physical mapping of the *Euglena gracilis*
    chloroplast DNA and ribosomal RNA gene region. Biochemistry
    17:284.
Guillemaut P, Steinmetz A, Burkard G, Weil JH (1975) Aminoacylation
    of tRNA[Leu] species from *E.coli* and from the cytoplasm,
    chloroplasts and mitochondria of *Phaseolus vulgaris* by
    homologous and heterologous enzymes. Biochim Biophys Acta
    378:64.
Guillemaut P, Weil JH (1982). The nucleotide sequence of the maize
    and spinach chloroplast isoleucine transfer RNA encoded in
    the 16S to 23S rDNA spacer. Nucl Acids Res 10:1653.
Hallick RB, Gray PW, Chelm BK, Rushlow KE, Orozco EM (1978).
    Euglena gracilis chloroplast DNA structure, gene mapping and
    RNA transcription. In Akoyunoglou G, Argyroudi-Akoyunoglou
    JH (eds) : "Chloroplast Development", Amsterdam, Elsevier,
    p 619.
Imbault P, Sarantoglou V, Weil JH (1979). Purification of the
    chloroplastic valyl-tRNA synthetase from *Euglena gracilis*

Biochem Biophys Res Commum 88:75.

Imbault P, Colas B, Sarantoglou V, Boulanger Y, Weil JH (1981).
    Chloroplast leucyl-tRNA synthetase from *Euglena gracilis*.
    Purification, kinetic analysis and structural characterization
    Biochemistry 20:5855.

Imbault P, Sarantoglou V, Weil JH (1982). Properties of purified
    chloroplastic and cytoplasmic valyl- and leucyl-tRNA
    synthetases from *Euglena gracilis*. Phytochemistry 21:1189.

Jenni B, Stutz E (1978). Physical mapping of the ribosomal DNA
    region of *Euglena gracilis* chloroplast DNA. Eur J Biochem
    88:127.

Keller M, Burkard G, Bohnert HJ, Mubumbila M, Gordon K,
    Steinmetz A, Heiser D, Crouse EJ, Weil JH (1980). Transfer
    RNA genes associated with the 16S and 23S rRNA genes of
    Euglena chloroplast DNA. Biochem Biophys Res Commun 95:47.

Knapp G, Ogden RC, Peebles CL, Abelson J (1979). Splicing og yeast
    tRNA precursors : Structure of the reaction intermediates.
    Cell 18:37.

Koch W, Edwards K, Kössel H (1981). Sequencing of the 16S-23S spacer
    in a ribosomal RNA operon of *Zea mays* chloroplast DNA reveals
    two splits tRNA genes. Cell 25:203.

Loughney K, Lund E, Dahlberg JE (1982). tRNA genes are found between
    the 16S and 23S rRNA genes in *Bacillus subtilis*. Nucl Acids
    Res 10:1607.

Malnoe P, Rochaix JD (1978). Localization of 4S RNA genes on
    chloroplast genome of *Chlamydomonas reinhardi*. Mol Gen Genet
    166:269.

Morgan EA, Ikemura T, Nomura M (1977). Identification of spacer tRNA
    genes in individual ribosomal RNA transcription units of
    E.coli. Proc Natl Acad Sci US 74:2710.

Mubumbila M, Burkard G, Keller M, Steinmetz A, Crouse EJ, Weil JH
    (1980). Hybridization of bean, spinach, maize and Euglena
    transfer RNAs with homologous and heterologous chloroplasts
    DNAs. Biochim Biophys Acta 609:31.

Orozco EM, Rushlow KE, Dodd JR, Hallick RB (1980). *Euglena gracilis*
    chloroplast ribosomal RNA transcription units. II. Nucleotide
    sequence homology between 16S-23S ribosomal RNA spacer and
    the 16S ribosomal RNA leader regions. J Biol Chem 255:10997.

Rawson JR, Kushner SR, Vapnek D, ALton NK, Boerma CL (1978).
    Chloroplast ribosomal RNA genes in *Euglena gracilis* exists
    as three clustered tandem repeats. Gene 3:191.

Sarantoglou V, Imbault P, Weil JH (1980). The use of affinity elution
    from blue dextran Sepharose by yeast tRNA$_2^{Val}$ in the complete
    purification of the cytoplasmic valyl-tRNA synthetase from
    Euglena gracilis. Biochem Biophys Res Commun 93;134.

Sarantoglou V, Imbault P, Weil JH (1981). Purification of *Euglena
    gracilis* cytoplasmic leucyl-tRNA synthetase. Plant Sci Lett.
    22:291.

Souciet G, Dietrich A, Colas B, Razafimahatratra P, Weil JH (1982).
    Purification and properties of chloroplast leucyl-tRNA

synthetase from a higher plant : *Phaseolus vulgaris* J Biol
        Chem, in press.
Steinmetz A, Gubbins EJ Bogorad L (1982). Nucleic Acids Res
        10, 3027-3037.
Weil JH (1979). Cytoplasmic and organellar tRNAs in plants. In Hall
        TC, Davies J (eds) : "Nucleic Acids in Plants", West Palm
        Beach, CRC Press, p 143.
Weil JH, Guillemaut P, Burkard G, Canaday J, Mubumbila M, Osorio ML,
        Keller M, Gloeckler R, Steinmetz A, Keith G, Heiser D,
        Crouse EJ (1981). Comparative studies on chloroplast transfer
        RNAs : tRNA sequences and tRNA gene localization in the rDNA
        units. In Akoyunoglou G (ed) : "Photosynthesis", Philadelphia,
        Balabian International Science, vol V, p 777.
Weil JH, Parthier B (1982). Transfer RNAs and aminoacyl-tRNA
        synthetases in plants. In Boulter D, Parthier B (eds) :
        "Encyclopedia of Plant Physiology, New Series", Heidelberg,
        Springer Verlag, vol 17, p 65.

STRUCTURE OF THE GENE *(tmpA)* FOR THE "32,000-M$_r$" THYLAKOID MEMBRANE POLYPEPTIDE OF *SPINACIA OLERACEA* AND *NICOTIANA DEBNEYI*

G. Zurawski[*], H.-J. Bohnert[**], P.R. Whitfeld and W. Bottomley

CSIRO, Division of Plant Industry, P.O. Box 1600, Canberra City, A.C.T. 2601 (Australia)

INTRODUCTION

One of the most rapidly labeled products of chloroplast protein synthesis is a polypeptide of Mr 32,000-36,000[1,2,3,4]. It is synthesized as a precursor of Mr 33,500-34,500[3,4] and does not accumulate in the organelle but is rapidly turned over[4]. Recently the polypeptide has been shown to be involved in the binding of the herbicides atrazine and DCMU and to be part of Photosystem II with a role in electron flow[5]. The gene *(tmpA)* for this polypeptide has been mapped on the chloroplast genome of a number of plant species. In spinach, as in most other plants so far studied, *tmpA* is located in the large single copy region of the chloroplast genome very close to the end of one of the inverted repeat regions[6].

RESULTS AND DISCUSSION

We have cloned the spinach chloroplast DNA fragment containing *tmpA* into both the plasmid pBR322 and the single stranded virus fd106. By hybridization of the fd clones containing *tmpA*, inserted in the two possible orientations, with chloroplast RNA, it was demonstrated that *tmpA* is transcribed towards the adjacent inverted repeat.

Analysis of the nucleotide sequence of part of the fragment revealed that there was one long open reading frame in the expected orientation. The deduced amino acid sequence (Fig. 1), beginning at the first methionine in the open reading frame would form a

* DNAX Research Institute, Palo Alto, Calif. 94304 USA.
** M.P.I. Züchtungsforschung, Cologne, F.R.G.

181

M T A I L E R R E S E S L W G R F C N W I T S T E N R L Y I G W F G
V L M I P T L L T A T S V F I I A F I A A P P V D I D G I R E P V S
G S L L Y G N N I I S G A I I P T S A A I G L H F Y P I W E A A S V
D E W L Y N G G P Y E L I V L H F L L G V A C Y M G R E W E L S F R
L G M R P W I A V A Y S A P V A A A T A V F L I Y P I G Q G S F S D
G M P L G I S G T F N F M I V F Q A E H N I L M H P F H M L G V A G
V F G G S L F S A M H G S L V T S S L I R E T T E N E S A N E G Y R
F G Q E E E T Y N I V A A H G Y F G R L I F Q Y A S F N N S R S L H
F F L A A W P V V G I W F T A L G I S T M A F N L N G F N F N Q S V
V D S Q G R V I N T W A D I I N R A N L G M E V M H E R N A H N F P
L D L A A I E A P S T N G

Figure 1.   The amino acid sequence derived from the nucleotide
            sequence of *tmpA* from the chloroplasts of
            S. oleracea and *N. debneyi*.

polypeptide of Mr 38,950. If, on the other hand, translation were
to commence at the second methionine, then the predicted molecular
weight would be closer to the 35,000 reported for the Mr of the
in vitro translation product of spinach chloroplast mRNA[7]. In
order to distinguish between the two possibilities the clone
containing *tmpA* was isolated from a bank, constructed from *Nicotiana
debneyi* chloroplast DNA, kindly provided by Dr. J.B. Langridge. The
nucleotide sequence of this gene showed over 95% homology with that
of spinach over the whole reading frame. The amino acid sequence
deduced from *tmpA* from *N. debneyi* was identical with that of

Table 1.   AMINO ACID COMPOSITION OF THE "32,000-M_r" POLYPEPTIDE
            FROM *SPINACIA OLERACEA* AND *NICOTIANA DEBNEYI*

Alanine	35	Leucine	31
Arginine	15	Lysine	0
Asparagine	22	Methionine	12
Aspartic acid	7	Phenylalanine	26
Cysteine	2	Proline	15
Glutamic acid	21	Serine	27
Glutamine	6	Threonine	17
Glycine	33	Tryptophane	10
Histidine	10	Tyrosine	12
Isoleucine	31	Valine	21

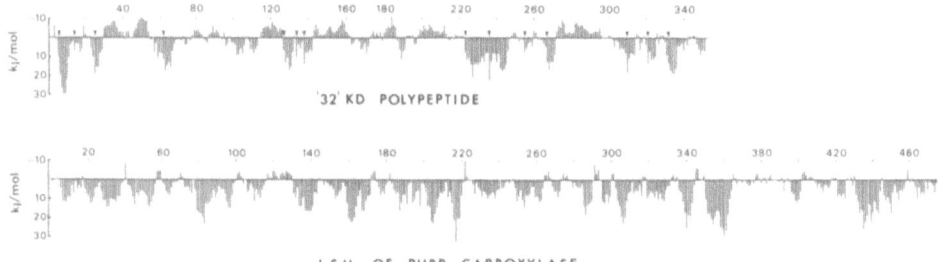

'32' KD POLYPEPTIDE

L.S.U. OF RUBP CARBOXYLASE

Figure 2. Estimated free energy of transfer of the amino acid
           residues in the "32,000-Mr" polypeptide of *S.*
           oleracea and *N. debneyi* from a helix in water to a
           helix in a non-polar solvent[8] compared with that of
           the large subunit of ribulose bisphosphate carboxylase
           from *S. oleracea*. Each line represents the value for
           each amino acid averaged with those of the two residues
           on either side. Arrows indicate the position of
           arginine residues in the "32,000-Mr" polypeptide.

spinach throughout the entire 353 amino acid residues. Since it
seems highly unlikely that such conservation would exist outside
the protein coding region it is concluded that translation begins
at the first methionine and that the molecular weight of the
primary translation product is, in fact, 38,950.

    Examination of the amino acid composition of the "32,000-Mr"
polypeptide of spinach and *N. debneyi* (Table 1) showed that, as
has been reported for the same polypeptide from *Spirodela*[4], it
contains no lysine. In addition, as would be expected in a
membrane protein, there is a high proportion of hydrophobic amino
acids. When the free energy of transfer of each amino acid
residue from a helix in water to a helix in a non-polar phase[8], is

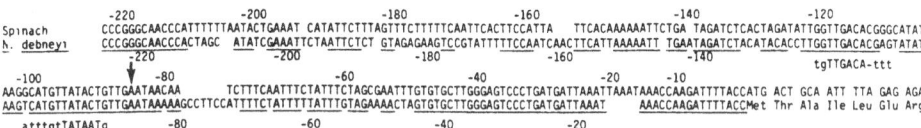

Figure 3. The sequences prior to the translation initiation sites
           of *tmpA* from *S. oleracea* (upper) and *N. debneyi* (lower).
           The '-10' and '-35' consensus sequence of *E. coli* genes[9]
           are shown below the *N. debneyi* sequence. The arrow
           indicates the site of transcription initiation in
           spinach. Conserved sequences are underlined.

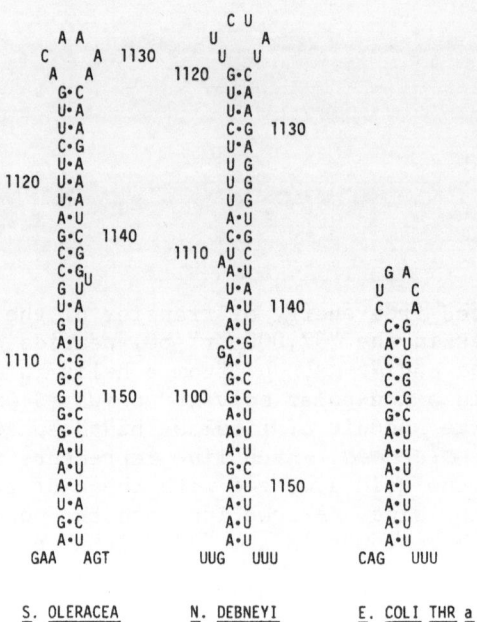

```
                                    C U
              A A              U      A
         C      A  1130       U   U
          A    A            1120  G•C
          G•C                     U•A
          U•A                     U•A
          U•A                     C•G  1130
          C•G                     U•A
          U•A                     U G
    1120  U•A                     U G
          U•A                     U G
          A•U                     A•U
          G•C  1140               C•G
          C•G               1110 A U C
          C•G U                   A•U
          G U U                   U•A              G A
          U•A                     A•U  1140     U      C
          G U                     A•U           C      A
          A•U                    G C•G             C•G
    1110  C•G                    G A•U             A•U
          G•C                     A•C             C•G
          G U  1150        1100  G•C             C•G
          G•C                     A•U             G•C
          G•C                     A•U             A•U
          A•U                     A•U             A•U
          A•U                     G•C             A•U
          A•U                     A•U  1150       A•U
          U•A                     A•U             A•U
          G•C                     A•U             A•U
          A•U                     A•U             A•U
         GAA    AGT            UUG   UUU        CAG   UUU

         S. OLERACEA           N. DEBNEYI       E. COLI THR a
```

Figure 4. Stem and loop structure immediately preceeding the
           transcription termination sites of *tmpA* in *S. oleracea*
           and *N. debneyi* in comparison with that of an *E. coli*
           gene[9]. The numbers indicate the position of the
           nucleotides relative to the methionine initiation codon.

integrated with those of the two amino acid residues on either
side, a pattern emerges of a number of hydrophobic regions
interspersed with hydrophilic ones. Fig. 2 shows this pattern in
comparison with a stroma-located polypeptide. The clustering of
the hydrophobic residues indicates that the polypeptide is not
completely embedded in the thylakoid membrane but that it is
partly exposed. This is in accord with the finding that trypsin
digestion of thylakoid membranes gives only partial cleavage of
the "32,000-Mr" polypeptide suggesting that a number of the
arginine residues are not accessible to the enzyme[5].

     The site of initiation of transcription of *tmpA* in spinach
was determined by S1 mapping to be about 86 bp prior to translation
initiation. Just upstream from this initiation site is a typical
procaryote-like Pribnow box, while around 20 bp further upstream
is a sequence resembling the consensus sequence of the -35 bp
region of *E. coli* promoters[9] (Fig. 3).

     The mRNA for *tmpA*, identified by Northern blots, is 1.24 kb
long. Based on this, it is estimated that transcription terminates
80-90 bp distal to the translation stop codon. Immediately before

this position the sequence codes for an RNA which is capable of forming a stable stem and loop structure analogous to those involved in transcription termination in procaryotic genes[9] (Fig. 4).

CONCLUSION

The nucleotide sequence of the genes *(tmpA)* coding for a chloroplast membrane protein associated with photosystem II from both *Spinacia oleracea* and *Nicotiana debneyi* have been determined. The derived amino acid sequences from the two plants are identical. This total conservation between species from two different families indicates that there are severe constraints on the evolution of the primary structure of this polypeptide. The molecular weight of 38,950 for the protein derived from its deduced amino acid sequence is higher than has been reported. This difference could be due to anomalous behaviour on gel electro-phoresis caused by its hydrophobic nature.

The elucidation of the amino acid sequence of the polypeptide should facilitate the isolation and purification of the protein from chloroplasts and assist in further clarification of its function.

REFERENCES

[1] G.E. Blair and R.J. Ellis, Protein synthesis in chloroplasts 1. Light-driven synthesis of the large subunit of Fraction 1 protein by isolated pea chloroplasts, *Biochim. Biophys. Acta* 319: 223 (1973).

[2] W. Bottomley, D. Spencer and P.R. Whitfeld, Protein synthesis in isolated chloroplasts : Comparison of light-driven and ATP-driven synthesis, *Arch. Biochem. Biophys.* 164: 186 (1974).

[3] A.E. Grebanier, D.M. Coen, A. Rich and L. Bogorad, Membrane proteins synthesized but not processed by isolated maize chloroplasts, *J. Cell Biol.* 78: 734 (1978).

[4] M. Edelman and A. Reisfeld, Characterization, translation and control of the 32,000 dalton chloroplast membrane protein in *Spirodela, in* "Chloroplast Development" G. Akoyunoglou and J.H. Argyroudi-Akoyunoglou, eds. Elsevier North-Holland, Amsterdam, New York (1978).

[5] K.E. Steinback, L. McIntosh, L. Bogorad and C.J. Arntzen, Identification of the triazine receptor protein as a chloroplast gene product, *Proc. Natl. Acad. Sci. USA* 78: 7463 (1981).

[6] A.J. Driesel, J. Speirs and H.-J. Bohnert, Spinach chloroplast mRNA for a 32,000 dalton polypeptide. Size and localization on the physical map of the chloroplast DNA, *Biochem. Biophys. Acta* 610: 297 (1980).

7   M.R. Hartley, A. Wheeler and R.J. Ellis, Protein synthesis in
     chloroplasts V Translation of messenger RNA for the large
     subunit of Fraction 1 protein in a heterologous cell-free
     system, *J. Mol. Biol.* 91: 67 (1975).

8   G. von Heijne, On the hydrophobic nature of signal sequences,
     Eur. J. Biochem. 116: 419 (1981).

9   M. Rosenberg and D. Court, Regulatory sequences involved in the
     promotion and termination of RNA transcription, *Ann. Rev.
     Genet.* 13: 319 (1979).

A COMPENDIUM OF CHARACTERISTICS FOR THE RAPIDLY-METABOLIZED

32 KD PROTEIN OF THE CHLOROPLAST MEMBRANE

Marvin Edelman, Jonathan B. Marder and Autar K.
Mattoo*

Dept. of Plant Genetics, Weizmann Institute of
Science, Rehovot, ISRAEL and *Plant Hormone
Laboratory, USDA-ARC, BARC-W, Beltsville, MD
20705, USA

Our studies have concentrated on a 32 kd protein
partially surface exposed at the photosynthetic membranes of
the aquatic angiosperm, **Spirodela oligorrhiza**. This protein
is encoded and translated within the chloroplast as a 33.5
kd precursor polypeptide. Processing to the 32 kd form
occurs **in vivo** on the membrane and commences only after
completion of the 33.5 kd polypeptide chain [28].
Polypeptide fragments, obtained following sequential
proteolyses by several enzymes, have been aligned to give a
proteolytic map of the 33.5 kd precursor protein. The short
maturation fragment was found at the end of the hydrophylic
portion of the molecule, which extends beyond the thylakoid
membrane. In comparisons involving rapidly-labelled 32 kd
polypeptides from chloroplast membranes of various
angiosperms and the alga Chlamydomonas, a broad distribution
and high degree of similarity was found at levels of
precursor maturation, membrane orientation and primary
structure [19]. On the other hand, a number of surface-
exposed thylakoid polypeptides exist, at various levels of
abundancy, with mobilities in SDS-polyacrylamide gels very
similar to that of the rapidly-metabolized 32 kd polypeptide
[1,13,16,21,23,30]. The protein we are studying is the
product of the "32 kd gene" mapping in the large, unique-
copy region of chloroplast DNA adjacent to one of the
inverted repeats [34]. A list of distinguishing
characteristics for the rapidly-metabolized 32 kd protein is
given in Table I. It is hoped that this will be of some help
to those faced with problems of polypeptide identification.

Table I. Some distinguishing characteristics for the rapidly-metabolized 32 kd protein.

Characteristic	Organism and references
DNA	
1. Gene maps just distal to one of the inverted repeats in the large single-copy region of chloroplast DNA.	Chlamydomonas [20], Oenothera [a], maize [2], mustard [18], Spirodela [34], spinach [6], tobacco [b]
2. Gene hybridizes to 14.5 S (500 kd) chloroplast RNA.	Chlamydomonas [20], spinach [6], Spirodela [34,b], tobacco [b]
3. Cloned gene linked to the 32 kd protein by _in vitro_ transcription /translation.	Chlamydomonas [20], maize [3], spinach [6], Spirodela [b], tobacco [b]
mRNA	
1. Poly A⁻., ~500 kd (14 S).	Chlamydomonas [20], Spinach [6], Spirodela [27,29], tobacco [37]
2. Associated with thylakoid-bound 70 S polysomes.	pea [11], tobacco [37]
3. Abundant transcript, accumulates during light-induced plastid maturation	maize [2], mustard [18], pea [31], spinach [32], Spirodela [8,36]

Characteristic	Organism and references
PROTEIN	
1. Major, rapidly-labeled thylakoid protein in mature light-grown plants: a) *in vivo*	Amaranthus [33], Brassica [21], Bromus [21], Chenopodium [21], Chlamydomonas [5,19], maize [14,19], pea [31], Solanum [21], spinach [32], Spirodela [9,19,28], tobacco [19]
b) *in organello*	Acetabularia [15], Euglena [35], lettuce [19], maize [13,14], pea [7,19,31,33], spinach [4,24,32], tobacco [17]
2. Low steady-state amount (rapid turnover)	Bromus [21], Chenopodium [21], pea [12], Solanum [21], spinach [32], Spirodela [8,10]
3. Remains tightly bound to thylakoid membrane after salt or EDTA washes.	pea [7], Spirodela [26]
4. Surface-exposed on membrane; mild trypsinization leaves characteristic embedded fragments (20 and 18 kd approx.)	Amaranthus [33], brassica [21], Bromus [19,21], Chenopodium [21], maize [13], pea [19,33], Solanum [19], Spirodela [19,22], tobacco [19]

(continued)

Table I (continued)

Characteristic	Organism and references
5. Highly-conserved partial-proteolytic (Cleveland) patterns.	Brassica [21], Bromus [21], Chenopodium [21], Chlamydomonas [19], lettuce [19], maize [13,19], pea [19], Solanum [21], Spirodela [19,28], tobacco [19]
6. Lacks lysine residues: a) [3H]-amino acid labelling	Spirodela [9,28]
b) decoded gene sequence	spinach [a]
7. Photoaffinity labels with azido-atrazine.	Amaranthus [25], pea [33]
8. Derives from a slightly larger precursor: a) in vivo	Spirodela [9,28]
b) in organello	lettuce [c], maize [13], pea [12,19]
c) in vitro	maize [2], Spirodela [9,28], tobacco [19]

a. H. Bohnert (personal communication).   b. R. Fluhr and M. Edelman (unpublished).
c. A.K. Mattoo, Z. Kahane and M. Edelman (unpublished).

REFERENCES

1. Astier, C. and Joset-Espardellier, F. (1981) FEBS Lett.
    129, 47-51.
2. Bedbrook, J.R., Link, G., Coen, D.M., Bogorad, L. and
    Rich, A. (1978) Proc. Natl. Acad. Sci. USA. 75,
    3060-3064.
3. Bogorad, L., Jolly, S.O., Kidd, G,. Link, G. and
    McIntosh, L. (1980) in: Genome Organization and
    Expression in Plants (ed. Leaver, C.J.), Plenum
    Press, New York pp. 291-304.
4. Bottomley, W., Spencer, D. and Whitfeld, P.R. (1974)
    Arch. Biochem. Biophys. 164, 106-117.
5. Chua, N-H., and Gillham, N.W. (1977) J. Cell Biol.
    74,441-452.
6. Driesel, A.J., Spiers, J. and Bonhert, H.J. (1980)
    Biochim. Biophys. Acta 610, 297-310
7. Eaglesham, A.R.J. and Ellis, R.J. (1974) Biochim.
    Biophys. Acta 335, 396-407.
8. Edelman, M., Mattoo, A.K. and Marder, J.B. (1982) in:
    Chloroplast Biogenesis (ed. Ellis, R.J.) Cambridge
    Univ. Press (in press)
9. Edelman, M. and Reisfeld, A. (1978) in: Chloroplast
    Development (eds. Akoyunoglou, G. and Argyroudi-
    Akoyunoglou, J.H.) Elsevier/North Holland,
    Amsterdam pp.641-652.
10. Edelman, M. and Reisfeld, A. (1980) in: Genome
    Organization and Expression in Plants (ed. Leaver,
    C.J.), Plenum Press, New York pp. 353-362.
11. Ellis, R.J. (1977) Biochim. Biophys. Acta, 463,
    185-215.
12. Ellis, R.J. (1981) Ann. Rev. Plant Physiol. 32,
    111-137.
13. Grebanier, A.E., Coen, D.M., Rich, A. and Bogorad, L.
    (1978) J. Cell Biol. 78, 734-746.
14. Grebanier, A.E., Steinback, K.E. and Bogorad, L. (1979)
    Plant Physiol. 63, 436-439.
15. Green, B. (1980) Biochim. Biophys. Acta 609, 107-120.
16. Kuwabara, T. and Murata, N. (1979) Biochim. Biophys.
    Acta 581, 228-236.
17. Lescure, A-M. (1980) Plant Sci. Lett. 19, 181-191.
18. Link, G. (1982) Planta 154, 81-86.
19. Hoffman-Falk, H., Mattoo, A.K., Marder, J.B., Edelman,
    M. and Ellis, R.J. (1982) J. Biol. Chem. 257,
    4583-4587.

20. Malnoe, P., Rochaix, J.D., Chua, N-H. and Spahr, P.F.
     (1979) J. Mol. Biol. 133, 417-434.
21. Mattoo, A.K., Marder, J.B., Gressel, J. and Edelman, M.
     (1982) FEBS Lett. 140, 36-40.
22. Mattoo, A.K., Pick, U., Hoffman-Falk, H and Edelman, M.
     (1981) Proc. Natl. Acad. Sci. USA. 78, 1572-1576.
23. Metz, J. and Bishop, N.I. (1980) Biochem. Biophys. Res.
     Commun. 94, 560-566.
24. Morgenthaler, J.J. and Mendiola-Morgenthaler, L. (1976)
     Arch. Biochem. Biophy. 172, 51-58.
25. Pfister, K. Steinback, K.E., Gardner, G. and Ar.tzen,
     C.J. (1981) Proc. Natl. Acad. Sci. USA. 78, 981-985.
26. Reisfeld, A., Gressel, J., Jakob, K.M. and Edelman, M.
     (1978) Photochem. Photobiol. 27, 161-165.
27. Reisfeld, A., Jacob, K.M. and Edelman, M. (1978) in:
     Chloroplast Development (eds. Akoyunoglou, G. and
     Argyroudi-Akoyunoglou, J.H.) Elsevier/North Holland,
     Amsterdam pp.669-674.
28. Reisfeld, A., Mattoo, A.K. and Edelman, M. (1982) Eur.
     J. Biochem. 124, 125-129.
29. Rosner, A., Reisfeld, A., Jakob, K.M., Gressel, J. and
     Edelman, M. (1977) in: Acides Nucleiques et Synthese
     des Proteines chez les Vegetaux (eds. Bogorad, L.
     and Weil, J.H.) pp. 305-311. C.N.R.S., Paris.
30. Shochat, S., Owens, G.C., Hubert, P. and Ohad, I.
     (1982) Biochim. Biophys. Acta (in press).
31. Siddell, S.G. and Ellis, R.J. (1975) Biochem. J. 146,
     675-685.
32. Silverthorne, J. and Ellis, R.J. (1980) Biochim.
     Biophys. Acta 607, 319-330.
33. Steinback, K.E., McIntosh, L., Bogorad, L. and Arntzen,
     C.J. (1981) Proc. Natl. Acad. Sci. USA. 78,
     7463-7467.
34. Van Ee, J.H. (1981) Ph.D Thesis (Univ. Amsterdam),
     Amsterdam, Holland.
35. Vasconcelos, A.C. (1976) Plant Physiol. 58,719-721.
36. Weinbaum, S.A., Gressel, J., Reisfeld, A. and Edelman,
     M. (1979) Plant Physiol. 64, 828-832.
37. Wollgiehn, R., Lerbs, S. and Munsche, D. (1978)
     Biochem. Physiol. Pflanz. 173, 60-69.

ORGANIZATION AND STRUCTURE OF THE GENES FOR THE β AND ε SUBUNITS

OF SPINACH AND PEA CHLOROPLAST ATPase

P.R. Whitfeld, G. Zurawski[*] and W. Bottomley

CSIRO, Division of Plant Industry, P.O. Box 1600
Canberra City, A.C.T. 2601, Australia

INTRODUCTION

Chloroplast ATPase (CF_1) is composed of five subunits, three of which (α,β and ε) are synthesized within the chloroplast (see (1) for references) and coded by chloroplast genes (2). The γ and δ subunits are synthesized in the cytoplasm and are presumed to be coded by nuclear genes (see (1) for references). The genes for the β and ε subunits map close to the gene *(rbcL)* for the large subunit of ribulose bisphosphate carboxylase but the gene for the α subunit is located some 40 kb away on the spinach chloroplast DNA (cpDNA) map (2). In this paper we report the results of our investigations into the structure and organization of the genes for the β and ε subunits of ATPase from *Spinacia oleracea* and *Pisum sativum* chloroplasts.

RESULTS AND DISCUSSION

In spinach cpDNA the *rbcL* gene lies at one end of *BamH1* fragment 3 (BF3) (3). When sequences from BF3 adjacent to the 5' end of *rbcL* were hybridized to size fractionated spinach chloroplast RNA bound to diazotized paper, three high molecular weight bands (2.4, 2.6, 2.8 kb) were detected (Fig. 1). The three species were shown to be transcribed from the same region of BF3 and from the same DNA strand, the different sizes being attributable to differences at the 5' end of the RNA. It is not known whether they reflect the existence of several transcription start sites or post-transcriptional processing of the RNA. Only one RNA species

---

* DNAX Research Institute, Palo Alto, Calif. 94304 U.S.A.

(2.4 kb) was detected when pea chloroplast RNA was hybridized with the same probe (Fig. 1). These experiments showed that the region adjacent to *rbcL* was transcriptionally active and that the direction of transcription of the large RNAs was divergent with respect to transcription of *rbcL* (3). The organization of this region in spinach and pea thus resembles the organization of the region in maize cpDNA that codes for *rbcL* and an adjacent 2.2 kb RNA (4).

Transcription-translation in an *in vitro E. coli* S30 system of the 2 kb region adjacent to *rbcL* on BF3 yielded a number of poly-peptides. The largest of these products co-migrated with the β subunit of ATPase on 2-dimensional gel analysis (5). The smaller products probably resulted from premature termination of translation.

The sequence of the segment of BF3 encoding the large RNA transcript was determined (5). There was only one open reading large enough to code for the 52000-M_r β subunit of ATPase. The derived amino acid composition of the 498 residue protein agreed closely with the composition determined (6) for the β subunit of spinach chloroplast ATPase. Furthermore, the deduced amino acid sequence showed 67% homology with the sequence of the β subunit of *E. coli* ATPase (7) and it was concluded that this DNA sequence was the *atpB* gene.

A second open reading frame in this sequence had the same polarity as *atpB* but was read in a different reading frame and was identified as the gene for the ε subunit of ATPase *(atpE)* on the following grounds. The size and derived amino acid composition of this 134 residue protein is very similar to the size and composi-tion determined (6) for the ε subunit of spinach chloroplast ATPase. The deduced amino acid sequence also has significant homology (26%) with the sequence of the ε subunit of *E. coli* ATPase (7). Finally it is known that the ε subunit gene maps close to *atpB* (2).

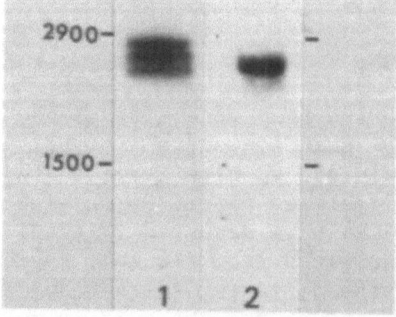

Fig. 1.   Hybridization of sequences adjacent to *rbcL* to size-frac-
          tionated chloroplast RNA from 1, spinach and 2, pea. Auto-
          radiograph of a 'Northern blot'. The numbers indicate the
          positions to which chloroplast ribosomal RNAs migrated.

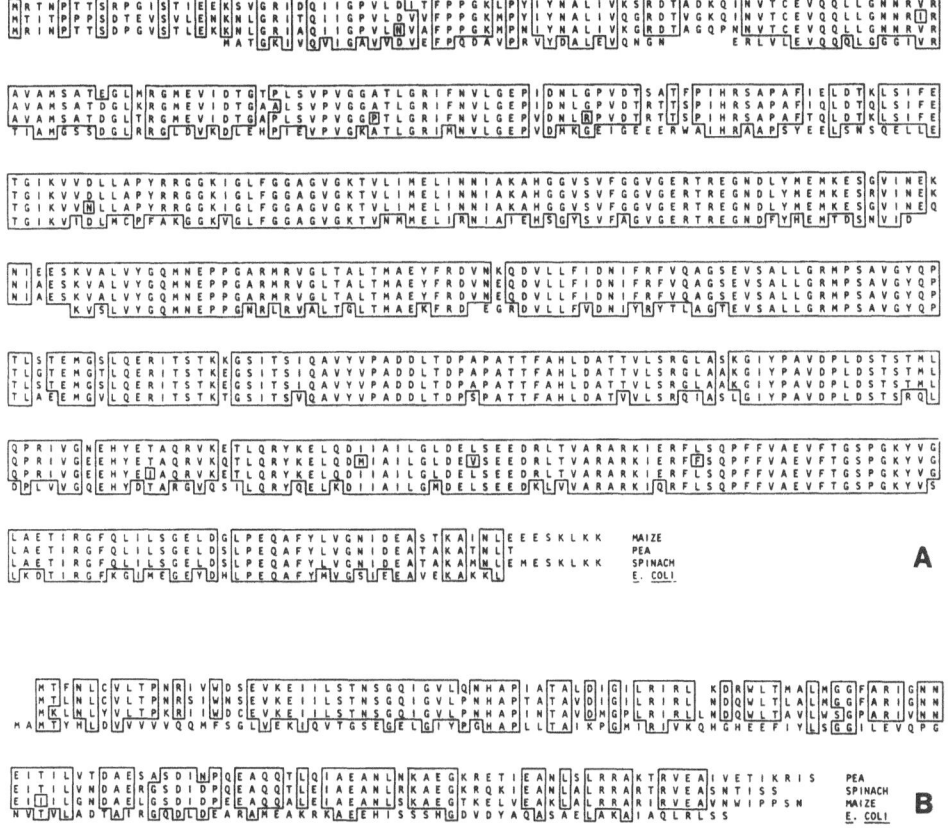

Fig. 2.   Comparison of the amino acid sequences of A, the β subunit
          and B, the ε subunit of ATPase from spinach, pea and maize
          (8) chloroplasts and from *E. coli* (7).

Analysis of the equivalent region of pea cpDNA showed the
genes for the β subunit and the ε subunit to contain 491 and 136
codons respectively.   The deduced amino acid sequences of the β
and ε subunits from spinach and pea are compared in Fig. 2 with the
corresponding sequences from maize chloroplast (8) and *E. coli* (7)
ATPases.   82% of the β subunit residues are conserved between the
three plant species, the pea and maize being the most divergent
(85% homology) and the spinach and pea being the most conserved
(89%).   Analysis of the variation in the level of homology along
the molecule shows the amino terminal third and the extreme carboxyl
end are subject to fewer constraints in sequence specificity than
elsewhere in the molecule.   This is particularly apparent in the
comparison with the sequence of the *E. coli* protein (Fig. 2A).

In the case of the ε subunit, the pea and maize sequences also are least conserved (67% homology) and the spinach and pea sequences the most conserved (81%) with 64% of all residues being conserved between the three plant species. Here also the homology is least at the carboxyl end of the molecule (Fig. 2B). The divergence of the spinach and pea amino acid sequences at the carboxyl terminus can be seen to result from the deletion of a 5 bp and a 6 bp nucleotide sequence each of which occurs as a direct repeat in the pea sequence but is present in only one copy in the spinach sequence (Fig. 3).

The greater conservation of the β subunit relative to that of the ε subunit probably reflects a basic difference in the roles the two subunits play in the ATPase complex. The β subunit is involved in the catalytic reaction and has sites for binding Mg^{++} and nucleotides. Constraints on its amino acid sequence may therefore be fairly severe. The ε subunit on the other hand has only a structural and perhaps regulatory role and constraints on its sequence appear to be far less demanding.

The coding regions assigned to the β and ε subunits of spinach ATPase have four nucleotides in common. The third nucleotide (A) of the terminal lysine codon together with the TG of the TGA stop codon of the β subunit comprise the ATG methionine translation initiation codon of the ε subunit (Fig. 4). Although the β and ε subunit genes of maize chloroplast ATPase also overlap (8), this arrangement is not a feature of the organization of these genes from all species. The β and ε subunit genes of pea are separated by 20 bp (Fig. 4). Comparison of the spinach and pea nucleotide sequences across the junction shows that overall they are highly conserved and the basis for the different amino acid sequence lies simply in the fact that in spinach one copy of a 5 bp sequence (ACTTA) which occurs as a direct tandem repeat in pea has been deleted (Fig. 4). This removes the stop codon which functions in pea and translation continues for another 7 codons in spinach before another stop codon is reached.

```
ε SUBUNIT THR  ARG  VAL  GLU  ALA  SER                          ASN  THR  ILE  SER  SER  END
SPINACH   A C·A·C·G·A·G·T·C·G·A·G·G·C·T·A·G·C·                  A A·T·A·C·G·A·T·T·C·T·T·C·G·T·A·A·C·C·A·G·T·C
PEA       A C·A·C·G·A·G·T·A·G·A·G·G·C·T·A·T·C·G·T·A·G·A·G·A·C·T·A·T·C·A·A·G·A·G·G·A·T·C·T·C·C·T·A·A·    C A A G T T
ε SUBUNIT THR  ARG  VAL  GLU  ALA  ILE  VAL  GLU  THR  ILE  LYS  ARG  ILE  SER  END
```

Fig. 3.   Nucleotide and amino acid sequence at the carboxyl terminus of the ε subunit of spinach and pea chloroplast ATPase. Sequences are aligned to maximize the homology. The arrows denote two sequences each of which occurs as a direct repeat in pea but only once in spinach.

```
                                                    MET   THR   LEU  ASN  ε SUBUNIT
β SUBUNIT  MET  ASN  LEU       GLU  MET  GLU  SER  LYS  LEU  LYS  LYS  END
SPINACH    A T G·A A C·T T A·        G A A·T|G·G A G|A G C·A A A·T T A·A A G·A A A·T G·A C C·T T A·A A T·
PEA        A C G·A A C·T T A·A C T·T A G·A A A T|G G A G|A A C A A A T T C A A G A A·A T G·A C T·T T T·A A T·
β SUBUNIT  THR  ASN  LEU  THR  END                        MET   THR   PHE   ASN  ε SUBUNIT
```

Fig. 4.   Nucleotide and amino acid sequences across the junction of
           the β and ε subunits of spinach and pea showing the overlap-
           ping translation stop/start codons in the spinach sequence.
           The sequences have been aligned to maximize the homology. The
           arrows denote a 5 bp sequence which occurs as a direct repeat
           in pea. A possible ribosome binding site is boxed with a
           broken line.

     In both spinach and pea, sequences specific to the *atpE* gene
hybridize to the same large RNA species as do sequences specific
for the *atpB* gene. No indication of a smaller RNA species
hybridizing to *atpE* sequences was seen. Thus the two genes are
co-transcribed into a single RNA and, although we have not
explicitly demonstrated that both subunits are translated from the
same RNA species, it would seem highly probable that the
transcript is functioning as a dicistronic mRNA in the chloroplast.
In the case of spinach, ribosomes translating the *b* subunit may
traverse the overlapping stop/start codons without dissociating from
the mRNA but, in the case of pea, ribosomes must bind to the mRNA
between the β and ε coding regions and it is interesting to note
that there is a Shine-Dalgarno (9) sequence (GGAG) located 14
nucleotides prior to the ε subunit initiation codon in both pea
and spinach (Fig. 4).

     S1 nuclease mapping of the 5' ends of *atpB* shows that the
untranslated leader sequence is 454 bp in spinach and 351 bp in pea.
Compared to the extensive homology in the protein coding regions,
the 5' untranslated sequences are poorly conserved. However, a
48 bp sequence (-42 to +6 relative to the transcription
initiation point) is well conserved (85% homology). This 48 bp
segment includes sequences which are similar to the consensus
sequence of *E. coli* promoters (Pribnow box and '-35' recognition
site) (10) lending support to our previous contention (3) that the
sequences to which chloroplast RNA polymerase binds probably
resemble those recognized by *E. coli* polymerase.

CONCLUSION

     Analysis of a 2.4 kb region of spinach and pea cpDNA adjacent
to the 5' end of *rbcL* has shown that it contains the genes for the
β and ε subunits of chloroplast ATPase. The two genes are
cotranscribed into a dicistronic RNA and the translation stop/start
codons overlap in the case of the spinach genes but not in the
case of the pea genes. Comparison of the spinach and pea protein

sequences shows the β subunits have 89% homology while the ε
subunits have 81% homology.

REFERENCES

1.   Ellis, R.J., Chloroplast proteins : synthesis transport and
     assembly. *Annu. Rev. Plant Physiol.* 32: 111 (1981).
2.   Westhoff, P., Nelson, N., Bünemann, H. and Herrmann, R.G.,
     Localization of genes for coupling factor subunits on the
     spinach plastid chromosome. *Current Genet.* 4: 109 (1981).
3.   Zurawski, G., Perrot, B., Bottomley, W. and Whitfeld, P.R.,
     The structure of the gene for the large subunit of ribulose
     1,5-bisphosphate carboxylase from spinach chloroplast DNA.
     Nucleic Acids Res. 9: 3251 (1981).
4.   Link, G. and Bogorad, L., Sizes, locations and directions
     of transcription of two genes on a cloned maize chloroplast
     DNA sequence. *Proc. Natl. Acad. Sci. USA* 77: 1832 (1980).
5.   Zurawski, G., Bottomley, W. and Whitfeld, P.R., Structure
     of the genes for the β and ε subunits of spinach chloroplast
     ATPase indicates a dicistronic mRNA and an overlapping
     translation stop/start signal. *Proc. Natl. Acad. Sci. USA*
     In Press.
6.   Binder, A., Jagendorf, A. and Ngo, E., Isolation and
     composition of the subunits of spinach chloroplast coupling
     factor protein. *J. Biol. Chem.* 253: 3094 (1978).
7.   Saraste, M., Gay, N.J., Eberle, A., Runswick, M.J. and
     Walker, J.E., The atp operon : nucleotide sequence of the
     genes for the γ,β and ε subunits of *Escherichia coli* ATP
     synthase. *Nucleic Acids Res.* 9: 5287 (1981).
8.   Krebbers, E.T., Larrinua, I.M., McIntosh, L., and Bogorad, L.,
     The maize chloroplast genes for the β and ε subunits of the
     photosynthetic coupling factor CF_1 are fused. *Nucleic Acids
     Res.* 10: 4985 (1982).
9.   Shine, J. and Dalgarno, L., Determinant of cistron specificity
     in bacterial ribosomes. *Nature* 254: 34 (1975).
10. Rosenberg, M. and Court, D., Regulatory sequences involved
     in the promotion and termination of RNA transcription.
     Annu. Rev. Genet. 13: 319 (1979).

CHLOROPLAST EF-Tu IS CODED IN SPINACH CHLOROPLAST DNA

Orio Ciferri, Orsola Tiboni and Giuseppe Di Pasquale

Institute of Microbiology and Plant Physiology
University of Pavia, Pavia, Italy

INTRODUCTION

Chloroplasts contain elongation factors for protein synthesis different from the corresponding factors involved in cytoplasmic and mitochondrial protein synthesis[1]. Previously, we have demonstrated that chloroplast elongation factor G is synthesized in the organelle in <u>Chlorella vulgaris</u>[2] and that this factor, as well as elongation factor Tu ($EF-Tu_{chl}$), are synthesized in spinach chloroplasts[3]. In addition, preliminary results were presented suggesting that the two elongation factors are coded in spinach chloroplast DNA[4]. We present now a more rigorous evidence that $EF-Tu_{chl}$ is coded in the organellar DNA.

RESULTS

When spinach chloroplast DNA is trascribed and translated <u>in vitro</u> in a system from <u>E. coli</u>, a number of radioactive bands may be separated by SDS-polyacrylamide gel electrophoresis. As shown in Fig. 1 (lanes 2 and 3), one of these bands has the same mobility of the large subunit of ribulose-1,5-bisphosphate carboxylase (LS) whereas another migrates in the same position of authentic $EF-Tu_{chl}$ (Tu). The intensity of the radioactive bands depends on the amount of chloroplast DNA present in the reaction mixture and, furthermore, such bands are absent from the control

199

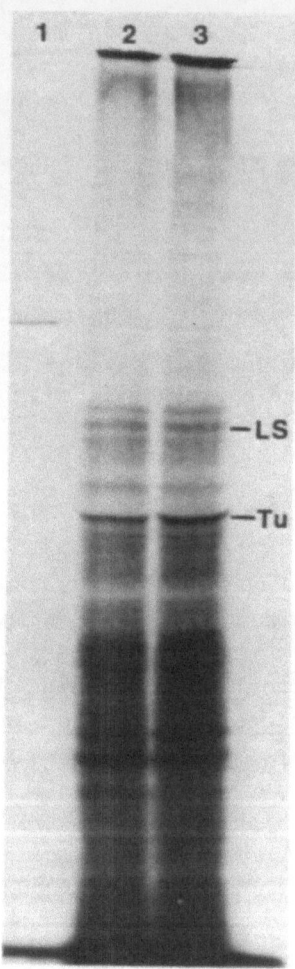

Fig. 1 <u>Autoradiograph of labelled peptides synthesized on tran-
scription/translation of spinach chloroplast DNA</u>
    Chloroplast DNA was transcribed and translated <u>in vitro</u> in a
system from <u>E. coli</u> in the presence of [^{35}S]-methionine. The
products were separated by electrophoresis in 10% polyacrylamide
gels in the presence of SDS.
1. preincubated <u>E. coli</u> extract, no addition
2.   "   "   "   + 2 µg of spinach chloroplast DNA
3.   "   "   "   + 4 µg of spinach chloroplast DNA

in which no chloroplast DNA was added to the pre-incubated E. coli extract (Fig. 1, lane 1). It is important to stress that if the E. coli extract is not pre-incubated with micrococcal nuclease, a heavily radioactive band with the same mobility of EF-Tu$_{chl}$ is evident even if no chloroplast DNA is added. This band is that of the endogenously-synthesized E. coli EF-Tu. Since the two factors have the same molecular weight[5], it is impossible to separate the two proteins by gel electrophoresis (see also Fig. 2, lanes 1 and 2).

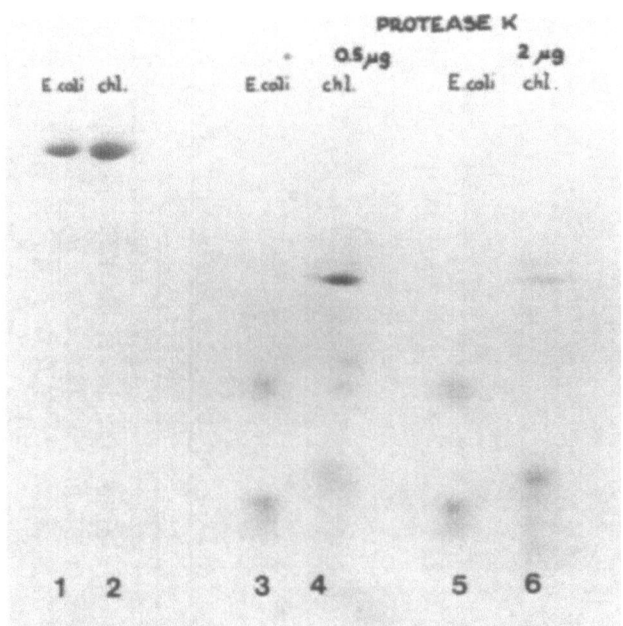

Fig. 2 Maps of the partial proteolytic digestion of EF-Tu from E. coli and spinach chloroplasts.

    Purified, unlabelled EF-Tu from E. coli and spinach chloroplasts were digested with protease K as reported[6].

1. untreated E. coli EF-Tu (2 μg)
2. untreated EF-Tu$_{chl}$ (4 μg)
3,5. digested E. coli EF-Tu
4,6. digested EF-Tu$_{chl}$

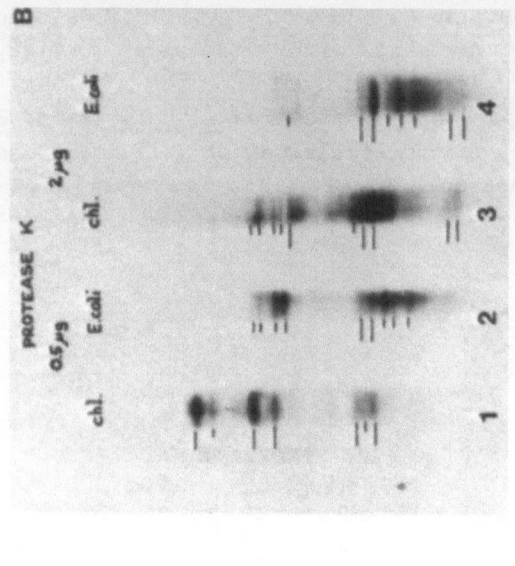

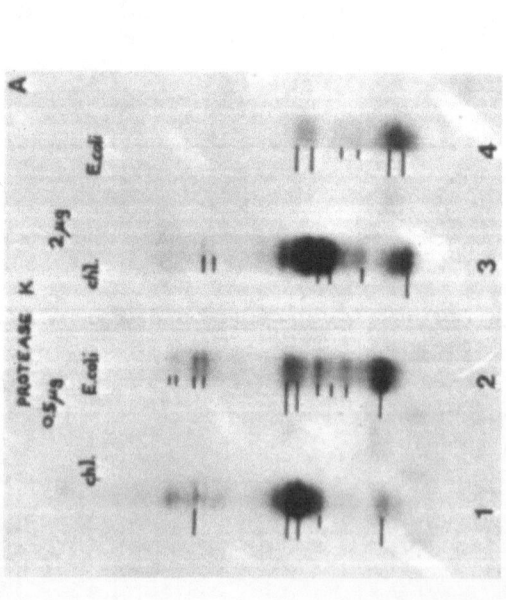

Fig. 3 Partial proteolytic maps of E. coli EF-Tu and EF-Tu chl synthesized in vitro in the presence of labelled methionine or leucine.

Labelled EF-Tu from either E. coli or spinach chloroplasts synthesized in a E. coli system was recovered and digested with protease K as reported.
A.[S^{35}]-labelled proteins: 1,3. EF-Tu$_{chl}$;2,4. E. coli EF-Tu
B.[H^3]-labelled proteins: 1,3. EF-Tu$_{chl}$;2,4. E.coli EF-Tu
    Long and short bars correspond to the major or minor bands stained with Coomassie blue.

Partial proteolytic digestion of the purified, unlabelled EF-Tu from E. coli and spinach chloroplasts reveals that they are different proteins. When digested with protease K, E. coli EF-Tu gives rise to 4 prominent peptide bands (Fig. 2, lanes 3 and 5) whereas in the case of EF-Tu$_{chl}$ 6 to 8 bands are evident. The majority of the peptide bands produced on digestion of EF-Tu$_{chl}$ have mobilities that differ from those of the bands observed in the case of E. coli EF-Tu. Thus it is possible to compare the peptide profiles obtained from the two EF-Tu synthesized in vitro. (It must be born in mind that the same mobility of the two proteins precludes for EF-Tu$_{chl}$ the possibility of comparing the radioactive and the stain profiles in the same experiment). As depicted in Fig. 3, the patterns of radioactive bands produced by digestion of the two EF-Tu are different one from the other but show a good correlation with the stained pattern obtained digesting the authentic, unlabelled proteins. This is evident when either [S^{35}]-methionine (Fig. 3A) or [H^3]-leucine (Fig. 3B) were utilized as labelled amino acid. The incomplete match between some radioactive and stained bands may be due to the presence of radioactive proteins contaminating the labelled EF-Tu synthesized in vitro. In addition, it must be remembered that the digestion of labelled EF-Tu$_{chl}$ was always performed in the presence of the large excess of the unlabelled E. coli EF-Tu present in the extracts.

CONCLUSIONS

The above reported data confirm for EF-Tu$_{chl}$ our previous findings that chloroplast elongation factors are synthesized and coded in spinach chloroplasts[3,4]. Recently it has been reported that also in Euglena gracilis EF-Tu$_{chl}$ is synthesized in the organelle[7]. Further, presumptive evidence for a chloroplastic codification of EF-Tu$_{chl}$ in Chlamydomonas reinhardii has been also presented[8].

ACKNOWLEDGEMENTS

This work was supported by grants from Consiglio Nazionale delle Ricerche.

REFERENCES

1. O. Ciferri, O. Tiboni, M.L. Munoz-Calvo and G. Camerino, Protein synthesis in plants: specificy and role of the cytoplasmic and organellar systems, in "Nucleic acids and protein synthesis in plants", L. Bogorad and J.H. Weil, eds., p. 155 Plenum, New York, 1977.
2. O. Ciferri, and O. Tiboni, Evidence for the synthesis in the chloroplast of elongation factor G, Plant Sci. Lett. 7: 455 (1976).
3. O. Ciferri, G. Di Pasquale and O. Tiboni, Chloroplast elongation factors are synthesized in the chloroplast, Eur. J. Biochem. 102: 331 (1979).
4. O. Ciferri, O. Tiboni, G. Di Pasquale and D. Carbonera, Site of synthesis and codification of chloroplast elongation factors, in "Genome organization and expression in plants", C.J. Leaver, ed., Plenum, New York, p. 373 (1980).
5. O. Tiboni, G. Di Pasquale, and O. Ciferri, Purification of the elongation factors present in spinach chloroplasts, Eur. J. Biochem. 92: 471 (1978).
6. D. W. Cleveland, S. G. Fisher, and M. W. Kirschner, and U. K. Laemmli, Peptide mapping by limited proteolysis in sodium dodecyl sulfate and analysis by gel electrophoresis J. Biol. Chem. 252: 1102 (1977).
7. L. L. Spremulli, Chloroplast elongation factor Tu: evidence that it is the product of a chloroplast gene in Euglena, Arch. Biochem. Biophys. 214: 734 (1982).
8. J. C. Watson, and S. J. Surzycki, Extensive sequence homology in the DNA coding for elongation factor Tu from Escherichia coli and the Chlamydomonas reinhardtii chloroplast, Proc. Natl. Acad. Sci. U.S.A. 79: 2264 (1982).

CHLOROPLAST GENES AND TRANSFORMATION IN CHLAMYDOMONAS

J.-D. Rochaix, M. Dron, M. Rahire,
J.-M. Boissel and J. van Dillewijn

Départements de Biologie Moléculaire
et Biologie Végétale
Université de Genève, 1211 Geneva, Switzerland

The green unicellular alga Chlamydomonas reinhardii is particularly well suited for studying the function of the chloroplast genome since this organism can be manipulated with ease both at the biochemical and genetic level. Indeed, C. reinhardii is to date the only organism in which an analysis of chloroplast gene recombination is feasible. Most of the numerous chloroplast mutants which have been isolated are affected in some photosynthetic function or are resistant to antibiotics which inhibit translation on chloroplast ribosomes. Several of these mutations have been mapped and a chloroplast linkage group has been established (cf. Gillham, 1978). During the last years several chloroplast genes have been identified and localized on the chloroplast DNA restriction map of C. reinhardii (cf. Rochaix, 1981). They include the genes coding for chloroplast rRNAs, several tRNAs and the genes coding for abundant chloroplast polypeptides such as the large subunit of ribulose bisphosphate carboxylase (LS), several thylakoid polypeptides and elongation factor Tu (Watson and Surzycki, 1981). While biochemical techniques are powerful for isolating and characterizing genes of this sort, other methods may be required for studying chloroplast genes which are poorly expressed. Coupling the genetic and biochemical studies appears to be a promising new approach in this respect. However, two important conditions will have to be fulfilled before this approach becomes feasible. First, the physical and genetic maps of the chloroplast genome need to be correlated; and second, a method has to be developed to introduce chloroplast genes, or at least their products, into chloroplasts. Here we wish to review some recent work in our laboratory which bears on these two problems.

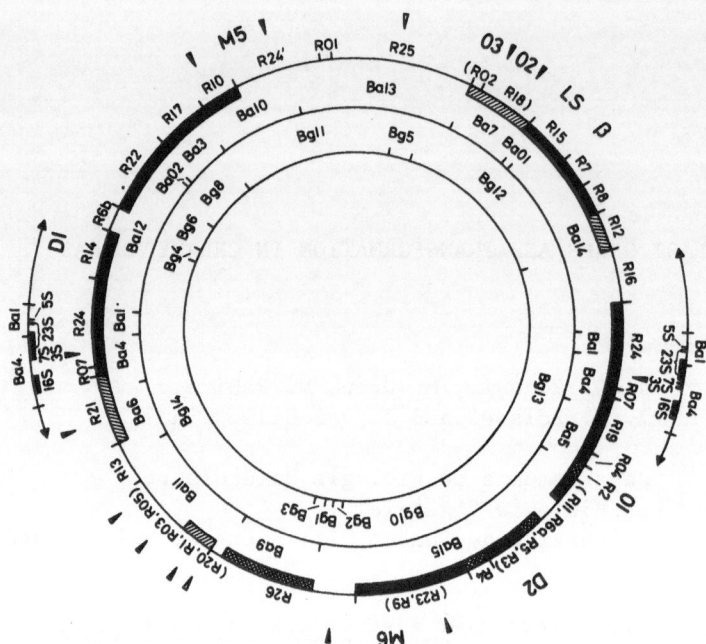

Fig. 1.   Restriction map of the chloroplast genome of C. reinhardii.
The EcoRI, BamHI and BglII fragments are shown on the outer,
middle and inner circles, resp. (Rochaix, 1978). The two
ribosomal regions are indicated. The locations of the genes
coding for LS, β subunit of coupling factor and the membrane polypeptides D1, D2, M5 and M6 are shown. The latter
two assignments are still tentative (Malnoë and Rochaix,
unpublished results). 01, 02 and 03 denote three putative
chloroplast replication origins (cf text).

The LS gene of C. reinhardii: a first correlation site between the
genetic and physical maps of the chloroplast genome.

        The chloroplast genome of C. reinhardii consists of 190 kb
circles. Fig. 1 shows the physical map of this genome with the genes
which have been identified to date. The two ribosomal regions oriented in opposite direction on the map contain – in the order of transcription – the genes of 16S, 7S, 3S, 23S and 5SrRNA (Rochaix and
Malnoë, 1978; Rochaix and Darlix, 1982). It is noticeable that the
chloroplast ribosomal units of C. reinhardii display two unusual
features, as compared with other plants. First, the 23SrRNA gene
contains an 870 bp intron, and two small rRNA genes coding for 3S
and 7S RNA are present near the 5' end of the 23SrRNA gene. In contrast to higher plants there is no 4.5SrRNA gene between the 23S
and 5SrRNA genes.

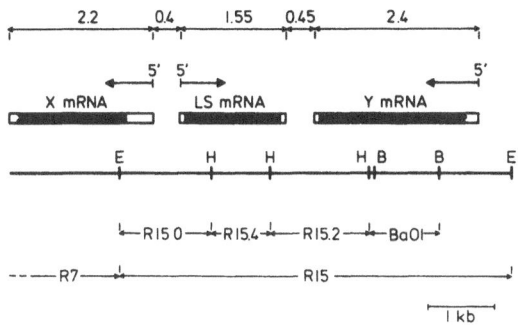

Fig. 2. Transcriptional
organization of
the LS gene
region of
C. reinhardii.

Recently we have examined the transcriptional organization and
the sequence of a 4 kb region of the chloroplast genome of C.
reinhardii (Fig. 2, Dron, Rahire and Rochaix, 1982). The region includes the LS gene and portions of two neighbouring genes X and Y
which are oriented in opposite direction relative to the LS gene.
The transcripts of the LS, X and Y genes are 1.6, 2.2 and 2.4 kb,
resp. We have noticed some limited amino acid sequence homology
between the N terminal part of X and the βATP synthase of E. coli
(Saraste et al, 1981). This is compatible with our earlier mapping
studies (Rochaix, 1981) and with the results obtained by others
(Westhoff et al., 1981; Jolly et al., 1981). The 5' untranslated
regions of the chloroplast mRNAs are variable in size: 51 ± 3 and
430 ± 10 bases for LS and X, resp. These regions are AT rich. The
410 bp spacer between the LS and X genes contains several repetitive
elements of the type TATTT(ATA). Sequences which are highly related
to the bacterial Pribnow box and the −35 box are found upstream from
the transcription initiation sites of the LS and X genes. Homologues
of the bacterial Shine-Dalgarno sequence can be found in the vicinity
of the AUG initiation codons (fig. 3). It is striking that the Shine-
Dalgarno sequence of the LS mRNA is unusually distant from the AUG
initiation codon (17 bases) and that the intervening bases can be
folded into a stem-loop structure (fig. 3).

The LS gene codes for a polypeptide of 475 amino acids whose
sequence diverges 13 to 14% from the LS amino acid sequences of
maize and spinach (McIntosh et al., 1980; Zurawski et al., 1981).
The corresponding gene sequences differ 23 to 25% from each other.
Most of the nucleotide differences occur in the third position of
the codons and in the 3' terminal portion of the gene. Only 40 different codons are used in the LS gene of C. reinhardii. The three
catalytic sites (Schloss et al., 1978), and the CO_2 activator
region (Lorimer, 1981) of the LS polypeptide have been highly conserved between C. reinhardii, maize and spinach.

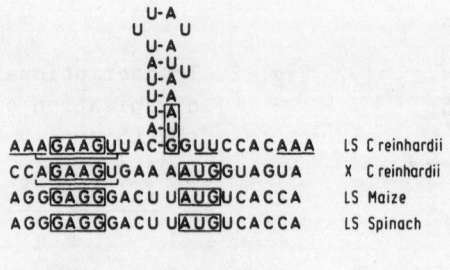

Fig. 3. Comparison of Shine-Dalgarno sequences of several chloroplast genes. The data of maize and spinach are from McIntosh et al. (1980) and Zurawski et al. (1981). The lower part of the figure shows the base complimentarity between the Shine-Dalgarno sequences of the LS gene of C. reinhardii and the 3' end of 16S rRNA.

Recently Spreitzer and Mets (1980) have isolated a uniparental mutant of C. reinhardii which appears to be specifically affected in LS. It has been shown that this mutation is linked to other uniparental markers of the chloroplast genetic map. (Mets and Geist, unpublished observations). In order to prove that this mutation is indeed located within the LS gene, a comparative sequence analysis of the entire wild type LS gene sequence and of the active domains of the mutant LS gene was performed. The latter was cloned and provided by L. Mets. It was found that the mutation is a single base-pair substitution in a region of the LS gene which corresponds to the first active domain of LS (fig. 4, Dron et al., 1982). The change involves a GC to AT transition so that the gly residue at position 171 is converted into an asp residue. The amino acid change is compatible with the observation that the mutant LS has a lower isoelectric point than the wild-type polypeptide (Spreitzer and Mets, 1980). This sequence analysis therefore establishes a first correlation site between the genetic and physical maps of the chloroplast genome of C. reinhardii.

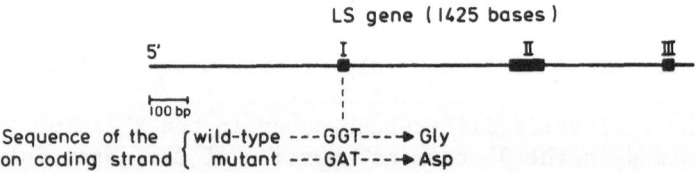

Fig. 4. Comparative sequence analysis of wild-type and a mutant LS gene of C. reinhardii. The LS gene with its active domains is represented by a horizontal line. The location and sequence of the mutated codon are shown.

Transformation in Chlamydomonas

We have recently been able to transform C. reinhardii, using
the arg 7 locus for selection (Rochaix and Van Dillewijn, 1982).
This locus codes for argininosuccinate lyase (Hudock, 1963) the
last enzyme of the arginine biosynthetic pathway, which converts
argininosuccinate into arginine and fumarate. Initially the yeast
plasmid pYearg4 (Clarke and Carbon, 1978), which carries the corresponding yeast locus, was used for transforming the cell wall deficient strain cw15 arg 7 (Davies and Plaskitt, 1971; Gillham, 1965).
Stable transformants containing integrated yeast DNA sequences could
be recovered, although with a low efficiency (of the order of 10^{-6}
transformants/treated cell).

The next step was to construct suitable transformation vectors.
Since no free plasmids (except chloroplast and mitochondrial DNA)
have been found in C. reinhardii, the following strategy was used
for constructing autonomously replicating plasmids (fig. 5). The
2.7 kb HindIII fragment of pYearg4 which carries the yeast arg 4
locus (Clarke and Carbon, 1978) and EcoRI treated pBR322 were made
flush ended with DNA polymerase and joined together by blunt end
ligation. The new plasmid pJD2 was used to clone HindIII and MboI
fragments from the nuclear, chloroplast and mitochondrial genomes

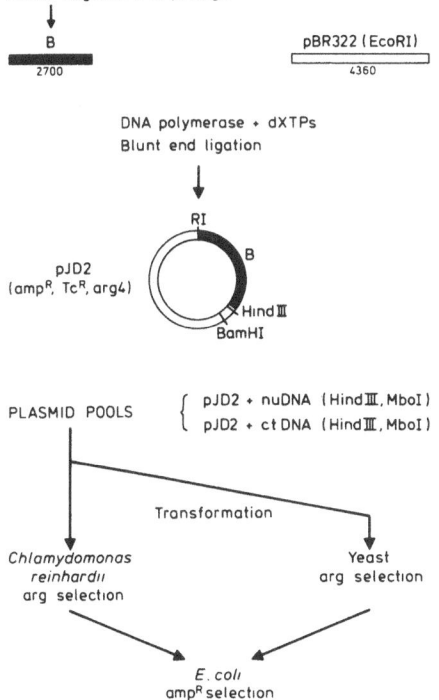

Fig. 5.
Strategy used for
constructing auto-
nomously replicating
plasmids in
C. reinhardii

of C. reinhardii. The insertion of these fragments into pJD2 was
checked by the loss of tetracycline resistance. Pools of about 100
hybrid plasmids were prepared and used for transforming C. reinhardii
using the arginine selection. The DNA of several transformants was
examined for the presence of free plasmids by Southern blot hybridization and by transformation of E. coli using either ampicillin or
arginine selection. Fig. 6 displays the hybridization results
obtained with two transformants. It can be seen that shortly after
the transformation event (slots a'+, a'⁻) the cells contain a large
amount of free plasmids of different sizes. At later times however
(slots b'+, b'⁻) the amount of free plasmids diminishes considerably
and only one major type of plasmid can be detected which is only
slightly larger than the pJD2 plasmid. Similar results were obtained
with the other transformant (cf. slots c'+, c'⁻ and d'+, d'⁻). These
data indicate that considerable deletions occur in these free plasmids. It is puzzling that the deleted DNA regions include mainly
C. reinhardii nuclear DNA and, to a much smaller extent, bacterial
DNA sequences of the plasmid.

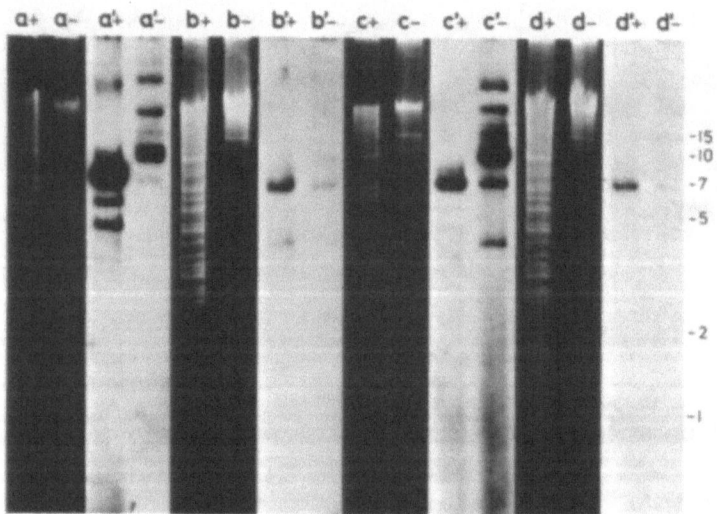

Fig. 6.   Free plasmid sequences in transformants of C. reinhardii.
          The DNAs of transformants I and II were extracted after
          25 (lanes a and c, resp.) and 60 generations (lanes b and
          e, resp.) after transformation. The EcoRI treated and un-
          digested DNAs were electrophoresed on agarose gels and
          stained with ethidium bromide (lanes + and -, resp.). The
          DNAs were transferred to nitrocellulose sheets (Southern,
          1975) and hybridized with ³²P-labelled pJD2 plasmid (lanes
          '+ and '-,). Sizes are indicated in kb.

Chloroplast and mitochondrial transformation is not yet feasible. However, Zakian (1981) has shown that a small mitochondrial
restriction fragment of Xenopus laevis which contains the mitochondrial DNA replication origin is able to promote autonomous replication in yeast. Since chloroplast replication origins may exhibit the
same behavior, hybrid plasmids consisting of pJD2 and chloroplast
DNA fragments were used to transform an arg 4 mutant of yeast (arg 4
in yeast corresponds to arg 7 in C. reinhardii). Yeast transformants
could be obtained readily; the DNAs from several of them were isolated and used to transform E. coli (usually by selection for ampicillin resistance) in order to recover the free plasmids. The latter
can be ordered into three distinct classes according to their hybridization patterns with chloroplast DNA. The first class (O1) contains a 400 bp MboI fragment which hybridizes to the EcoRI fragment
R2 (fig. 7d) and BamHI fragment Ba5. The second class (O2) contains
a 3 kb HindIII fragment which hybridizes to the chloroplast EcoRI
fragment R18 (fig. 7b) and BamHI fragment Ba7. The third class (O3)
contains a 450 bp MboI fragment which hybridizes to the EcoRI fragments RO2, R18 and R25 (fig. 7c) and BamHI fragment Ba7. The locations of these putative chloroplast replication origins is shown on
the physical chloroplast DNA map of Fig. 1. Similar attempts with
mitochondrial DNA have produced hybrid plasmids all of which contain at least one of the chloroplast DNA fragments belonging to the
three classes mentioned. It may be that the mitochondrial replication origin is located at or near the ends of the linear mitochondrial DNA molecules, a region we have not yet cloned.

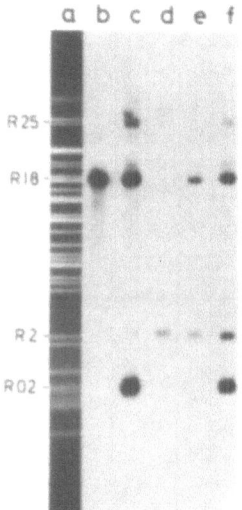

Fig. 7.
Chloroplast restriction fragments promoting
autonomous replication in yeast. Hybrid plasmids containing chloroplast HindIII and MboI
fragments were ^{32}P-labelled and hybridized
with a total chloroplast EcoRI digest. Lanes
b, c and d correspond to the three classes of
plasmids mentioned in the text. Lanes e and
f correspond to composite plasmids (i.e. containing DNA fragments of more than one class).

ACKNOWLEDGEMENTS

We thank J. Erickson for helpful comments. This work was supported by grant 3.659.80 from the Swiss National Science Foundation.

REFERENCES

Clarke, L. and Carbon, J., 1978, J. Mol. Biol., 120:517.

Davies, D.R. and Plaskitt, A., 1971, Genet. Res. 17:33.

Dron, M., Rahire, M. and Rochaix, 1982, submitted for publication.

Dron, M., Rahire, M., Rochaix, J.D. and Mets, L., 1982, submitted for publication.

Gillham, N.W., 1965, Genetics, 52:529.

Gillham, N.W., 1978, Organelle Heredity, Raven Press, New York.

Hudock, G., 1973, Biochem. Biophys. Res. Comm. 10:133.

Jolly, S.O., McIntosh, L., Link, G. and Bogorad, L., 1981, Proc. Nat. Acad. Sci. USA, 78:6821.

Lorimer, G.H., 1981, Biochemistry, 20:1236.

McIntosh, L., Poulsen, C. and Bogorad, L., 1980, Nature, 288:556.

Rochaix, J.D., 1978, J. Mol. Biol., 126:597.

Rochaix, J.D., 1981, Experientia, 37:323.

Rochaix, J.D., and Malnoë, 1978, Cell, 15:661.

Rochaix, H.D. and Darlix. J.L., 1982, J. Mol. Biol., in press.

Rochaix, J.D. and van Dillewijn, J., 1982, Nature, 296:70.

Saraste, M., Gray, N.J., Eberle, A., Runswick, M.J. and Walker, J.E., 1981, 9:5287.

Schloss, J.V., Stringer, C.D. and Hartman, F.C., 1978, J. Biol. Chem., 253:5707.

Southern, E.M., 1975, J. Mol. Biol., 95:51.

Spreitzer, R.J. and Mets, L., 1980, Nature, 285:114.

Watson, J.C. and Surzycki, S.J., 1982, Proc. Nat. Acad. Sci. USA, 79:2264.

Westhoff, P., Nelson, N., Bünemann, H. and Herrmann, R.G., 1981, Current Genet., 4:109.

Zakian, V., 1981, Proc. Nat Acad. Sci. USA, 78:3129.

Zurawski, G., Perrot, R., Bottomley, W. and Whitfeld, P.R., 1981, Nucl. Acids Res., 9:3251.

THE IN VIVO TRANSCRIPTIONAL ACTIVITY OF THE BARLEY

CHLOROPLAST GENOME

Carsten Poulsen

Department of Physiology
Carlsberg Laboratory
DK-2500 Copenhagen Valby, Denmark

INTRODUCTION

Well characterized genes localized on chloroplast DNA* include those for the large subunit of ribulose bisphosphate carboxylase[1,2,3] and the photogene 32[1,4,5]. Also located on chloroplast DNA are the genes for the α-, β- and ε-subunits of the CF_1 ATP synthetase and the photosystem II associated chlorophyll$_a$-proteins 2 and 3[6]. Work on the localization of the genes for chlorophyll$_a$-protein 1 of photosystem I[7] and cytochrome f[8] is in progress. The genes for chloroplast ribosomal 16S, 23S, 5S and 4.5S RNSs have been extensively mapped[1,9,10] as have genes for many chloroplast tRNA species[1,11,12].

The genes mentioned occupy a minor part of the cpDNA coding capacity. I have therefore attempted to map the number of transcripts which can be identified by hybridization of cloned chloroplast DNA fragments to filterbound barley chloroplast RNA. The experiments have been carried out with plastid RNA from dark grown seedlings and seedlings greened for various length of time. The results will be described in more detail in a forthcoming publication[13].

THE BARLEY CHLOROPLAST GENOME

Purified barley chloroplast DNA was isolated and cleaved with restriction endonucleases. HindIII fragments were cloned in the bacterial plasmid pBR322[14] and PstI fragments in pBR325[14]. All

---

*Abbreviations: LS: large subunit, kbp: kilobasepair(s), kb: kilobase(s), cpDNA: chloroplast DNA, cpRNA: chloroplast RNA.

recombinant PstI plasmids and many HindIII plasmids containing
cpDNA sequences were then mapped with the aid of single, double
and triple digestions using combinations of the four restriction
enzymes PstI, SalI, PvuII and HindIII. A comparison of the number
and sizes of fragments obtained by restriction of barley cpDNA
with PstI and SalI to the published patterns for maize[15] and
wheat cpDNA[9] revealed a high degree of similarity, particularly
with the wheat cpDNA. This allowed the construction of a preliminary map. The data obtained from the PstI clones were integrated
into the map, whereafter it was further fitted to results from
single, double and triple digests of intact barley cpDNA with
PstI, SalI and PvuII. Positions of some of the cloned HindIII
fragments were integrated according to their size and content of
sites for the other three restriction enzymes. Identical RNA hybridization patterns of HindIII fragments isolated from the PstI
clones allowed additional localization. This final map allowed
the assignment of most HindIII fragments obtained from intact
cpDNA. The resulting tentative restriction endonuclease map is
shown in Figure 1. Like most other higher plant cpDNAs the circular
molecule contains a large inverted repeat. It is bordered by a
SalI site towards the small single copy region and by a PvuII site
towards the large single copy region. The approximate size of the
inverted repeat is 20 kbp and the overall size of the chloroplast
genome 133 kbp which is slightly smaller than the wheat cpDNA[9].
In terms of overall physical structure the barley and wheat cpDNAs
are very similar. However, the two PstI sites separating the P3,
P10 and P12 fragments in wheat are absent in barley. Size summation
of these wheat fragments gives 21,1 kbp, whereas the single corresponding fragment in barley is only 19 kbp (as estimated by addition of subfragments). This missing sequence may account for the
difference in size between the two genomes. That this region is
rather different in the two genomes is further supported by the
fact that the S6 (SalI) fragment and one of the three S5 fragments
of the wheat cpDNA appears as a fused 14 kbp fragment in barley.
In addition, the barley SalI fragment corresponding to S7 in wheat
appears to be smaller (5,7 kbp) and the wheat cpDNA fragments P7
and P11 are found as a single fragment in the barley cpDNA. The
largest Pst I fragment in wheat, P1, seems in barley to be split
into a 19 kbp and a 14 kbp fragment. The two barley Pst I fragments
corresponding in position to P8 and P9 in wheat have a reduced size.

HYBRIDIZATION OF cpDNA SEQUENCES WITH FILTERBOUND CHLOROPLAST RNAs

     Barley seedlings were grown in the dark for six days whereafter
they were illuminated for 0 or 8 hours in white light. From 100 g
batches of leaves the plastids, representing two different developmental stages were isolated. The purified plastids were lysed in
buffer containing 5 M guanidinium rhodanide. Four ml of 20,000 x
g supernatant of the lysis mixture was loaded on each of four
cushions containing 1 ml of sterile 5,7 M CsCl. The RNA was spun

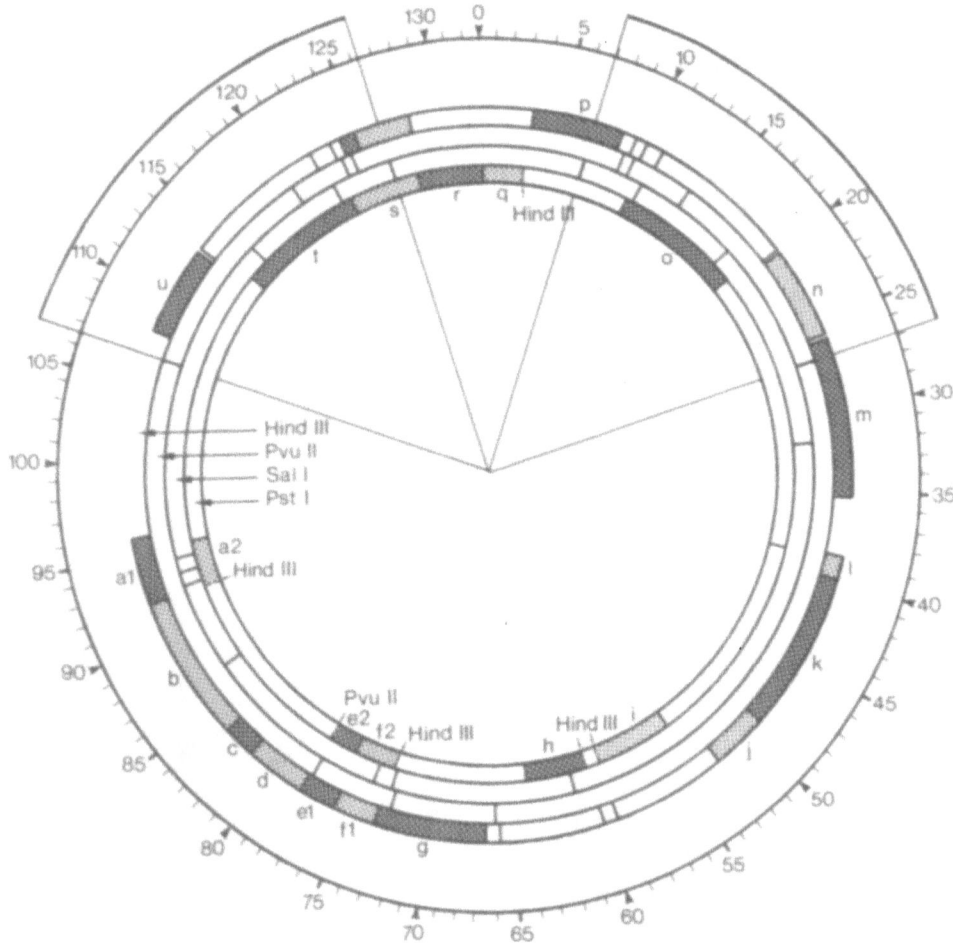

Figure 1. Tentative restriction endonuclease map of the barley chloroplast genome. The outer circle provides a scale for the size of the genome in kilobasepairs (kbp). The cloned restriction fragments which have been used for identification of transcripts are shaded and designated with small letters.

through the cushions in a SW50 rotor in a Beckman ultracentrifuge (16 hours, 37,000 rpm, 20°C). Supernatants were discarded and the RNA pellets redissolved in sterile H_2O and stored at -18°C. Aliquots of the RNA preparations containing six μg of RNA were electrophoresed in 1,5% agarose gels containing 6% formaldehyde. The separated RNA molecules were blotted onto DBM-paper as described by Alwine et al.[17]. After blotting, the RNA bound to the filters was hybridized with specific ^{32}P-cpDNA probes according to Alwine et al.[17] with the modifications suggested in the Schleicher and

Schull "Transabind" prescription.   After hybridization filters were
washed and autoradiographed.

     For the hybridizations 22 different cpDNA restriction fragments
covering about 118 of the 133 kbp in the barley chloroplast genome
were used. The position and nature of the fragments designated a
to u are shown in Figure 1. The DNA fragments were isolated after
separation on agarose gels and nick-translated. Hybridization at
43°C-44°C to filterbound RNA from etioplasts and from plastids
greened for 8 hrs were carried out with 0,1 μg of ^{32}P-DNA.

IN VIVO TRANSCRIPTS

     The RNA preparations revealed similar band patterns after
ethidium bromide staining of samples run on denaturing agarose gels
The 16S rRNA and two fragments of the 23S rRNA were the predominant
species. Similar fragmentation has been observed with the 23S rRNA
of other species such as wheat[3] and maize (McIntosh and Poulsen,

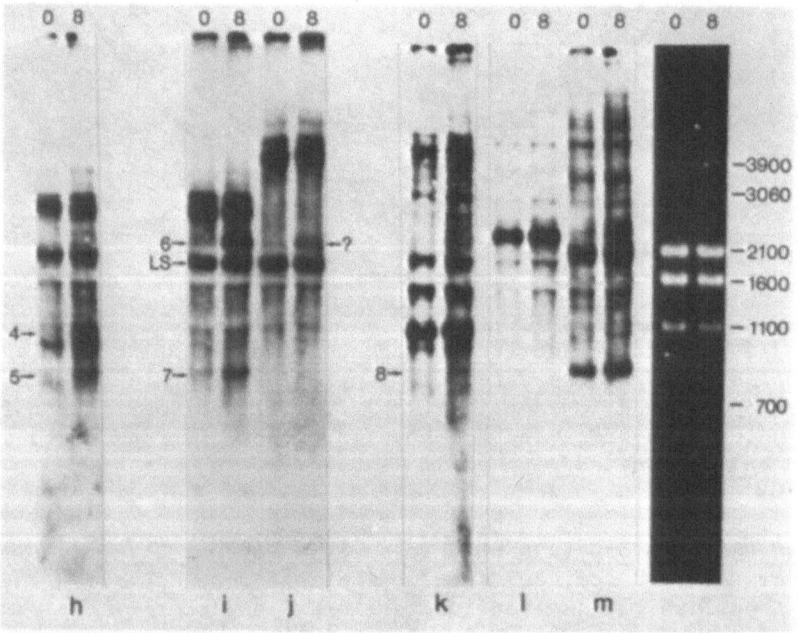

Figure 2. Hybridization of six ^{32}P-labelled cpDNA restriction
fragments to filterbound cpRNA. A gel strip with ethidium bromide
stained cpRNA bands and a size scale is given to the right of the
autoradiographs. 0 = dark grown seedlings; 8 = eight hr greened
seedlings.

unpublished). Furthermore, traces of the 25S cytoplasmic rRNA and
of apparently intact 23S rRNA could be seen. The RNA preparation
procedure did not allow the co-isolation of significant amounts of
the small rRNAs and tRNAs. All other RNA species could only be seen
as a background smear.

The hybridizations of filterbound RNAs with the radioactive
cpDNA probes, followed by autoradiography of the washed filters,
have led to the following observations: 1) All cpDNA fragments gave
unique hybridization patterns, with the exception of two pairs of
fragments originating from the inverted repeat. 2) Certain regions
of the genome showed hybridization with a surprisingly high number
of transcripts. 3) A little less than half of all hybridizing RNA
species had a hypothetical coding capacity of more than 1000 amino
acids. 4) Since about equal amounts of rRNAs were run in the different tracks of gels used for the "Northern" blots, it can be concluded that very little variation in quantity of most RNA species is
observed between samples from etioplasts and greened plastids. 5)
Only a few RNA species are synthesized preferentially or exclusively in the light. Most of these conclusions are examplified in
Figure 2, which shows the hybridizations of filter bound RNA from
0 hour and 8 hours greened plastids with the cpDNA fragments h,
i,j,k,l and m. The 4.5 kbp fragment h hybridizes with at least
seven species of RNA, which are all smaller than 3 kb. Two of the
RNA species (marked 4 and 5) with sizes of about 1 and 0,75 kb,
respectively, lack in the etioplast sample, but are prominent in
plastids after 8 hours greening. These two transcripts thus identify two photogenes. A third light induced transcript (0.85 kb) might
be hidden below the major transcript located in the gel between 4
and 5. In addition there is a unique transcript of 1.9 kb and at
least two transcripts of 2.7-2.9 kb. The latter also seem to hybridize with the 5.0 kbp fragment i, which is separated from h by a
0.6 kbp HindIII fragment. The fragment i is part of a 6.0 kbp Hind
III fragment. This fragment hybridizes with pZmC3711[1,2] which contains the LS gene of maize and part of the DNA encoding a 2.2 kb
transcript (Poulsen and McIntosh, unpublished). The hybridization
of cpRNA with i identifies these two transcripts (marked LS and 6
in Figure 2). In analogy with this region of the wheat[3] and maize[1,2]
cpDNAs, it is expected that i hybridizes only with the 5' end of
the LS mRNA of 1750 nucleotides, but with the entire 2.2 kb transcript. Interestingly, this transcript is light-induced. A smaller
transcript of 750 nucleotides marked 7, is synthesized preferentially in the light. A transcript of comparable size was found in wheat
by Koller et al.[3]. The 3.5 kbp fragment j apparently hybridizes
with the 3' end of the LS transcript and with at least three transcripts in the 4 kb size class. These are also seen in the hybridization pattern obtained with the 9.0 kbp fragment k. There are at
least 12 transcripts hybridizing with this cpDNA fragment. Of
these, four are possibly major species of mRNAs (900-1800 nucleotide
region). There are three minor species in the 600-900 nucleotide
region of which at least one is light induced (8). The small frag-

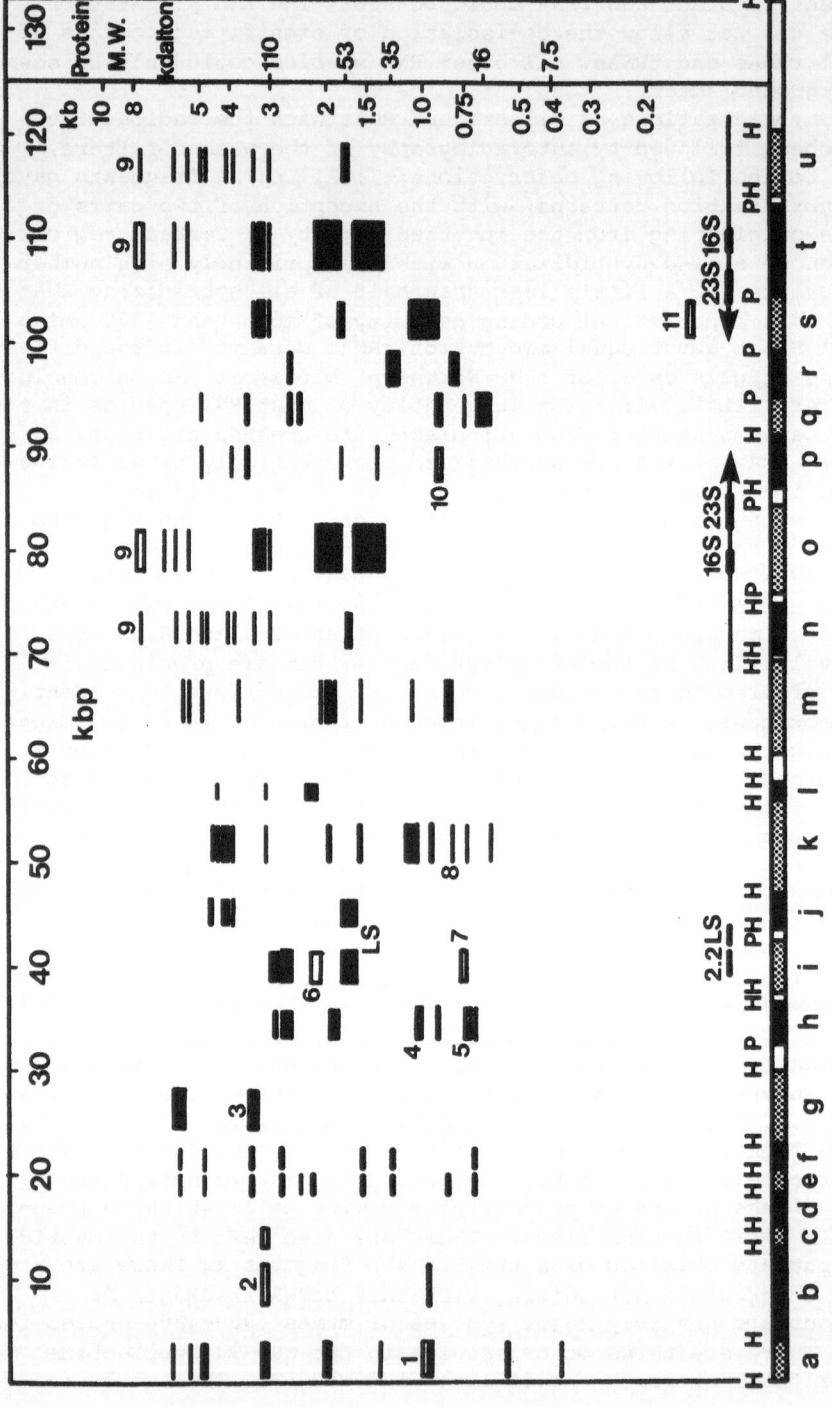

Figure 3. Transcript map of the barley cpDNA. The restriction fragments a to u used for hybridization are arranged along the linearized physical map. H = HindIII; P = PstI. Ordinate: the size of the transcripts in kilobases (kb) and the expected molecular weights of proteins translated from the RNA. Hybridization intensities are indicated by the thickness of the lines. Eleven light induced transcripts are numbered 1-11.

ment l (1.5 kbp) hybridizes predominantly with one transcript of 2.4 kb, which thus must extend beyound the edge of the fragment towards m. The hybridization of chloroplast RNAs with the 9.0 kbp fragment m also appears very complex. However, there are no indications for light induced transcripts and the transcript of about 850 nucleotides is the dominant one.

A transcript map of the barley cpDNA is presented in Figure 3. The diagram includes the data of Figure 2, comprising the 32 to 70 kbp region. Many of the weakest hybridizing species have not been included in the diagram. The map underlines the conclusions mentioned above and reveals the following additional points: 1) The symmetric positions of the large rRNAs are clearly exhibited within the inverted repeat regions. 2) There are a total of at least 11 light induced transcripts, of which one (9) is very large and covers the rRNA cistrons. At the other extreme is the transcript (11) containing less than 200 nucleotides. Of the nine remaining light induced transcripts two (2 and 3) are either polycistronic mRNAs or mRNAs for very large polypeptides (more than 1000 amino acids). 3) For the very large transcripts it cannot be excluded that a given transcript hybridizes with more than one DNA segment even if these occupy physically quite separate regions of the cpDNA. 4) If all hybridizing species shown in Figure 3 are unique transcripts, more than 90 RNA molecules are transcribed from the 118 kbp fraction of the barley cpDNA analyzed. 5) The 4-18 kbp region of the barley cpDNA (Figure 3) which is significantly different from the wheat chloroplast genome exhibits a low transcriptional activity.

The large number of transcripts observed and the big size of many transcripts suggest that the following questions should be investigated: Are there several transcription-initiation sites on both DNA strands within limited regions of the genome such as the a and the e+f region ? Do chloroplasts contain an RNA processing and splicing system, which is present in etioplasts and in developing plastids ? Are larger transcripts which hybridize to the same cpDNA fragment as smaller ones precursors for the latter ?

REFERENCES

1. L. Bogorad, S.O. Jolly, G. Link, L. McIntosh, C. Poulsen, Z. Schwarz and A. Steinmetz, Studies of the maize chloroplast chromosome, in: "Biological chemistry of organelle formation", T. Bücher, W. Sebald and H. Weiss, eds., Springer-Verlag, Berlin, Heidelberg, New York (1980).
2. L. McIntosh, C. Poulsen and L. Bogorad, Chloroplast gene sequence for the large subunit of ribulose bisphosphate carboxylase of maize, Nature 288:556-560 (1980).
3. B. Koller, H. Delius and T.A. Dyer, The organization of the chloroplast DNA in wheat and maize in the region containing the LS gene, Eur. J. Biochem. 122: 17-23 (1982).

4. K.E. Steinback, L. McIntosh, L. Bogorad and C.J. Arntzen, Identification of the triazine receptor protein as a chloroplast
   gene product, Proc. Natl. Acad. Sci. USA, 78:7463-7467 (1981).
5. G. Link, Phytochrome control of plastid mRNA in mustard
   (Sinapis alba L.) (1982).
6. D. von Wettstein, Chloroplast and nucleus: conterted interplay
   between genomes of different cell organelles. The Emil Heitz
   Lecture, in: "International Cell Biology 1980-1981", H.G.
   Schweiger, ed., SpringerVerlag, Berlin, Heidelberg (1981).
7. R. Nechushtai, N. Nelson, A.K. Mattoo and M. Edelman, Site of
   synthesis of subunits to photosystem 1 reaction center and
   proton-ATPase in Spirodela, FEBS lett. 125:115-119 (1981).
8. A. Doherty and J.C. Gray, Synthesis of cytochrome f by isolated
   pea plastids, Eur. J. Biochem. 98:87-92 (1979).
9. C.M. Bowman, B. Koller, H. Delius and T.A. Dyer, A physical
   map of wheat chloroplast DNA showing the locations of the
   structural genes for the ribosomal RNAs and the large subunit
   of ribulose 1,5-bisphosphate carboxylase, Mol. Gen. Genet.
   183:93-101 (1981).
10. F. Takaiwa and M. Sugiara, The complete sequence of a 23-S rRNA
    from tobacco chloroplasts, Eur. J. Bio. chem. 124:13-19 (1982).
11. A.J. Driesel, E.J. Crouse, K. Gordon, H.J. Bohnert, R.G. Herr-
    mann, A. Steinmetz, M. Mubumbila, M. Keller, G. Burkard and
    J.H. Weil, Fractionation and identification of spinach chloro-
    plast tRNAs and mapping of their genes on the restriction map
    of chloroplast DNA, Gene 6:285-306 (1979).
12. Z. Schwarz, S.O. Jolly, A.A. Steinmetz and L.Bogorad, Overlap-
    ping divergent genes in the maize chromosome and in vitro
    transcription of the gene for tRNA$_{His}$, Proc. Natl. Acad. Sci.
    USA 78:3423-3427 (1981).
13. C. Poulsen, Carlsberg Res. Commun. in preparation.
14. X. Soberon, L. Covarrubias and F. Bolivar, Construction
    of new cloning vehicles. IV. Deletion derivatives of pBR322
    and pBR325, Gene 9:287-305 (1980).
15. J.R. Bedbrook and L. Bogorad, Endonuclease recognition sites
    mapped on Zea mays chloroplast DNA, Proc. Natl. Acad. Sci.
    USA 73:4309-4313 (1976).
16. E.M. Southern, Detection of specific sequences among DNA frag-
    ments separated by gel electrophoresis, J. Mol. Biol. 98:503-
    517 (1975).
17. J.C. Alwine, D.J. Kemp, B.A. Parker, J. Reiser, J. Renart,
    G.R. Stark and G.M. Wahl, Detection of specific RNAs or speci-
    fic fragments of DNA by fractionation in gels and transfer to
    diazobenzyloxymethyl paper, in: "Methods in Enzymology", vol.
    68, R. Wu, ed. (1980).
18. P.W. Rigby, M. Dieckmann, C. Rhodes and P. Berg, Labeling
    deoxyribonucleic acid to high specific activity in vitro by
    nick translation with DNA polymerase I, J. Mol. Biol. 113:237-
    251 (1977).

CHLORPHYLL a/b BINDING PROTEINS AND THE SMALL SUBUNIT OF RIBULOSE

BISPHOSPHATE CARBOXYLASE ARE ENCODED BY MULTIPLE GENES IN PETUNIA

Pamela Dunsmuir and John Bedbrook*

CSIRO Division of Plant Industry
Canberra City, Australia

SUMMARY

There are at least sixteen chorophyll a/b binding protein coding
sequences in the nuclear genome of the diploidized Mitchell haploid
Petunia line. These genes can be classified into at least five distinct
families based on the relatedness of the nucleotide sequence which
encodes the 60, C-terminal amino acids of the peptide. There is as
much as 10% nucleotide divergence and 5% amino acid sequence
divergence between the genes of different families in this region. For
two of the families we find that two closely related genes are adjacent
and in both examples the two genes are in an inverted orientation with
respect to each other such that the 5' ends of the genes are opposed.
At least one gene from four of the families is transcribed. The 3'
untranslated sequences of the genes are divergent between families yet
well conserved within a single family.

The multiple genes for the small subunit peptide of ribulose (-1,5-)
bisphosphate carboxylase (SSU) can be also be divided into four families
based on the relatedness of the coding sequences. We have found
evidence for linkage between two SSU genes and for the transcription
of at least one gene from each family.

Our data suggest that there may be at least five different chlorophyll
a/b binding peptides, and four different small subunit peptides for
ribulose (-1,5-) bisphosphate carboxylase in the petunia leaf chloroplast.

*.Advanced Genetic Sciences Inc.
P.O. Box 3266 Berkeley Cal.
U.S.A.

INTRODUCTION

Two major chloroplast proteins-the small subunit (SSU) of ribulose
(-1,5-) bisphosphate carboxylase, and the chlorophyll a/b binding
protein (Cab) of the thylakoid light harvesting complex, are encoded by
nuclear genes (Kawashima and Wildman 1972,Von Wettstein 1981).
It is well established for both SSU and Cab polypeptides, in pea,
spinach, and chlamydomonas, that the mRNAs are translated on
cytoplasmic polyribosomes to yield precursor peptides (containing 45-50
additional N-terminal amino acids) which undergo post translational
transport into intact chlorplasts, followed by, or coupled
with proteolytic cleavage to produce mature peptides in the chloroplast
(Cashmore,1976: Dobberstein et al., 1977; Chua, N.-H. & Schmidt, 1979;
Highfield and Ellis, 1978, Schmidt et al., 1979). The mature SSU
peptide is combined with the chloroplast encoded large subunit peptide
to form the holoenzyme ribulose (-1,5-) biphosphate carboxylase. The
mature Cab peptides are non-convalently bound with chlorophylls a and
b, which are synthesized in the chloroplast, and incorporated into the
thylakoid membrane (Boardman et. al, 1978). We show here that both
SSU and Cab proteins are specified by multiple genes. Many of the
individual genes differ in nucleotide sequence. Further several of these
different genes for both SSU and Cab polypeptides are transcribed in
petunia leaves.

RESULTS AND DISCUSSION

In order to understand the structure and expression of the Cab and SSU
genes we have focused our attention on the Mitchell Petunia strain.
This plant has a low C value (IN = 1 pg) is a doubled haploid and thus
genetically homozygous (Mitchell, 1979), and is amenable to
propagation from protoplast culture. We isolated five Cab and five SSU
cDNA clones from the set constructed using Petunia leaf poly A+RNA
(Figure 1). The alignment of these cDNAs with respect to each other
and to the end of the mRNA has been determined from DNA sequence
analyses and comparison with the published sequence for the SSU
mRNA in pea (Bedbrook et al., 1980) and Cab mRNA sequence in pea
(Coruzzi et al., 1982)

Although several of the Cab cDNA clones have a number of conserved
restriction endonuclease cleavage sites, no single site is present in all
five examples. Thus each cDNA is unique on the basis of physical
mapping. For the SSU cDNA clones, pSSU 117 and pSSU 71 differ by
virtue of EcoRI and Hpa II sites, and pSSU 51 may be distinguished from
these by a Hinfl site. Although pSSU 103 and pSSU 41 are not
distinguished by unique restriction enzyme cleavage sites, they do
differ at the nucleotide sequence level from the other SSU cDNAs
(Dunsmuir and Bedbrook, submitted).

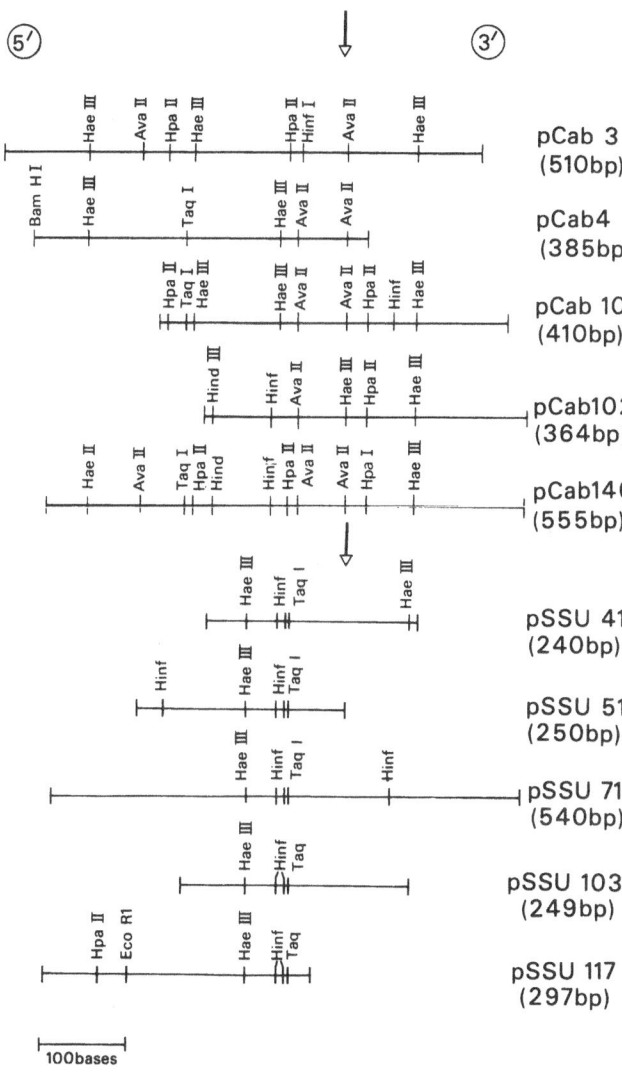

FIGURE 1

Restriction endonuclease cleavage site maps for Petunia cDNA clones.
The vertical arrow indicates the translation termination points.

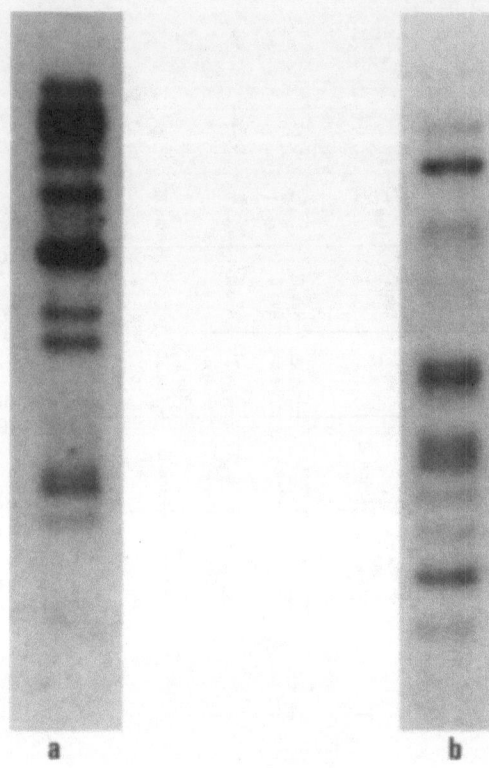

FIGURE 2.

Petunia DNA digested with EcoRI and hybridized with (a) pCab146
cDNA (b) pSSU117 cDNA.

On the basis of these characterized cDNA clones we expect that at
least five different Cab peptide genes and four different SSU peptide
genes are transcribed in green leaf tissue.

The autoradiographs of Figure 2 illustrate that a petunia Cab cDNA
probe hybridizes to fourteen EcoRI fragments, labelled A-M and
ranging in size from 17 kb to 1 kb, and a petunia SSU cDNA probe
hybridizes to twelve EcoRI fragments, labelled A-L and ranging in size
from 12kb to 2kb in the Petunia Mitchell DNA. To isolate and
characterize these hybridizing genomic sequences in petunia DNA we
cloned nuclear DNA partially digested with EcoRI into the lambdoid
phage vector Charon 28 (Rimm et al., 1980). Petunia cDNAs for Cab

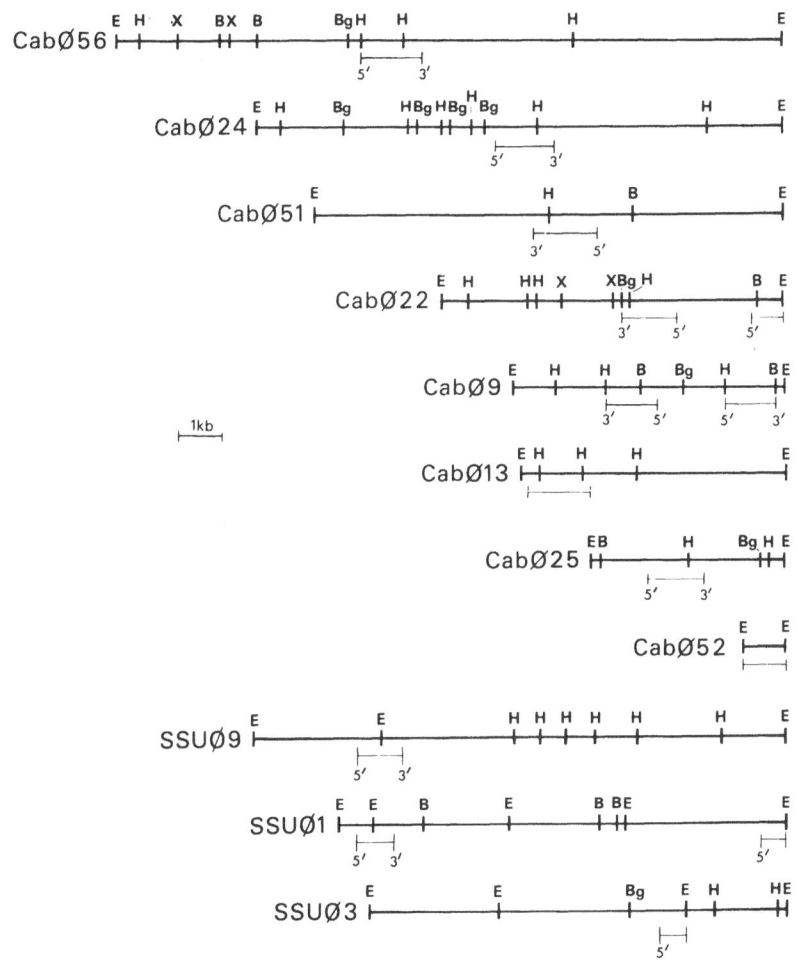

FIGURE 3.

Restriction endonuclease maps of Petunia nuclear fragments cloned in Charon 28 phage. Sites are abbreviated, E-EcoR1, B-BamH1, H-Hind III, Bg-Bgl II and X-Xhol. Regions corresponding to Cab and SSU coding sequences are indicated under the maps.

and SSU were used as probes to identify the recombinant phage containing the corresponding genomic coding regions (Benton & Davis, 1977). To localize the regions of these genomic fragments which correspond to the Cab and SSU genes we initially hybridized a cDNA clone (of known length) corresponding to the 3' end of the coding region, to recombinant phage DNAs digested with appropriate enzymes and transferred to nitrocellulose (Southern, 1975). A comparison between these 3' end hybridizations, and hybridizations using full length cDNA probes allowed us to determine the direction of transcription and also make some estimate of the extent of homology between the Cab or SSU transcripts and the cloned fragment - these are designated in Figure 2 . The restriction endonuclease cleavage site differences within the hybridizing regions on the different cloned Cab and SSU nuclear fragments indicated that there are sequence differences between the multiple genes. Cab phage fragments 9 and 22, and the SSU phage fragment 1, each have two separate regions which hybridize to the corresponding cDNA probes.

In an attempt to correlate the different Cab and SSU cDNA clones with the different nuclear genes we compared the stability of the hybrids formed between each cDNA, and the known set of genomic EcoRI fragments under stringent, and normal hybridization conditions. For every cDNA example the hybridization profile under more stringent conditions is composed of only a subset of the fragments which hybridize under normal conditions (data not shown). Further, each cDNA probe hybridized best with a unique subset of genomic fragments implying that each cDNA is most closely related to a specific non-overlapping subset of the nuclear genes. These results were corroborated by analogous hybridizations between different cDNAs and cloned genomic fragments. Since we know that each of the cloned fragments encompasses a complete coding sequence for the Cab peptide, these results indicate that the set of Cab genes could be subdivided into distinct families based on their relatedness to particular cDNA clones.

Data from restriction endonuclease mapping, nucleotide sequence analyses, and high stringency hybridization experiments on the Cab and SSU cDNA clones, and cloned nuclear fragments are assembled in Table I where the different genes are categorized into families based on the relatedness of the peptide coding regions.

The family of Cab 146, corresponds to the genes of nuclear fragment F, cloned in Cab ∅22, which we known encompasses 2 distinct genes (Figure 3). The Cab 102 family contains genes on the nuclear fragments A (Cab ∅ 56), B (Cab∅24), C (Cab∅51), I (Cab∅25) and K (no genomic clone isolated). Each of these cloned fragments encompasses a single coding region and although we have not yet isolated the genomic fragment K, we assume from its relative hybridization intensity that it also contains a single gene. Thus the Cab 102 family comprises 5 separate genes. We do not know which nuclear fragment relates

TABLE 1

Designation of Cab and SSU gene families in the Petunia genome.

Gene family	EcoR1 genomic fragments	Phage fragments	Number of genes per family	Relatedness* of coding sequences to selected clone
Cab 146	F	22	2	100
Cab 10	G	9	2	91
Cab 102	A,B,C,I,K	56,24,51, 25	5	89
Cab 3	D,J,K	No clone	3	91
X	E,H,M,N	13,52	?	?
SSU 117	B,E,K	1,3	3	100
SSU 41	E	No clone	?	93
SSU 51	B,C,D,F,H I,L	No clone	?	?
SSU 71	D	9	?	?

* The sequences compared are those encoding the 60 N terminal amino acids. All Cab clones were compared to pCab 146, and SSU clones were compared to pSSU 117.

specifically to cDNA clone 102 nor whether the genes are identical in sequence. The Cab 10 family corresponds to the genes on nuclear fragment G (CabØ9). The two complete genes on Cab Ø9 hybridize equally well to the cDNAs Cab 10, and Cab 4 under stringent conditions. The fourth family, Cab 3 is composed of the genes on fragments D, J and L however these genomic clones have not been isolated. The hybridization intensity of these fragments indicates that they each contain a single region.

The nuclear fragments H (CabØ13), and N (CabØ52) cannot be ascribed to any of the known Cab families on the basis of high stringency hybridization experiments with the characterized cDNA probes, however from experiments with total leaf cDNA as a probe to Cab phage DNA we know that the genes of fragments H and N are transcribed. Cab Ø13 appears to contain a complete coding region and Cab Ø52 contains part of a gene, thus we postutlate that there is at least one additional Cab gene family which is composed of a minimum of two genes. We have no infomation relating to the expression of the genes of fragments E and M which we have not isolated.

We have sequenced each of the Cab cDNA clones (Dunsmuir and Bedbrook, submitted) and these data are summarised in Table 1. The cDNA clones Cab 4 and Cab 3 are more closely related to the Cab 146 clone with 16 nucleotide changes in the common region, 15 of which are silent third codon position chages. For the Cab 102 cDNA, 14 of the 20 nucleotide differences are silent.

The SSU cDNA clones also classify the nuclear genes into distinct families however we have cloned only six of the SSU genomic EcoRI fragments, thus it is not possible to specify the number of genes of each family except for the SSU 117 family. This SSU gene family contains 3 genes, two of which are contained in the SSU Ø1 (genomic fragments B and K) and the third in fragment E (SSUØ3). The analysis of the SSU genes is complicated by the presence of EcoRI sites internal to a number of the nuclear gene sequences. Although we do not yet have as extensive data relating to the SSU genomic fragments as we do for the Cab genes, the evidence is strongly suggestive that like the Cab genes, the nuclear genes which code for the SSU peptide may be classified into discrete gene families which are represented in the leaf mRNA population and, if translated would specify distinct peptides.

Nucleotide sequence analysis demonstrated as much as 10% sequence divergence between different Cab cDNAs when a region encoding the C-terminal 60 amino acids of the peptide was compared. The 3' untranslated sequence from a representative of each of the four defined gene families encoding the chlorphyll a/b binding protein have also been determined (Dunsmuir and Bedbrook submitted). We find that there is extreme sequence divergence (greater than 60% if consecutive bases are compared) between these regions in the different genes. The 3' untranslated regions of the Cab cDNAs 146 and 10 each have a sequence A-A-T-A-A, 11 and 22 basepairs respectively from the poly A tail - such a sequence may be the signal for poly A addition (Proudfoot and Brownlee, 1976). In spite of the extreme divergence between the 3' untranslated regions in the different cDNA clones, there are two sequences which are conserved in every gene. At approximately thirty five base pairs from the translation termination signal is the 20 nucleotide sequence TTGTTT^G/CXTGGCCTTCTA^A/TA, and at about ninety nucleotides from the translation termination is the 7 base sequence TTTGTTT.

In order to test whether the 3' untranslated regions of the Cab genes within any one family are conserved we have isolated the 3' untranslated regions from the Cab cDNA clones 10, 102 and 146 (which define 3 distinct families) and used these sequences as hybridization probes to petunia genomic DNA. The 3' untranslated sequence of Cab cDNA 102 hybridizes to the geonomic fragments A, B, C, I and K -the identical fragments to those defined as the Cab 102 gene family by high stringency hybridization of the entire Cab 102 cDNA. Similarly the 3' untranslated regions from Cab 146, and Cab 10 cDNA hybridize only to the genomic fragments of the Cab 146 family and Cab 10 family respectively. It should be noted that while the subcloned 3' untranslated sequences hybridize the same subset of genomic fragments at normal stringency as do the entire cDNA sequences at high stringency, the 3' untranslated sequences do not contribute substantially to the high stringency hybridization because of their very high AT sequence bias. These data demonstrate that the 3' untranslated regions from genes of different families are divergent in sequence, but these same regions are sufficiently conserved between members within any particular family to allow specific cross hybridization. This result strengthens the gene family classification system presented in Table 1 based upon the relatedness of Cab gene coding sequences. As yet we do not have direct nucleotide sequence comparisons for the 3' untranslated regions of genes within the same family.

We conclude then, that both the chlorophyll a/b binding protein of the light harvesting complex and the small subunit of ribulose bisphosphate carboxylase are encoded by multiple expressed genes. Each set of genes is divisible into families based on their sequence relatedness to independent cDNA clones and at least one member of each family is transcribed in Petunia leaf tissue.

REFERENCES

Boardman, N.K., Anderson, J.M., and Goodchild, D.J. (1978). Current Topics in Bioenergetics 8; 35-109.
Bedbrook, J.R., Smith, S.M., and Ellis, R.J. (1980). Nature 287: 692-697.
Cashmore, A.R. (1976). J.Biol.Chem. 251: 2848-2853.

Chua, N.-H., and Schmidt, G.W. (1979). Proc. Natl. Acad. Sci. USA
75:6110-6114.
Coruzzi, G., Broglie, A., Cashmore, A, and Chua,N.-H. (1982)
J.Biol.Chem, (in press)
Dobberstein, B.G., Blobel, G., and Chua, N.-H. (1977) Proc, Natl. Acad.
Sci. USA 74: 1082-1085.
Dunsmuir, P. and Bedbrook, J. (1982) Submitted.
Highfield, P.E., and Ellis, R.J. (1978). Nature 271:420-424.
Kawashima, N., and Wildman, S.G. (1972). BBA 262:42-49.
Mitchell, A.Z. (1979). Anther Culture in Petunia. Thesis B.A.(Hons)
Harvard University.
Proudfoot, N.J., and Brownlee, G.G. (1976). Nature 263: 211-214.
Rimm, D.L., Horness, D., Kucera, J., and Blattner, F.R. (1980). Gene
12: 301-309.
Schmidt, G.W., Devilliers-Thiery, A., Desruisseaux, H., Blobel, G., and
Chua, N.-H. (1979). J.Cell Biol. 83:615-622.
Southern, E.M. (1975).J.Mol.Biol. 98:503-517.
Von Wettstein, D. (1981). Int. Cell Biol. 250-272.

BIOCHEMICAL GENETICS OF NITROGEN FIXATION

Winston J. Brill

Department of Bacteriology and
Center for Studies of Nitrogen Fixation
University of Wisconsin
Madison, Wisconsin 53706
U.S.A.

INTRODUCTION

This chapter will introduce the subject of nitrogen fixation and will stress the biochemical aspects. Subsequent papers on nitrogen fixation in this volume will focus on the molecular biology and regulation of the system in several different organisms. For a more detailed background, the reader may want to consult one or more reviews dealing with the Rhizobium-legume symbiosis[1,2,3,4,5,6,7] or those dealing with the biochemistry of nitrogen fixation in free-living bacteria[3,6,8,9]. Both the biochemistry and molecular biology of nitrogen fixation are quite complex and breakthroughs in one area of nitrogen fixation research frequently impact on other areas.

NITROGENASE

Bacteria as diverse as Azotobacter, Clostridium, Anabaena, Klebsiella, Rhizobium, Frankia and Azospirillum have nitrogenases with essentially the same properties. Nitrogenase is composed of two component proteins, component I and component II. Component I is composed of two different subunits, both of which have very similar molecular weights and amino acid compositions. Component II contains only one kind of subunit. Component I contains approximately 36 atoms of iron and component II has four iron atoms. Component I also contains two molybdenum atoms. As a demonstration of the similarity between nitrogenases from different bacteria, many component I proteins can complement in vitro component II from other nitrogen-fixing bacteria.

Reduction of nitrogen to ammonia occurs on component I. The
role of component II is to reduce component I. The reduction of
nitrogen gas to ammonia requires 12 to 24 ATP, which are converted
to ADP. A side reaction of all nitrogenases is the reduction of
protons to yield hydrogen gas. This seems to be a wasteful reaction since it utilizes ATP as well as electrons. Some organisms
have a hydrogenase that recoups electrons or ATP from hydrogen gas
oxidation.

Another feature common to all nitrogenases is that they are
all very labile to oxygen. Organisms that fix nitrogen either do
so under anaerobic conditions (such as Clostridium, a strict anaer-
obe) or have a mechanism to protect nitrogenase from irreversible
oxygen damage. In the case of some cyanobacteria, a filament of
vegetative cells will include some specialized cells called heterocysts. These heterocysts contain active nitrogenase and do not
have the oxygen-forming reactions of photosynthesis. Rhizobium
within nodules are surrounded by leghemoglobin, a plant-coded
protein that tightly binds oxygen and presumably keeps free oxygen
from reaching nitrogenase. Klebsiella, unlike Clostridium, can
grow on fixed nitrogen compounds aerobically; however, Klebsiella
will not fix nitrogen in the presence of oxygen. In fact, oxygen
represses nitrogenase synthesis.

Nitrogenases from all organisms examined are capable of reducing other compounds besides nitrogen gas. These compounds have
triple bonds between carbon and nitrogen (e.g., cyanide) or carbon
and carbon (e.g., acetylene). The latter reaction is the basis of
an extremely convenient method for assaying nitrogenase.
Acetylene, which is quite water soluble, is reduced to ethylene,
which is not very water soluble. Both are gases, which can be
quantitated with high sensitivity within a minute or two by gas
chromatography. Samples of pure nitrogenase, a crude extract,
whole bacteria, root systems, or soil samples can easily be assayed
for nitrogenase activity by injecting acetylene in a closed system,
incubating the system, and then taking a gas sample with a syringe
and determining the amount of ethylene formed. The quantity of
ethylene produced is an index of the amount of nitrogen that would
have been fixed.

The molybdenum in component I is in the form of a cofactor
(FeMo-co) that is the active site of nitrogenase. FeMo-co contains, for each molybdenum atom, eight iron atoms and six acid-
labile sulfides. This cofactor is responsible for the electron
paramagnetic resonance signal that is associated with nitrogenase
activity. FeMo-co, itself, is capable of catalyzing the reduction
of acetylene to ethylene without the presence of the apoprotein.
No ATP or component II is required for this reaction, which is 8%

of the rate of acetylene reduced by the enzyme on the basis of
molybdenum concentration.

Before studies of the genetics of nitrogen fixation began to
yield data, one might have predicted that there are approximately
three genes that are specific for nitrogen fixation (nif genes)--
two for the two component I subunits and one for component II. It
was surprising, therefore, when fine-structure mapping and complementation studies with Klebsiella pneumoniae showed that there are
at least seventeen nif genes. Figure 1 shows the order of genes
and the functions of many of their products. The two subunits of
component I are coded by contiguous genes (nifD, nifK) sharing the
same operon with nifH, the gene coding for component II. The fact
that the structural genes are on one operon guarantees that the
components are synthesized in the optimum proportion of each other.
It is known, for instance, that an excess of component I inhibits
nitrogen fixation.

Component II, synthesized by nifH, is inactive. Certain
protein modifications are required to make component II active.
For instance, the product of nifM is necessary for formation of
active component II. Nothing is known yet about the nature of such
modifications. They could involve synthesis and incorporation of
the iron-sulfur center.

A specific electron-transport pathway is associated with
nitrogenase. Two genes, nifF and nifJ, produce proteins that are
required for in vivo nitrogen fixation but are not required for
nitrogenase activity in vitro when dithionite is added as a nitrogenase reducing agent. The nifJ product is a pyruvate dehydrogenase that reduces a flavoprotein coded by nifF. This
flavoprotein, in turn, reduces component II, which then reduces
component I.

The nifRLA operon is responsible for the regulation of nif
expression. The nifA product acts as a positive regulatory effec-
tor that turns on expression of all of the other six operons, but
is necessary for transcription of its own operon. In the presence
of excess fixed nitrogen, the nifRLA operon is not expressed;
therefore, no nifA product is available to induce synthesis of the
other operons. Regulation of nif expression by oxygen is provided
by the nifL gene product. In the presence of oxygen, the nifL
protein prevents the nifA protein from activating transcription of
the other nif operons. Oxygen, besides repressing nitrogenase
synthesis, also causes the messenger RNAs of all of the operons
except nifRLA to be extremely unstable (J. Collins, unpublished
results). An interesting observation, yet to be explained, is that
the nifA product either catalyzes the reaction that converts 6-
cyanopurine to a purple pigment or else regulates a non-nif gene
responsible for that reaction. This observation has been useful

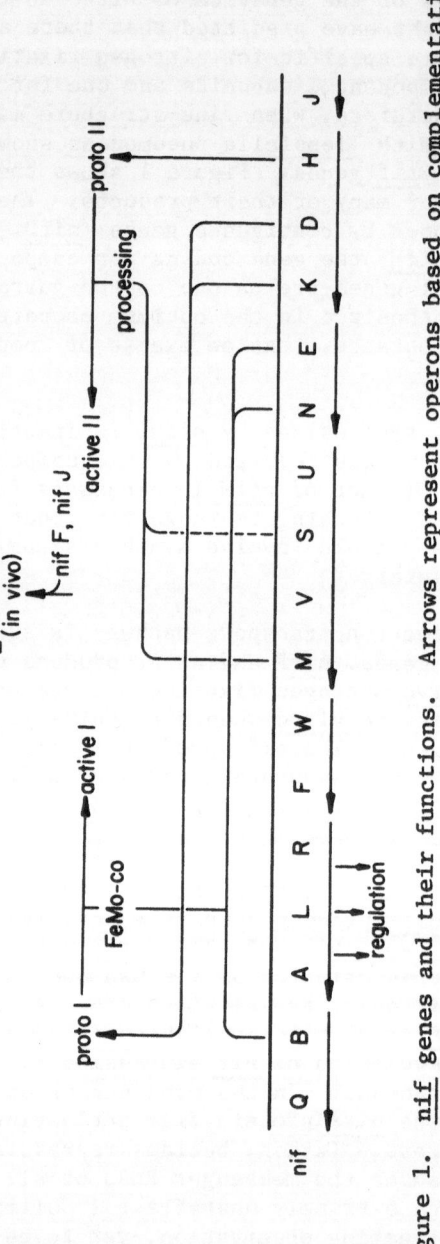

Figure 1. nif genes and their functions. Arrows represent operons based on complementation analyses with polar mutations.

for isolating derepressed mutants.

Temperature also plays a regulatory role. K. pneumoniae fixes nitrogen optimally at 30°C, but is unable to fix nitrogen at 37°C. The organism will grow well at 37°C when fixed nitrogen is available. The temperature-sensitive step seems to be the function of the nifA product, which is unable to turn on transcription of any of the other operons at the higher temperatures. Many wild-type strains of K. pneumoniae are temperature-sensitive for nitrogen fixation. This indicates that temperature control has some important selective advantage.

Most of the nif-coded proteins have been identified. Even though many of these proteins have not been purified, we know that some of them have an effect on expression of others. For instance, most mutations in nifE cause the nifN protein to be unstable in vivo and most mutations in nifN cause the nifE protein to be unstable. This result can be explained by the fact that the two proteins normally are found as a complex. The same phenomenon is observed with the nifK and nifD proteins. Even the component II (nifH) structure has an effect on the stability of the component I proteins.

Very little is known about genes other than nifK, nifD, and nifH and nif-related proteins other than components I and II in other nitrogen-fixing bacteria. A crude genetic map ordering some nif mutations has been initiated in Azotobacter vinelandii. It will be interesting to compare the biochemical steps and the genes responsible for these steps in other organisms. Will nif be simpler or more complicated in Rhizobium than in Klebsiella? Also, once the Klebsiella nif genes are genetically engineered into a cereal plant, will the plant's cytoplasm be suitable for the various modifications of the nif-coded proteins and will the high iron, molybdenum, electron, and ATP requirements be compatible with a healthy plant cell?

RHIZOBIUM-LEGUME SYMBIOSIS

As far as application of nitrogen fixation to agriculture, most interest is focused on the Rhizobium-legume system. As subsequent chapters will point out, knowledge of the organization of the K. pneumoniae nif genes has aided studies on the molecular biology of nif in Rhizobium strains. With the exception of nifK, nifD, and nifH, no other genes in Rhizobium analogous to the K. pneumoniae nif genes have been detected. All of the nif genes necessary for nitrogen fixation are coded by the Rhizobium since certain strains can fix nitrogen in the absence of the host plant; however, these strains are unable to assimilate the fixed nitrogen and are, therefore, unable to grow with nitrogen as the sole nitrogen source.

The most interesting aspect of nitrogen fixation in this pro-
karyote-eukaryote relationship is the establishment of the
symbiosis, itself. Certain Rhizobium species nodulate specific
hosts, but there are many cases in which the normal host range of a
Rhizobium species is bridged. Even though millions of rhizobia may
bind to a root, only a few nodules are formed. Some root hair
cells are infected via an invagination in which the rhizobia multiply. This infection thread courses through internal cells into the
cortex of the root. At some stage, the infection thread opens into
a plant cell and the bacteria multiply within that cell and begin
to invade neighboring cells. The rhizobia are enclosed in packets
of plant membrane within the plant cell. The bacteria in these
membranes are not capable of division and are considered to be dead
cells; however, these are the cells that contain the active nitrogenase and fix nitrogen for the plant. Living rhizobia, necessary
for perpetuation of the species from one season to the next, remain
in the infection threads.

Each legume synthesizes several species of globin that react
with Rhizobium-synthesized heme. Leghemoglobin surrounds the
rhizobia in the infected cells. No leghemoglobin has been detected
in any other plant tissue. A major question, yet to be solved, is
how the Rhizobium induces the plant to synthesize leghemoglobin.
There is no evidence yet of the different globins playing different
roles. Currently, my laboratory is examining these questions with
the use of mutants defective in globin synthesis.

There seems to be some role of plant lectins in the symbiosis.
Correlations between Rhizobium species binding to the lectins of
their host plants have been made; however, certain lectin-less
soybeans are still nodulated normally by R. japonicum. Fixed
nitrogen compounds do not repress nitrogenase synthesis in Rhizobium, but rather prevent initiation of nodule formation. There is
some indication that the root lectin is unavailable to the Rhizobium in the presence of excess fixed nitrogen and therefore nodules
will not be formed until the plant is limited for nitrogen.
Virtually nothing is known about the biochemical details of any of
the plant-bacteria reactions leading to a nitrogen-fixing nodule.

A problem with the use of Rhizobium inoculants in agriculture
is that strains added to the seed are frequently not the strains
that end up in the nodule. There are many cases of indigenous
strains outcompeting strains that are superior under greenhouse or
laboratory conditions. In my laboratory, J. Handelsman and R.
Ugalde have recently shown that R. meliloti spontaneously mutates
at high frequency from a wild type that binds the alfalfa lectin
very tightly (high titer) to a mutant that is less effective in
lectin recognition activity (low titer). The strains cannot be
distinguished from one another by visual examination of cloning
types. The interesting observation is that the low-titer

derivatives always outcompete the high-titer strains in experiments in which the two strains are mixed in the plant inoculum. The biochemical difference between the two types of strains is the activity of galactose incorporation into a large water-insoluble polymer. The involvement of plasmids with these differences is currently being examined.

The Rhizobium-legume symbiosis is certainly one of the most challenging systems to study. It is important in world agriculture, it should yield techniques and concepts that may be applied to other nitrogen-fixing symbioses and it may yield information relevant to plant-pathogen interactions. Standard biochemical techniques have not yet yielded a great deal of information. Hopefully, examination of mutants that produce defective nodules or those unable to form nodules will be useful for understanding the biochemical steps involved. My laboratory is studying a large collection of such mutants of R. meliloti and R. japonicum. Another approach that may be valuable would be to introduce Rhizobium genes into free-living bacteria. For instance, we were able to use transformation to put Rhizobium lectin-binding genes from R. trifolii and R. japonicum into Azotobacter vinelandii. The resulting Azotobacter strains were able to bind the lectin and attach to root hairs of the legume (clover or soybean) normally the host of the donor Rhizobium strain.

REFERENCES

1. W. D. Bauer, Infection of legumes by rhizobia, Ann. Rev. Plant Physiol. 32:407 (1981).
2. J. E. Beringer, N. Brewin, A. W. B. Johnston, H. M. Schulman, and D. A. Hopwood, The Rhizobium-legume symbiosis, Proc. R. Soc. London Ser. B 204:219 (1979).
3. W. J. Brill, Biochemical genetics of nitrogen fixation, Microbiol. Rev. 44:449 (1980).
4. W. J. Broughton, Control of specificity in legume-Rhizobium associations, J. Appl. Bacteriol. 45:165 (1978).
5. F. B. Dazzo, Bacterial attachment as related to cellular recognition in the Rhizobium-legume symbiosis, J. Supramol. Struct. and Cell. Biochem. 16:29 (1981)
6. G. P. Roberts and W. J. Brill, Genetics and regulation of nitrogen fixation, Ann. Rev. Microbiol. 35:207 (1981).
7. E. L. Schmidt, Initiation of plant root-microbe interactions, Annu. Rev. Microbiol. 33:335 (1979).
8. F. M. Ausubel and F. C. Cannon, Molecular genetic analysis of Klebsiella pneumoniae nitrogen fixation (nif) genes, Cold Spring Harbor Symposium of Quantitative Biology 45:487 (1980).
9. L. E. Mortenson and R. N. F. Thorneley, Structure and function of nitrogenase, Annu. Rev. Biochem. 48:387 (1979).

NITROGEN-CONTROL OF THE nif REGULON IN Klebsiella pneumoniae

M.J. Merrick, A. Alvarez-Morales, J. Clements, R. Dixon and M. Drummond

A.R.C. Unit of Nitrogen Fixation, University of Sussex Brighton, BN1 9RQ, England

INTRODUCTION

The prospect of manipulating nitrogen-fixing systems so as to reduce the demand for nitrogenous fertiliser in agriculture is frequently discussed in the context of plant genetic engineering. Klebsiella pneumoniae has become the model system for analysis of genetic and biochemical control of nitrogen fixation and a detailed understanding of the genetic control systems which regulate the nif regulon in K. pneumoniae is of considerable importance for future genetic manipulation of this complex gene cluster.

Nitrogen fixation in K. pneumoniae is repressed by ammonia and certain amino acids, and recent studies in our laboratory have demonstrated that this 'nitrogen-control' is exerted at two levels. A general nitrogen-control system, analogous to the ntr (gln) system of Salmonella typhimurium[1] and Escherichia coli,[2] coordinates the synthesis of enzymes required for assimilation of a wide variety of nitrogen sources. This general control is mediated by the products of the ntrA, B and C genes which are responsible for regulation of the glnA (glutamine synthetase) gene, the hutUH (histidine) operon, several amino acid transport operons and the nifLA operon. Nif-specific control is in turn mediated by the products of the nifLA operon.

Our recent studies have been directed towards a dissection of the relative contributions of the ntrA,B,C and nifLA systems to nitrogen-control of the nif regulon. These studies reveal an intriguing similarity between the ntrBC and nifLA systems, and comparison of the promoter sequences of genes under the control of either or both systems lends further support to the hypothesis

239

that ntrBC and nifLA are related both in evolutionary terms and in
their modes of action.   Such studies also have important
implications for research designed to obtain expression of the nif
regulon in other organisms.

GENERAL NITROGEN-CONTROL OF THE NIF REGULON

In 1974 Magasanik et al.[3] proposed a model for nitrogen-control
in which it was postulated that the enzyme glutamine synthetase (GS)
could function as a transcriptional activator for several nitrogen
assimilation operons such as those responsible for utilisation of
histidine and proline.   Studies of mutations affecting GS expression
in K. pneumoniae then led Streicher et al.[4] and Tubb[5] to propose that
GS also regulated expression of the nif gene cluster.   However in
the last five years genetic studies of nitrogen control in
S. typhimurium, E. coli, K. aerogenes and K. pneumoniae have led to
the emergence of a different model[6] for regulation of nitrogen
assimilation in which GS is no longer considered to be a regulatory
protein, and instead the products of three genes ntrA, ntrB and
ntrC are proposed to mediate nitrogen control.   We have studied
these three genes in K. pneumoniae and shown that they are primarily
responsible for transcriptional control of the nifLA operon.

The glnA ntrB ntrC gene cluster from K. pneumoniae was cloned
on a 12 kb HindIII fragment into plasmid pACYC184 to give plasmid
pGE100.[7]   This plasmid and a number of its derivatives (Fig. 1)
were studied by complementation analysis and by in vitro
transcription/translation in order to locate particular genes and

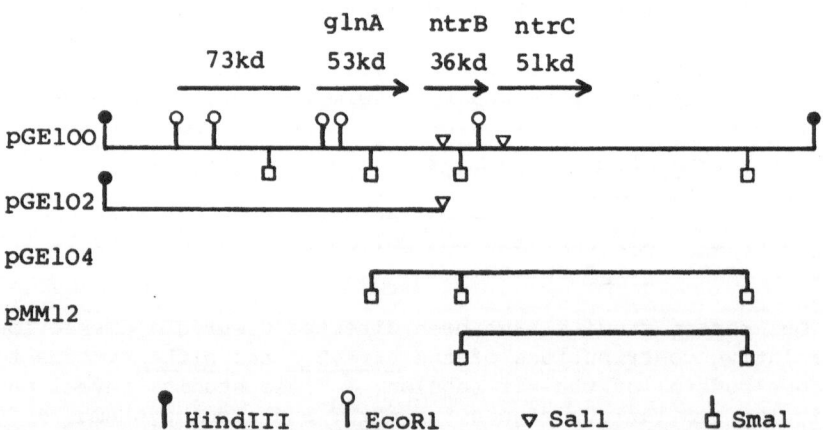

Fig. 1. Plasmid pGE100 and derivative clones.

identify their products.   Using two-dimensional polyacrylamide gel electrophoresis pGE100 was shown to direct synthesis of five polypeptides (molecular weights 73, 53, 51, 39, 36 kd) from the 12 kb cloned fragment.[7]   Subsequent analysis allowed us to locate the genes coding for most of these polypeptides (Fig. 1) and suggested, by analogy with data from E. coli and S. typhimurium that the 53 kd, 36 kd and 51 kd polypeptides were respectively the glnA, ntrB and ntrC products of K. pneumoniae.   Complementation analysis was consistent with these allocations.   Only pGE100 and pGE102 complemented glutamine auxotrophs to prototrophy in agreement with our prediction that the 53 kd polypeptide is the GS monomer produced from glnA.   The 36 kd and 51 kd polypeptides were synthesised from a 3 kb region previously defined as glnR.[8]   In E. coli and S. typhimurium the analogous region comprises ntrB and ntrC with products of 36 kd and 54 kd respectively.[1]

We have shown that of the genes in the glnA ntrB ntrC cluster only ntrC is required for activation of the nif regulon [see UNF1838 (pMM12), Table 1].   However activation by the ntrC product from pMM12 is not observed in an ntrA⁻ strain.   As ntrC is expressed from a constitutive promoter (that of the kan gene) on pMM12, ntrA is not required for ntrC transcription and we therefore conclude that the ntrA product is required for activity of the ntrC product.

Table 1.   Complementation analysis of pGE100 and derivative plasmids

Recipient strain			Plasmid					
	-		pGE100 glnA$^+$ntrB$^+$C$^+$		pGE104 ntrB$^+$C$^+$		pMM12 ntrC$^+$	
	N_2[a]	NH_4[b]	N_2	NH_4	N_2	NH_4	N_2	NH_4
UNF619 glnA$^+$ntrB$^+$C$^+$	100	<0.1	72	<0.1	78	<0.1	122	16
UNF1828 ntrC⁻	3	<0.1	88	<0.1	79	<0.1	nd	nd
UNF1838 Δ(glnA ntrBC)	<0.1	<0.1	96	<0.1	92	135	64	59
UNF1748 ntrA⁻	<0.1	<0.1	nd	nd	<0.1	<0.1	<0.1	<0.1

[a] Nitrogenase activity as % of derepressed (N_2) UNF619.

[b] Nitrogenase activity in repressed conditions (20 mM NH_4^+) as % of UNF619 (N_2).   nd - not done.

Comparison of the data obtained with pGE100 (glnA$^+$,ntrB$^+$,ntrC$^+$) and pGE104 (ntrB$^+$C$^+$) in strains UNF1828 (ntrC$^-$) and UNF1838 (glnA ntrB ntrC)Δ indicates that a functional glnA gene is required in order to obtain ammonia repression of the nif regulon.   This is consistent with the occurrence of point mutations in glnA which allow ammonia constitutive expression of nif.[9,10]   Such strains (GlnAC$^-$) have very low glutamate dehydrogenase levels and cannot therefore assimilate ammonia via either the GS or GDH pathways. Consequently the cells are always subject to a marked nitrogen limitation and are not able to generate the metabolic signal for ammonia repression.

The precise role of ntrB in nif regulation has not yet been determined.   However by analogy with data from S. typhimurium[1] and E. coli[11] ntrB might be expected to mediate ammonia repression of nifLA probably by acting in concert with ntrC.

To summarise, our present data indicate that activation of transcription at p nifLA requires the products of ntrC and ntrA, whilst repression probably requires the ntrB and ntrC products together with a functional glnA gene to generate the metabolic signal for repression.   In strains in which nifA is expressed constitutively from a foreign promoter ntr control of nif is overridden, suggesting that all ntr control is exerted at p nifLA. In support of this we have demonstrated that ntrC cannot activate transcription of the nifHDKY operon (M. Merrick, unpublished).

In a detailed analysis of the nifLA promoter we have now defined those regions in the promoter which are required for ntrC activation.[12]   Full promoter activity requires a region of at least 150 bp upstream of the transcriptional start site and the level of expression is progressively reduced as this upstream sequence is deleted.   However, 7% of full promoter activity is retained in a deletion extending to nucleotide -28 and this level of activity is still ntrC dependent and subject to ammonia control. The retention of some positive control in deletions removing the -35 region of the nifLA promoter tends to preclude binding of the activator molecules to an upstream site as the sole mechanism of transcriptional activation at this promoter.   It is possible that activation occurs by a mechanism involving direct contact between the activator and RNA polymerase as has been proposed for the cat[13] and λP$_{RM}$ promoters.[14]

NIF-SPECIFIC CONTROL OF THE NIF REGULON

In the absence of ntrC activation of p nifLA we found that the nifA gene product is able to autogenously activate at its own promoter;[12] a feature which further extends the analogy between the nifA and ntrC gene products.   With this in mind we examined the relationship between ntrA and nifA and found that, as with ntrC, the ntrA gene product is required if the nifA gene product is to be functionally active.   Using plasmids which constitutively produce either nifA product (pMC71A) or ntrC product (pMM14) we found that whereas either plasmid can complement an ntrC mutation and activate pnifLA neither plasmid allows activation in an ntrA⁻ strain (Table 2).

Previous experiments to study nif-specific regulation of the nif regulon have shown that the nifA product acts as a transcriptional activator at all other nif promoters[15] and that the nifL product acts as a nif-specific repressor in response to ammonia and amino acids[16] although at lower levels of fixed nitrogen than those required for nifLA repression.   Consequently we can now construct a model (Fig. 2) in which the products of ntrA, ntrB, ntrC, nifL and nifA act in concert to produce a regulatory cascade which controls very precisely the level of expression of the nif regulon.

CONCLUSION

The similarities between ntrBC and nifLA are considerable. Both gene pairs comprise an operon in which the product of the first gene is a repressor and that of the second is an activator. In both cases the activator is dependent upon the product of a third gene, ntrA, for activity.   The activator proteins are very similar in molecular weight (51-55 kd) and both are basic proteins of similar pI.   Finally in the case of pnifLA either ntrC or nifA can function to promote transcription.

Table 2. Failure of nifA and ntrC gene products to activate nifLA transcription in an ntrA⁻ mutant.[a]

Plasmid genotype	Recipient genotype		
	ntr⁺	ntrA⁻	ntrC⁻
(nifL::lac)	507	8.3	12.8
(nifL::lac)(nifA^c)	365	14.5	194
(nifL::lac)(ntrC^c)	462	10.5	445

[a] Activation by nifA or ntrC products from multicopy plasmids was assessed by measuring β galactosidase activity (standard units) from a nifL::lac fusion on plasmid pMF182, under derepressed conditions.

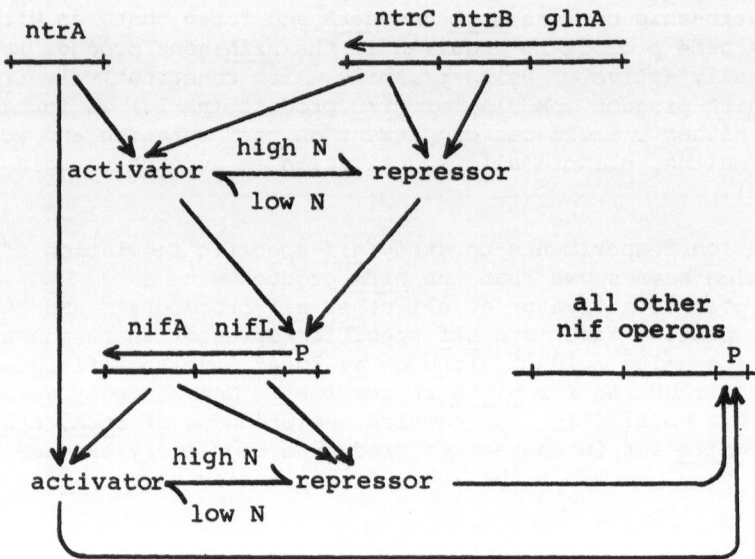

Fig. 2.   Proposed model for nitrogen control of the nif gene
           cluster.   Repression may be mediated by ntrB/C and
           nifL/A protein complexes.   Both the ntrC and nifA
           products require ntrA product for activity.

Comparison of sequences upstream of genes regulated by ntrC
or nifA has revealed a region of substantial homology located
between 50 and 100 nucleotides upstream of the ATG initiation codon
of these genes (Table 3).   In this comparison the nifH sequence
lacks homology at the downstream end which may reflect the absence
of ntr mediated control at this promoter.   Whilst the precise
significance of those common sequences is unknown they do lend
further support to the concept of an evolutionary and functional
relationship between ntrC and nifA.

Finally, it is clear that in any future consideration of the
expression of the K. pneumoniae nif regulon in other organisms the
nifA-specific requirement for ntrA product dictates that in its
present form the nif regulon will not be expected to function under
nifA control unless a compatible ntrA gene product is present in
the cell.   Such considerations highlight the utility of the
Klebsiella pneumoniae nif regulon as a model system for our
understanding of and future manipulation of the nitrogen fixation
process.

Table 3. Homologous sequences in regions upstream of
          genes under ntrC or nifA control

Organism	Gene	Homologous sequence
S. typhimurium	argTr	5'-tTAAcGtcGaAtcGtTTTtGC-3'
S. typhimurium	dhuA	5'-AcAAGGtaGaAttGcTTT-GC-3'
E. coli	glnA	5'-AaAAGttgGCACaGaTTTcGC-3'
K. pneumoniae	nifL	5'-ATAAGGgcGCACgG-TTT-GC-3'
K. pneumoniae	nifH	5'-ATAAacagGCACgGcTggtat-3'

REFERENCES

1. N. McFarland, L. McCarter, S. Artz, and S. Kustu,
    Nitrogen regulatory locus 'glnR' of enteric bacteria
    is composed of cistrons ntrB and ntrC: Identification
    of their protein products, Proc. Natl. Acad. Sci. USA
    78:2135 (1981).
2. G. Pahel, D.M. Rothstein, and B. Magasanik, Complex
    glnA-glnL-glnG operon of Escherichia coli, J. Bact.
    150:202 (1982).
3. B. Magasanik, M.J. Prival, J.E. Brenchley, B.M. Tyler,
    A.B. Deleo, S.L. Streicher, R.A. Bender, and C.G. Paris,
    Glutamine synthetase as a regulator of enzyme synthesis,
    Curr. Top. Cell. Regul. 8:119 (1974).
4. S.L. Streicher, K.T. Shanmugam, F. Ausubel, C. Morandi,
    and R.B. Goldberg, Regulation of nitrogen fixation in
    Klebsiella pneumoniae: evidence for a role of glutamine
    synthetase as a regulator of nitrogenase synthesis,
    J. Bact. 120:815 (1974).
5. R.S. Tubb, Glutamine synthetase and ammonium regulation
    of nitrogenase synthesis in Klebsiella, Nature,
    251:481 (1974).
6. M.J. Merrick, A new model for nitrogen control, Nature,
    297:362 (1982).
7. G. Espin, A. Alvarez-Morales, F. Cannon, R. Dixon, and
    M. Merrick, Cloning of the glnA, ntrB and ntrC genes
    of Klebsiella pneumoniae and studies of their role in
    regulation of the nitrogen fixation (nif) gene cluster,
    Mol. Gen. Genet. (in press) (1982).

8. F.J. de Bruijn, and F.M. Ausubel, The cloning and
    transposon Tn5 mutagenesis of the glnA region of
    Klebsiella pneumoniae: Identification of glnR, a gene
    involved in the regulation of the nif and hut operons,
    Mol. Gen. Genet. 183:289 (1981).

9. K.T. Shanmugam, I. Chan, and C. Morandi, Regulation of
    nitrogen fixation. Nitrogenase-derepressed mutants of
    Klebsiella pneumoniae, Biochim. Biophys. Acta, 408:101
    (1975).

10. J.M. Leonardo, and R.B. Goldberg, Regulation of nitrogen
    metabolism in glutamine auxotrophs of Klebsiella
    pneumoniae, J. Bact. 142:99 (1980).

11. Y-M. Chen, K. Backman, and B. Magasanik, Characterisation
    of a gene, glnL, the product of which is involved in
    the regulation of nitrogen utilisation in Escherichia
    coli, J. Bact. 150:214 (1982).

12. M. Drummond, J. Clements, M. Merrick, and R. Dixon,
    Positive control and autogenous regulation at the nifLA
    promoter in Klebsiella pneumoniae, (submitted for
    publication).

13. S.F.J. Le Grice, and H. Matzura, Binding of RNA polymerase
    and the catabolite gene activator protein within the cat
    promoter in Escherichia coli, J. Mol. Biol. 150:185
    (1981).

14. D.K. Hawley, and W.R. McClure, Mechanism of activation of
    transcription initiation from the λP_{RM} promoter, J. Mol.
    Biol. 157:493 (1982).

15. R. Dixon, R.R. Eady, G. Espin, S. Hill, M. Iaccarino,
    D. Kahn, and M. Merrick, Analysis of regulation of
    Klebsiella pneumoniae nitrogen fixation (nif) gene
    cluster with gene fusions, Nature, 286:128 (1980).

16. M. Merrick, S. Hill, H. Hennecke, M. Hahn, R. Dixon, and
    C. Kennedy, Repressor properties of the nifL gene
    product in Klebsiella pneumoniae, Mol. Gen. Genet.
    185:75 (1982).

LOCALIZATION AND MOLECULAR GENETIC ANALYSIS OF SYMBIOTIC NITROGEN FIXATION GENES IN RHIZOBIUM MELILOTI

A. Kondorosi[*o], Z. Banfalvi[*], W. J. Broughton[o],
T. Forrai[*], G. B. Kiss[*], E. Kondorosi[*o], C. Pankhurst[o],
G. Randhawa[*], Z. Svab[*] and E. Vincze[*]

[*]Biological Research Centre, Hung. Acad.Sci. P.O.B.521
H-6701 Szeged, Hungary
[o]Max-Planck Institut für Züchtungsforschung, Abt. Schell
D-5000 Köln, FRG

INTRODUCTION

The soil bacterium Rhizobium meliloti fixes molecular nitrogen after establishment of a symbiotic association with the plant host Medigaco sativa. Certain genes coding for the development of this symbiosis reside in the bacterium, others are carried by the plant partner. This study was devoted to localize and identify symbiotic nitrogen fixation genes in the bacterium Rhizobium meliloti strain 41.

LOCALIZATION OF SYMBIOTIC MUTATIONS

In order to localize symbiotic genes in R. meliloti first a rather general approach was taken. We performed a random mutagenesis of the wild type R. meliloti 41 (AK631), isolated symbiotically defective mutants and then determined the location of mutations in the R. meliloti genome.
Two symbiotic phenotypes that are readily recognizable are the ability to form nodules (Nod$^+$) and the ability to fix molecular nitrogen within the nodules (Fix$^+$). Table 1 shows that after nitrosoguanidine (NTG) or Tn5 mutagenesis (using the suicide plasmid technique of Beringer et al., 1978) both Nod$^-$ and Fix$^-$ mutants were obtained. The number of Fix$^-$ mutants was much higher than that of the Nod$^-$, suggesting that the number of genes involved in the fixation process is higher.
There are a number of stages of nodule development which are recognizable by light or electronmicroscopy (Vincent, 1980). On

Table 1.   Isolation of symbiotic mutants of <u>Rhizobium</u> <u>meliloti</u> 41

Mutagenic treatment	Number of colonies screened	Mutants Nod$^-$	Fix$^+$
NTG	3900	2	42
Tn5	4550	3	15

this basis both Nod$^-$ and Fix$^-$ mutants could be assigned into several classes. For instance, some Nod$^-$ mutants evoked root hair
curling while others were unable to do so. These studies are in
progress in our laboratory.

In order to visualise the arrangement of symbiotic genes, we
wanted to localize symbiotic mutations on the chromsomal linkage
map of R.meliloti 41. This linkage map has earlier been constructed using R68.45-promoted chromosome mobilization (Kondorosi et al.
1977, 1980). In 5 mutants the <u>fix</u> alleles were localized on 4 different chromsomal regions, but in 6 other mutants the <u>fix</u> mutations and the <u>nod</u> mutations tested did not map onto the chromosome
(Forrai et al., submitted for publication).

We reported earlier (Banfalvi et al., 1981) that R. meliloti
41 harbours two large indigenous plasmids (megaplasmids; pRme4l<u>a</u>
and pRme4l<u>b</u>). Several lines of evidence have indicated that pRme
4l<u>b</u> codes for some nodulation and nitrogen fixation (<u>nif</u>) genes
(Banfalvi et al., 1981; Rosenberg et al., 1981). For instance,
Nod$^-$ mutants isolated after growth of AK631 at elevated temperature had deletions in this plasmid and some had lost the <u>nif</u> structural genes. The <u>nifH</u> and <u>nifD</u> structural genes of AK631 have been
cloned (Banfalvi et al., 1981) and the nucleotide sequences of
<u>nifH</u> and part of <u>nifD</u> have been determined from which the amino
acid sequences of the nitrogenase polypeptides were deduced (Török and Kondorosi, 1981). The size of the <u>nifH</u> gene product was
about the same (34000 d) when it was expressed from a strong E.co-
<u>li</u> promoter in E.coli minicells (Svab and Kondorosi, manuscript).
This cloned region (pID1 on Figure 1) was shown to hybridize specifically to pRme4l<u>b</u> (Banfalvi et al., 1981).

Using a ^{32}P-labelled DNA fragment carrying Tn5 as a hybridization probe, it was shown that in 5 extrachromosomally located
Tn5-induced Fix$^-$ and 1 Nod$^-$ mutants tested the Tn5 was located on
pRme4l<u>b</u>. In 4 of the 5 Fix$^-$ mutants the Tn5 was localized on a
12.8 kb <u>Bam</u>H1 fragment carrying the <u>nifH,D</u> genes.

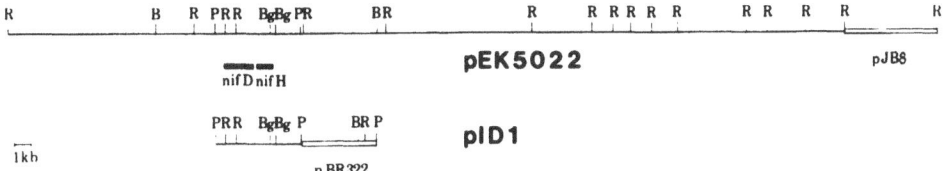

Figure 1. R.meliloti nif clones used in this study (from Kondorosi et al., submitted). The map shows only the EcoRI(R)
sites and some of the BamHI(B), BglII(Bg) and PstI(P)
sites. The detailed map of pID1 and the nucleotide sequences of nifH and part of nifD have been reported
(Banfalvi et al., 1981; Török and Kondorosi, 1981).

MOBILIZATION OF THE MEGAPLASMID CARRYING NODULATION AND NITROGEN
FIXATION GENES INTO OTHER RHIZOBIA AND AGROBACTERIUM

      We observed that the megaplasmid (pRme41b) exhibited a very
low level of self-transmissibility. To increase its transfer frequency we made it susceptible to mobilization with the P-1 type
plasmid pJB3JI (obtained from J. Beringer) by inserting the mobilization (mob) region of RP4 into it. First the mob region together with the kanamycine resistance marker (from a recombinant clone
p1011, kindly provided by R. Simon) was inserted in vitro into a
fragment of pRme41b cloned into pBR322. The recombinant plasmids
so formed (pAK11 and pAK12) were then mobilized into R.meliloti.
Since these recombinant plasmids were unable to replicate in R.me-
liloti, selection for kanamycin resistant derivatives allowed the
isolation of pRme41b::pAK11 and pRme41b::pAK12 cointegrates. It
was shown that in the majority of the recombinants pAK11 or pAK12
were integrated into the homologous fragment of pRme41b.
      The pRme41b cointegrates were transferred into nod - nif
deletion mutants of R.meliloti 41 where it was shown that both
Nod$^+$ and Fix$^+$ phenotypes could be restored. The cointegrates were
also transferred into two other Rhizobium strains (Rhizobium sp.
PN4003, Pankhurst, 1977; and NGR234, Trinick, 1980) and into Agrobacterium tumefaciens. The Rhizobium strains and A.tumefaciens
carrying pRme41b formed nodules of variable size on Medicago sativa roots, indicating that at least the early steps of nodulation of M.sativa are coded by pRme41b and are expressed in these
bacteria. Although the transconjugants contained the nif region,
as demonstrated by hybridization with a cosmid clone carrying a
49 kb segment of pRme41b containing the nif gene cluster (pEK

5022, Figure 1), the nodules did not fix N_2 (Kondorosi et al., submitted for publication).

CONSTRUCTION OF R-PRIME PLASMIDS CARRYING SYMBIOTIC GENES OF R.MELILOTI

Previous studies on symbiotic genes of R.meliloti indicated that some of these genes are clustered (Banfalvi et al., 1981; Rosenberg et al., 1981; Ruvkun et al., 1982). We thought that transmissible R-prime plasmids carrying sets of symbiotic genes might be valuable for further studies. In vivo - constructed R-primes carrying R.meliloti chromosomal regions have been already reported (Johnston et al., 1978; Kiss et al., 1980; Kondorosi et al., 1980). In these studies the ability of R68.45 to interact with the chromosome was exploited. Symbiotic genes, however, have not been identified on these R-primes.

In our experiments R-primes were derived from strains containing Tn5-induced symbiotic mutations. Since Tn5 is unable to transpose into new sites in R.meliloti (Meade et al., 1982; Forrai et al., submitted), transfer of kanamycin resistance into E.coli could be followed, providing a simple and efficient way to isolate R-primes.

Such R-primes were generated from both the chromosome and from the megaplasmid. Several R-primes from the megaplasmid were shown to hybridize with the cloned nif region. When these R-primes were transferred into different Nod$^-$ deletion mutants, the Nod$^+$ phenotype was restored. The plasmids were introduced also into A. tumefaciens and the transconjugants formed small nodules on M.sativa. The smallest R-prime of this type was 128 kb. From its physical analysis we concluded that nodulation and nitrogen fixation genes of the megaplasmid are clustered on less than a 70 kb DNA segment. With the help of a R.meliloti 41 gene library, made in cosmid vehicle pJB8, the physical map of these R-primes covering a 250 kb region of the megaplasmid, can now be determined.

EXPRESSION OF SYMBIOTIC GENES

We observed that only a relatively small region of the megaplasmid is transcribed actively in the nitrogen-fixing nodules. In these experiments RNA was isolated from nodules and from vegetatively grown bacteria, labelled with ^{32}P and hybridized to various R-primes or cosmid clones.

Fig. 2 shows that when RNA from vegetatively grown bacteria was used, numerous hybridizing fragments were observed, even in the case of the nif cosmid clone. The nif structural genes, however, did not express, as expected. When RNA from the nodules was hybridized, about a 20 kb region conferring the nif structural genes hybridized. This also suggests that in this DNA region several fix (probably nif) genes are clustered. This clustering was

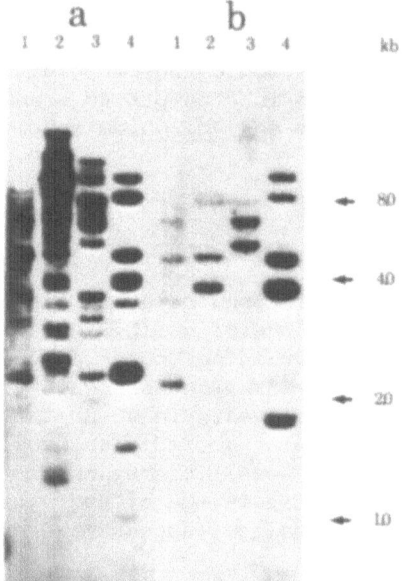

Figure 2.   Hybridization of ^{32}P-labelled RNA from vegetatively
            grown bacteria (a) and from nodules (b) to EcoRI-diges-
            ted R.meliloti DNA clones. Lanes 1 and 2: R-primes from
            the megaplasmid; 3: R-prime from the chromosome; 4: pEK
            5022 (Fig.1).

observed for two other R.meliloti strains as well (Ausubel et al.,
this volume; Corbin et al., 1982).

R-primes carrying other megaplasmid regions showed little
hybridization with nodule RNA. On Fig.2 /lane 3 a chromosomal R-
prime contains two EcoR1 fragments which hybridize to nodule RNA.
Tn5 mutagenesis indicated that at least one of these fragments
carries symbiotic genes. This gene maps between the pur-1 and cys-
46 chromosomal markers.
       Our studies suggest that hybridization of labelled nodule
RNA to R.meliloti gene library might be useful to fish out genes
expressing in the nodules.

CONCLUSIONS

       Genes coding for early functions of nodulation, the nif
structural genes and some other fix (probably nif) genes are clustered on about a 70 kb region of the megaplasmid. Transfer of
this region into other Rhizobium species or into Agrobacterium
resulted in Nod[+] Fix[-]nodules.
       Other fix genes were localized at four different chromosomal

regions. We assume that some of these genes are different or not present in other rhizobia or in Agrobacterium. This implies that some chromosomal fix genes would exhibit plant host specificity, which should be considered in attempts to transfer symbiotic nitrogen-fixing ability from one Rhizobium species to other bacterial species.

ACKNOWLEDGEMENTS

The work performed in Szeged was partially supported by O.M. F.B. grant No. 13017/FPI. One of us (G.S.R.) was recipient of a fellowship from the Int. Training Course of the Hungarian Academy of Sciences. Part of this work was done when three of us (A.K., E. K. and C.E.P.) were on one years leave at the Max-Planck-Institut für Züchtungsforschung, Köln, as recipients of fellowships from EMBO, from the Max-Planck-Gesellschaft and from the Alexander-von-Humboldt-Stiftung, respectively. We are very grateful to Prof. J. Schell for generous hospitality, support and critical discussions.

REFERENCES

Banfalvi, Z., Sakanyan, V., Koncz, C., Kiss, A., Dusha, I., Kondorosi, A. (1981) Mol. Gen. Genet. 184:334
Beringer, J.E., Beynon, J.L., Buchanan-Wollaston, A.V., Johnston, A.W.B. (1978) Nature (Lond.) 276:633
Corbin, D., Ditta, G., Helinski, D.R. (1982) J. Bacteriol. 149:221
Forrai, T., Vincze, E., Banfalvi, Z., Kiss, G.B., Randhawa, G.S., Kondorosi, A. (1982) submitted
Johnston, A.W.B., Bibb, M.J., Beringer, J.E. (1978) Mol. Gen. Genet. 165:323
Kiss, G.B., Dobo, K., Dusha, I., Breznovits, A., Orosz, L., Vincze, E., Kondorosi, A. (1980) J. Bacteriol. 141:121
Kondorosi, A., Kiss, G.B., Forrai, T., Vincze, E., Banfalvi, Z. (1977) Nature (Lond.) 264:525
Kondorosi, A., Vincze, E., Johnston, A.W.B., Beringer, J.E. (1980) Mol. Gen. Genet. 178:403
Kondorosi, A., Kondorosi, E., Pankhurst, C.E., Broughton, W.J., Banfalvi, Z. (1982) submitted
Meade, M.H., Long, S.R., Ruvkun, G.B., Brown, S.E., Ausubel, F.M. (1982) J. Bacteriol. 149:114
Pankhurst, C.E. (1977) Can. J. Microbiol. 23:1026
Ruvkun, G.B., Sundaresan, V., Ausubel, F.M. (1982) Cell 29:551
Rosenberg, C., Boistard, P., Denarie, J., Casse-Delbart, F.L. (1981) Mol. Gen. Genet. 184:326
Török, I., Kondorosi, A. (1981) Nucl. Acids Res. 9:5711
Trinick, M.J. (1980) J. Appl. Bacteriol. 49:39
Vincent, J.M. (1980) in: "Nitrogen Fixation 2", W.E. Newman, W.H. Orme-Johnson, eds, University Park Press, Baltimore.

CONSERVATION OF THE REGULATORY MECHANISMS REGULATNG THE EXPRESSION OF NITROGEN FIXATION GENES IN <u>R. meliloti</u> AND <u>K. pneumoniae</u>

Frederick M. Ausubel, David W. Ow and
Venkatesan Sundaresan

Department of Molecular Biology
Massachusetts General Hospital
Boston, Massachusetts 02114, USA

INTRODUCTION

The free-living nitrogen fixing bacterium <u>Klebsiella</u> <u>pneumoniae</u> reduces N_2 to NH_4^+ under conditions of NH_4^+ starvation and low O_2 tension. The reduction of N_2 is carried out by the enzyme complex nitrogenase which is comprised of polypeptides encoded by genes <u>nifH</u>, <u>nifD</u> and <u>nifK</u>. These three genes are organized into an operon transcribed in the direction <u>nifH</u> to <u>nifK</u> and are located within a cluster of at least 17 <u>nif</u> genes which are grouped into 7-8 transcription units. One of these operons, the <u>nifLA</u> operon, codes for regulatory proteins (for review, see ref. 1). The <u>nifA</u> product is involved in the activation of all of the other <u>nif</u> operons, while the <u>nifL</u> product is involved in the repression of these operons (2-7).

Recent studies of nitrogen assimilation in enteric bacteria (including <u>K. pneumoniae</u>) have shown that the process is under the control of a central regulatory system. Three genes, <u>glnF</u> (or <u>ntrA</u>), <u>glnL</u> (or <u>ntrB</u>), and <u>glnG</u> (or <u>ntrC</u>) have been identified as the regulatory elements in this process. Under conditions of NH_4^+ excess, various operons involved in nitrogen assimilation [e.g. <u>hut</u> (histidine utilization); <u>put</u> (proline utilization); etc.] are repressed by <u>glnG</u> in concert with <u>glnL</u>, and under conditions of NH_4^+ starvation they are activated by <u>glnG</u> in concert with <u>glnF</u> (for review, see ref. 8). The <u>K. pneumoniae</u> <u>nif</u> genes are also under the control of the <u>gln</u> (or <u>ntr</u>) regulatory system due to the fact that the <u>nifLA</u> regulatory operon is itself regulated by <u>glnG</u> (<u>ntrC</u>) (9,10).

In this paper we review recent data from our laboratory which demonstrate that the nifA gene can substitute for the glnG gene in a variety of genetic complementation tests (11). In addition, we review data which show that the nifA gene, like the glnG (ntrC) gene, requires glnF (ntrA) in order to mediate its regulatory effect (11,12). These results, and others described below, suggest that the nifA gene has evolved directly from the glnG gene.

In contrast to K. pneumoniae, the bacterium Rhizobium meliloti does not reduce nitrogen in the free-living state but only in symbiosis with its host plant alfalfa. Recently, our laboratory has described the cloning and characterization of the nifHDK genes from R. meliloti (13,14). We showed that the R. meliloti nifH and nifD genes share considerable sequence homology with their K. pneumoniae counterparts and that the operon organization of the nifHDK genes is the same in the two species (14). Here we summarize recent data from our lab which demonstrate that the regulatory proteins and DNA sequences which regulate nifHDK expression have also been conserved between the two species (15). Thus the K. pneumoniae nifA gene product specifically activates the R. meliloti nifH promoter and this activation requires the glnF gene product (12,15). In contrast to the K. pneumoniae nifH promoter, however, the R. meliloti nifH promoter can also be activated by the E. coli glnG (ntrC) gene (12). This latter finding supports the conclusion, stated above, that the nifA and glnG genes are evolutionarily related.

In conjunction with the above studies, we have determined the DNA sequences and transcriptional start points of three promoters: K. pneumoniae nifL and nifH and R. meliloti nifH (15,16). A comparison of these promoter sequences (all of which are activated by the nifA gene product) reveals striking sequence homologies in the -10 and -35 sequences.

Structure of the nifHDK and nifLA Promoters

The DNA sequences of the K. pneumoniae nifL promoter and the K. pneumoniae and R. meliloti nifH promoters are shown in Figure 1. Because the amino acid sequences of the nitrogenase polypeptides have been highly conserved in evolution, it was possible to identify and clone the R. meliloti nifHDK genes on the basis of DNA homology to previously cloned K. pneumoniae nifHDK genes (17). The approximate location of the R. meliloti nifH gene promoter was determined using Tn5 mutagenesis and partial DNA sequencing data which localized the R. meliloti nifH gene on cloned DNA fragments (13,14). The translational initiation codons of the two nifH genes were determined by comparing the DNA sequences of the two genes with the known amino acid sequences of nifH polypeptides from several species (14,18). The transcriptional start points of the two nifH genes was determined by the S1 nuclease mapping procedure of Berk and Sharp (19) using RNA isolated from derepressed K. pneumoniae

```
            -30         -20                55 bp          +70
             .           .             .                   .
nifL:   CACGCCGATAAGGGCGCACG GTTTGCA TG-------CACAGGAGTTTGCGATG
                                                   SD        Met


            -30         -20               . 52 bp    +60      +70
             .           .                           .         .
Rm nifH: TTTAGACGGCTGGCACGAC TTTTGCA CG-------ACAAAGGAAGCAAGATG
                                                   SD        Met


            -30         -20               . 12 bp    +20      +30
             .           .                           .         .
Kp nifH: CAGGCACGGCTGGTATGTT CCCTGCA CT-------CAGGAGAAGTCACCATG
                                                   SD        Met
```

Fig. 1. Promoter sequences of the K. pneumoniae nifH and nifL genes
        and the R. meliloti nifH gene.

cells or alfalfa nodules (15).

The K. pneumoniae nifL promoter region was initially delimited
by generating a set of deletions in vitro extending from a
restriction endonuclease site within and near the 5' end of the nifL
gene (16). [The location of the nifL gene had been determined
previously by physically mapping insertion mutations within the
gene.] The resulting set of nifL deletion plasmids was tested for
complementation of a nifA⁻ mutation. Because none of the deletions
used for this analysis extended into the nifA gene, a Nif⁻ phenotype
could be attributed to the deletion of regions required for nifL
transcription or translation. The presumptive promoter region was
then sequenced and the transcriptional initiation point was
determined as above using the S1 nuclease mapping procedure with in
vivo mRNA. The ATG translational initiation codon was identified by
aligning the DNA sequences with unpublished N terminal amino acid
sequence data provided by M. Chance and W.H. Orme-Johnson.

In order to readily monitor the activity of gln (ntr) and nif
regulatory proteins on the nifH and nifL promoters, we constructed a
variety of gene fusions as described below. The overall strategy
underlying these studies was to construct E. coli strains carrying
two compatible recombinant plasmids. One plasmid produced either
the nifA or the glnG gene product under the influence of a strong
promoter. The second plasmid carried the promoter whose activation
we wished to monitor fused translationally to the E. coli lacZ gene.
The advantage of using E. coli as the host strain for these studies
is the availability of a large number of mutant strains carrying

256   F. M. AUSUBEL ET AL.

well characterized lesions in gln (ntr) regulatory genes (8). By
monitoring the production of beta-galactosidase, we could thus
determine the ability of either glnG (ntrC) or nifA to activate one
of the three promoters in a genetically defined system.

The activity of the nifH promoters was monitored by constructing
translational nifH::lacZ fusions using lacZ from E. coli (20).
These "lac" fusions were carried on plasmid pBR322; The 1st and 29th
codons of K. pneumoniae and R. meliloti nifH respectively were fused
to the 8th codon of lacZ (15). The activity of the nifL promoter
was also monitored with a lacZ translational fusion at approximately
the 60th codon of nifL (11,16). This latter fusion was derived from
a plasmid which carries an internal nifL deletion on a low copy
plasmid vector derived from the broad host-range plasmid RK2.
Insertion of a lacZ fragment from plasmid pMC1403 (20) yielded the
nifL-lacZ in-frame fusion (pDO531).

NifA gene product was produced in E. coli using both
constitutive and inducible nifA overproducing plasmids. The
constitutive nifA overproducing plasmid (pGR397) (21) consisted of a
transcriptional fusion between the kanamycin promoter of pACYC177
and nifA. An inducible nifA overproducing plasmid (pDO516) was also
constructed which placed nifA transcriptionally fused to the
lacPO$_{UV5}$ promoter [the UV5 mutation renders the lac promoter
insensitive to glucose repression (11)]. Repression of the lacPO$_{UV5}$
promoter on the multicopy plasmid pDO516 was accomplished by the use
of a repressor-overproducing gene lacI^Q on an episome. In this
latter strain, nifA transcription is only "switched on" in the
presence of a lac inducer such as isopropyl-beta-D-galactoside
(IPTG).

In addition to the gene fusions described above which were
constructed in our laboratory, we also made use of two additional
fusions which allowed us to either produce the glnG product
constitutively in E. coli or to monitor the activity of the glnALG
promoter. λ gln101 contains the glnA promoter transcriptionally
fused to lacZ and cloned in phage lambda (22) and plasmid pGln53
contains the glnA promoter transcriptionally fused to glnG (23).
(The latter plasmid produces glnG constitutively in the presence of
NH$_4^+$ due to the deletion of the glnL gene which is required for
repression of the glnALG promoter.)

nifA Product Activates its Own Promoter and Substitutes for glnG
Product

We tested the validity of the current model that gln (ntr)
control elements regulate nif expression through the nifLA operon by
monitoring beta-galactosidase synthesis from the nifL-lacZ fusion
(pDO531) in various K. pneumoniae and E. coli strains containing
different gln (ntr) mutations. These experiments showed: 1) that a

plasmid containing only glnG⁺ (pGln53) is sufficient (and necessary) to activate the nifL promoter in an E. coli host carrying a gln(ALG) deletion, 2) that NH_4^+ does not repress the activation of nifL by constitutively produced glnG product in the absence of glnL, and 3) that glnF is required for glnG mediated activation of nifL (11).

Although the nifA gene product may not be required for nifLA transcription, it is conceivable that activation of this operon may be enhanced by the nifA gene product and thereby alleviate the requirement for high levels of glnG and possibly glnF gene products. In fact, we found that the constitutive production of the nifA product activated the nifL promoter in the absence of the glnALG operon (11).

Because we discovered that the nifA gene product activated a promoter also activated by glnG (namely its own promoter), we examined the possibility that the nifA product activates the glnA promoter (and thereby mediates the production of higher levels of glnG proteins and consequently higher levels of nifL and nifA proteins). We found a wild-type level of activation from the glnA promoter in a glnG⁻ mutant strain carrying a nifA plasmid. glnF was required for this activation. Thus it appears that nifA can substitute for glnG with apparently the same requirement for glnF as previously reported for glnG (11).

The finding that the nifA product can replace the glnG product in activating both its own promoter and that of the glnALG operon prompted us to investigate whether the nifA product can activate other genes positively controlled by glnG such as those governing the catabolism of certain amino acids. We found that an E. coli glnG⁻ strain recovered the ability to use arginine or proline as sole nitrogen source when harboring the nifA overproducing plasmid pGR397. We concluded that the nifA product can replace the glnG gene product in the activation of these glnG positively controlled genes (11).

Activation of the K. pneumoniae nifH Promoter

Activation of the K. pneumoniae nifH promoter in a glnALG deletion strain required only nifA product and was independent of NH_4^+ (15). As above, nifA activation of the nifH promoter required glnF (12). Constitutive production of glnG product, either in the presence or absence of NH_4^+ failed to activate K. pneumoniae nifH (12).

Activation of the R. meliloti nifH Promoter

Examination of the DNA sequences of the R. meliloti and K. pneumoniae nifH promoters shown in Fig. 1 reveals that neither promoter exhibits good homology to the E. coli consensus sequences at -10 and -35 which are required for recognition by RNA polymerase. This is consistent with the model that the nifH promoters require activator proteins for transciption.

The consensus sequences (based on data for E. coli RNA polymerase) are TTGACA at -35 and TATAAT at -10. Although the K. pneumoniae and R. meliloti nifH promoters show poor homology to these consensus sequences, they show surprisingly good homology to each other (8 bp at -32 and 5 bp at -10). The conservation of ACGGCTGG (located at -25 to -32) is particularly interesting since this region of certain promoters has been found to be involved in recognition by activator proteins. This observation raised the intriguing possibility that the K. pneumoniae nifA gene product might be able to activate the R. meliloti nifH promoter.

In fact, utilizing the promoter fusion plasmids described above, we made the following observations concerning the activation of the R. meliloti nifH promoter: 1) The R. meliloti nifH promoter is activated by K. pneumoniae nifA carried on a multicopy plasmid in E. coli at about 50% of the level of the K. pneumoniae nifH promoter (15). 2) Activation of the R. meliloti nifH promoter requires glnF (12).   3) In contrast to the K. pneumoniae nifH promoter, the R. meliloti nifH promoter is activated by glnG and this activation requires glnF (12).

The results reported in this section, in light of the results reported above that nifA can substitute for glnG, are consistent with the general model that gln (or ntr) regulation of nif expression evolved in a common ancestor of K. pneumoniae and R. meliloti and has been conserved in evolution. The data in this section also support the model that nifA evolved from glnG probably to mediate more stringent control on nif derepression in K. pneumoniae.

Comparison of Promoter Sequences Activated by nifA/glnG

Fig. 1 shows the structure of three promoters activated by K. pneumoniae nifA. Two of these promoters are also activated by E. coli glnG. All three also require glnF for activation. A comparison of these promoter sequences with the structure of three other promoters involved in nitrogen assimilation [the dhuA (histidine transport) and agrTr (arginine transport) promoters of Salmonella typhimurium and the glnA (glutamine synthetase) promoter of E. coli] reveals a presumptive consensus sequence of TTTTGCA at the -15 region for the promoters activated by nifA (16). This conclusion must be qualified because we have not demonstrated directly that nifA can activate the dhuA and argTr promoters, although this seems likely because nifA substitutes for glnG in the activation of the aut (arginine utilization), hut (histidine utilization), and put (proline utilization) genes (see above). A second qualification is that the transcriptional start points of the dhuA, argTr, and glnA promoters have not been determined. Therefore we cannot be certain that the presumptive consensus sequence (TTTTGCA) lies in the -15 region of each promoter although this seems likely because all of these promoter regions contain at least six out of seven basepairs of homology with TTTTGCA. Moreover, the dhuA and the glnA sequences share 8 basepairs (TTTTGCAC) and 12 basepairs (CTTTTGCACGAT) of homology with the R. meliloti nifH sequence respectively.

Among the six promoters that we compared, only the K. pneumoniae nifH promoter failed to respond to the glnG product. The -15 region of this promoter, which only responds to nifA, contains CCCTGCA instead of TTTTGCA. Because the K. pneumoniae and R. meliloti promoters share an 8 bp sequence (ACGGCTGG) in the -30 region, however, which is not shared by the other promoters, it is possible that strong activation by nifA requires the 8 bp sequence in conjunction with the common TGCA sequence in the -15 region.

A summary of the results presented in this paper are shown in diagrammatic form in Fig. 2. This figure reveals an interesting symmetry in the regulation of genes involved in nitrogen assimilation and helps to explain the evolutionay origin of the complex circuitry which regulates nif gene expression. Similar and related experiments are presented in this volume by Merrick et al. (24).

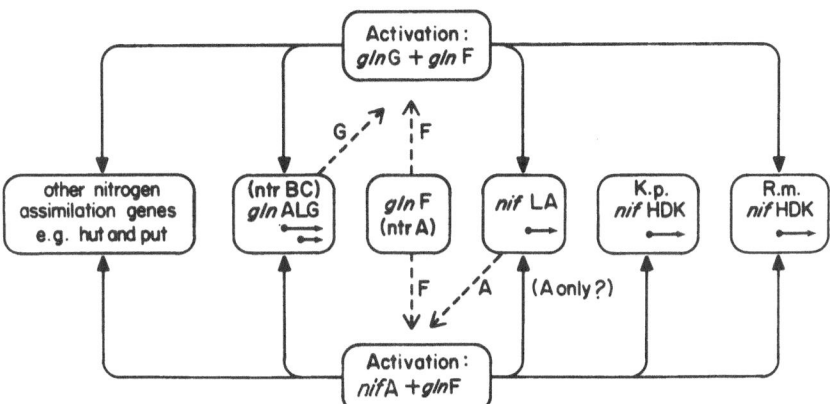

Fig. 2. Circuitry of nif control.

ACKNOWLEDGMENTS

    We thank W.H. Orme-Johnson and M. Chance for unpublished data on
the protein sequence of nifL; D. Rothstein for the DNA sequence of
the glnA promoter; B. Magasanik, G. Pahel, R. Bueno, J. Brosius, R.
Cate, W. Herr and G. Ruvkun for helpful discussions, and R. Hyde for
preparing the manuscript. This work was supported by NSF grants
#8104492 and #8104193 and USDA grant #59-2253-1-1-722-0. D.W.O. was
supported by a National Research Award in Biochemistry.

REFERENCES

1. F.M. Ausubel, S.E. Brown, F.J. de Bruijn, D.W. Ow, G.E. Riedel,
   G.B. Ruvkun and V. Sundaresan, Molecular cloning of nitrogen
   fixation (nif) genes from Klebsiella pneumoniae and Rhizobium
   meliloti, in: "Genetic Engineering," J.K. Setlow and A.
   Hollaender, eds., Plenum Press, New York (1982).

2. G.P. Roberts and W.J. Brill, Genetics and regulation of nitrogen
   fixation, Ann. Rev. Microbiol. 35:207 (1981).

3. R. Dixon, R.R. Eady, G. Espin, S. Hill, M. Iaccarino, D. Kahn
   and M. Merrick, Analysis of regulation of Klebsiella
   pneumoniae nitrogen fixation (nif) gene cluster with gene
   fusions, Nature 286:128 (1980).

4. S. Hill, C. Kennedy, E. Kavanagh, R.B. Goldberg and R. Hanau,
   Nitrogen fixation gene (nifL) involved in oxygen regulation of
   nitrogenase synthesis in K. pneumoniae, Nature 290:424 (1981).

5. M. Merrick, S. Hill, H. Hennecke, M. Hahn, R. Dixon and C.
   Kennedy, Repressor properties of the nifL gene product in
   Klebsiella pneumoniae, Molec. gen. Genet. 185:75 (1982).

6. V. Buchanan-Wollaston, M.C. Cannon and F.C. Cannon, The use of
   cloned nif (nitrogen fixation) DNA to investigate
   transcriptional regulation of nif expression in Klebsiella
   pneumoniae, Molec. gen. Genet. 184:102 (1981).

7. V. Buchanan-Wollaston, M.C. Cannon, J.L. Beynon and F.C. Cannon,
   Role of the nifA gene product in the regulation of nif
   expression in Klebsiella pneumoniae, Nature 294:776 (1981).

8. B. Magasanik, Genetic control of nitrogen assimilation in
   bacteria, Ann. Rev. Genetics 16:135 (1982).

9. F.J. de Bruijn and F.M. Ausubel, The cloning and transposon Tn5
   mutagenesis of the glnA region of Klebsiella pneumoniae:
   identification of glnR, a gene involved in the regulation of
   the nif and hut operons, Molec. gen. Genet. 183:289 (1981).

10. G. Espin, A. Alvarez-Mornales and M. Merrick, Complementation analysis of glnA-linked mutations which affect nitrogen fixation in Klebsiella pneumoniae, Molec. gen. Genet. 184:213 (1981).

11. D.W. Ow and F.M. Ausubel, The nifA gene which regulates the Klebsiella pneumoniae nif gene cluster can substitute for the nitrogen regulatory gene glnG, Nature, in press.

12. V. Sundaresan, D.W. Ow and F.M. Ausubel, Activation by gln regulatory proteins of the nifHDK promoters from K. pneumoniae and R. meliloti, submitted.

13. G.B. Ruvkun and F.M. Ausubel, A general method for site directed mutagenesis in prokaryotes: construction of mutations in symbiotic nitrogen fixation genes of Rhizobium meliloti, Nature 289:85 (1981).

14. G.B. Ruvkun, V. Sundaresan and F.M. Ausubel, Directed transposon Tn5 mutagenesis and complementation analysis of Rhizobium meliloti symbiotic nitrogen fixation genes, Cell 29:551 (1982).

15. V. Sundaresan, J.D.G. Jones, D.W. Ow and F.M. Ausubel, Conservation of nitrogenase promoters from Rhizobium meliloti and Klebsiella pneumoniae, submitted.

16. D.W. Ow, V. Sundaresan, D. Rothstein, S. Brown and F.M. Ausubel, A comparison of glnG and nifA regulated promoters, submitted.

17. G.B. Ruvkun and F.M. Ausubel, Interspecies homology of nitrogenase genes, Proc. Natl. Acad. Sci. USA 77:191 (1980).

18. V. Sundaresan and F.M. Ausubel, Nucleotide sequence of the gene coding for the nitrogenase iron protein from Klebsiella pneumoniae, J. Biol. Chem. 256:2808 (1981).

19. A.J. Berk and P.A. Sharp, Sizing and mapping of early adenovirus mRNAs by gel electrophoresis of S1 endonuclease-digested hybrids, Cell 12:721 (1977).

20. M.J. Casadaban, J. Chou and S.N. Cohen, In vitro gene fusions that join an enzymatically active beta-galactosidase segment to amino-terminal fragments of exogenous proteins: Escherichia coli plasmid vectors for the detection and cloning of translational initiation signals, J. Bacteriol. 143:971 (1980).

21. G.E. Riedel, S.E. Brown and F.M. Ausubel, Nitrogen fixation in Klebsiella pneumoniae is inhibited by certain multicopy hybrid

nif plasmids, J. Bacteriol., in press.

22. K. Backman, Y.M. Chen and B. Magasanik, Physical and genetic characterization of the glnA-glnG region of the Escherichia coli chromosome, Proc. Natl. Acad. Sci. USA 78:3743 (1981).

23. Y.M. Chen, K. Backman and B. Magasanik, Characterization of a gene, glnL, the product of which is involved in the regulation of nitrogen utilization in Escherichia coli, J. Bacteriol. 150:214 (1982).

24. M. Merrick et al., this volume (1983).

NODULE-SPECIFIC INDUCTION OF HOST GENES IN YELLOW LUPIN

A. B. Legocki, A. Konieczny, C. Madrzak, P. Stróżycki,
A. Wolánski and R. Kierzek[*]

Department of Biochemistry, Univeristy of Agriculture
60-637 Poznań, Wolyńska 35
*Institute of Bioorganic Chemistry, Polish Academy of
Sciences 61-704 Poznań, Noxkowskiego 12, Poland

There is a substantial progress in our knowledge about genetic
contribution of host plant to the process of symbiotic association
between legume plants and Rhizobium species. This progress has been
initiated recently by an elegant series of papers published by
D.P.S. Verma concerning identification and synthesis in vitro of
about 20 nodule-specific soybean polypeptides (nodulins).[1,2] These
studies revealed that soybean nodulins account for 7-11% of the total
nodule proteins and that they represent a class of 12-20kd polypeptides. The most abundant nodule-specific protein is leghaemoglobin.
The organization of leghaemoglobin genes in soybean has been proposed
recently.[3,4,5]

Here we summarize our recent studies on expression of nodule-
specific host genes in lupin plant. This work is a continuation of
our earlier studies on translation of poly(A)-containing RNA and
poly(A)-lacking RNA from lupin root nodules.[6,7]

I. Identification of lupin nodulins

In order to demonstrate the presence of de novo synthesized
nodule-specific lupin proteins we compared 2D electrophoretic
patterns of soluble proteins synthesized in vivo in root nodules
and in uninfected roots. Although the majority of polypeptides were
common for both tissues, we could detect a group of distinct polypeptides (nodulins) which were restricted to root nodules (Fig. 1).
They were detected by immunoelectrophoresis using lupin nodule-
specific sera. Lupin nodulins were found also among in vitro made
products directed by nodule mRNA (Fig. 2). According to our estima-

263

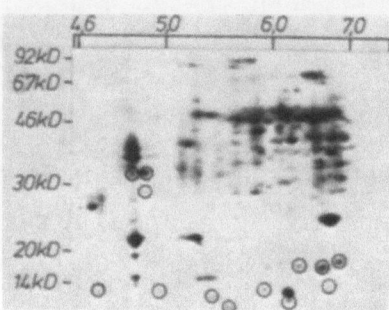

Fig. 1. Autoradiogram of gel electrophoresis of lupin nodule proteins
        labeled by reductive methylation. Nodule-specific polypep-
        tides are indicated (O).

tion, a group of lupin nodulins accounts for 10-12% of total soluble
nodule proteins. We started to purify lupin nodulins on preparative
scale using column chromatography on octylo-Sepharose and immunoaffinity chromatography on IgG-BioGel P300 column. These data will
be published elsewhere.

II. cDNA - mRNA hybridization studies

     The appearance of nodule specific polypeptides was confirmed in
soybean by cDNA - mRNA hybridization analysis. This method was proven
to be very useful for demonstration changes in the sequence concentration of mRNA population as a result of infection of the host plant
by Rhizobium species.[8] We performed similar studies with lupin mRNA
and applied for reverse transcription of poly(A)-RNA a synthetic
15-deoxy-nucleotide fragment: 5'-TGCTGCGTCTTT(GTC)CAT-3' specific
for two known C-terminal regions of lupin leghaemoglobins. The cDNA
transcript primed with synthetic fragment was expected to be enriched
with leghaemoglobin sequences. A preliminary identification of these
enriched sequences was obtained from reassociation analysis (Fig. 3)
and hybrid-arrested translation.

III. Radioimmunological screening for detection of cloned lupin
     sequences

     Since we are using plasmid vectors for cloning lupin nodule
sequences it was useful, having specific antibodies against lupin
proteins, to work out immunoscreening method for selection of those

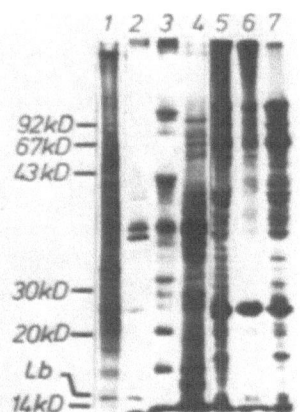

Fig. 2. SDS-gel electrophoresis of soluble cytoplasmic proteins
        synthesized in vivo (1-4) and in vitro in wheat germ
        system (5-7). Total nodule proteins (1), nodulins precipi-
        tated with anti-nodulin serum (2), uninfected root (3)
        and uninfected root proteins precipitated with anti-root
        serum (4), proteins were ^{3}H-labeled by reductive methylation,
        and ^{35}S-methionine-labeled translation products derived
        from translation of nodule mRNA before (5) and after
        immunoprecipitation with antinodulin (6) or anti-nodule (7)
        sera were autoradiographed.

transformants in which the expression of cloned plant sequences
occurs. The procedure is based on earlier findings that the
expressed hybrid polypeptide derived from sequence cloned to region
encoding for penicilinase, bacterial secretory protein is also
transported outside E. coli transformants. It involves the following
steps:

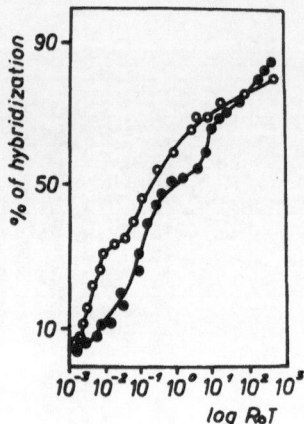

Fig. 3. Hybridization of cDNA primed by synthetic fragment (O)
and cDNA primed by oligo (dT)12-18 (●) with nodule
mRNA. Preparation of cDNA and reassociation conditions
will be published elsewhere (C. Mądrzak, R. Kierzek,
A. B. Legocki, manuscript in preparation).

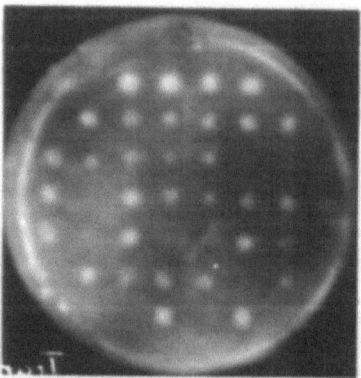

Fig. 4. Autoradiograph illustrating radioimmunodetection of lupin
antigens expressed in selected E. coli HB101 transformants.

a) Cloning lupin dscDNA to pBR 322 (G-C tailing, Pst 1 site, HB101).
b) Selection of recombinants (Tet^R, Amp^S), growth on agar plates 24h at 37°C and covering the plates with agar.
c) Transfer secretory hybrid bacterial-plant polypeptides on nitro-cellulose sheet by electrophoretic blotting.
d) Incubation with antiserum against lupin nodule proteins followed by incubation with ^{125}I IgG fraction for nodule proteins and auto-radiography.

From 1300 cDNA transformants about 30 clones were selected which gave a positive immunochemical response (Fig. 4). It was possible for selected transformants to detect on rocket immuno-electrophoresis plant polypeptides released to liquid medium. This simple immunoscreening procedure should significantly facilitate further structural work on organization of nodulin genes in lupin.

ACKNOWLEDGEMENTS

This work was carried out as Projects 09.7.1 and MR II.7 of the Polish Academy of Sciences.

REFERENCES

1. R.P. Legocki and D.P.S. Verma, A nodule-specific plant protein (Nodulin-35) from soybean. Science, 205:190 (1979).
2. R.P. Legocki and D.P.S. Verma, Identification of "nodule-specific" host proteins (nodulins) involved in the development of Rhizobium-legume symbiosis, Cell 20:153 (1980).
3. E. Truelsen, K. Gausing, B. Jochimsen, P. Jørgensen and K.A. Marcker, Cloning of soybean leghaemoglobin structural gene sequences synthesized in vitro, Nucl. Acids Res., 6:3061 (1979).
4. D. Sullivan, N. Brisson, B. Goodchild, D.P.S. Verma and D.Y. Thomas, Molecular cloning and organization of two leghaemoglobin genomic sequences of soybean, Nature 289:516 (1981).
5. O. Wiborg, J.J. Hyldig-Nielsen, E.Ø. Jensen, K. Paludan and K.A. Marcker, The nucleotide sequences of two leghaemoglobin genes from soybean, Nucl. Acids Res. 10:3487 (1982).
6. A. Konieczny and A.B. Legocki, Isolation and in vitro translation of leghaemoglobin mRNA from yellow lupin root nodules, Acta Biochim. Polon. 25:379 (1978).
7. A. Konieczny and A.B. Legocki, Translation and characterization of poly(A)-lacking RNA from lupin root nodules, Acta Biochim. Polon. 28:83 (1981).
8. S. Auger, D. Baulcombe and D.P.S. Verma, Sequence complexities of the poly(A)-containing mRNA in uninfected soybean root and the nodule tissue developed due to the infection by Rhizobium, Biochim. Biophys. Acta. 563:496 (1979).

A SEARCH FOR NODULIN GENES OF SOYBEAN

D.P.S. Verma, F. Fuller, J. Lee, P. Künstner,
N. Brisson, and T. Nguyen

Department of Biology
McGill University
Montreal, Canada

INTRODUCTION

The development of root nodule organs and eventual symbiotic
nitrogen fixation in a legume–Rhizobium association is the result of
complex genetic interactions between the two organisms. Data accumulated over 4 decades has shown that the host plays an important
role in this process. The influence of the host plant is observed
at all levels: recognition and acceptance of the rhizobial strain;
temporal regulation of nodule development; the number, size and
gross morphology of nodules; the intracellular organization and
structure of nodule cells; and finally the activity of the functional nodule (see Nutman, 1981; Verma, 1981; Verma and Long, 1982).
These processes are regulated in part by a number of host genes, and
several plant mutants have been isolated from various species which
exhibit specific perturbations of nodule development and efficiency
in fixing atmospheric nitrogen (Caldwell & West, 1977; Nutman,
1981). However, the exact number and function of these genes is not
known. Using molecular and immunological techniques, we have
attempted to identify some of the host genes and their products
which may be involved in the development of this symbiotic state.
The antibodies raised against soluble proteins of soybean root
nodules, when adsorbed with uninfected (control) root proteins and
reacted to the ^{35}S-methionine labelled in vitro translation products
of host polysomes, yielded a group of polypeptides which have been
termed nodulins (Legocki and Verma, 1980). Some of these proteins,
including nodulin-35 (Legocki and Verma, 1979), appear to be induced
in parallel with leghemoglobins (Lbs) and have been implicated in
the process of symbiosis (Verma, 1980).

A molecular probe for nodule-specific sequences, developed by
kinetic fractionation of total nodule cDNA, when hybridized to RNA
from uninfected and infected tissues indicated that nodule-specific
sequences may be present in the middle abundant fraction of the
nodule poly(A) + RNA (Auger and Verma, 1981). In order to understand
the molecular basis of interactions between a legume host and its
microsymbiont, Rhizobium, we attempted to isolate genes encoding
nodule-specific proteins of soybean. A cDNA library, constructed
from nodule-mRNA, was screened for nodule-specific sequences and
yielded several clones varying in abundance. These clones were
shown to be of host origin (see below) and were used for screening
two genomic libraries of soybean. Several genomic clones representing "nodulin" and leghemoglobin genes have been isolated. Two of
the Lb genes have been fully characterized at the nucleotide
sequence level, and we have shown that, in addition to the normal
genes, there are pseudo and truncated genes in the leghemoglobin
gene family in soybean. It appears that three of the Lb genes are
linked but no linkage to Lb genes has been observed for two nodulin
genes tested so far.

MODULATION OF HOST GENES DURING ROOT NODULE DEVELOPMENT

It is now well established that a number of host genes are
induced following infection of the plant by Rhizobium. Leghemoglobin, one of the major host gene products, appears in nodules
several days prior to the nitrogenase, and its mRNA sequences are
detected in all ineffective nodules tested (Verma et al., 1981a).
This indicates that the induction of Lb is independent of nitrogenase function. The level of induction, however, appears to depend
upon the specific strain of Rhizobium. Similar kinetics of induction is followed by several other nodule-specific sequences (Verma
et al., 1981b). Figure 1 summarizes our current understanding of
the modulation of various host genes following infection of the
plant by Rhizobium. Several evidences suggest that concomitant with
the induction of leghemoglobins and other nodule-specific sequences
there occurs a repression of some host sequences. The latter
mechanism may include regulation of the host defence mechanism,
since a normal response of a host to an invading pathogen is to
destroy it before it becomes parasitic. In addition, plant growth
hormones known to be produced by Rhizobium (see Libbenga and Bogers,
1974) appear to play an important role in the development of root
nodule symbiosis. We have shown (Auger and Verma, 1981) that there
is a subset of sequences which is common to both root and nodule
tissues but is more abundant in nodules, and its concentration can
be modulated by treatment with plant hormones (indole-acetic acid,
IAA). One such sequence is translated into a small molecular weight
peptide which can be induced by treatment of root with IAA alone
(Verma et al., 1982). The precise function of these genes can only

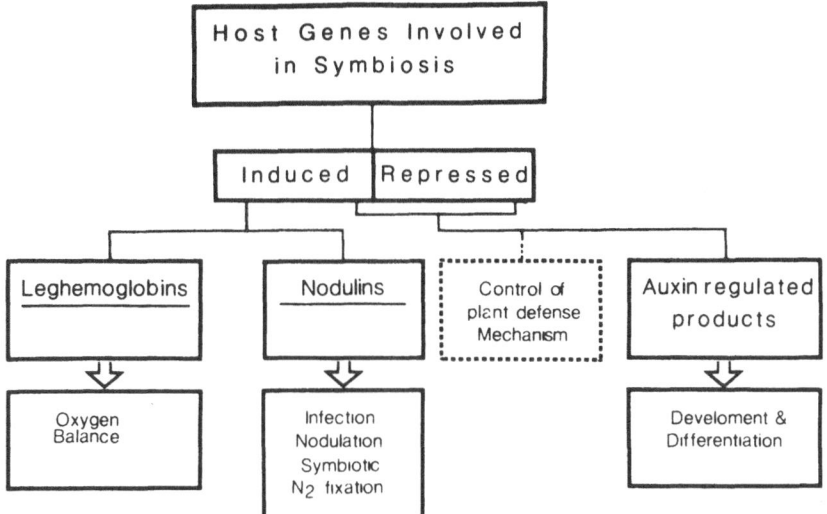

Figure 1. Various groups of host genes that appear to be involved
           in the development of root nodule symbiosis and their
           possible functions.

be studied once they are isolated and their products are fully
characterized.

MOLECULAR CLONING OF NODULE-SPECIFIC SEQUENCES

Development of a Soybean Nodule cDNA Library

     In order to isolate genes coding for nodulins and to study the
mode of induction of individual nodulin mRNAs, a library of cDNA
clones was prepared from poly(A) + RNA isolated from 21 day nodules.
Out of 6,000 ampicillin-sensitive clones, 25 were picked at random
and DNAs from these clones were dot-blotted onto nitrocellulose
paper and hybridized separately to nodule cDNA and root cDNA probes.
Thirteen clones hybridized well with the nodule probe but not with
the root probe. Five of these hybridized to a leghemoglobin genomic
clone, Ch4GmLb11 (Sullivan et al., 1981). Of the remaining 12
clones, one hybridized well to both root and nodule probes while one
hybridized weakly to the root probe. No hybridization of either
probe to the other 10 clones was detectable, indicating that the
sequences contained within them were of too low an abundance in the
cDNA population to be detected.

     The entire library was screened in a similar fashion by in
situ colony hybridization. About 600 clones (10%) hybridized above

Table 1. Characterization of some Nodule-specific Clones of Soybean

Clones Used as Probes	Approximate Size (bp)	Specification	Number of Clones Hybridized	Percentage	
				Total Library	Nod$^+$ cDNA Library
#23	510	Hybridize to pLb14 and GmLb11	900	15.0	–
#14	180	Cross-hybridize in colony hybridization and dot-blot assay	195	3.3	15.1
#15	700		295	4.9	22.9
#25	900		280	4.7	21.7
#45	370		62	1.0	4.8
#60	450		67	1.1	5.2

Controls on filters were: E. coli (strains DH1, K802 and DP50; E. coli containing pBR322; pLb14 (contain Lb cDNA sequence); clone 023 (contain sequences for rRNA); clone 59 and clone 60. Rhizobium japonicum (strains 61A76 and 61A24) and 61A76 DNA.

background to the root cDNA probe and were removed from the library. Of the remaining clones, about 2,300 (38% of the library) hybridized above background to the nodule cDNA probe. About 900 of these hybridized to a probe prepared by nick translation of the isolated insert DNA from a leghemoglobin cDNA clone, pLb23 (Table 1).Thus, the remaining 1,400 clones represented nodule-specific sequences.

Preliminary Characterization of Nodule-specific Clones

The 1,400 nodule-specific cDNA clones were further characterized by hybridization against nick translated, isolated insert DNAs from a subset of nodule-specific clones. The results are depicted in Table 1. Clones 14, 15 and 25 each hybridized to about 200 to 300 clones. Since the amount of overlap in colonies detected with each of these probes was very high, it seemed likely that these 3 clones contained different length copies of the same mRNA sequence. This is also indicated by the fact that the clone 15 probe cross-hybridizes intensely to isolated plasmid DNAs from clones 14 and 25. Two other clones, 45 and 60, hybridized to 62 and 67 distinct clones respectively. One of the clones hybridizing weakly to root cDNA, hybridized to about 15 clones in the nodule-specific library, indicating that some clones representing common sequences, which are in low abundance in nodule tissue, are represented in this library. In total, then, about 450 clones in the nodule-specific library have been identified in this manner, with about 950 yet to be characterized.

The fraction of the cDNA library represented by each clone is also depicted in Table 1. This number should be roughly equivalent to the mole fraction of poly(A) + RNA that each clone represents. Quantitative hybridizations of isolated cloned insert DNAs to increasing amounts of total polysomal RNA from root or nodule tissue (Fuller and Verma, manuscript in preparation) are in good agreement with the values indicated in Table 1. Normalizing to a value of 1 for clone 23 (leghemoglobin), clones 25 and 15 independently gave nearly the same results of about 0.30 mole fraction each, while clones 45 and 60 gave about 0.05 and 0.02 mole fractions respectively. No hybridization to root polysomal RNA, mitochondrial DNA or rhizobial DNA was observed for any of these clones, and their host origin was confirmed by hybridization to soybean genomic DNA (see below).

HOST ORIGIN OF THE CLONED NODULE-SPECIFIC SEQUENCES

Since RNA isolated from nodule tissue may be contaminated by sequences from bacteroids, the origin of the cloned sequences that appear to be specific to nodules was determined by direct hybridization with soybean genomic DNA. DNAs from Rhizobium (strain 61A76)

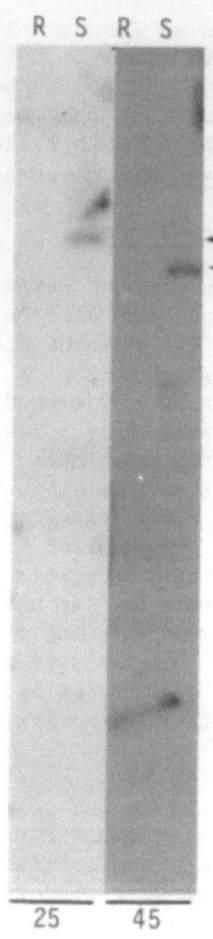

Figure 2. Hybridizations of clones 25
and 45 to EcoRI digested
soybean (s) and Rhizobium
japonicum (R) DNAs. Note
a single-band each corresponding to 7.0 and 5.8 kb fragment
hybridize to clones 25 and 45
in soybean genomic DNA only.

and uninfected soybean tissue (embryonic axes) were digested with
restriction enzyme EcoRI, and following electrophoresis, the DNA
fragments were transferred to nitrocellulose paper (Southern Blots)
and hybridized with ^{32}P-labelled DNA from clones 25 and 45. The
data in Figure 2 show that only one EcoRI fragment each in soybean
DNA hybridizes while there is no hybridization of these clones with
the Rhizobium DNA. These sequences do not appear to be reiterated
like leghemoglobins and are present on distinct EcoRI fragments of
5.8 and 7 kb in length. The host origin of several other nodule-
specific clones has been similarly determined. These results are
consistent with the earlier observations using a nodule-specific
cDNA probe which was hybridized in kinetic experiments with soybean
DNA (Auger and Verma, 1981).

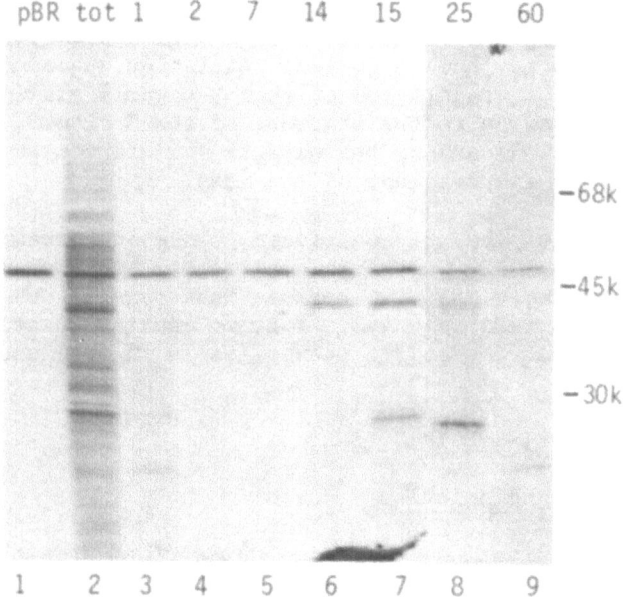

Figure 3. Hybrid-released translation of cloned nodule-specific
           sequences. Nodule RNA was hybridized to clones 1, 2, 7,
           14, 15-25, and 60, and hybrid-released fractions were
           translated in a rabbit reticulosyte lysate system using
           ^{35}S-methionine. Lanes 1 and 2 are pBR322 control and
           total translation product. The common band in the middle
           of the gel represents system background.

CHARACTERIZATION OF THE PRODUCT ENCODED BY CLONED SEQUENCES

     In order to determine if any of these clones indeed represent
mRNAs which encode nodulins (nodule-specific proteins), a positive
selection (hybrid-released) translation experiment was performed.
Isolated plasmid DNAs from various clones were denatured and fixed
to the nitrocellulose paper. Nodule total polysomal RNA was then
hybridized to each of these, and the nitrocellulose disks were
washed at high stringency. RNA/DNA hybrids were denatured by
boiling in water and the released RNA was translated in a rabbit
reticulocyte lysate in the presence of ^{35}S-methionine. Figure 3
depicts the autoradiograph of the resultant polypeptides after SDS-
polyacrylamide gel electrophoresis. Clones 14, 15, and 25 all
select a mRNA(s) encoding a polypeptide which appears as a doublet
at 44 and 43.5 kilo Daltons. In addition, clones 25 and 15 appear

to select a mRNA which encodes a 28.5 KD product. This may be the
result of selection and translation of a degradation product of the
parent mRNA which may have a correct initiation sequence but no
termination codon. Translation of such RNA would yield a truncated
polypeptide. Clone 14 is the shortest of the 3 clones, probably
corresponds to the 3' end of the mRNA, and would not be expected to
hybridize to a 5' end fragment of the mRNA.

In addition to these three clones, clone 60 corresponds to a
polypeptide of 23.7 KD. Although none of the other clones appear to
select a translatable mRNA, we believe that this is due to the
limited amount of mRNA selected. Further characterization of these
products using nodule-specific antibodies is in progress.

ISOLATION OF NODULE-SPECIFIC GENES

Genes Encoding Leghemoglobins

General Organization. Leghemoglobins (Lbs) are the most
abundant (25-30%) nodule-specific proteins. Earlier molecular
hybridization experiments (Baulcombe and Verma, 1978) had revealed
that the Lbs are encoded in the plant genome by a small family of
sequences, and about 10 EcoRI fragments from genomic DNA were found
to contain these sequences (Sullivan et al., 1981). We have isolated
several of these fragments from EcoRI and AluI-HaeIII genomic
libraries of soybean and have characterized two fragments at the
nucleotide sequence level (Brisson and Verma, 1982). The 11.5 kb
EcoRI fragment contained one complete Lb gene representing Lbc$_3$, as
well as a partial ψ Lb gene separated by 2.5 kb of intergenic
region. The 4 kb fragment contains a truncated sequence corresponding to the last exon of the normal Lb gene. We have recently
isolated an overlapping fragment that contains the rest of the ψ Lb
gene (Lee, unpublished data). Using flanking regions of these fragments, several clones have been isolated from an AluI-HaeIII library
which span about 28 kb around the 11.5 kb EcoRI fragment. Detailed
mapping in Figure 4 shows that there is no other Lb gene in the
vicinity of about 25 kb on the 3' end of the 11.5 kb EcoRI fragment.
Four other clones, representing 2 distinct gene regions which are
different from those described by Hyldig-Nielsen et al. (1982) and
Wiborg et al. (1982), have been isolated. These fragments do not
show any linkage at this stage of analysis; however, it is possible
that the intergenic regions are very large and thus would require
extensive "walking" on the chromosome.

Intragenic Structure and Evolution of Leghemoglobin Genes. There
are four major and four minor leghemoglobins present in soybean
nodules. While the major components are encoded by distinct genes,
the minor components appear to arise by post-translational

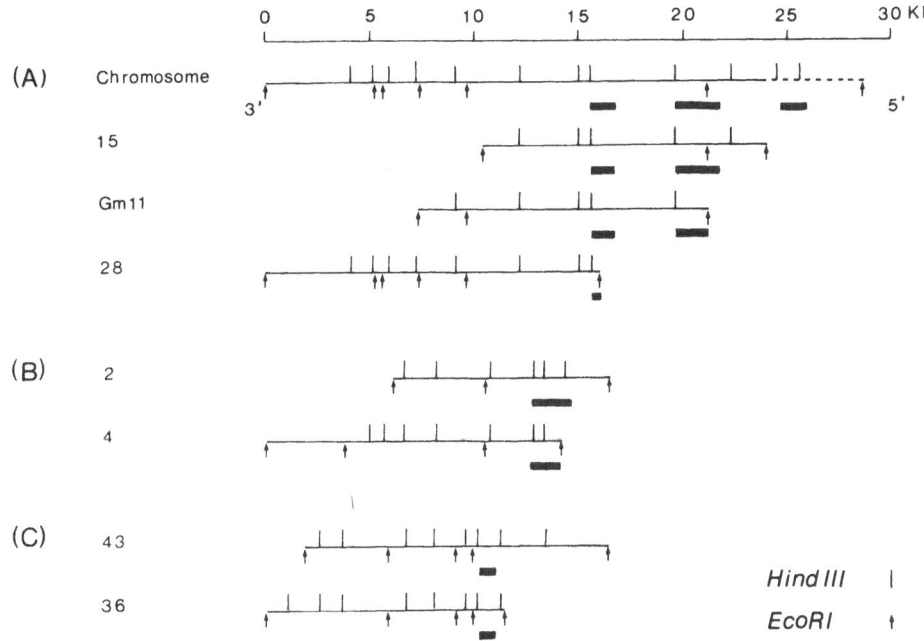

Figure 4. Linkage of three leghemoglobin genes and the isolation of
           genomic fragments representing two other Lb regions. (A)
           Chromosomal map around the 11.5 kb EcoRI fragment. (B) &
           (C), Restriction map of 4 genomic fragments isolated from
           an AluI-HaeIII library. The dotted region on the chromo-
           somal map is deduced from Hyldig-Nielsen (1982).

modifications of each of the major components (Whittaker et al.,
1981). Genes representing all major components have been isolated
(Brisson and Verma, 1982; Hyldig-Nielsen et al., 1982; Wiborg et
al., 1982). The Lbc_3 gene present on an 11.5 kb EcoRI genomic fragment spans 1200 nucleotides and is interrupted at 3 places (amino
acid positions 32-33, 68-69 and 103 - 104). The positions of the
intervening sequences are the same as in the other three leghemoglobin genes isolated so far. Thus, there is an extra intervening
sequence in this gene as compared to animal globin genes. The intervening sequences, as well as 5' and 3' flanking regions of Lb genes,
contain consensus sequences found in other eucaryotic genes.

The nucleotide sequence analysis of the second gene located
2.5 kb away on the 11.5 kb EcoRI fragment showed that this gene is

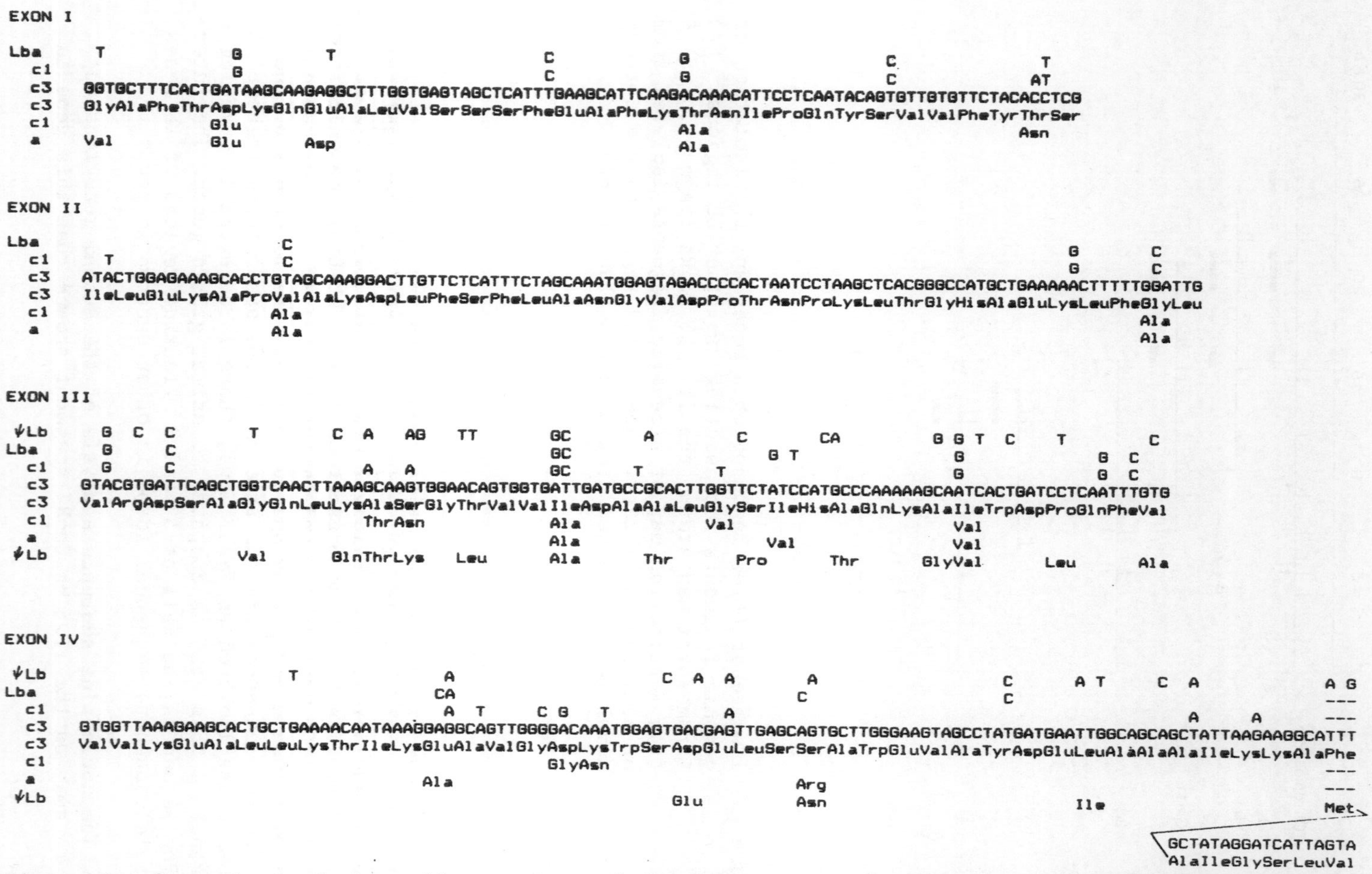

Figure 5. Comparison of the coding regions of the 3 Lb genes and that of a ψ Lb gene of soybean (see Lbc_3 and ψ Lb, Brisson and Verma, 1982; Lba and Lbc_1, Hyldig-Neilson et al., 1982).

incomplete, representing only exons 3 and 4. The coding sequence does not terminate at the normal position as in other Lbs, but an extra 6 amino acids, including methionine, are encoded at the 3' end of the molecule. The latter has not been found in any of the soybean leghemoglobins characterized to date. Thus, this sequence may represent a pseudo gene (ψ Lb). Figure 5 shows the comparison of the entire coding sequences of three different legitimate leghemoglobin genes and a ψ Lb gene. Sequence divergence values for different classes of nucleotide substitutions indicate that the amount of substitution at replacement sites is approximately the same for the three Lb gene comparisons. The silent substitution values are 6-8 times higher than the replacement values. However, the ratio of silent/replacement substitutions drops significantly when the coding sequences of ψ Lb is compared with the ones from the legitimate Lb genes. This provides some additional evidence that the ψ Lb sequences is in fact that of a pseudogene.

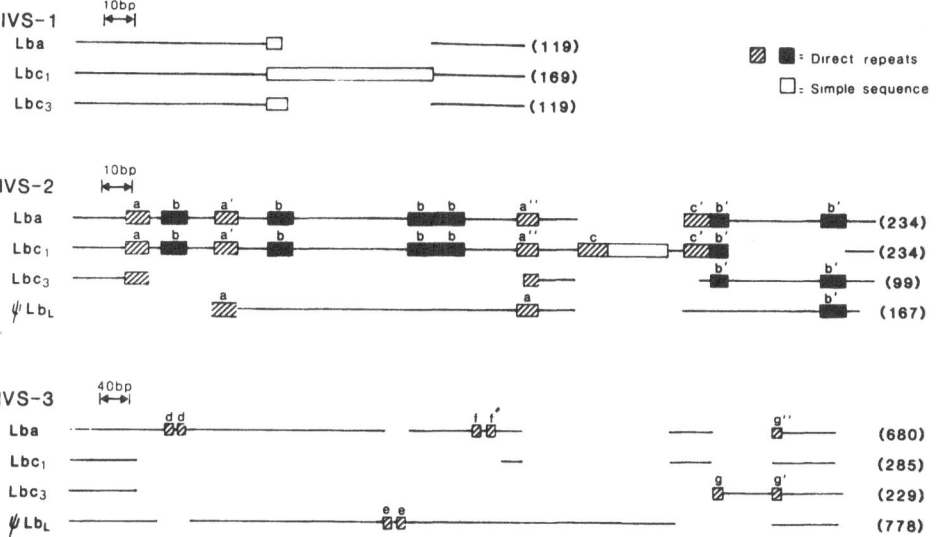

Figure 6.   Relationship between introns of various soybean leghemo-
            globins (see Fig. 5 for refs.). The length of the introns
            is indicated in parentheses. Homologous regions are shown
            by thin lines, and boxes indicate the location of various
            repeated sequences. Repeat a = TAAAATTA, a' = TAAGATTA,
            a" = TAAATTTC, b = TATTTTA, b' = TATTTTT, c = TGGTAATTA,
            c' = TGATAATTA, d = CAATCTTAAAA, e = TTGATTA,
            f = AGTTCAATATATATTCATTT, f' = AGTACAATATATTTTCATTT,
            g = TTTCGTACT, g' = TTATGTACT and g" = TTACGTACT.

The occurrence of deletions and insertions in the intervening
sequences is associated with repeated sequences (Figure 6). The
first additional stretch of sequence present in Lba, as compared to
the ψ Lb sequence, consists primarily of a direct repeat of the 14
bp sequence d. Similarly, additional stretches in ψ Lb, Lba and
Lbc$_3$ are flanked by the direct or near direct repeats e, f/f' and
g/g', respectively. Inverted repeat sequences, a feature common to
both procaryotic and eucaryotic transposons, are also found in the
Lb plant introns. This suggests that mobile genetic elements may
play a role in affecting heterogeneity in introns. Similar events
in goat globins have been postulated to be mediated by transposons
(Schon et al., 1981).

The amount of sequence divergence found between the leghemoglobin proteins within a species is considerably less than that
found between the Lb proteins of different species. A similar
situation is observed among the duplicated pairs of α and β globin
genes in animal genomes. This may be indicative of concerted evolution, i.e. the tendency of gene families to evolve in unison (Zimmer
et al., 1980). The rate at which replacement substitutions accumulate in a gene appears to be relatively constant, and it can serve
as a molecular clock for estimating the time that has elapsed since
various gene pairs diverged. By comparison with the rate of
accumulation of replacement substitutions in animal globin genes
(Efstratiadis et al., 1980), it can be estimated that the duplications which gave rise to the different Lb genes in soybean, or the
last time these duplicated genes were corrected against one another,
took place between 30 and 50 million years ago. However, the
sequence divergence between the soybean and lupin leghemoglobin proteins is nearly 50% (Hunt et al., 1978), a figure comparable to what
is observed between α and β globin proteins. Thus it appears that
the Lb genes may be evolving faster.

Nodulin Genes

Screening of the 2 (EcoRI and AluI-HaeIII) genomic libraries of
soybean with cDNA clones 25 and 45 yielded several recombinant
phages which may contain genes for these 2 nodule-specific sequence.
The frequency at which positive plaques were obtained is low but
similar for both genes, further indicating that they may be present
in only a few copies. This is consistent with the data in Figure 2
where only 1 EcoRI band hybridizing as unique sequence to each clone
was obtained. Hybridization of clone 25 with Lb genomic fragments
was negative, indicating that this gene is not closely linked with
Lb. Further characterization of nodulin genes, including general
organization and nucleotide sequence determination, may indicate
some common regulatory sequences which are responsible for their
coordinate induction following infection of the plant by Rhizobium.

Classical biochemical approaches to purify nodulins for their further characterization have so far been unsuccessful. However, attempts are being made to obtain monoclonal antibodies for these proteins which may assist in their purification and intracellular localization and thus provide some clue for their possible function(s) in root nodule symbiosis.

SUMMARY AND OVERVIEW

Evidence is presented which suggests that a number of host genes may be involved in the process of symbiotic nitrogen fixation. In addition to leghemoglobins, these genes encode a group of nodule-specific proteins, nodulins. Using molecular cloning we have isolated several cDNA clones representing these sequences. Moreover, we have obtained two genomic clones for nodulins and several for leghemoglobins. Chromosomal "walking" around the leghemoglobin gene locus showed that three Lb genes may be linked together. However, the sequences represented by 2 nodulin clones are not linked to the Lb genomic fragments isolated to date. Comparison of various Lb genes of soybean show a very similar structure in their coding regions while the lengths of the intervening sequences vary greatly. Several interesting features were found in the intervening sequences of these genes, including the presence of transposon type sequences. Based on the fraction of nucleotide substitutions in these genes, it appears that they have either been duplicated very recently or they are undergoing a kind of sequence correction. In addition to the normal genes, other sequences representing pseudo and truncated genes were also found in the Lb gene family.

What is the function of the nodule-specific genes in symbiosis and how are they regulated following infection of the plant by Rhizobium? These questions are fundamental to the understanding of the molecular basis of interactions between the host and the micro-symbiont. The role of leghemoglobins, the major nodule-specific product, is now well understood. However, the role of the nodulins is at present obscured. Most likely these gene products either: (a) are structural components of the nodule, or (b) are directly involved in facilitating nitrogen fixation, as is leghemoglobin, or (c) regulate expression of host and/or endosymbiont genes related to maintenance of nodule function. Since most of the nodule-specific sequences appear to be induced prior to nitrogenase in bacteroids, it is also likely that some nodulins play an important role in the establishment of symbiosis. The availability of specific molecular probes for nodulin encoding sequences (cDNA and genomic clones) and for nodulins in the form of monoclonal antibodies (experiments in progress) will now allow us to analyze the function of nodulins and the regulation of their syntheses in detail. Isolation of Rhizobium and plant mutants which affect specific stages of nodule development should further facilitate this analysis. It should also now be possible to determine whether any nodule-specific genes are present in the non-legume germ plasm which could aid in manipulation of the symbiotic nitrogen-fixation potential.

ACKNOWLEDGEMENTS

This work was supported by research grants from the National Sciences and Engineering Research Council of Canada and the Quebec Ministry of Education. The AluI-HaeIII library was kindly provided by R. Goldberg. We wish to thank Ms. Diane Longtin for maintaining various cultures, Mr. S. Purohit for his help in characterization of the cDNA library and Miss Yvette Mark for typing this manuscript. F.F. was supported in part by a NATO Post-doctoral Fellowship.

REFERENCES

Auger, S., and Verma, D.P.S., 1981. Biochem., 20:1300-1306.

Baucombe, D., and Verma, D.P.S., 1978, Nucl. Acid Res., 5:4141-4153.
        Brisson, N., Pombo-Gentile, A., and Verma, D.P.S., 1982, Can. J. Biochem., 60:272-278.

Brisson, N., and Verma, D.P.S., 1982, Proc. Nat. Acad. Sci., USA, 79:4055-4059.

Brown, G., Brisson, N., Fuller, F., and Verma, D.P.S., 1982, (Manuscript submitted).

Caldwell, B.E. and Vest, H.G., 1977, In: "A Treatise on Dinitrogen Fixation," R.W.F. Hardy and W.S. Silver, eds., Wiley-Interscience Pub., N.Y., pp. 557-576.

Efstratiadis, A., Posokony, J.W., Maniatis, T., Lawn, R.M., O'Connell, C., Spritz, R.A., De Riel, J.K., Forget, B.G., Weissman, S.M., Slightom, J.L., Blechl, A.E., Smithies, O., Baralle, F.E., Shoulders, C.C. and Proudfoot, N.J., 1980, Cell 21:653-668.

Hunt, L.T., Hurst-Caldrone, S., and Dayhoff, M.D., 1978, In: "Atlas of Protein Sequence and Structure 5," Supp. 3:229-251.

Hyldig-Nielsen, J.J., Jensen, E.O., Palndan, K., Wilborg, O., Garrett, R., Jorgensen, O.P., and Marker, K.A., 1982, Nucl. Acid. Res. 10:689-701.

Legocki, R.P., and Verma, D.P.S., 1979, Science, 205:190-193.

Legocki, R.P., and Verma, D.P.S., 1980, Cell, 20:153-163.
        Libbenga, K.R. and Bogers, R.J., 1974, In: "The Biology of Nitrogen Fixation," A. Quispel, ed., North-Holland Pub., Amsterdam, pp. 430-472.

Nutman, P.S., 1981, In: "Current Perspectives in Nitrogen Fixation," A.H. Gibson and W.E. Newton, eds., Aust. Acad. Sci., Canberra, pp. 194-204.

Schon, E.A., Cleary, M.L., Haynes, J.R. and Lingrel, J.B., 1981, Cell, 27:354-369.

Sullivan, D., Brisson, N., Goodchild, B., Verma, D.P.S., and Thomas,
    D.Y., 1981, Nature, London, 289:516-518.
Verma, D.P.S., 1980, In: "Genome Organization and Expression in
    Plants", C.J. Leaver, ed., Plenum Pub. Corporation, New York,
    pp. 439-452.
Verma, D.P.S., 1981, In: "Molecular Biology of Plant Development,"
    H. Smith and D. Grierson, eds., Blackwell Pub., Oxford,
    pp. 437-466.
Verma, D.P.S., Haugland, R., Brisson, N., Legocki, R., and
    Lacroix, L., 1981a, Biochem. Biophys. Acta, 653:98-107.
Verma, D.P.S., Legocki, R.P., and Auger, S., 1981b, In: "Current
    Perspectives in Nitrogen Fixation," A.H. Gibson and W.E.
    Newton, eds., Aust. Acad. Sci., Canberra, pp. 205-208.
Verma, D.P.S., and Long, S., 1982, Int. Review of Cytology, K. Jeon,
    ed., in press.
Verma, D.P.S., Bewley, D., Auger, S., Fuller, F., Purohit, S.K. and
    Künstner, P., 1982, In: "Genetic Engineering: Application to
    Agriculture," L.W. Owens, ed., USDA, Symposium VII, in press.
Whittaker, R.G., Lennox, S., and Appleby, C.A., 1981, Biochem. Int.,
    3: 117-124.
Wiborg, O., Hyldig-Nielson, J.J., Jensen, E.O. Paludan, K., and
    Marcker, K.A., 1982, Nucl. Acid Res., 10:3487-3494.
Zimmer, E.A., Matin, S.L., Beverley, S.M., Kan, Y.W., and Wilson,
    A.C., 1980, Proc. Nat. Acad. Sci., USA, 77:2158-2162.

ORGANIZATION AND TRANSCRIPTION OF NITROGEN FIXATION

GENES IN THE CYANOBACTERIUM ANABAENA

Robert Haselkorn, Steven J. Robinson and Douglas Rice

Department of Biophysics and Theoretical Biology
University of Chicago, Chicago, Ill. 60637 USA

The mechanisms for protection of nitrogen fixation enzymes from inactivation by oxygen appear to be as richly varied in the cyanobacteria as they are in the bacteria. An extra challenge to the cyanobacteria is provided by one property they all share: photosynthetic evolution of oxygen in the light. For many species of cyanobacteria, both unicellular and filamentous, this feature means that nitrogen fixation is principally a laboratory phenomenon, made possible by experimental inhibition of photosystem II and continuous removal of oxygen. Under these circumstances nif gene expression is formally regulated like that of Klebsiella: repressed by either oxygen or combined nitrogen (ammonia, nitrate, urea or amino acids). For other species, capable of differentiating heterocysts at regular intervals along filaments, aerobic nitrogen fixation is accomplished by restricting such activity to the anaerobic internal milieu of the heterocyst[1]. In such species, both differentiation and nif gene expression are repressed by combined nitrogen sources. Finally, some unicellular and filamentous cyanobacterial species have recently been shown to fix nitrogen under aerobic conditions without the benefit of morphologically evident structures, such as heterocyst walls, to protect against oxygen[2,3]. These species are particularly puzzling because, unlike Azotobacter which can fix nitrogen aerobically by consuming oxygen through vigorous respiration, the cyanobacteria evolve oxygen photosynthetically.

We have concentrated our efforts for the past decade on the regulation of heterocyst differentiation and the organization of the nif genes in Anabaena, a member of the second class described above[4-8]. We were initially attracted to this system because it presented a significant set of problems that could be approached using the techniques introduced for the study of bacterial virus infection, with which we were familiar. In fact, examination of the proteins synthesized at various stages of Anabaena heterocyst differentiation by using acrylamide gel electrophoresis, originally described by Hosoda and Levinthal for T4 infection of E. coli[9], was the first application of this methodology to a problem in prokaryotic development[5].

Those early studies produced two important results. First, under aerobic conditions, the nitrogenase proteins are synthesized only in heterocysts in Anabaena[4]. Second, the heterocyst develops from a vegetative cell by a succession of activations of sets of genes[5]. In this respect, the analogy with bacterial virus infection is particularly apt. In the absence of indications of significant transactions at the DNA level during heterocyst differentiation, the likely regulatory processes involve a transcription cascade. Because there are no systems of genetic analysis for any nitrogen-fixing cyanobacterium yet, we turned to recombinant DNA methods in order to obtain probes with which to study these transcriptional processes.

Before describing those studies, it is worth mentioning that the requisite genetic system may be attainable in the near future. Anabaena mutants that are defective in heterocyst development have been isolated[10,11]. Selectable antibiotic resistance markers have been described. Anabaena strains harbor a large number of small plasmids, as yet cryptic. It should be possible to construct transformation vectors by cloning antibiotic resistance genes into the endogenous plasmids and then to use these to clone developmental genes by complementation of the developmental mutants. However, this remains the program for the future. To date, we have only studied the genes for which cloned probes are already on hand.

We have cloned representatives of three classes of genes important in heterocyst differentiation and nitrogen fixation. These are the nif genes, which code for the structural components of nitrogenase;[6-8] the gln A gene, which codes for the enzyme glutamine synthetase;[12] and the rbc A gene, which codes for the large subunit of ribulose bisphosphate carboxylase[13]. During induction of nitrogenase, provoked by starvation for combined nitrogen, the activity of glutamine synthetase increases slightly while that of RuBP carboxylase disappears entirely. These changes are correlated with parallel changes in the corresponding messenger RNA levels.

The protocol for the cloning was similar in all three cases. Restriction enzyme fragments were first identified by hybridization of blots of total Anabaena DNA using cloned heterologous probes. In the case of the nif genes, these were the structural genes for nitrogenase (nif K, nif D) and nitrogenase reductase (nif H) from Klebsiella, cloned by Cannon, Riedel and Ausubel[14]. In each case the probe identified one or more fragments in Eco RI or Hind III digests of Anabaena DNA whose size dictated the appropriate λ library of total Anabaena DNA from which the cloned fragment could be isolated. Physical mapping, subcloning of fragments into plasmid vectors and, in some cases, nucleotide sequence determination followed[6-8,12,13,15].

Current information on the Anabaena nif genes is summarized in Figure 1 and compared there with the nif gene organization of Klebsiella. The Klebsiella genes are defined in terms of mutations that result in the absence

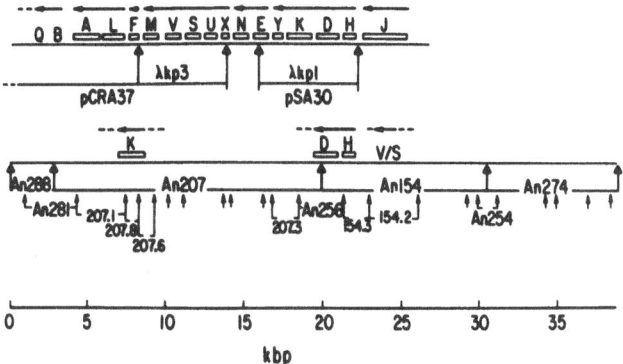

Fig. 1.   Comparison of the physical map of the nif genes of Klebsiella
            (above) and of Anabaena (below). Data for Klebsiella are from
            reference 16 and many others cited therein.   Boxes indicate
            protein sizes where they are known. Transcripts are shown by
            arrows but the only origin known precisely is for Anabaena nif H
            (this work). Thin vertical arrows on the Anabaena map locate
            HindIII sites;   thicker arrows   locate EcoRI sites.   HindIII
            subfragments of the Anabaena DNA with clone numbers are
            transcribed during nitrogenase induction; those without numbers
            are not transcribed (see reference 8).

of polypeptides of known function or, in the case of ts mutants, that result in
the production of polypeptides with altered isoelectric point. For Anabaena,
we do not have the appropriate mutants. However, in addition to the primary
identification of the gene by hybridization with specific Klebsiella probes, we
have used the cloned Anabaena DNA (in recombinant λ or in plasmids) to
direct the synthesis of proteins in UV irradiated E. coli, and then precipitated
the corresponding protein with antibody raised against partially purified
Anabaena nitrogenase subunits. Finally, Anabaena genes nif H[7] and nif K[15]
have been completely sequenced and nif D is nearly done. Each sequence
codes for a product of the size and properties (e.g., number and placement of
cysteine residues) expected for the relevant protein.

    The physical map has several unexpected features. In Klebsiella, the
three structural genes nif K, D and H are co-transcribed. This conclusion is
based on the polarity of insertion mutations in nif H and nif D. In Anabaena,
only nif D and nif H are cotranscribed. That conclusion is based on the
characterization of messenger RNA from Anabaena cells induced for
nitrogenase (shown below) and on the map of (Fig. 1). The gene nif K is
separated from nif D by 11 kbp. Transcripts corresponding to most of that 11
kbp are absent from the RNA prepared from induced cells[8]. On the other

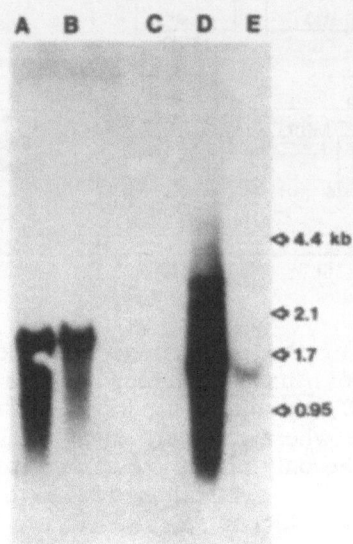

Fig. 2.   Northern blot hybridization detects three species of nif H
messenger RNA in Anabaena. Total RNA was prepared from cells
grown with NH3 (c) or induced anaerobically for nitrogenase (a
and d) or induced and then aerated for 45 min (b and e). Each
RNA preparation was glyoxal-denatured, electrophoresed, blotted,
and hybridized with labeled nif H DNA (pAn154.3; see Fig. 1 and
reference 7) (lanes c,d,e) or with labeled gln A DNA (pAn509,
containing a 1.4 kbp fragment within the gene for glutamine
synthetase; see reference 12) (lanes a,b). The latter serves as
control for the quality of the RNA from aerated cells. Mobility
of nucleic acid fragments of known sizes (in kb) are shown at
right.

hand, the RNA contains a 2.8 kb species identified by a nif H probe (Figure
2). Since the nif H gene contains only 900 bp and its transcript initiates
135 bp upstream (see below), this species must include the nif D gene as well.

There are more differences between Anabaena and Klebsiella nif gene
organization. The only other Anabaena nif gene we were able to identify by
hybridization with cloned Klebsiella DNA is either nif V or nif S, genes which
code for an unknown function required for "maturation" of nitrogenase.
These genes map to the left of nif K in Klebsiella but to the right of nif H in

G AG AC C CT S1

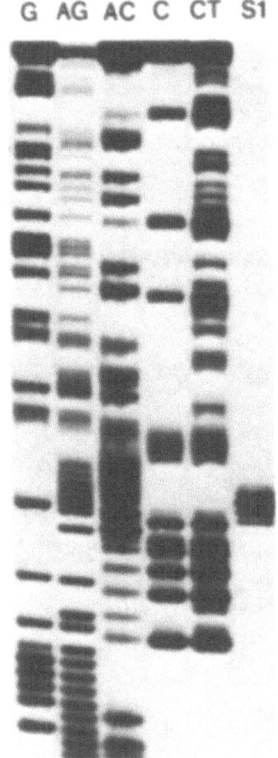

Fig. 3.   Determination of the origin of the Anabaena nif H transcript. A
^{32}P-labeled single-stranded DNA fragment, corresponding to
nucleotides -55 to -193 of the template strand for transcription
(the complement of the sequence in Figure 4), was annealed with
RNA from cells induced for nitrogenase, then digested with
nuclease S1 and analyzed by gel electrophoresis. A portion of the
undigested DNA fragment was subjected to base-specific
degradation procedures and analyzed in the other lanes (G, A+G,
A>C, C, C+T).

Anabaena (Fig. 1)[8]. In Klebsiella all of the nif genes are clustered within
20 kbp; there is virtually no space between the genes. We have cloned over
40 kbp of Anabaena DNA in four contiguous Eco RI fragments, but the
combined sizes of subfragments that are transcribed during nitrogenase
induction (Figure 1) is only 15 kbp[8]. It is likely that other nif genes lie
outside the region already cloned.

```
              -180                          -160
    TAACACCCAAAAGAACTTTCACAACTACATAACGAACCCATCATGAAC


         -140      ⬇       ⇩        -120                    -100
    ACTAATTCTACTGGTTTTTCTGTGGAGCGATCGCCCCCTCTTCGGCGACTG
                             Sau3a


              -80                          -60
    TTCTACATAACCCCTCACAGCCATAGCTCAAACAGGCGTGAGATCCAAAC
                                           Sau3a


         -40                      -20                      1
    ACAAAGACCGACCAACTAACCAACCAATTGCAGGAAAAGAGAACA  ATG


    ACT GAC GAA AAC ATT AGA CAG ATA GCT TTC etc.
```

Fig. 4.   Nucleotide sequence of the HincII DNA fragment containing the
            origin of transcription of Anabaena nif H. The open arrow shows
            the origin indicated by S1 nuclease protection; the solid arrow
            indicates the probable origin.

       Each of the small Hind III fragments of Anabaena DNA from the nif
region shown in Figure 1 was labeled and hybridized with RNA prepared from
cells induced anaerobically for nitrogenase. The qualitative result of these
experiments was that only two of the fragments, in addition to those already
known (by Southern hybridization with Klebsiella probes) to contain nif DNA,
were found to be transcribed. The others, including most of the region
between nif K and nif D, appear to be silent[8].

       The RNA complementary to the probe pAn154.3, which contains all of
Anabaena nif H, about 800 bp of 5'-flanking sequence, and about 100 bp of nif
D, was then examined in detail by Northern blot hybridization and by S1
nuclease protection. The former experiments are shown in Figure 2. The
messages containing nif H are found principally in three size classes, 3.2, 2.6
kb and 1.4 kb, which are seen only in the RNA prepared from induced cells.
These messages are absent from cells grown with NH_3 and they disappear
rapidly from anaerobically induced cells to which O_2 has been admitted
(Figure 2). The latter result explains in part why aerobic nitrogen fixation
requires heterocyst differentiation in Anabaena: the nif H gene is not
transcribed or its transcript is not stable in the presence of O_2.

       The message sizes are of interest as well. S1 nuclease protection
experiments show no RNA transcript on the 5' side of nif H before position
-135 in pAn154.3 (S. J. Robinson, unpublished). Therefore the message
species must have the same origin (at -135) and differ in their site of
termination or processing. The 3.2 and 2.6 kb species could encompass nif H
and nif D (135 + 900 + 1500 bp) while the smaller message would have to

terminate early in the nif D gene. Partial readthrough of a termination signal in nif D would allow the nif H protein to be made in greater abundance than the nif D protein, even though both genes are transcribed from the same promoter.

The nature of that promoter was determined by S1 nuclease protection, shown in Figure 3, of a DNA fragment cut from pAn154.3 with HincII and Sau 3A. The nif H message can be seen to originate just before a sequence of 5 A's, which corresponds to 5 U's on the message strand. The complete sequence of the HincII fragment is shown in Figure 4, with the apparent origin of transcription indicated by an open arrow. Because the stretch of A-U pairs is vulnerable to S1, we believe the true origin of transcription may be at the G indicated by the solid arrow. If that is so, then the sequences centered at -145 and -170 should be compared to the consensus "-10" and "-35" sequences of E. coli and B. subtilis. Those sequences are underlined in Figure 4. For strong promoters they should be TATAAT and TTGACA, respectively. The actual sequences observed, as well as nearby sequences, correspond to very strong down mutations in E. coli phage promoters (P. Youderian, personal communication). In addition, the Hinc II DNA fragment is not strongly transcribed in vitro by either E. coli or Anabaena RNA polymerase (C. Richaud, unpublished). All of these results suggest that the Anabaena nif H promoter is activated for transcription in vivo, perhaps by the Anabaena equivalent of the Klebsiella nif A protein.

To summarize: the structural genes for nitrogenase and nitrogenase reductase have been cloned from Anabaena and physically mapped. The map differs from that of Klebsiella in several ways, including the insertion of 11 kbp between nif K and nif D in Anabaena. One nif RNA transcript has been studied in detail and shown to originate from a site in the Anabaena chromosome that lacks good correspondence with a typical prokaryotic strong promoter, suggesting the possibility of a need for positive activation. The nif H message is unstable or repressed or both under aerobic conditions. This feature is sufficient to account for the need for heterocyst differentiation in order for Anabaena to fix nitrogen aerobically.

ACKNOWLEDGMENT

This research was supported by grant GM 21823 from the United States Public Health Service, grant 5901-0410 from the United States Department of Agriculture/Sciences and Education Administration through the Competitive Grants Office, a postdoctoral fellowship from the American Cancer Society to S.J.R. and a predoctoral traineeship from the NIH to D.R.

REFERENCES

1.   R. Haselkorn, Heterocysts, Annu. Rev. Plant Physiol. 29: 319 (1978).
2.   J. T. Wyatt and J. K. G. Silvey, Nitrogen fixation by Gloeocapsa, Science 165: 908 (1969).

3.   L. J. Stal and W. E. Krumbein, Aerobic nitrogen fixation in pure cultures of a benthic marine Oscillatoria, FEMS Microbiol. Lett. 11: 295 (1981).

4.   H. Fleming and R. Haselkorn, Differentiation in Nostoc muscorum: nitrogenase is synthesized in heterocysts, Proc. Natl. Acad. Sci. USA 70: 2727 (2973).

5.   H. Fleming and R. Haselkorn, The program of protein synthesis during heterocyst differentiation in nitrogen-fixing bluegreen algae, Cell 3: 159 (1974).

6.   B. J. Mazur, D. Rice and R. Haselkorn, Identification of bluegreen algal nitrogen fixation genes by using heterologous DNA hybridization probes, Proc. Natl. Acad. Sci. USA 77: 186 (1980).

7.   M. Mevarech, D. Rice and R. Haselkorn, Nucleotide sequence of a cyanobacterial nifH gene coding for nitrogenase reductase, Proc. Natl. Acad. Sci. USA 77: 6476 (1980).

8.   D. Rice, B. J. Mazur, and R. Haselkorn, Isolation and physical mapping of nitrogen fixation genes from the cyanobacterium Anabaena 7120, J. Biol. Chem. in press (1982).

9.   J. Hosoda and C. Levinthal, Protein synthesis by E. coli infected with bacteriophage T4D, Virology 34: 709 (1968).

10. T. C. Currier, J. F. Haury and C. P. Wolk, Isolation and preliminary characterization of auxotrophs of a filamentous cyanobacterium, J. Bacteriol. 129: 1556 (1977).

11. M. Wilcox, G. Mitchison and R. J. Smith, Mutants of Anabaena cylindrica altered in heterocyst spacing, Arch. Microbiol. 103: 219 (1975).

12. R. Fisher, R. Tuli and R. Haselkorn, A cloned cyanobacterial gene for glutamine synthetase functions in E. coli but the enzyme is not adenylylated, Proc. Natl. Acad. Sci. USA 78: 3393 (1981).

13. S. E. Curtis and R. Haselkorn, Characterization of a cloned cyanobacterial gene for the large subunit of RuBP carboxylase. DNA 1: 203 (1982).

14. F. C. Cannon, G. E. Riedel and F. M. Ausubel, Overlapping sequences of K. pneumoniae nif DNA cloned and characterized, Mol. Gen. Genet. 174: 59 (1979).

15. B. J. Mazur and C.-F. Chiu, Sequence of the gene coding for the β subunit of dinitrogenase from Anabaena, Proc. Natl. Acad. Sci. USA in press (1982).

16. F. M. Ausubel and F. C. Cannon, Molecular genetic analysis of K. pneumoniae nitrogen fixation genes, Cold Spring Harbor Symp. Quant. Biol. 45: 487 (1980).

OLIGOSACCHARINS: NATURALLY OCCURRING CARBOHYDRATES WITH BIO-

LOGICAL REGULATORY FUNCTIONS

Peter Albersheim, Alan G. Darvill, Michael McNeil, Barbara S. Valent, Janice K. Sharp, Eugene A. Nothnagel, Keith R. Davis, Noboru Yamazaki, David J. Gollin, William S. York, William F. Dudman and Janet E. Darvill and Anne Dell[*]

Department of Chemistry, Campus Box 215, University of Colorado, Boulder, Colorado 80309 USA
[*]Imperial College of Science and Technology, Department of Biochemistry, London SW7 2AZ, England

INTRODUCTION

Complex carbohydrates have many functions but, until recently, their functions were thought to be limited to serving as structural polymers and energy reserves. It is now well established that complex carbohydrates play an important role in biological recognition. In their role as recognition agents, complex carbohydrates are: receptors for phage and bacteriocins; specific surface antigens that can determine the pathogenicity of microbes, and the mating type, the blood group type, and tissue type of eukaryotic cells; highly specific receptors in eukaryotes for viruses, bacteria, hormones, and toxins; and determinants of where glycoproteins go within cells, when they are secreted, and when they are taken up. We have now come to recognize that certain complex carbohydrates are chemical messengers, that they are, in fact, biological regulatory molecules. Results of research in our laboratory have led us to believe that these chemical messengers are especially important in regulating growth, development, reproduction, and disease resistance in plants.

It has been known for some six years that oligoglucoside fragments of a major structural polysaccharide of fungal cell walls can elicit plant cells to accumulate phytoalexins (antibiotics). The enzymes that catalyze the synthesis of the phytoalexins are themselves synthesized _de novo_ in response to the elicitor[1,2,3,4]. The synthesis of phytoalexins by plants appears to be a general defense mechanism against potential pathogens[5].

Recognition of the biological activity of the fungal wall oligoglucosides did not, in itself, lead us to consider that fragments of plant cell wall polysaccharides might possess biological activity. This was true even though we were discovering hitherto unexpected structural complexities in plant cell wall polysaccharides, complexities that were far beyond those anticipated if these polysaccharides were serving a purely structural role[6,7,8]. The connection between biologically active carbohydrates and plant cell wall polysaccharides was made when it was discovered that bacteria can elicit the accumulation of phytoalexins in plant tissues by injuring plant cells and, in doing so, causing the release of a fragment of a plant cell wall polysaccharide that elicits the synthesis of phytoalexins[9,10]. This "endogenous elicitor," the first-to-be-recognized biologically active carbohydrate derived from plant cell walls, was shown to be a fragment of a pectic polysaccharide[10].

The second biologically active carbohydrate found to be present in plant cell walls was also determined to originate within a pectic polysaccharide. In this case, the biologically active carbohydrate is a molecule that induces the de novo synthesis in plants of proteins possessing the ability to inhibit the digestive proteinases of insects and bacteria[11]. A highly purified preparation of the pectic polysaccharide, rhamnogalacturonan I, extracted from the walls of sycamore cells grown in suspension culture induces the synthesis of the proteinase inhibitors in tomato leaves. The sycamore cell wall polysaccharide preparation was shown to be chemically related to a tomato leaf polysaccharide preparation possessing similar proteinase inhibitor-inducing activity[12].

The discovery that fragments of the wall polysaccharides of plant cells are regulatory molecules can be considered analogous to the discovery that peptide hormones in animals originate as portions of larger inactive polypeptides[13]. For example, several peptide hormones synthesized in the pituitary gland originate in a common precursor polypeptide called pro-opiocortin. A 16,000 dalton fragment of the precursor polypeptide is released by enzymatic hydrolysis, and the remaining polypeptide is cleaved to produce the hormones corticotropin and β-lipotropin. The corticotropin can be further cleaved to yield, among other peptides, α-melanotropin, a corticotropin-like intermediate peptide, and the β-lipotropin can be cleaved to yield γ-lipotropin, β-melanotropin, and β-endorphin. This processing of polypeptides and of fragments of polypeptides to yield a variety of regulatory molecules is strictly analogous to the process we envision to occur in cell walls, in which polysaccharides are cleaved to yield regulatory molecules.

We now call naturally occurring carbohydrates with biological regulatory functions "oligosaccharins." It appears that the endogenous elicitor and the proteinase inhibitor-inducing factor are just two examples of a variety of oligosaccharins with diverse activities. Our laboratory is now focussing much of its effort on confirming and extending the oligosaccharin hypothesis. A discussion of evidence in support of the existence of oligosaccharins is the primary topic of this lecture.

OLIGOSACCHARINS: NATURALLY OCCURRING CARBOHYDRATES WITH BIOLOG-
ICAL REGULATORY FUNCTIONS

The Purification and Structural Characterization of a Glucan Oligosaccharide Elicitor of Phytoalexins

The cell walls of Phytophthora megasperma f.sp. glycinea elicit the accumulation of phytoalexins in soybean[1,14]. Partial acid hydrolysis of the fungal cell walls yields literally hundreds of different β-glucan oligosaccharides, of which only a few possess elicitor activity.   In an effort to learn what structural requirements distinguish active from inactive glucan oligosaccharide elicitors, we have been working hard to purify elicitor-active and -inactive glucan oligosaccharides.   This knowledge will allow the chemical synthesis of relatively large quantities of an active glucan oligosaccharide elicitor that will then be used in experiments designed to determine how the oligoglucoside elicitor triggers phytoalexin accumulation.

The separation of a large number of neutral, similarly sized oligoglucosides to obtain a pure oligoglucoside elicitor has required the use of high-resolution gel filtration, normal-phase liquid chromatography, a PAC carbohydrate column, and reversed-phase liquid chromatography (RPLC) on 5 μ C-18 columns.   RPLC yields striking separations.   An oligoglucoside mixture, purified first by high-resolution gel filtration and eluting as one of several peaks on the PAC carbohydrate column, was separated into approximately 50 components by chromatography on two tandem Supelco Spherisorb-5 C-18 reversed-phase columns.   Only one of these components (a heptasaccharide as determined by fast atom bombardment mass spectrometry) has elicitor activity.   One nano-gram of the highly purified elicitor-active component elicits phytoalexins when applied to a soybean cotyledon.   The elicitor-active component eluting from the tandem Supelco Spherisorb-5 C-18 columns is still contaminated with inactive oligoglucosides. Chromatography of the most-purified component from the Supelco columns on tandem reversed-phase C-18 columns with different chromatography properties (Altex Ultrasphere ODS) appears to result in a pure oligoglucoside elicitor.

Inactive as well as active oligoglucosides from the complex mixture produced by partial hydrolysis of the mycelial walls are being purified and structurally characterized in order to determine the structural features which result in biological activity. The tentative structures of one active and three inactive heptaglucosides have been obtained using less than 25 μg of each of their permethylated derivatives. This was made possible by a micro methylation method developed in our laboratory (unpublished results of Thomas Waeghe). Combined gas chromatographic-mass spectrometric analysis, with selected-ion monitoring to enhance sensitivity, is being used to determine the structure of overlapping peralkylated oligosaccharide alditol fragments derived from the heptaglucosides[15,16]. We hope soon to confirm the structures of the active and inactive heptaglucosides.

The Purification and Structural Features of the Endogenous Elicitor of Phytoalexins

A major breakthrough, which led to the oligosaccharin hypothesis, was the discovery that a fragment of a plant cell wall polysaccharide is itself an elicitor of phytoalexins. The endogenous elicitor[17] has been purified from the mixture of oligosaccharides produced by partial acid hydrolysis of citrus pectin and, in separate experiments, from the mixture of oligosaccharides produced by partial acid hydrolysis of soybean cell walls. The predominant chemical component of the most purified preparation from both sources is an α-1,4-oligogalacturonide. This was established by glycosyl-residue composition-analysis, glycosyl-linkage composition-analysis, NMR analysis, and susceptibility of the biologically active material to hydrolysis by a highly purified α-1,4-endopolygalacturonase. Fast atom bombardment-mass spectrometric analysis established that the predominant chemical species of the most purified fraction is an α-1,4-dodecagalacturonide, an oligogalacturonide containing 12 galacturonosyl residues.

The endogenous elicitor can be inactivated by treatment with either a purified endopolygalacturonase or a purified polygalacturonic acid lyase[17]. The specific elicitor activities of the most highly purifed preparations were similar whether they were purified from the partial hydrolysate of citrus pectin or that of soybean cell walls. Thus, the endogenous elicitor is a molecule highly rich in α-1,4-galacturonic acid. The question remains as to whether the α-1,4-dodecagalacturonide is the elicitor. It is possible that a modified oligogalacturonide could copurify with the α-1,4-dodecagalacturonide and be the active component. The best approach to determining whether the α-1,4-dodecagalacturonide is the active elicitor is to synthesize it chemically.

The presence of the endogenous elicitor in plant cell walls raises the interesting question of the role this elictor plays in host-pathogen interactions. Recent experiments have shown that the bacterial pathogen Erwinia carotovora secretes polygalacturonic acid lyase, an enzyme that, when applied to soybean cotyledons, elicits phytoalexin accumulation. Further, this polygalacturonic acid lyase will release heat-stable pectic oligosaccharide elicitors from either citrus pectin or purified soybean cell walls. Similar results have been obtained by C.A. West and his co-workers, using another host-pathogen system. They have found that an endopolygalacturonase, a pectic-degrading enzyme secreted by the fungus Rhizopus stolonifer, can elicit the production of the phytoalexin casbene in castor beans[18,19]. They have also shown that the endopolygalacturonase can release a heat-stable elicitor (pectic oligosaccharide) from isolated cell walls of castor bean[20]. It seems likely that these enzyme-released heat-stable elicitors contain the oligosaccharin that we call the endogenous elicitor.

Abiotic treatments that injure plant cells, e.g., partial freeze-thawing, also elicit phytoalexin accumulation in plant tissue[5]. Such treatments may elicit phytoalexin accumulation by activating a plant enzyme that releases the endogenous elicitor from the cell wall. Evidence exists for the presence in injured plant cells of an enzyme that can release a heat-stable elicitor from plant cell walls[21]. The discoveries of a constitutive elicitor in extracts of injured plant tissues[22,23,24], of the chemical nature of the endogenous elicitor[10,17], and of an enzyme that can activate the endogenous elicitor by releasing it from covalent attachment in the cell wall, provide an explanation for the manner in which microbes, as well as such abiotic elicitors as heavy metals, UV light, and partial freezing, can result in accumulation of phytoalexins in plant tissues.

An Oligosaccharin That Inhibits the Incorporation of ^{14}C-Leucine into Polymers of Sycamore Cells and That Could Be Involved in the Hypersensitive Resistance Response

An important mechanism by which plants resist microbial invasion is known as the hypersensitive response. This response involves the death of the first plant cell or cells contacted by an invading microorganism. The "sacrifice" of the plant cells appears to result in the slowing down of the microorganism's growth. Although the ultrastructural changes that take place during the hypersensitive response have been studied in detail[25], the biochemical events that occur are not understood.

Results from several different lines of research suggested to us that plant cell walls are likely to contain an oligosaccharin that is responsible for initiating the hypersensitive response. It has been well documented that invading microbes secrete cell wall-degrading enzymes[26,27], and we reasoned that the action of such enzymes could result in the release of an oligosaccharin capable of initiating the hypersensitive response. It has also been observed that exposure to purified pectic-degrading enzymes will kill plant cells, although it is not known why the cells die[28,29,30,31]. We took this observation as additional evidence of the existence of an oligosaccharide fragment capable of initiating the hypersensitive response, a fragment released from the cell walls by pectic-degrading enzymes. Furthermore, it is well known that, when making protoplasts from plant cells, it is neces-

sary to plasmolyze the cells before treating them with the microbial enzymes that digest the cell walls. Without plasmolysis, the
cells die when exposed to the enzymes. The requirement for plasmolysis has been interpreted as the prevention of osmotic bursting
of the fragile protoplasts. The requirement for plasmolysis could
also be interpreted as a means of preventing the killing of the
plant cells by oligosaccharide fragments of the walls released by
the protoplast-forming enzymes. In other words, plasmolysis could
render ineffective the sites of attachment or transport of the
death-inducing oligosaccharides, and thus protect the protoplasts
until the wall fragments are washed away. These observations,
considered together, encouraged us to look at cell wall fragments
for an oligosaccharin capable of initiating the hypersensitive
response.

We have obtained evidence that such an oligosaccharin does
exist in the mixture of fragments produced by partial acid hydrolysis of sycamore cell walls. Initially, we assayed visually,
using vital dyes, for the ability of the wall fragments to kill
suspension-cultured sycamore cells. The acid-released fragments
did appear to cause cell death. However, it was extremely difficult to quantitate this activity. In an effort to quantitate
better the effect of the wall fragments on the sycamore cells, we
developed an assay to measure the incorporation of ^{14}C-leucine
into acid-precipitable polymers of the suspension-cultured sycamore cells and to determine the effects of cell wall fragments on
this incorporation. This bioassay had previously been used to
measure phytotoxicity of various chemicals[32].

We have determined, using the ^{14}C-leucine incorporation
assay, that the acid-released fragments of sycamore cell walls can
completely inhibit the ability of the cells to incorporate ^{14}C-
leucine into acid-precipitable polymers. Relative to a control
sample, where no fragments were added, a 2-hour preincubation of
cultured cells with 400 µg/ml of acid-released cell wall fragments
followed by a 3-hour incubation with ^{14}C-leucine resulted in 85%
inhibition of ^{14}C-leucine incorporation; 500 µg/ml of fragments

resulted in 98% inhibition. Similar preparations of fragments of starch, citrus pectin, and larch galactan failed to inhibit the incorporation of ^{14}C-leucine into the polymers of sycamore cells. The ability of the wall fragments to inhibit protein synthesis is destroyed by hydrolysis in 2N trifluoroacetic acid at 121° C for 2 hours. This is the result expected if the active component is an oligosaccharide. We believe the physiological effect seen upon adding the fragments to the cells is of great interest whether or not the effect is related to the hypersensitive response.

An Oligosaccharin that Inhibits Flowering in Lemna gibba G3 (Duckweed)

The effect of day length on flowering in Lemna has been widely studied[33]. Lemna gibba G3 requires long day lengths in order to flower. We have been carrying out experiments to determine whether acid- or base-released fragments of the walls of suspension-cultured sycamore cells, a dicot, affect flowering in Lemna, a monocot. Our experiments show that the acid-released fragments will inhibit flowering in Lemna gibba G3.

The inhibition of flowering has been investigated using Lemna grown under inductive conditions (continuous light) for a period of 11 to 13 days. Approximately 50% of the Lemna flower under such conditions. The addition of acid-released cell wall fragments at 0.05-0.1 mg/ml results in almost complete inhibition of flowering and an approximate doubling of the number of Lemna fronds, that is, the acid-released fragments stimulate vegetative growth. This is evidence that the inhibition of flowering does not result from a toxic effect but, rather, represents a change in the morphogenetic state of the plant.

An Oligosaccharin Inhibitor of 2,4-D-Stimulated Growth of Pea-Epicotyl Segments

An oligosaccharin present in the fragments produced by base-catalyzed partial degradation of isolated walls of suspension-cultured sycamore cells inhibits, at 1 mg/ml, 2,4-D-stimulated growth of pea-epicotyl segments. This oligosaccharin, which was partially purified by gel filtration chromatography, has a molecular weight of between 1,000 and 5,000. Further purification of this oligosaccharin proved too difficult due to the extremely complex composition of the base-released wall fragments. However, we appear to have discovered a source of a wall fragment inhibitor of 2,4-D-promoted growth that is more amenable to study.

Xyloglucan is a well-characterized polysaccharide of cell walls that is known to be solubilized by base. Therefore, it seemed possible that the fragment of cell walls that inhibits 2,4-D-stimulated growth of pea epicotyls could be contained within xyloglucan. This possibility led to the isolation, by methods previously described, of xyloglucan from the mixture of polysaccharides secreted into the culture medium by suspension-cultured sycamore cells. The isolated xyloglucan was treated with a β-1,4-endoglucanase isolated from Tricoderma viride[34]. Among the major enzymic digestion products are a heptasaccharide and a nonasaccharide. The nonasaccharide differs from the heptasaccharide by possessing a fucosyl-α-1,2-galactosyl disaccharide α-linked to O-2 of the first xylosyl side chain of the heptasaccharide. At a concentration of between 10 and 20 µg/ml, the nonasaccharide inhibits approximately 75% of the 2,4-D-stimulated growth of etiolated pea-stem segments. At a similar concentration, the heptasaccharide does not inhibit the 2,4-D-stimulated growth. This result, albeit preliminary, is very exciting because it offers the possibility of a well-defined example of the structural specificity required for oligosaccharin activity.

UNDERSTANDING RHIZOBIUM-LEGUME INTERACTIONS

The polysaccharides secreted by rhizobia have been studied in considerable detail[35,36,37,38,39]. It has been widely suggested that the rhizobial polysaccharides play an important biological role in rhizobia/legume symbioses. We have undertaken extensive structural studies of the acidic polysaccharides secreted by the rhizobia in an attempt to ascertain whether these polysaccharides participate in the establishment of symbiotic relationships.

The structures of the acidic polysaccharides secreted by nine strains of four Rhizobium species have been elucidated in our laboratory[40,41,42,43,44,45]. The complete structures of the polysaccharides have been determined except for the identities and positions of base-labile substituents. Our studies have shown that four different strains of a single Rhizobium species (R. phaseoli) each secrete an acidic polysaccharide with a unique structure[40,42,43,44]. However, each of the polysaccharides secreted by the R. phaseoli strains has an identical sequence of six glycosyl residues, including the entire four-glycosyl residue repeating-sequence of the backbone of the polysaccharides. The glycosyl sequences of the polysaccharides differ in the outer regions of the side chains. If these polysaccharides participate in recognition between the plant and the microbe, bean plants (the host of R. phaseoli) could recognize all of these polysaccharides by identifying structural features within the six-glycosyl residue portion common to the polysaccharides secreted by the four R. phaseoli strains.

Our studies have also shown that different Rhizobium species may secrete polysaccharides that have identical structures except for the possibility of differently substituted base-labile O-acyl groups[45]. In particular, the acidic polysaccharides secreted by two strains of R. trifolii, two strains of R. leguminosarum, and one strain of R. phaseoli have identical glycosyl sequences, anomeric configurations, and locations of pyruvic acid substituents. If different Rhizobium species do, in fact, secrete exactly the same acidic polysaccharides, these acidic polysaccharides could not be important in recognition. For this reason, the structurally similar polysaccharides secreted by the R. trifolii, R. leguminosarum, and R. phaseoli strains have been examined by ¹H-NMR in an effort to compare their base-labile O-acyl substituents. Our initial experiments have shown that the acidic polysaccharides secreted by strains of each of the three different Rhizobium species do indeed differ in the chemical nature, quan-

tity, and/or location of their O-acyl substituents. The ^{1}H-NMR
data suggest that the O-acyl substituents of the otherwise identical polysaccharides may include O-acetyl, O-succinyl, and O-lactyl
groups. Thus, these polysaccharides do have have sufficiently
unique structures to participate in the specific recognition that
is so characteristic of the interactions between legumes and
rhizobia.

It has been reported[35] that mature root hairs of soybeans are
not normally infected by rhizobia. Rather, only root hairs that
have developed in the presence of homologous (symbiotic) Rhizobium
can be infected. Other experiments of that laboratory suggest
that oligosaccharides derived from Rhizobium exopolysaccharides
stimulate the development of infectible root hairs in the legume
host in the absence of homologous Rhizobium[35]. There are also
preliminary reports that plant roots secrete enzymes that will de-
grade Rhizobium exopolysaccharides[46]. We propose to determine
whether legume roots have enzymes that can specifically depolymer-
ize the acidic polysaccharides secreted by symbiont rhizobia but
not the acidic polysaccharides secreted by nonsymbiont rhizobia.
If specific depolymerization is observed, we would determine
whether the resulting oligosaccharides can stimulate, in a host-
specific manner, the development of root hairs capable of being
infected by rhizobia. The long-term goal of both the structural
and enzymatic studies is to determine whether the polysaccharides
secreted by the rhizobia are, in fact, converted to biologically
active oligosaccharides that are capable of altering the metabolism of receptive plant cells.

Another polysaccharide secreted by both Rhizobium and Agrobacterium species is a β-2-linked glucan[47,37,48,49]. The biological purpose of this unusual polysaccharide, which is secreted
only by the Rhizobiaceae, bacteria that cause cell proliferation
in their host plants, remains unknown. We have confirmed our
earlier structural characterization of this molecule suggesting
that the molecule was circular[49]. Fast atom bombardment-mass
spectrometric analysis of the β-2-linked glucan yields molecular

ions consistent with a family of macrocyclic molecules composed of from 18 through 23 glucosyl residues. Analysis of these β-glucans by ^{13}C-NMR confirms the macrocyclic structure and suggests that there are no ends on the molecules, indicating that the structure is a full circle rather than a circle with a tail. Could this unusual complex carbohydrate be biologically active?

CONCLUDING THOUGHTS

Plant scientists have discovered what appear to be five primary hormones--auxins, gibberellins, cytokinins, abscisic acid, and ethylene--each of which affects many different physiological functions of plants. By comparison, animals are known to possess hundreds of different hormones, of which only a relatively few appear to be primary hormones. Most of the animal hormones are more specific than those of plants in terms of the physiological functions that they regulate; many of the hormones are peptides. Although it has been more or less apparent that many secondary hormones exist in plants, the origin and nature of these hormones have remained unknown. The discovery that regulatory molecules are stored in the polymers of the walls of the plant cells not only offers the possibility of specific ways for controlling plant growth, but it also encourages experimentation to determine whether these wall fragment regulatory molecules are active in vivo.

The noncellulosic polysaccharides of plant cell walls set a new standard for structural complexity. The only known mechanism for the synthesis of polysaccharides requires catalysis by a unique enzyme for each glycosyl residue that possesses a unique structural position or configuration within the polysaccharide. The enzymes involved in the synthesis of the activated monosac-charide precursors, the enzymes that catalyze the polymerization (the glycosyl transferases), the enzymes involved in modification of polysaccharides, such as those involved in the synthesis of methyl, acetyl, or feruloyl esters[50], and the enzymes that cleave polysaccharides into defined fragments, add up to an enormous

array of enzymes.   Indeed, we calculate that the synthesis and
metabolism of the polysaccharides of plant cell walls requires
hundreds, perhaps well over a thousand, different enzymes.   It is
no wonder that no cell wall polysaccharide has been synthesized in
vitro, and that the complete structure of a noncellulosic cell
wall polysaccharide has yet to be described.

There is a real possibility that different plant cells have,
within their primary cell walls, structurally related yet structurally unique polysaccharides.   This would demand that different
cells possess different arrays of enzymes for the synthesis of
these polysaccharides.   It is also possible that different cells
produce different sets of enzymes for releasing oligosaccharins.
It is likely that different cells have different oligosaccharin
receptor proteins.   All such enzymes and receptors offer exciting
targets for genetic modifications aimed at regulating physiological processes in plants.   But, before these targets can be regulated or their genes transferred from one plant to another, the
targets must be biochemically defined.

ACKNOWLEDGEMENTS

Supported by the U.S. Department of Energy (Contract No. DE-AC-
76ERO-1426) and The Rockefeller Foundation (#RF 78049).

REFERENCES

1. P. Albersheim and B. S. Valent, Host-pathogen interactions in
        plants. Plants, when exposed to oligosaccharides of fungal
        origin, defend themselves by accumulating antibiotics, J.
        Cell Biol. 78:627-643 (1978).
2. R. A. Dixon and C. J. Lamb, Stimulation of de novo synthesis
        of L-phenylalanine ammonia-lyase in relation to phytoalexin
        accumulation in Colletotrichum lindemuthianum elicitor-
        treated cell suspension cultures of French bean (Phaseolus
        vulgaris), Biochem. Biophys. Acta 586:453-463 (1979).

3. J. Ebel, A. R. Ayers, and P. Albersheim, Host-pathogen inter-
    actions XII. Response of suspension-cultured soybean cells
    to the elicitor isolated from Phytophthora megasperma var.
    sojae, a fungal pathogen of soybeans, Plant Physiol.
    57:775-779 (1976).

4. H. Ragg, D. N. Kuhn, and K. Hahlbrock, Coordinated regulation
    of 4-coumarate:CoA ligase and phenylalanine ammonia-lyase
    mRNAs in cultured plant cells, J. Biol. Chem. 256:10061-
    10065 (1981).

5. J. A. Bailey and J. W. Mansfield, eds., "Phytoalexins,"
    Halsted Press, John Wiley and Sons, New York (1982).

6. A. Darvill, M. McNeil, P. Albersheim, and D. P. Delmer, The
    primary cell walls of flowering plants, in: "The Biochem-
    istry of Plants," N. E. Tolbert, ed., Academic Press, New
    York, 1:91-162 (1980).

7. M. McNeil, A. G. Darvill, and P. Albersheim, The structural
    polymers of the primary cell walls of dicots, in: "Progress
    in the Chemistry of Organic Natural Products," W. Herz, H.
    Grisebach and G. W. Kirby, eds., Springer-Verlag, Vienna
    and New York, 37:191-249 (1979).

8. M. McNeil, A. G. Darvill, and P. Albersheim, Structure of
    plant cell walls XII. Identification of seven differently-
    linked glycosyl residues attached to C-4 of the 2,4-linked
    L-rhamnosyl residues of rhamnogalacuronan I, Plant
    Physiol., in press (1982).

9. K. R. Davis, G. Lyon, A. G. Darvill, and P. Albersheim,
    unpublished results.

10. M. G. Hahn, A. G. Darvill, and P. Albersheim, Host-pathogen
    interactions XIX: The endogenous elicitor, a fragment of a
    plant cell wall polysaccharide that elicits phytoalexin ac-
    cumulation in soybeans, Plant Physiol. 68:1161-1169 (1981).

11. C. A. Ryan, Proteinase inhibitors in plant leaves: A bio-
    chemical model for pest-induced natural plant protection,
    TIBS July:148-150 (1978).

12. C. A. Ryan, P. Bishop, G. Pearce, A. G. Darvill, M. McNeil,
    and P. Albersheim, A sycamore cell polysaccharide and a

chemically related tomato leaf polysaccharide possess similar proteinase inhibitor-inducing activities, Plant Physiol. 68:616-618 (1981).

13. K. Docherty and D. F. Steiner, Post-transitional proteolysis in polypeptide hormone biosynthesis, Ann. Rev. Physiol. 44:625-638 (1982).

14. A. R. Ayers, J. Ebel, B. Valent, and P. Albersheim, Host-pathogen interactions X. Fractionation and biological activity of an elicitor isolated from the mycelial walls of Phytophthora megasperma var. sojae, Plant Physiol. 57:760-765 (1976).

15. M. McNeil, A. G. Darvill, P. Åman, L.-E. Franzén, and P. Albersheim, Structural analysis of complex carbohydrates using high performance liquid chromatography, gas chromatography and mass spectrometry, Meth. Enzymol. 83:3-45 (1982).

16. B. S. Valent, A. G. Darvill, M. McNeil, B. K. Robertsen, and P. Albersheim, A general and sensitive chemical method for sequencing the glycosyl residues of complex carbohydrates, Carbohydr. Res. 79:165-192 (1980).

17. E. A. Nothnagel, M. McNeil, and P. Albersheim, Host-pathogen interactions XXII: A galacturonic acid oligosaccharide from plant cell walls elicits phytoalexins, in preparation (1982).

18. S.-C. Lee and C. A. West, Polygalacturonase from Rhizopus stolonifer, an elicitor of casbene synthetase activity in castor bean (Ricinus communis L.) seedlings, Plant Physiol. 67:633-639 (1981).

19. S.-C. Lee and C. A. West, Properties of Rhizopus stolonifer polygalacturonase, an elicitor of casbene synthetase activity in castor bean (Ricinus communis L.) seedlings, Plant Physiol. 67:640-645 (1981).

20. R. J. Bruce and C. A. West, Elicitation of casbene synthetase activity in castor bean. The role of pectic fragments of the plant cell wall in elicitation by a fungal endopolygalacturonase. Plant Physiol. 69:1181-1188 (1982).

21. G. Lyon and P. Albersheim, Host-pathogen interactions XXI. Extraction of a heat-labile elicitor of phytoalexin accumulation from frozen soybean stem, Plant Physiol. 70:406-409 (1982).

22. J. A. Hargreaves, Investigations into the mechanism of mercuric chloride stimulated phytoalexin accumulation in Phaseolus vulgaris and Pisum sativum, Physiol. Plant Pathol. 15:279-287 (1979).

23. J. A. Hargreaves, A possible mechanism for the phytotoxicity of the phytoalexin phaseollin, Physiol. Plant Pathol. 16:351-357 (1980).

24. J. A. Hargreaves and J. A. Bailey, Phytoalexin production by hypocotyls of Phaseolus vulgaris in response to constitutive metabolites released by damaged bean cells, Physiol. Plant Pathol. 13:89-100 (1978).

25. R. K. S. Wood, ed., "Active Defense Mechanisms in Plants," Plenum Press, New York, pp. 1-19 (1982).

26. P. Albersheim, T. M. Jones and P. D. English, Biochemistry of the cell wall in relation to infective processes, Ann. Rev. Phytopath. 7:171-194 (1969).

27. E. T. Reese, Degradation of polymeric carbohydrates by microbial enzymes, in: "Recent Advances in Phytochemistry," F.

38. T. L. Graham, Recognition in Rhizobium-legume symbioses, in: "International Review of Cytology," Academic Press, Supp. 13:127-148 (1981).

39. P.-E. Jansson, L. Kenne, B. Lindberg, H. Ljunggren, J. Lönngren, U. Rudén and S. Svensson, Demonstration of an octasaccharide repeating unit in the extracellular polysaccharide of Rhizobium meliloti by sequential degradation. J. Amer. Chem. Soc. 99:3812-3815 (1977).

40. P. Åman, L.-E. Franzén, A. G. Darvill, M. McNeil and P. Albersheim, Structural elucidation of the acidic extracellular polysaccharide secreted by Rhizobium phaseoli 127K38, Carbohydr. Res. 103:77-100 (1982).

31. R. K. S. Wood, "Physiological Plant Pathology," Blackwell Scientific Publications, Oxford (1967).

32. A. Breiman and E. Galun, Plant protoplasts as tools in quantitative assays of phytotoxic compound from culture filtrates of Phytophthora citrophthora, Physiol. Plant Pathol. 19:181-191 (1981).

33. W. S. Hillman, Experimental control of flowering in Lemna. I. Photoperiodism in L. pepusilla 6746, Am. J. Bot. 46:466-473, (1959).

34. W. D. Bauer, K. Talmadge, K. Keegstra, and P. Albersheim, The structure of plant cell walls II. The hemicellulose of the walls of suspension-cultured sycamore cells, Plant Physiol. 51:174-187 (1973).

35. W. D. Bauer, Infection of legumes by rhizobia, in: "Annual Review of Plant Physiology," 32:407-449 (1981).

36. R. W. Carlson, in: "Ecology of Nitrogen Fixation," Vol. II, W. J. Broughton, ed., Oxford University Press, London and New York, in press, (1982).

37. W. F. Dudman, The Role of Surface Polysaccharides in Natural Environments, in: I. Sutherland, ed., "Surface Carbohydrates of the Prokaryotic Cell," Academic Press, London, pp. 357-414 (1977).

47. R. A. Dedonder, and W. Z. Hassid, The enzymatic synthesis of a β-1,2-0-linked glucan by an extract of Rhizobium japonicum, Biochem. Biophys. Acta, 90:239-248 (1964).

48. P. A. J. Gorin, J. F. T. Spencer and D. W. S. Westlake, The structure and resistance to methylation of 1-2-β-glucans from species of Agrobacteria, Can. J. Chem. 39:1067-1073 (1961).

49. W. S. York, M. McNeil, A. G. Darvill and P. Albersheim, Host-symbiont interactions VIII: β-2-linked glucans secreted by fast growing species of Rhizobium, J. Bacteriol. 142:243-248 (1980).

41. P. Åman, M. McNeil, L.-E. Franzén, A. G. Darvill and P. Alber-
    sheim, Host-symbiont interactions IX.   Structural eluci-
    dation, using H.P.L.C.-M.S. and G.L.C.-M.S., of the acidic
    extracellular polysaccharide secreted by Rhizobium meliloti
    strain 1021, Carbohydr. Res. 95:263-282 (1981).

42. W. F. Dudman, L.-E. Franzén, J. E. Darvill, M. McNeil, A. G.
    Darvill and P. Albersheim, The structure of the acidic
    polysaccharide   secreted   by   Rhizobium   phaseoli   strain
    127K36, in preparation (1982).

43. W. F. Dudman, L.-E. Franzén, M. McNeil, A.G. Darvill and P.
    Albersheim, Host-symbiont interactions XII. The structure
    of the acidic polysaccharide secreted by Rhizobium phaseoli
    strain 127K87, in preparation (1982).

44. L.-E. Franzén, W. F. Dudman, M. McNeil, A. G. Darvill and P.
    Albersheim, Host-symbiont interactions XII. The structure
    of the acidic polysaccharide secreted by Rhizobium phaseoli
    strain 127K44, in preparation (1982).

45. B. Robertsen, P. Åman, A. G. Darvill, M. McNeil and P. Alber-
    sheim, Host-symbiont interactions V. The structure of the
    acidic extracellular polysaccharides secreted by Rhizobium
    leguminosarum and Rhizobium trifolii, Plant Physiol.
    67:389-400 (1981).

46. K. E. Fjellheim and B. Solheim, personal communication, quoted
    in W. D. Bauer, Infection of legumes by rhizobia, in:
    "Annual Review of Plant Physiology," 32:407-449 (1981).

    A. Loewus and V. C. Runeckles, eds., Plenum Pub. Corp, New
    York, 11:311-367 (1977).

28. H. G. Basham and D. F. Bateman, Killing of plant cells by
    pectic enzymes: the lack of direct injurious interaction
    between pectic enzymes or their soluble reaction products
    and plant cells, Phytopathology 65:141-153 (1975).

29. M. S. Mount, D. F. Bateman, and H. G. Basham, Induction of
    electrolyte loss, tissue maceration, and cellular death of
    potato tissue by an endopolygalacturonate trans-eliminase,
    Phytopathology 60:924-931 (1970).

30. R. K. S. Wood, Killing of protoplasts by plant pathogens, in:
    "Current Topics in Plant Pathology," Z. Király, ed.,
    Akadémiai Kiadó, Budapest, pp. 107-115 (1977).

50. S. C. Fry, Phenolic components of the primary cell wall. Feru-
    lolylated disaccharides of D-galactose and L-arabinose from
    spinach polysaccharide, Biochem. J. 203:493-504 (1982).

EARLY MOLECULAR EVENTS IN THE PHYTOALEXIN DEFENSE RESPONSE

Chris Lamb[1,2], John Bell[1,2], Paul Norman[1,2], Mike
Lawton[2,3], Richard Dixon[4], Pat Rowell[5] and John Bailey[5]

[1]Salk Institute, PO Box 85800, San Diego, Ca 92138, USA
[2]Department of Biochemistry, University of Oxford, UK
[3]Washington University, St. Louis, Mo, USA
[4]Royal Holloway College, University of London, Uk
[5]Long Ashton Research Station, University of Bristol, UK

INTRODUCTION

This chapter deals with recent studies on the biochemistry of
disease resistance expression in Phaseolus vulgaris L., paying
particular attention to the regulation of phytoalexin accumulation.
Advantages of this system for biochemical studies are: (a) The
disease resistance profile of P vulgaris has been characterised
genetically to some extent (Meiners, 1981) and physiologically
(Bailey, 1981). In particular, different cultivars (eg. Kievit,
Immuna, Red Kidney) undergo highly specific interactions with
physiological races of Colletotrichum lindemuthianum (eg. β,δ,γ)
the causal agent of anthracnose disease of P. vulgaris. (b) The
physiology of this interaction has been extensively studied using
hypocotyls, the organ which together with leaves is the natural
site of attack by C. lindemuthianum. There is strong evidence that
the differential accumulation of the isoflavonoid derivative
phaseollin and other structurally related phytoalexins such as
phaseollidin, phaseollinisoflavan and kievitone in resistant and
susceptible interactions plays a crucial role in the specificity of
host resistance (Bailey, 1981). (c) Detailed study of the effects
of phytoalexin inducing agents on phenylpropanoid metabolism in
P. vulgaris hypocotyls indicates that accumulation of phytoalexins
is a specific event, and the levels of most other phenylpropanoid
products (eg. hydroxycinnamic acids) remain roughly constant
relative to untreated control tissue (Rathmell and Bendall, 1971).
(d) High molecular weight glycan elicitors including a β-3 linked
glucan, which are capable of inducing a hypersensitive response and
phytoalexin accumulation in P. vulgaris have been isolated from

313

cell walls and culture filtrates of <u>C. lindemuthianum</u> (Anderson-Prouty and Albersheim, 1975).

Plant cell cultures can provide aseptic, relatively homogenous cell populations growing under precisely defined conditions (Dixon, 1980). Early work with suspension cultures centred on the development of optimal conditions for the induction of phaseollin accumulation by elciitors (Dixon and Fuller, 1976, 1978). Furthermore, [^{14}C]phenylalanine incorporation studies indicated that phaseollin was synthesised <u>de novo</u> from phenylalanine during elicitor-induced phaseollin accumulation and it is probable that control of synthesis is an important regulatory element in phytoalexin accumulation (Moesta and Grisebach, 1981) .

INDUCTION OF ENZYMES OF PHYTOALEXIN BIOSYNTHESIS

Phenylalanine is the precursor for a wide variety of phenylpropanoid compounds including lignin, coumarins, flavonoids and esters of hydroxycinnamic acids in addition to isoflavonoid-derivatives such as phaseollin (Camm and Towers, 1977). A central pathway from phenylalanine via cinnamic acid and 4-coumaric acid to 4-coumaroyl-CoA has been elucidated and 4-coumaroyl-CoA is a key intermediate from which branch pathways originate associated with the biosynthesis of particular groups of phenylpropanoid compounds (Hahlbrock and Grisebach, 1979). The enzymes of the central pathway: phenylalanine ammonia-lyase (PAL, EC 4.3.1.5), cinnamic acid 4-hydroxylase (C4H, EC 1.14.13.11) and 4-coumarate:CoA ligase (4CL EC 6.2.1.12) have been well characterised. Unfortunately with the exceptions of chalcone synthase (CHS)- the first enzyme of the branch pathway specific for flavonoid/isoflavonoid biosynthesis (Kreuzaler et al., 1979), chalcone isomerase (CHI, EC 5.5.1.6) (Dixon et al., 1982) and dimethylallyl pyrophosphate : dihydroxypterocarpan dimethylallyl transferase (Zähringer et al., 1978), relatively little is known of the enzymology of the later stages of the synthesis of isoflavonoid-derived phytoalexins.

In cell cultures of <u>P. vulgaris</u>, PAL, C4H, 4CL and CHS activities are present only at relatively low levels. Following treatment with elicitors there are marked and rapid increases in the activities of these enzymes concomitant with the onset of phytoalexin accumulation (Dixon and Bendall, 1978). In the cases of PAL and CHS these increases are only transient and there is a subsequent rapid decay to basal activity levels. In contrast, CHI is present at relatively high levels in control cultures and responds only sluggishly to elicitor treatment (Dixon and Lamb, 1979). On this basis it is probable that elicitor induction of PAL, C4H, 4CL and CHS activities is a key element in the control of phytoalexin accumulation in this system. It should be noted that unlike the case of fine control there is no theoretically rigorous criterion for the identification of specific sites of coarse control (Kacser and Burns, 1973). However, detailed studies of the regulation of flavonoid production in cell cultures of Petroselinum hortense and chlorogenic acid in disks of Solanum tuberosum, cases where the enzymology of the pathways is well characterised, strongly suggest that PAL is the primary control site (Hahlbrock et al., 1976; Lamb and Rubery 1976a) although secondary control points have been implicated at the first stage in the respective branch pathways (Schröder et al., 1977; Lamb, 1977). It is probable that a similar situation obtains with respect to regulation of phytoalexin accumulation in P. vulgaris and hence attention has been focussed on the molecular mechanisms underlying the marked but transient increases in PAL and CHS activities following elicitor treatment.

DENSITY LABELLING ANALYSIS OF THE INDUCTION OF PAL BY ELICITOR

Initially the induction of PAL activity was investigated using comparative density labelling (Dixon and Lamb, 1979; Lamb and Dixon, 1978). Growth of cultures in a defined medium lacking exogenous amino acids allows enzyme density labelling with ^{2}H from ^{2}H$_2$O. The basis of the comparative density labelling technique is to apply the density label to the tissue in the presence and absence of elicitor and to compare rates of incorporation of ^{2}H into assayable enzyme protein, by analysis of the equilibrium distribution of enzyme activity in CsCl density gradients (Lamb and Rubery, 1976b). At all stages PAL extracted from elicitor-treated cultures was heavier than enzyme from comparable control cultures. In contrast, the activity level and rate of labelling of the internal control enzyme acid phosphatase was unaffected by elicitor treatment. Hence the observed differences in the rate of labelling of PAL can be ascribed to elcitor induced changes in the turnover of the enzyme rather than changes in the turnover of the amino acid pools. It was concluded that elicitor caused an increase in the rate of de novo synthesis of PAL and that this was an early event in the phytoalexin defense response.

This analysis, using CsCl as a density gradient solute provided only semi-quantitative data which furthermore was dependent on the assumption that PAL and acid phosphatase were synthesised from the same pool of amino acids. CsCl is far from ideal as a solute for these purposes and recently KBr has found favour in protein density labelling studies (Fourcroy, 1978). The theoretical advantages of KBr were exploited to re-investigate the transient increase in PAL activity during elicitor-induced phytoalexin accumulation (Lawton et al., 1980). The resolution of labelled and unlabelled PAL in this system was sufficient to allow quantitative analysis of the relative proportions of light, unlabelled, pre-existing PAL and heavy, labelled, newly-synthesised PAL without assumptions about or measurement of the specific activity of label in the amino acid pool from which PAL was synthesised.

The induction of phaseollin accumulation by elicitor heat-released from cell walls of C. lindemuthianum is markedly suppressed at supra-optimal elicitor concentrations (Dixon and Lamb, 1979). Similarly, the induction of PAL activity is highly dependent on elciitor concentration, with induction occurring in two discrete elicitor concentration ranges, at an intermediate concentration and at supra-optimal elicitor concentrations, no induction of PAL activity was observed (Lawton et al.,1980). Using the high resolution KBr gradients it was possible to show that at low elicitor concentrations there was no stabilisation of enzyme relative to no-elicitor controls and that the induction of PAL activity was entirely a result of stimulation of the rate of de novo synthesis of the enzymne. In contrast, at higher elicitor concentrations, the increase in PAL activity was accompanied by a marked stabilisation of the enzyme in vivo, and the rapid but transient increase in enzyme activity was achieved by a programme of reciprocal changes in the rate constant for de novo enzyme synthesis and the rate constant for removal of enzyme activity. An interesting sidelight was that by analysis of the equilibrium distribution of the labelled component of the total population of PAL molecules it was possible to show directly that elicitor had no effect on the turnover of label in the amino acid pools from which PAL itself was synthesised.

Although density labelling uniquely among in vivo protein labelling techniques can provide simultaneous quantitative estimates of the amounts of both labelled, newly synthesised PAL and unlabelled, pre-existing PAL, without assumptions about or measurememnt of the specific activity of label in the amino acid pools from which the enzyme was synthesised, the technique has a number of important limitations (Lamb and Rubery, 1976b). First, quantitative data are only obtainable in favourable cases where the enzyme is stable in high concentrations of solute and is of high molceular weight so that labelled and unlabelled species are extensively resolved. Second, the technique measures the ratio of labelled to unlabelled enzyme and is therefore not applicable to studies requiring short pulses of label for detailed analysis of the early stages of rapid regulatory responses. Third, the information obtained is essentially kinetic rather than molecular. Putative inactive or processed forms of the enzyme are not monitored and the technique cannot be extended to study protein synthesis in vitro.

DIRECT IMMUNOPRECIPITATION OF IN VIVO LABELLED PAL AND CHS

To overcome these limitations, elicitor-induced changes in the rates of synthesis of both PAL and CHS have been measured by

direct   immunoprecipitation   of   enzyme   subunits   pulse-labelled
in vivo   with   [^{35}S]methionine   (Lawton   et al.,   1982a).
[^{35}S]Methionine-labelled   polypeptides   with   molecular   weights of
77,000 and 42,000 were immunoprecipitated by antiserum to PAL   and
CHS respectively. These polypeptides were identified as PAL and CHS
subunits by (a) co-migration with authentic PAL and CHS subunits in
SDS-polyacrylamide   gel   electrophoresis,   (b) the close correlation
in   immunotitration   experiments   between   immunoprecipitation   of
enzyme   activity   and   of   radioactivity   in   the   putative   enzyme
subunits isolated by immunoprecipitation and SDS-polyacrylamide gel
electrophoresis   and   (c)   by comparison of the peptide maps of the
immunoprecipitated   putative   enzyme   subunits   and   authentic   enzyme
subunits.

     Elicitor caused marked but transient increases in the rate of
incorporation of [^{35}S]methionine into   immunoprecipitable   PAL   and
CHS subunits as a proportion of incorporation of radioactivity into
total cellular protein. Incorporation into PAL and CHS subunits can
account for up to 0.5% and 1.0% respectively of total incorporation
of radioactivity into protein. Taken   with   the   observation   from
density   labelling   that   elicitor   treatment   does   not   alter the
turnover of amino acid pools in this system,   it   was   possible   to
conclude   that   these   changes   in incorporation of [^{35}S]methionine
into immunoprecipitable PAL and CHS subunits represented changes in
the   rates   of   synthesis   of these enzymes, thereby confirming the
conclusions drawn from density labelling experiments with respect
to PAL and extending the analysis to CHS, the first enzyme specific
to the flavonoid/isoflavonoid   branch   pathway   of   phenylpropanoid
biosynthesis.

     Increased   rates of synthesis of both enzymes can be observed
10-20 minutes after elicitor treatment (ie. within the labelling
period of 20 minutes) and the patterns of induction of PAL and CHS
are broadly similar with   respect   to   elicitor   concentration   and
time, maximum rates of synthesis being attained between 2.5 and 3.0
h after elicitor treatment. Within this   overall   co-ordination,
small but distinct differences between the enzymes were observed in
(a) the elicitor concentrations giving maximum induction of   enzyme
activity,   (b) the elicitor concentrations giving maximum induction
of enzyme synthesis and (c) the precise timing   of   maximum   enzyme
synthesis,   with   that for CHS occurring 20-30 minutes earlier than
that for PAL.

     The data from these experiments provide further evidence   for
the   importance   of   enzyme   synthesis   in   the   regulation of the
activity levels of PAL and CHS. However, for a given rate of enzyme
synthesis, induction of PAL and CHS activities is more efficient at
high elicitor concentrations. This may reflect the operation   under
certain circumstances of post-translational control of the activity
levels of these enzymes as   implicated   for   PAL   by   the   previous

density labelling experiments (Lawton et al., 1980) and for CHS by radio-immunoassay studies in light-induced parsley cell cultures (Schröder & Schäfer, 1980).

Nothing is known of the molecular mechanisms underlying putative elicitor-mediated post-translational control of PAL and CHS levels in P. vulgaris cell cultures. However, it is worth noting that in epicotyl sections of Pisum sativum, density labelling studies have shown that exogenous supplies of cinnamic acid, the immediate product of PAL activity, cause a rapid decay in the cellular level of PAL by a dual mechanism involving not only inhibition of de novo production of the enzyme, but also marked stimulation of the rate of removal of pre-existing PAL (Shields et al., 1982). Furthermore, studies using the potent and specific inhibitor of PAL, α-aminooxy-β-phenylpropionic acid, to generate phenocopies of mutants deficient in PAL activity, have shown that this dual control mechanism also operates in vivo following endogenous production of cinnamic acid. This response seems particularly well-suited for study of post-translational control of PAL at the molecular level.

IN VITRO SYNTHESIS OF PAL AND CHS

In order to elucidate the molecular mechanisms underlying elicitor-induced increases in PAL and CHS synthesis in vivo, changes in the activity levels of the mRNAs encoding these enzymes have been investigated by indirect immunoprecipitation with protein A-sepharose of [^{35}S]methionine-labelled enzyme subunits synthesised in vitro in a mRNA-dependent rabbit reticulocyte lysate translation system (Lawton et al., 1982b). The product of in vitro synthesis immunoprecipitated by anti serum to CHS is identical in terms of subunit molecular weight and peptide map to the equivalent subunit synthesised in vivo. In the case of PAL, the in vitro product is somewhat smaller (73,000 daltons) compared to the in vivo product (77,000 daltons). However, there is extensive identity between the respective peptide maps and it is probable that the smaller product reflects premature termination of the in vitro translation process. Increased polysomal mRNA activities encoding the two enzymes can be observed rapidly following elicitor treatment (Fig. 1) and there is a close correlation between the induction of polysomal mRNA activity and the induction of enzyme synthesis in vivo, with respect to both the kinetics of induction and the dependence on elicitor concentration. The data show that elicitor stimulation of PAL and CHS synthesis in vivo is largely if not entirely a result of increased polysomal activity of the mRNAs encoding these enzymes. Furthermore, the marked increases in polysomal mRNA activities encoding PAL and CHS represent increased activities of these specific messages as a proportion of total cellular mRNA activity, thus indicating that elicitor does not increase these polysomal mRNA activities by stimulation of selective recruitment

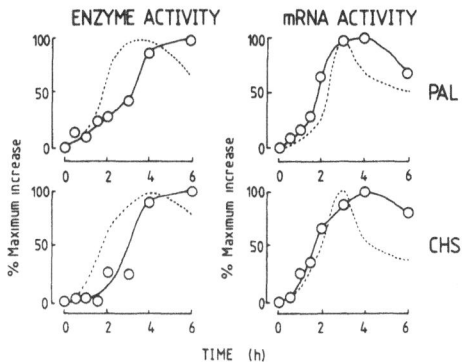

Fig. 1 Elicitor induction of PAL and CHS enzyme and mRNA activity. For comparison, hatched lines denote mRNA activities in left hand panels and rates of enzyme synthesis in vivo in right hand panels.

from the total pool of cellular mRNA.

SPECIFICITY OF ELICITATION

Natural elicitor preparations from culture filtrates and cell walls of a number of different fungi cause marked induction of PAL and CHS synthesis both in vivo and in vitro (Lawton et al., 1982a,b). That this is the case for the elicitor present in culture filtrates of Phytophthora megasperma f.sp. glycinea is of particular interest since previous results have shown that, whilst this elicitor preparation causes marked and rapid induction of PAL activity and synthesis in cell suspension cultures of Petroselinum hortense, there is, in contrast to the situation in P. vulgaris, no elicitor-mediated induction of CHS synthesis or activity (Hahlbrock et al., 1981). Although a proportion of cells in P. hortense cultures turn yellowish-brown and die following elicitor treatment there is no accumulation of isoflavonoid-derived phytoalexins and recently it has been shown that elicitor induces accumulation of furanocoumarin phytoalexins (Tietjen and Matern, personal communication). Hence CHS induction is not required in response to elicitor in P. hortense. Furthermore, elicitor totally inhibits light-mediated induction of CHS synthesis associated with flavonoid pigment production in this system. Hence elicitor seems to cause not only marked and rapid stimulation of the production of enzymes of phytoalexin biosynthesis but also, where appropriate, inhibition of the synthesis of other enzymes, so as to divert the flux of material within the phenylpropanoid metabolic system.

Elicitor can also exert negative effects in P. vulgaris cells as judged by 2D gel electrophoretic comparisons of the polypeptide products encoded by polysomal mRNA from elicitor-treated and control cultures (Lamb et al., unpublished). Whilst there are 30 or more polypeptides whose polysomal mRNA activities are enhanced by elicitor, there are at least 3 with markedly decreased activities.

It is of considerable interest to identify as many as possible of the polypeptides whose mRNA activities are under elicitor control. Preliminary data suggest that not all may be associated with the phytoalexin defense response. Thus elicitor markedly and rapidly increases the activities of two polysomal mRNAs encoding polypetides that are immunoprecipitated by antiserum to P. vulgaris seed lectin (phytohaemagglutinin). In these experiments in vitro synthesised proteins were labelled with [^{3}H]leucine because the seed lectin is methionine deficient. Furthermore, in vivo labelling experiments have shown a marked increase in the rates of synthesis of certain membrane bound polypeptides and polypeptides present in the culture medium following elicitor treatment of P. vulgaris cell cultures. Similarly elicitor causes· a marked increase in activity, as a proportion of total polysomal mRNA activity, of those polysomal mRNAs that encode polypeptides that in vitro are co-translationally processed by and inserted accross canine pancreatic microsomes. Hence in elicitor-treated cells there may be, as in wounded cells, a marked stimulation of protein synthesis associated with the endo-membrane system. The function of these polypetides and their ultimate site of accumulation in the intact system remain to be established.

TRANSMISSION OF ELICITATION

In addition to infection and natural elicitors isolated from fungal cell walls and culture filtrates, phytoalexin accumulation can also be induced by a wide range of structurally unrelated, unnatural elicitors such as heavy metal salts, anti-metabolites, polyamines, autoclaved RNase and DNase, chloroform, detergents and localised freezing and thawing of tissue. Detailed physiological studies have established a strong correlation between localised necrosis and the induction of phytoalexin accumulation (Bailey, 1981). Recently endogenous elicitors have been detected, one of which appears to be a fragment of a host cell wall pectic polysaccharide (Albersheim, this volume; Bailey, 1981). It has been postulated that external elicitors or the living fungus might induce phytoalexin accumulation by causing release of endogenous elicitor activity. In this model, the action of unnatural elicitors could be explained by the release of endogenous elicitor following localised cell death. Cell death might also be involved in the action of natural elicitors although other possible mechanisms are (a) that natural elicitors are cell wall degrading enzymes that cause release of endogenous elicitor by their enzyme action and (b) that natural elicitors trigger the activation of cell wall degrading enzymes in the host, leading to the release of endogenous elicitor. Certain wall degrading enzymes appear to be toxic to plant cells (Bailey, 1981) and recently the enzymic activity of a fungal endopolygalacturonase has been shown to be required for this molecule to act as an elicitor (see Albersheim, this volume, for review).

All of these models imply a transmission of the elicitation signal either (a) from host cell wall to the cell surface of the same cell or (b) an intercellular transmisson. Treatment of P. vulgaris cell cultures or hypocotyl tissue with the macromolecular, unnatural elicitor autoclaved RNase does indeed release a factor that is able to transmit the elicitation signal from cells in direct contact with this elicitor across a dialysis membrane. This leads to induction of PAL activity and phytoalexin accumulation in cells not in direct contact with the macromolecular elicitor which cannot itself penetrate the membrane (Lamb et al., 1980; Dixon et al., 1982). The diffusible elicitation signal is probably not a breakdown product of the external elicitor but rather a product of the plant cells directly exposed to the external elicitor. These data may indicate a causal sequence of events which involve a transmissible factor of host origin operating between an external elicitor and the induction of PAL activity and phaseollin accumulation in distant cells. It is not yet clear whether the same or a similar factor is involved in the transmission of the elicitation signal from the exterior to the interior of cells in direct contact with the RNase.

There is a lag of 2 h between the induction of PAL activity in cells directly in contact with RNase and those separated by the dialysis membrane. An internal elicitor can be obtained by autoclaving P. vulgaris cell walls and this elicitor preparation, as with RNase, can elicit PAL activity not only in directly exposed cells but also in cells separated by a dialysis membrane. However, unlike elicitation with RNase, there is no difference in the rapidity of PAL induction in these two sets of cells and furthermore the elicitor can itself cross the dialysis membrane. These results are consistent with the idea that this internal elicitor is the transmissible signal produced or released following treatment with RNase, but there is no direct evidence for this yet.

Interestingly, the natural elicitor heat-released from cell walls of C. lindemuthianum is unable to release a factor that can transmit the elicitation signal accross a dialysis membrane to

cells not in contact with this elicitor. These observations do not
rule out local intercellular transmission of the elicitation signal
in response to this natural elicitor, or of course, the involvement
of a factor of host origin in transmitting the signal from the
exterior to the interior of individual cells. Nonetheless, there is
an indication that natural and unnatural elicitors may have
differing initial modes of action although it should be noted that
as with natural elicitors, the increase in PAL and CHS activities
in response to RNase involves stimulation of de novo synthesis of
these enzymes (Lawton et al., 1982a).

REGULATION OF PHYTOALEXIN ACCUMULATION IN INFECTED TISSUE

        Phytoalexin accumulation is not restricted to incompatible
interactions alone and specificity appears to be associated with
quantitative rather than qualitative differences, depending on the
timing, magnitude and duration of phytoalexin accumulation in
different specific interaction types (Bailey, 1981). Theoretical
studies have demonstrated that simultaneous reciprocal changes in
the rates of enzyme synthesis and removal enhance the flexibility
and rapidity of changes in enzyme amount during enzyme accumulation
(Paskin and Meyer, 1977). In the present case it is possible to
speculate that the ability of elicitor to regulate the level of PAL
by reciprocal modulation of enzyme production and removal may be
crucial in determining the magnitude and duration of the
phytoalexin defense response and hence the specificity of
phytoalexin action.

        However, although it is clear that in some systems
race-specific resistance may be wholly or partially expressed in
cultured plant cells, a major criticism of the application of
tissue culture methods to the study of phytoalexin induction
concerns the problem of extrapolation of results to the intact
host:pathogen interaction (Dixon, 1980). For example, production of
glyceollin in callus cultures of different cultivars of Glycine max
in response to P. megasperma f.sp. glycinea was qualitatively
different to that of the intact plant (Keen and Horsch, 1972).
Similarly, spatial interactions such as those involved in the
intercellular transmission of the elicitation signal may be
considerably different in the intact tissue compared to cell
culltures.

        These considerations have prompted us to commence study of
the regulation of gene expression in race:cultivar specific
interactions   between   C. lindemuthianum   and   hypocotyls   of
P. vulgaris. In the incompatible interaction following application
of spores to the unwounded surface of host hypocotyls (a natural
infection site) there is a period of 2-3 days during which the
spores germinate and the fungus penetrates the cuticle. Immediately
the surveillance mechanisms of the plant cell detect the presence

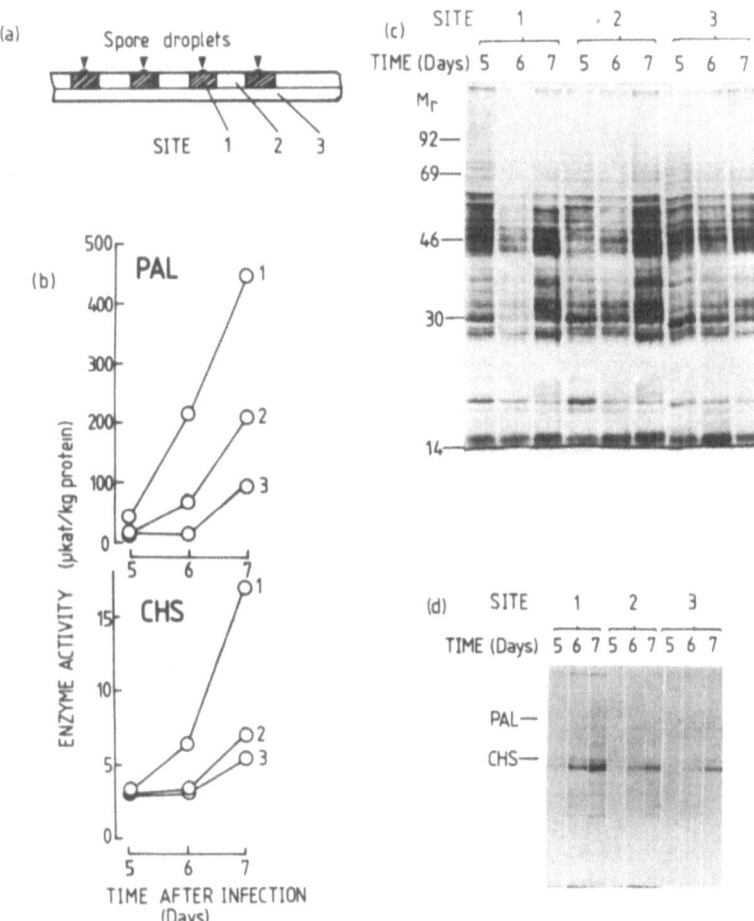

Fig. 2   Biochemical   changes   in   a   compatible   interaction: (a)
Biological source of samples; (b) Changes in PAL   and   CHS
activities;   (c)   General   changes   in   polysomal   mRNA
activities; (d)   Changes   in   polysomal   mRNA   activities
encoding PAL and CHS.

of the fungus and there is a hypersensitive response in the
initially infected cells leading to marked but localised
accumulation of phytoalexins and restriction of further fungal
growth. In contrast in the compatible interaction the surveillance
mechanism of the plant cells apparently does not operate, the
infected cells remain alive and the fungus is able to undergo
extensive biotrophic intercellular growth. After a further 4-5 days
(ie. 6-7 days from spore innoculation) widespread host cell death
and development of watery, spreading anthracnose lesions occurs.
Although there is marked phytoalexin accumulation at this stage, it
is too late to prevent further growth of the fungus and eventually
the whole hypocotyl rots and the plant dies.

So far our biochemical analysis has been largely limited to a
compatible interaction (Fig. 2). At the onset of phytoalexin
accumulation and formation of anthracnose lesions there are very
pronounced increases in PAL and CHS activities in the directly
infected region. Furthermore, increases in enzyme activity are also
observed in regions of the tissue distant from the initial site of
infection and which remain apparently healthy at this stage.
Concomitantly, there are changes in polysomal mRNA activities as
judged by the polypeptide products synthesised in a heterologous
mRNA-dependent translation system. It is not yet possible to
identify fully which of these products are encoded by the host or
pathogen genomes, but indirect immunoprecipitation studies have
shown induction of mRNA activities encoding PAL and CHS at the time
of rapid increase in enzyme activity at the onset of phytoalexin
accumulation. These observations suggest that in the intact system
the basic biochemical mechanisms governing phytoalexin accumulation
are similar to those operating in the elicitor-mediated induction
of phytoalexin accumulation in cell suspension cultures. However,
an interesting difference in detail is that in the intact
compatible interaction expression of the PAL gene occurs slightly
earlier than that of the CHS gene as judged by the timing of the
increase in the respective enzyme and mRNA activities whereas the
order is reversed in elicitor-treated cell cultures. In an
incompatible interaction, induction of enzyme activity occurs much
earlier and is localised to the immediate site of attempted
infection. Experiments to monitor changes in the mRNA activities
encoding PAL and CHS in an incompatible interaction are currently
in progress.

CONCLUSION

The rapid and marked induction of synthesis of the enzymes of
phytoalexin biosynthesis in P. vulgaris represent an excellent
system for study of the molecular mechanisms governing co-ordinate
control of plant gene expression by the environment and future
work will in part be directed toward further analysis, using
recombinant DNA techniques, of the structure, function and

expression of genes involved in plant defense. It is becoming apparent that there may be extensive intercellular communication associated with the expression of plant defense mechanisms and our recent studies using intact hypocotyls and cells separated by dialysis membranes suggest that these will be useful model systems for molecular analysis.

ACKNOWLEDGEMENTS

We thank Professor Dr. K. Hahlbrock (Freiburg) for his interest in this work and for providing antisera. We acknowledge support from the SERC, ARC, British Council, EMBO and The Queen's College, Oxford.

REFERENCES

Bailey, J.A., 1981, Physiological and biochemical events associated with expression of resistance to disease, in, "Active Defense Mechanisms in Plants", Wood, R.K.S., ed., pp 39–65, Plenum, New York.

Camm, E.E. and Towers, G.H.N., 1977, Phenylalanine ammonia-lyase, Prog. Phytochem., 4, 169–188.

Dixon, R.A., 1980, Plant tissue culture methods in the study of phytoalexin induction, in "Tissue Culture Methods for Plant Pathologists", Ingram, D.S. and Helgson, J.P. eds., pp 185–196, Blackwell, Oxford.

Dixon, R.A. and Bendall, D.S., 1978, Changes in the levels of enzymes of phenylpropanoid and flavonoid synthesis during phaseollin production in cell suspension cultures of Phaseolus vulgaris, Physiol. Plant Pathol., 13, 295–306.

Dixon, R.A. and Fuller, K.W., 1976, Effects of synthetic auxin levels on phaseollin production and phenylalanine ammonia-lyase (PAL) activity in tissue cultures of Phaseolus vulgaris L., Physiol. Plant Pathol., 9, 299–312.

Dixon, R.A. and Fuller, K.W., 1978, Effects of growth substances on non-induced and Botrytis cinerea culture filtrate induced phaseollin production in Phaseolus vulgaris cell suspension cultures, Physiol. Plant Pathol., 12, 279–288.

Dixon, R.A. and Lamb, C.J., 1979, Stimulation of de novo synthesis of L-phenylalanine ammonia-lyase in relation to phytoalexin accumulation in Colletotrichum lindemuthianum elicitor treated cell suspension cultures of French bean (Phaseolus vulgaris), Biochim. Biophys. Acta, 586, 453–463.

Dixon, R.A., Dey, P.M. and Whitehead, I.M., 1982, Purification and properties of chalcone isomerase from cell suspension cultures of Phaseolus vulgaris, Biochem. Biophys. Acta, 715, 25–33.

Dixon, R.A., Dey, P.M., Lawton, M.A. and Lamb, C.J., 1982, Phytoalexin induction in French bean: Intercellular transmission of elicitation in cell suspension cultures and hypocotyl sections, submitted for publication.

Fourcroy, P., 1978, Advantages of potassium bromide gradients for isopycnic centrifugation of proteins, Biochem. Biophys. Res. Commun., 84, 713-720.

Hahlbrock, K. and Grisebach, H., 1979, Enzymic controls in the biosynthesis of lignin and flavonoids, Ann. Rev. Plant Physiol., 30, 105-130.

Hahlbrock, K., Knobloch, K-H., Kreuzaler, F., Potts, J.R.M. and Wellmann, E., 1976, Co-ordinated induction and subsequent activity changes of two groups of metabolically interrelated enzymes. Light induced synthesis of flavonoid glycosides in cell suspension cultures of Petroselinum hortense, Eur. J. Biochem., 61, 199-206.

Hahlbrock, K., Lamb, C.J., Purwin, C., Ebel, J., Fautz, E. and Schäfer, E., 1981, Rapid response of suspension cultured parsley cells to the elicitor from Phytophthora megasperma var sojae. Induction of the enzymes of general phenylpropanoid metabolism, Plant Physiol., 67, 768-773.

Kacser, H. and Burns, J.A., 1973, The control of flux, Symp. Soc. Exp. Biol., 27, 65-104.

Keen, N.T. and Horsch, R., 1972, Hydroxyphaseollin production by various soybean tissues: A warning against use of "unnatural" host-parasite systems, Phytopathology, 62, 439-442.

Kreuzaler, F., Ragg, H., Heller, W., Tesch, R., Witt, I., Hammer, D. and Hahlbrock, K., 1979, Flavanone synthase from Petroselinum hortense. Molecular weight, subunit composition, size of messenger RNA, and absence of pantetheinyl residue, Eur. J. Biochem., 99, 89-96.

Lamb, C.J., 1977, Trans-Cinnamic acid as a mediator of the light stimulated increase in hydroxycinnamoyl-CoA : quinate hydroxycinnamoyl transferase, FEBS Lett., 75, 37-40.

Lamb, C.J. and Dixon, R.A., 1978, Stimulation of de novo synthesis of L-phenylalanine ammonia-lyase during induction of phytoalexin biosynthesis in cell suspension cultures of Phaseolus vulgaris, FEBS Lett., 94, 277-280.

Lamb, C.J. and Rubery, P.H., 1976a, Photocontrol of chlorogenic acid biosynthesis in potato tuber discs, Phytochemistry, 15, 665-668.

Lamb, C.J. and Rubery, P.H., 1976b, Interpretation of the rate of density labelling of enzymes with H_2O. Possible implications for the mode of action of phytochrome, Biochim. Biophys. Acta, 421, 308-318.

Lamb, C.J., Lawton, M.A., Taylor, S.J. and Dixon, R.A., 1980, Elicitor modulation of phenylalanine ammonia-lyase in Phaseolus vulgaris, Ann. Phytopathol., 12, 423-433.

Lawton, M.A., Dixon, R.A. and Lamb, C.J., 1980, Elicitor modulation of the turnover of L-phenylalanine ammonia-lyase in French bean cell suspension cultures, Biochim. Biophys. Acta, 633, 162-175.

Lawton, M.A., Dixon, R.A., Hahlbrock, K. and Lamb, C.J., 1982a,
    Rapid induction of phenylalanine ammonia-lyase and chalcone
    synthase synthesis in elicitor-treated plant cells,
    Eur. J. Biochem., in press.
Lawton, M.A., Dixon, R.A., Hahlbrock, K. and Lamb, C.J., 1982b,
    Rapid effects of elicitor on phenylalanine ammonia-lyase
    and chalcone synthase mRNA activities in bean cells,
    submitted for publication.
Meiners, J.P., 1981, Genetics of disease resistance in edible
    legumes, Ann. Rev. Phytopathology, 19, 189-209.
Moesta, P. and Grisebach, H., 1981, Investigation of the mechanism
    of phytoalexin accumulation in soybean induced by glucan or
    mercuric chloride, Arch. Biochem. Biophys., 211, 39-43.
Paskin, N. and Meyer, R.J., 1977, The role of enzyme degradation in
    enzyme turnover during tissue differentiation,
    Biochim. Biophys. Acta, 474, 1-11.
Rathmell, W.G. and Bendall, D.S., 1971, Phenolic compounds in
    relation to phytoalexin biosynthesis in hypocotyls of
    Phaseolus vulgaris, Physiol. Plant Pathol., 1, 351-362.
Schröder, J. and Schäfer, E., 1980, Radioiodinated antibodies, a
    tool in studies on the presence and role of inactive enzyme
    forms: Regulation of chalcone synthase in parsley cell
    cultures, Arch. Biochem. Biophys., 203, 800-808.
Schröder, J., Heller, W. and Hahlbrock, K., 1979, Flavanone
    synthase: simple and rapid assay for the key enzyme of
    flavonoid biosynthesis, Plant Sci. Lett., 14, 281-286.
Shields, S.E., Wingate, V.P. and Lamb, C.J., 1982, Dual control of
    phenylalanine ammonia-lyase production and removal by its
    product cinnamic acid, Eur. J. Biochem., 123, 389-395.
Zähringer, U., Ebel, J. and Grisebach, H., 1978, Induction of
    phytoalexin synthesis in soybean. Elicitor induced increase
    in enzyme activities of flavonoid biosynthesis and
    incorporation of mevalonate into glyceollin,
    Arch. Biochem. Biophys., 188, 450-455.

IDENTIFICATION AND USE OF cDNAS OF PHENYLALANINE AMMONIA-LYASE AND 4-COUMARATE:CoA LIGASE mRNAS IN STUDIES OF THE INDUCTION OF PHYTOALEXIN BIOSYNTHETIC ENZYMES IN CULTURED PARSLEY CELLS

David N. Kuhn, Joseph Chappell and Klaus Hahlbrock

Biologisches Institut II
Universität Freiburg
D-7800 Freiburg im Breisgau, FRG

In the present study, parsley suspension culture cells are treated with a cell wall preparation of Phytophthora megasperma var. glycinia and this interaction is considered as a model system for plant-fungal pathogen interactions with respect to phytoalexin biosynthesis. The relevance of this system for these studies can best be understood by a general discussion of phytoalexins and their biosynthesis in more intensively researched plant families, such as the Leguminosae.

Phytoalexins are compounds with antibiotic properties that accumulate in some plants after pathogen attack.[1] The production of phytoalexins is certainly not the only method that a plant has to resist disease, but phytoalexins are thought to play a necessary part in some plant's disease resistance response.[2] Phytoalexins fall into different chemical classes which correspond with plant taxonomic families. Pterocarpans, typical of the Leguminosae, are products of the shikimate-polymalonic biosynthetic pathway, which includes the enzymes phenylalanine ammonia-lyase (PAL), 4-coumarate:CoA ligase (4CL) and chalcone synthase (CHS).[3] The increase in activity of PAL upon interaction of a pathogen with a plant is well documented in a number of the Leguminosae, such as soybean[4] and pea[5]. The implication of these results is that the plant has induced the enzyme activities of the phytoalexin biosynthetic pathway in response to the invading growth of the pathogen.

Induction of phytoalexins and the enzymes involved in their synthesis can occur under a number of circumstances. Thses range from the meeting of the plant and pathogen in their natural surroundings to treatment of a wounded segment of a plant with heavy metals.[6] The study of the host-pathogen interaction is really that of two eukaryotes struggling for survival and is necessarily so complicated

in its natural form that it must be simplified to allow it to be
studied. One simplification is the sue of plant tissue culture
cells and a cell wall fraction (elicitor)[7] of the fungal pathogen.
Soybean tissue culture cells respond to Pmg elicitor by an increase
in PAL activity and production of the phytoalexin glyceollin, the
same compound produced by the whole plant in response to the live
pathogen.[8] In Nature, the pathogen may be able to counter the host's
response by degrading the phytoalexins or by simply overgrowing the
cells before sufficient phytoalexins can accumulate. However, in
the tissue culture-elicitor model system, the plant-pathogen interaction has been simplified to the plant's recognition of a fungal
cell wall component and its response to such a recognition. The
signal is rather unspecific in that a wide range of fungal and chemical elicitors induce the cells. However, the cells' response is
specific. They produce the same phytoalexins that are found in the
whole plant and these phytoalexins are representative of their taxonomic family.

        Accumulation of phytoalexins typical of the Umbelliferae has
been observed for parsley suspension cells treated with a Pmg elicitor.[9] PAL and 4CL , enzymes most probably involved in the biosynthesis of these phytoalexins, have been shown to increase in activity
prior to the accumulation of the phytoalexin.[10] These findings indicate the Pmg elicitor-parsley suspension culture cell system is a
representative model for the study of the host-pathogen interaction.
The use of parsley suspension culture cells is made even more attrac-
tive by the previous observation that PAL and 4CL, along with enzymes
involved in flavonoid biosynthesis are induced by irradiating the
cultures with UV light.[12,13] Hence, the parsley cell system affords
us the unique opportunity to study and compare two types of induction
for PAL and 4CL.

        To date, the response of parsley cells to the Pmg elicitor has
been characterized as the coordinated increase and decrease in enzyme
activity, de novo synthesis and mRNA translational activity for PAL
and 4CL.[10,11] To investigate the underlying mechanism for these
observed changes in mRNA translational activity, hybridization probes
for PAL and 4CL were necessary. These hybridization probes would
allow us to qualitatively measure the amounts of specific mRNA before
and after elicitor induction and enable us to determine whether the
increase in translational activity previously measured is due to an
increase in the amount of mRNA. An alternative explanation would be
that the observed changes in translational activity could be mediated
by an increase in the translational efficiency of existing mRNA.

        In addition to measuring changes in PAL and 4CL mRNA amounts,
we wanted to study in a more general way the effects of the elicitor
on protein and RNA synthesis in the cell. The goal of this approach
was to define more specifically the sequence of events following
elicitor treatment and to identify the earliest appearance of newly

synthesized elicitor specific proteins. This was accomplished by
characterizing de novo synthesized proteins at various times after
elicitor treatment by two dimensional gel electrophoresis.[14]

IDENTIFICATION OF cDNAS FOR PAL AND 4CL

Poly A+ RNA from induced cells was reverse transcribed and
cloned into the Pst1 site of pBR322 by G-C tailing.[15] Colonies
containing recombinant plasmids were screened for their ability to
hybridize to 32P-labelled RNA from UV light or Pmg elicitor induced
cells and uninduced cells. Those colonies showing more hybridization
with RNA from induced cells than with RNA from uninduced cells were
further screened by a modification of the hybrid selection translation procedure.[16] Plasmid DNA was isolated from chosen colonies and
covalently bound to DBM filters. These filters were then hybridized
against a mixture of poly A+ and polysomal RNA from induced cells
under non-stringent conditions (37°C, 16 h) to obtain the maximal
amount of hybridization possible. After hybridization, the nonhybridized RNA was washed away and the remaining RNA released with
boiling water, ethanol precipitated and translated in a micrococcal
nuclease treated rabbit reticulocyte lysate.[17] An aliquot of the
translation products were analysed on SDS-PAGE and those samples
with products of similar molecular weights to PAL (80 kd) or 4CL
(60 kd) were further challenged with anti-PAL and anti-4CL antibodies.
Figures 1 and 2 show examples of this procedure for identification
of cDNAs for 4CL and PAL.

Figure 1a shows a typical SDS-PAG of the products of a hybrid
selection translation experiment for pc4CL and pcH35, two cDNAs
from a cDNA library made from RNA from elicitor treated cells. pcH35
is a clone that hybridizes to an mRNA coding for an approximately
30 kd protein. It is presented as a positive control showing that
despite the background due to the non-stringent hybridization conditions, specific messages are clearly selected by the filter bound
pcDNAs. When increasing amounts of pc4CL are bound to the filter,
an increase in the strength of a protein band appearing at approximately 60 kd is seen up to 30 µg pDNA per filter. Figure 1b shows
the SDS-PAGE analysis of the antibody precipitation of the in vitro
translation products with anti-4CL antibody. The anti-4CL antibody
precipitate of the in vitro translation products of poly A+ RNA from
light induced cells is shown as the radioactive standard for 4CL.
Strong bands running at the same molecular weight as authentic 4CL
are seen for all the antibody precipitated translation products of
pc4CL but not for pcH35. Hence, pc4CL has been identified as a cDNA
complementary to an mRNA coding for 4CL. Figure 1c is a restriction
map of the inserted DNA of pc4CL. The Pst1 site closest to the
EcoR1 site of pBR322 was altered during cloning so that Pst1 is no
longer capable of excising the insert DNA. The cDNA insert in pc4CL
is approximately 450 base pairs and could account for 30% of the
coding region of 4CL mRNA.

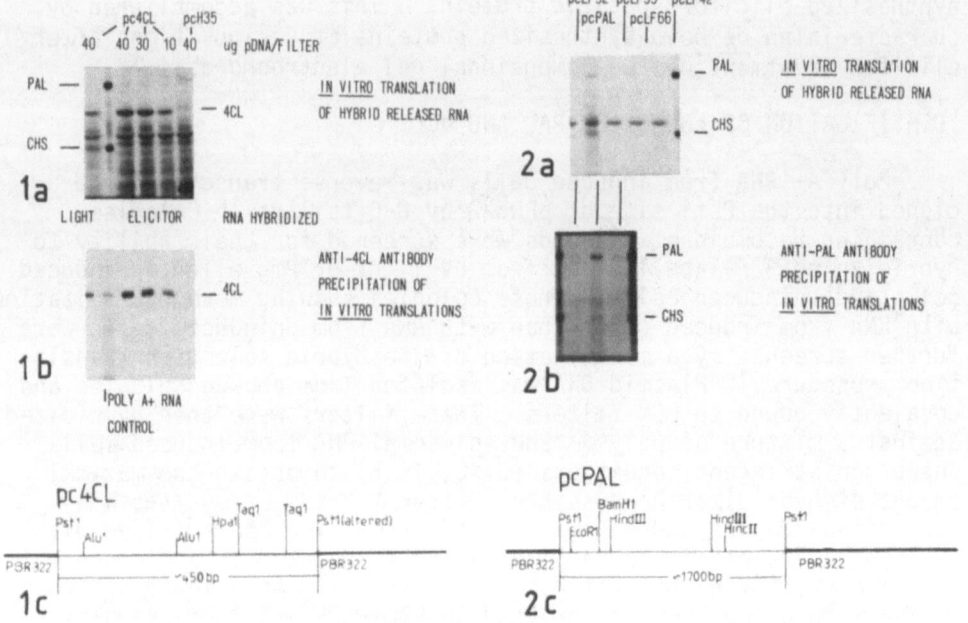

Figure 1. (a) SDS-PAG of hybrid selected translation products, (b) SDS-PAG of anti4CL antibody precipitation of products in (a), (c) restriction map of pc4CL.

Figure 2. (a) SDS-PAG of hybrid selected translation products, (b) SDS-PAG of anti-PAL antibody precipitation of products in (a), (c) restriction map of pcPAL.

Figure 2 illustrates a similar type of analysis for pcPAL. In 2a, the translation products of RNA from light induced cells selected by various pcDNAs are shown. Anti-PAL and anti-CHS antibody precipitates of translation products of poly A+ RNA from light induced cells are also shown for molecular weight comparison. The SDS-PAGE analysis of the anti-PAL antibody precipitates for the hybrid-selected translation products seen in 2a are shown in 2b. Therefore, as for 4CL, we have identified a cDNA complementary to an mRNA coding for a protein with the same molecular weight as PAL and precipitable by anti-PAL antibodies. In figure 2c, a restriction map of pcPAL is shown. The insert DNA is approximately 1700 base pairs and could account for 70% of the coding region of PAL mRNA. pcPAL and pc4CL are the first cDNAs identified for enzymes of the phenylpropanoid biosynthetic pathway, and along with pcCHS 15 are the first cDNAs identified for enzymes involved in phytoalexin biosynthesis.

USE OF pc4CL and pcPAL TO STUDY CHANGES IN mRNA LEVELS AFTER ELICITOR INDUCTION

Total RNA was isolated from parsley cells at 0,1,2,3,5,9 and 20 hours after elicitor treatment. RNA was electrophoresed on formaldehyde-agarose gels[18], transferred to nitrocellulose paper and hybridized against 32P nick translated labelled pc4CL or pcPAL. Strong hybridization was seen for both pc4CL and pcPAL with RNA from elicitor treated cells, but not with RNA from uninduced cells. Using E.coli rRNA and restricted DNA fragments as molecular weight standards on the gel, the molecular weight for 4CL mRNA was estimated at 0.8×10^6 daltons and that for PAL mRNA at 0.9×10^6 daltons. PAL mRNA had previously been estimated at 1.06×10^6 daltons by sucrose density centrifugation.[19] 4CL mRNA is approximately 2500 bases and PAL 2600 bases, both long enough to code for their respective proteins.

mRNA for 4CL and PAL increased to detectable levels within 1 hour after elicitor treatment. The amount of 4CL mRNA reached its maximum 3 hours after elicitor treatment and subsequently declined to control levels by 9 hours. This transient increase is in excellent agreement with the changes seen for the 4CL mRNA translational activity measured previously.[11] The amount of PAL mRNA increased slowly for the first 3 hours, then rose rapidly at 5 hours and reached a maximum at 9 hours after elicitor treatment. In contrast to the 4CL mRNA, the amount of PAL mRNA was high at 9 hours and remained at that elevated level even at 20 hours after elicitor treatment. These changes in the PAL mRNA levels do not correlate with similar changes in the PAL mRNA translational activity, which increases and decreases in a manner very similar to that of 4CL mRNA translational activity.

GENERAL RESPONSE OF PARSLEY SUSPENSION CULTURE CELLS TO Pmg ELICITOR

Cells treated with Pmg elicitor were analysed for changes in de novo synthesis of protein. Cells were pulse labelled with 35S methionine at various times after elicitor treatment and extracted for both protein and RNA. The extracted RNA was translated in a micrococcal nuclease treated rabbit reticulocyte lysate. Both in vivo and in vitro labelled proteins were analysed by two dimensional gel electrophoresis. Results from this analysis must be considered carefully, as the pattern of proteins from in vitro translations of RNA from uninduced cells is not consistent with the pattern of proteins from in vivo labelling of uninduced cells. However, by comparing uninduced,elicitor and light induced cells under the same conditions (in this case, in vitro labelling) several conclusions can be drawn. (Data is not presented here due to space and style considerations, but is in preparation for publication.)

First, 16 spots appear after elicitor treatment that are not present in the uninduced control. The absolute number of proteins is impossible to determine, as two dimensional gel analysis of antibody precipitates of in vitro translated PAL, 4CL and CHS have given more than one spot of the same molecular weight for each. Hence, it is not clear that the appearance of three new spots (as for CHS) signifies the appearance of three different proteins or one protein that has been modified by the rabbit system to change its pI. Since a meaningful quantitation of unknown spots is not possible, a more qualitative interpretation of the two dimensional gel electrophoresis data is presented here.

Second, the change in protein pattern is greater for elicitor than light induction. Elicitor induction causes not only more new spots to appear but, in general, decreases the intensity of a number of spots that remain constant in the uninduced or light induced cases. The light induction appears to add new spots without decreasing the intensity of spots found in the uninduced cell pattern.

Third, although two dimensional gel analysis on in vivo and in vitro labelled proteins does not produce patterns that are exactly the same, certain subsections of the patterns are alike. One of these subsections is a group of small (18 kd) acidic (pI 5.0-5.3) proteins that appear only after elicitor treatment of cells and are never seen in uninduced or light induced cells.

The characterization of elicitor induced proteins of unknown function by their position on a two dimensional gel supplies a means to identify cDNAs complementary to the mRNAs for these proteins. In the hybrid selection translation screening of the cDNA library made from RNA from elicitor induced cells, clones were found that selected mRNA for proteins varying in size from 16 to 55 kd. These in vitro translation products were further analysed by two dimensional gel electrophoresis and compared with the protein patterns from elicitor induced cells. Two cDNAs have been identified in this manner, one complementary to RNA coding for two proteins of approximately 18 kd with pI of 5.0-5.3 and the other for a 16 kd protein with pI of 5.5. These proteins are never seen in uninduced or light induced cells, unlike PAL and 4CL which are light induced. Hence, we have identified two cDNAs for RNAs that are specific to elicitor induced cells.

SUMMARY

Using the Pmg elicitor-parsley suspension culture system as a model for the study of plant-fungal pathogen interaction at the molecular level, we have attempted to answer several questions. Firstly, does the amount of mRNA for PAL and 4CL, two enzymes involved in the phytoalexin biosynthetic pathway, change after elicitor treatment and how does this change correlate with previously measured transient increases in PAL and 4CL mRNA translational activity? Secondly, what is the most immediate response of the cell to Pmg elicitor treatment and what new proteins or RNAs are synthesized immediately after induction?

Using the cDNAs for PAL and 4CL, identified by hybrid selection translation as described here, we observed increases in the amount of PAL and 4CL mRNA in elicitor treated cells. The increase in the amount of hybridizable RNA could be caused by either an increase in its transcription rate or a decrease in its rate of degradation. At present, we are attempting to measure the de novo synthesis rate of mRNA after induction, in order to distinguish between these two possibilities. In any case, the increase and subsequent decrease in 4CL mRNA and 4CL mRNA translational activity is consistent with a transient increase in the transcription of the 4CL gene. The slow increase and continued elevation of PAL mRNA levels does not correlate with the mRNA translational activity previously measured. However, PAL is also induced by UV light and under these conditions, PAL mRNA levels show a transient increase and are in agreement with mRNA translational activities. PAL is the first enzyme in the phenyl-propanoid biosynthetic pathway and may be under both transcriptional and translational control in elicitor treated cells. Hybrid selection translation of PAL mRNA from cells treated with elicitor for 9 hours or more will be done to determine the size of the translation product of this "late" mRNA and whether it can be precipated by anti-PAL antibodies. It is nonetheless clear that mRNA for PAL and 4CL increases to a detectable level by the first hour after treatment of cells with elicitor, so that induction of PAL and 4CL mRNAs is one of the first events in the cell's response.

In terms of newly synthesized proteins, we have identified a group of small, acidic proteins that are strictly elicitor induced and have identified cDNAs for two of them. With these cDNAs and those for 4CL and PAL, we will explore the changes that take place within minutes after elicitor treatment of cells.

REFERENCES

1. J. Kuc, Ann. Rev. Phytopathol., 10:207-232 (1972)
2. A. Ayers, B. Valent, J. Ebel and P. Albersheim, Plant Physiol 57:766-774 (1976)
3. A. Stoessl in "Phytoalexins", J.A. Bailey and J.W. Mansfield, eds., Blackie, Glasgow 1982
4. H. Börner and H. Grisebach, Arch Biochem Biophys 217:65-71 (1982)
5. D.C. Loschke, L.A. Hadwiger, J. Schröder and K. Hahlbrock, Plant Physiol 68:680-685 (1981)
6. J. A. Hargreaves Physiol Plant Pathol 15:279-287 (1979)
7. A. Ayers, J. Ebel, B. Valent and P. Albersheim, Plant Physiol 57:760-765 (1976)

8. J. Ebel, A. Ayers and P. Albersheim, Plant Physiol 57:775-779
    (1976)
9. K. G. Tietjen, D. Hunkler, E. Schaller, M. Weber and U. Matern,
    Eur J Biochem (submitted)
10. K. Hahlbrock, C.J. Lamb, C. Purwin, J. Ebel, E. Fautz and
    E. Schäfer Plant Physiol 67:768-773 (1981)
11. H. Ragg, D.N. Kuhn and K. Hahlbrock J Biol Chem 256:10061-65
    (1981)
12. J. Schröder, F. Kreuzaler, E. Schäfer and K. Hahlbrock
    J Biol Chem 254:57-65 (1979)
13. K. Hahlbrock et al, this volume
14. P. H. O'Farrell J Biol Chem 250:4007-4021 (1975)
15. F. Kreuzaler, H. Ragg, E. Fautz, D.N. Kuhn and K. Hahlbrock
    Proc Natl Acad Sci (USA) in press
16. R.P. Ricciardi, J.S. Miller and B.E. Roberts Proc Natl Acad
    Sci (USA) 76:4927-4931 (1979)
17. H.R.B. Pelham and R.J. Jackson Eur J Biochem 67:247 (1976)
18. J.R. Nevins and M.C. Wilson Nature 290:113-118 (1981)
19. H. Ragg and K. Hahlbrock Eur J Biochem 103:323-330 (1980)

WOUND-REGULATED SYNTHESIS AND COMPARTMENTATION OF

PROTEINASE INHIBITORS IN PLANT LEAVES

C. A. Ryan

Institute of Biological Chemistry and
Program in Biochemistry and Biophysics
Washington State University
Pullman, Washington 99164-6340

INTRODUCTION

The loss of agricultural crops because of plant pests is enormous. Estimates have been presented that over 30% of the potential yield of many crops is lost, either in the field or in storage, due to pest attacks. The recovery of even 5-10% of these losses could have major impacts on the political, social and economic aspects of food production in both developed and under-developed nations.

Within the past several years an increasing body of scientific data indicates that plants possess natural chemical defense systems that include an array of constitutive chemicals that discourage pest attacks. It is also recognized that chemicals involved in defense can be induced to accumulate in plant tissues as a result of environmental changes, including pest attacks.[1] At the practical level, natural defense systems have not been vigorously exploited to increase crop productivity, primarily because of the lack of a detailed understanding of their fundamental biochemical mechanisms. Most reports of pest induced natural plant protection are still phenomenological. Their occurrence has been recognized but we have limited knowledge of the biochemical basis for most of the known induced resistances.

An example of pest-induced synthesis of specific antinutrient proteins has been studied in our laboratory over the past several years.[2] The pest-induced synthesis and accumulation of proteinase inhibitors in leaves of Solanaceous plants has provided a convenient model system to study the nature of the chemical messengers released by pest attacks, and to study the fundamental mechanisms by which specific genes are regulated by these signals. In this chapter we briefly describe our biochemical research concerning two .insect-induced proteinase inhibitors in tomato plants and our progress in seeking the molecular events that regulate their synthesis and accumulation. This research has led us to hypothesize that a fundamental chemical communication system may be operating in plants that plays a central role in regulating defense mechanisms in diverse plant species or genera.[3,4] If such a mechanism is present then its value to agriculture could be highly significant, particularly in selecting or producing genetic strains with enhanced natural protective systems.

RESULTS AND DISCUSSION

Any severe mechanical wounding of leaves of tomato plants initiates a series of reactions which result in the synthesis and accumulation in leaf cells of the two proteinase inhibitors, called Inhibitors I and II.[2,5] A second wounding, within a few hours, results in a 2-3 fold increase in the rates of accumulation initiated by the first wound.[6] A putative wound hormone, called the proteinase inhibitor inducing factor, PIIF,[7-9] is released at the wound site and travels throughout the plant to initiate synthesis and accumulation of the two proteinase inhibitors in both the wounded leaves and in unwounded leaves distant from the wound site. We view this process as a primitive immune-like response in which the plant is responding to pest damage by producing powerful antinutrient proteins, the proteinase inhibitors, to help the plant discourage persistent or future pest attacks.[7] At present no direct evidence for the role of wound-induced proteinase inhibitors as protective agents has been reported, but trypsin inhibitors in diets of higher animals and insects have been shown to be highly detrimental, and if consumed for long periods, can be lethal.[10-12] The concentrations of proteinase inhibitors in varieties of legumes and grasses has been correlated with resistance to insects and fungi.[13,14] The roles of proteinase inhibitors in plants is not the subject of this review and the data has been discussed elsewhere.[2,15]

The two proteinase inhibitors that accumulate in leaves of wounded tomato leaves have been isolated and characterized. Inhibitor I has a molecular weight of 41,000 and is composed of subunits with molecular weights of about 8100.[5] It is, therefore, a pentamer in its native state. Each subunit possesses an active site specific for chymotrypsin, and the apparent K_i for the inhibition of chymotrypsin is about 10^{-9} M.[5] Inhibitor II has a molecular weight of about 23,000, is composed of two subunits, and strongly inhibits both trypsin and chymotrypsin with K_i values of about 10^{-8} and 10^{-7} M respectively.[5]

Recently, partial amino acid sequences of wound-induced tomato Inhibitors I and II have been determined.[16] Thirty of the residues at the N-terminal end of Inhibitor I were sequenced and 40 residues of Inhibitor II. The Inhibitor I sequence is homologous with that of potato Inhibitor I[17] and is clearly a member of the Potato I family of inhibitors.[20] Potato I has been shown to be homologous with two barley isoinhibitors[18] and an inhibitor from the leech, called eglin.[19] The relationships between these inhibitors represents the only unambiguous homologies between a plant and animal inhibitor reported to date. The similarities among the three inhibitors are remarkable. For example, 30% of the residues between potato I and barley C-1 are identical, whereas 46% of the residues between potato I and leech are identical. On an evolutionary scale, the common ancestor of a potato and a leech existed one billion years ago (Figure 1). On the other hand, barley and potato probably shared a common ancestor only 100 million years ago, when the angiosperms diverged. Yet a comparison of the sequences doesn't reflect these differences in the times of divergence. All three inhibitors have retained specificities directed toward chymotrypsin or elastase-like enzymes. When considering function as the evolutionary pressure for conservation of structure and activity, the data suggests that the chymotrypsin-elastase inhibitory specificities are probably a key factor in the high degree of structural integrity among the inhibitors.

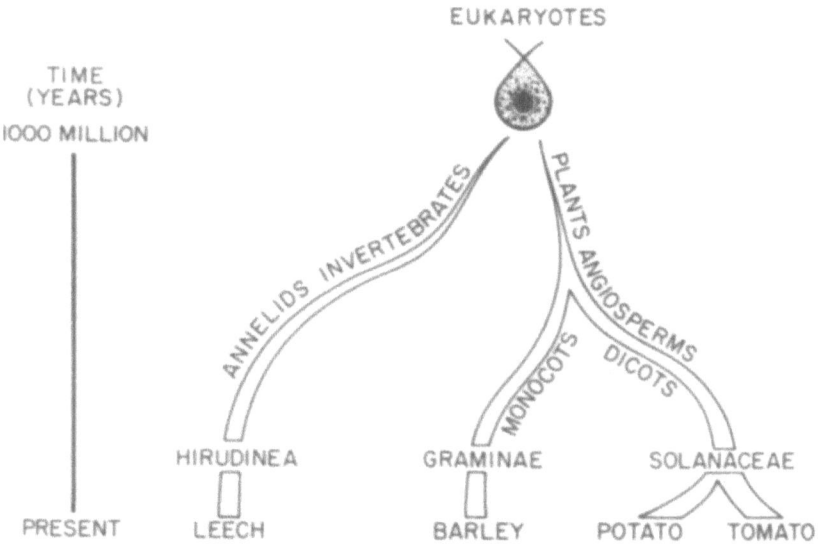

Fig. 1. Evolutionary relationships of Inhibitor I family.

The two inhibitors, Inhibitor I and II, that accumulate in
leaf cells of wounded tomato plants, are posttranslational products
of larger molecules that are synthesized from poly(A)$^+$ messenger
RNAs.[21] The two inhibitors are somehow sequestered in the central
vacuoles of the leaf cells where they have half lives of days or
weeks. Earlier evidence,[22] obtained by electron microscopy combined
with immunological identification, demonstrated that Inhibitor I
was compartmented in the central vacuole of tomato and potato leaf
cells. Recently we isolated central vacuoles from wounded tomato
plants and demonstrated that the majority of both Inhibitor I and
II could be accounted for within the vacuolar compartment.[23] Thus,
there appears to be a selective process for the vectoral synthesis
and compartmentation of the inhibitors into the central vacuole,
which has been likened to a giant lysosome.[24] In animal systems
lysosomal enzymes are thought to be synthesized on rough ER and
processed in the Golgi.[25] These events involve carbohydrate
additions to the proteins and specific segregation markers to
identify them as potential lysosomal proteins. Neither Inhibitor I
nor II are known to possess carbohydrates and their mode of synthesis
and transport into the vacuole is virtually unknown. Messenger RNA
has been prepared from leaves of wounded and unwounded tomato
plants and only leaves of wounded plants contain translatable mRNAs
specific for Inhibitors I and II.[21] Both proteins have been shown
to be translated in vitro in a reticulocyte lysate system as
preinhibitors, 2000-3000 daltons larger than those synthesized and
accumulated in vivo.[21] The preinhibitors may be important in the
process of compartmentalization of the inhibitors in the central
vacuole.

When young tomato plants are wounded, by chewing insects or by
a severe crushing of any type, the levels of total poly(A)$^+$ translatable mRNA for both proteinase Inhibitor I and Inhibitor II rise
rapidly during the first 4 hr after wounding.[6] This rise was
measured by quantifying the immunoprecipitates that can be recovered
specifically from electrophoretic gels after translation in a cell
free rabbit reticulocyte lysate system.[6,26] The analysis of
radioactivity ([^{35}S]methionine) incorporated into each inhibitor in
the gels could be used as a measure of the concentration of inhibitor
mRNAs present at various times following wounding. Translatable
mRNAs for Inhibitors I and II are present at near maximum levels
within 4 hr following a single wounding. The levels remain high
until 9 hr when they decrease to less than half their original
levels. In the same leaves, during the same time, the rates of in
vivo accumulation of Inhibitors I and II steadily increase during
the first 9 hr after wounding. By 14 hr the rates of accumulation
have reached a steady state rate that remains constant for several
hours.[26] This suggests that some shift in the cell is occurring at
about 9 hr that is reflected in both the in vitro translation of
mRNA and in the in vivo accumulation of inhibitors. The cause of

the shift in levels of translatable mRNA is unknown and could
reside in either some structural feature of the mRNAs themselves
that change their translational rates, or the differences could
result in changes in their rates of synthesis or degradation.
Nevertheless, the shift results in species of mRNA that are responsible for the more efficient steady state rate of synthesis of the
two inhibitors after 9 hr.

A second wounding of the leaves 9 hr after the initial wounding,
doubled the rate of accumulation of both Inhibitors I and II over
those of once wounded plants.[26] This second wound also resulted in
the maintenance of the mRNA levels already present at 9 hr so that
the decrease in translatable mRNA noted in singly wounded plants
did not occur. The second wound apparently provides more mRNA when
the plant's translational system is already operating at high
efficiency.

The specific messengers for the inhibitors could be further
enriched from total poly(A)[+] mRNA by centrifugation in 15-30%
sucrose gradients.[26] Inhibitors I and II mRNAs were identified in
fractions from the gradients using an in vitro reticulocyte lysate
translation system. Fractions containing Inhibitors I and II mRNA
were pooled together and recentrifuged in a 10-25% linear sucrose
gradient. A pooling of the region of the second sucrose gradient
containing the two inhibitor mRNA species provided a mRNA preparation
containing a 15-fold enrichment of the specific mRNA for Inhibitor
I and a 5-fold enrichment of Inhibitor II mRNA. This mRNA was
utilized for experiments to prepare cDNAs for cloning.

Cloning of the mRNAs enriched in Inhibitors I and II messages
is underway to provide specific cDNAs for use as hibridization
probes to study the early events of Inhibitors I and II mRNA
synthesis and processing in response to wounding. Such clones can
also be employed to probe a library of tomato genes for the inhibitor
genomics so that the structural features of the genes be studied
and the molecular basis for the regulation of gene expression in
response to stress can be explored.

The wound-induced expression of the two proteinase inhibitors
is mediated by a putative wound hormone, called PIIF, the proteinase
inhibitor inducing factor. Within about one and a half to two
hours following wounding of a tomato leaflet a signal is transported
throughout the plants that initiates the simultaneous synthesis of
Inhibitors I and II.[2] The factor is apparently transported through
the phloem, since phloem destruction by a hot air stream, leaving
the xylem intact, blocks the signal from leaving a wounded leaf.
Recent data suggests that a reaction at the wound site may be
occurring that builds up a gradient of the signal that moves out of
the leaf with a maximum at about 120 min.[26]

A pectic fraction has been isolated from tomato leaves that is active in inducing proteinase inhibitor accumulation in detached tomato leaves.[27] The fragment elutes from Sephadex G-25 with an apparent MW of about 5000 daltons. Its monosaccharide composition upon acid hydrolysis is rich in galacturonic acid residues and is generally similar to pectic substances associated with plant cell walls.[4] A highly pure cell wall pectic polysaccharide isolated from sycamore cell walls called RG1, MW $\sim$200,000,[28] is also a highly active inducer of Inhibitor I and II synthesis in detached tomato leaves. Other pectic-like substances also exhibit activity, such as citrus pectin and polygalacturonic acid, but none are as highly active on a weight basis as the tomato PIIF or RG1.

PIIF-active oligosaccharides could be hydrolyzed from polysaccharide tomato PIIF using an endo α1-4,galacturonase obtained from the fungus Rhizopus stolonifer.[3] Active oligosaccharides could also be released from isolated tomato leaf cell walls by an endopolygalacturonase partially purified from tomato plants. It was suggested that oligosaccharides, released from plant cell wall pectic polysaccharides by either endogenous or exogenous endopolygalacturonases at a wound or infection site, may have hormone-like roles in regulating plant defense responses in unwounded tissues many centimeters away from the site of release.[3] It should also be noted that the conversion of tomato PIIF into small oligosaccharides by fungal endopolygalacturonase required pectinesterase. This implies that the latter enzyme may play a role in the process of PIIF release in vivo and that demethylation of cell walls or their products may be additional levels of control of the formation or release of active PIIF.[3]

The cumulative evidence supports a hypothesis wherein oligosaccharides arise from the degradation of the plant cell wall by hydrolytic enzymes that either are activated during wounding or are introduced by invading pests. These oligosaccharides themselves, or a product induced by their presence, could then be transported rapidly through the plant vascular system to target cells where they induce the synthesis and accumulation of proteinase inhibitor proteins. We suggest that this process may be a common feature of plants to communicate information.

Pectic substances have been found to be involved in triggering antifungal phytoalexin accumulation in legumes. West has reported[29] that an "endogenous elicitor" can be released from castor beans by the action of a pure endo α1-4,endopolygalacturonase. The enzyme activity is necessary for elicitation of the phytoalexin casbene, and the enzyme can release pectic fragments from castor bean cell walls that act as the elicitors. Tomato PIIF as well as citrus pectin and polygalacturonic acid were also found to elicit casbene synthesis in castor beans.

Recently Albersheim has reported[31] that pectic substances isolated from cell walls of tobacco, wheat, sycamore and soybeans by partial acid hydrolysis are elicitors of the phytoalexin glycinol in soybean cotyledons. In addition, partial acid hydrolysis of other pectic materials including RG1 were elicitors of the phytoalexin. More recently we have found that tomato PIIF elicits synthesis of another isoflavonoid phytoalexin, pisitin, in pea pods.[32]

Table 1. A Summary of Pectic Fragments that Evoke Responses in Plant Tissues

Pectic Fragment Origin	Plant Tissues	Response (Synthesis)
Tomato	Tomato Leaves	Proteinase Inhibitors[3]
Sycamore	Tomato Leaves	Proteinase Inhibitors[4]
Citrus	Tomato Leaves	Proteinase Inhibitors[4]
Tomato	Potato Leaves	Proteinase Inhibitors[34]
Tomato	Alfalfa Leaves	Proteinase Inhibitors[35]
Castor Beans	Castor Bean Seedlings	Casbene[30]
Tomato	Castor Bean Seedlings	Casbene[30]
Citrus	Castor Bean Seedlings	Casbene[30]
Soybeans	Castor Bean Seedlings	Casbene[30]
Soybeans	Soybean Cotyledons	Glycinol[31]
Tobacco	Soybean Cotyledons	Glycinol[31]
Sycamore	Soybean Cotyledons	Glycinol[31]
Wheat	Soybean Cotyledons	Glycinol[31]
Tomato	Pea Pods	Pisitin[32]

The most interesting aspect of these observations is that casbene is a diterpene and glycinol and pisitin are isoflavonoids.[33] Diterpenes and isoflavonoids are synthesized by entirely different pathways. Thus, the pectic substances are regulating two different biosynthetic pathways for phytoalexins as well as regulating proteinase inhibitor synthesis. Table 1 summarizes our present knowledge of various pectic fragments that regulate these systems in various plants.

The most intriguing possibility stemming from these cumulative studies is that a common fundamental chemical communication system

may be operating in plants, triggered by pectic fragments released
during pest attacks. The possibility arises that at least some of
the many pest induced natural defense processes that have been
recognized may involve similar mechanisms of the control of gene
expression. If this is the case then the system would offer
molecular biologists involved in genetic engineering in plants, a
potential mechanism for regulating engineered genes. Such possibilities, of course, must await further studies of fundamental mechanisms of action of the pectic fragments and full understanding of
the breadth of the system in nature. It is clear, however, that
natural plant protection and its basic biochemical mechanisms,
encompassing informational molecules, receptor systems and the
regulation of gene expression in response to pest attacks, provides
an exciting and significant frontier for scientists from diverse
disciplines to interact with a common goal, that is, to help feed
our fellow man.

ACKNOWLEDGMENTS

The author gratefully acknowledges the contributions of his
students and colleagues to this research. The technical assistance
of Joel Bryant and Greg Pearce has been invaluable. The research
was supported in part by grants from the National Science Foundation,
the U. S. Department of Agriculture, Cooperative States Research
Service and the Rockefeller Foundation.

REFERENCES

1. D. Rhodes, Evolution of plant chemical defense against herbivores, in: "Herbivores, Their Interaction with Secondary
Plant Metabolites," G. A. Rosenthal and D. H. Janzen,
eds., Academic Press, New York (1979).
2. C. A. Ryan, Wound-regulated synthesis and vacuolar compartmentation of proteinase inhibitors in plant leaves, in:
"Current Topics in Cellular Regulation," Vol. 17, B.
Horecker and E. Stadtman, eds., Academic Press (1980).
3. P. Bishop, D. J. Makus, G. Pearce and C. A. Ryan, Proteinase
inhibitor-inducing factor activity in tomato leaves
resides in oligosaccharides enzymically released from cell
walls, Proc. Natl. Acad. Sci. 78:3536 (1981).
4. C. A. Ryan, P. Bishop, G. Pearce, A. G. Darvill, M. McNeil and
P. Albersheim, A sycamore cell wall polysaccharide and a
chemically related tomato leaf polysaccharide possess
similar proteinase inhibitor-inducing activities, Plant
Physiol. 68:616 (1981).
5. G. Plunkett, D. F. Senear, G. Zuroske and C. A. Ryan, Proteinase
Inhibitor I and II from leaves of wounded tomato plants:

purification and properties, Arch. Biochem. Biophys. 213:463 (1982).

6. C. E. Nelson and C. A. Ryan, Temporal shifts in the apparent in vivo translational efficiencies of tomato leaf proteinase Inhibitors I and II mRNAs following wounding, Biochem. Biophys. Res. Commun. 94:355 (1980).

7. T. R. Green and C. A. Ryan, Wound-induced proteinase inhibitor in plant leaves: a possible defense mechanism against insects, Science 175:776 (1972).

8. T. R. Green and C. A. Ryan, Wound-induced proteinase inhibitor in tomato leaves: some effects of light and temperature on the wound response, Plant Physiol. 51:19 (1973).

9. C. A. Ryan, Assay and biochemical properties of the proteinase inhibitor inducing factor, a wound hormone, Plant Physiol. 54:328 (1974).

10. S. Applebaum, Physiological aspects of host specificity in the Bruchidae. I. General considerations of developmental compatibility, J. Insect. Physiol. 10:783 (1964).

11. D. H. Janzen, H. B. Juster and E. A. Bell, Toxicity of secondary compounds to the seed-eating larvae of the bruchid beetle Callospobruchus maculatus, Phytochemistry 16:223 (1970).

12. I. Liener and M. L. Kakade, Protease inhibitors, in: "Toxic Constituents of Plant Foodstuffs," I. E. Liener, ed., Academic Press, New York (1969).

13. A. M. Yamaleeva, V. K. Musinov, R. F. Isaev, A. A. Yamaleeva and V. I. Krivchenko, Activity of protease inhibitors and resistance of wheat to the causal agent of hard smut. Sel'skozyaistvennaya Biologiya 15:143 (1980).

14. M. Angharad, R. Gatehouse, J. A. Gatehouse, P. Dobie, A. M. Kilminster and D. Boulter, Biochemical basis of insect resistance in Vigna anguiculata, J. Sci. Food Agr. 30:948 (1979).

15. C. A. Ryan, Proteolytic enzymes and their inhibitors in plants, Ann. Rev. Plant. Physiol. 24:173 (1973).

16. K. Titani, K. Walsh and C. A. Ryan, in preparation.

17. M. Richardson and L. Cossins, Chymotryptic Inhibitor I from potato: the amino acid sequences of subunits B, C and D, FEBS Lett. 52:1610 (1974).

18. I. Svendsen, I. Jonassen, J. Hejgaard and S. Borsen, Amino acid sequence homology between a serine protease inhibitor from barley and potato Inhibitor I, Carslberg Res. Comm. 45:389 (1980).

19. U. Seemuller , M. Eulitz, H. Fritz and A. Strobl, Structure of the elastase-cathpsin G. inhibitor from the leech Hirudo medicinalis. Hoppe-Seyler's Z. Physiol. Chem. 361:1841 (1981).

20. M. Laskowski and I. Kato, Protein inhibitors of proteinases, Ann. Rev. Biochem. 49:593 (1980).

21. C. E. Nelson and C. A. Ryan, In vitro synthesis of pre-proteins

of two vacuolar compartmented proteinase inhibitors that accumulate in leaves of wounded tomato plants, Proc. Natl. Acad. Sci., 77:1975 (1980).

22. L. K. Shumway, J. M. Rancour and C. A. Ryan, Vacuolar protein bodies in tomato leaf cells and their relationship to chymotrypsin Inhibitor I protein, Planta 93:1 (1970).

23. M. Walker-Simmons and C. A. Ryan, Immunological identification of proteinase Inhibitors I and II in isolated tomato leaf vacuoles, Plant Physiol. 60:61 (1977).

24. P. L. Matile, Zellkmopartimentierung am beispiel der pflanzeichen vakuole, Naturwissenschaften 66:343 (1979).

25. A. Hasilik and E. F. Neufeld, Biosynthesis of lysosomal enzymes in fibroblasts. synthesis as precursors of higher molecular weight, J. Biol. Chem. 255:1937 (1980).

26. C. Nelson, M. Walker-Simmons, D. Makus, G. Zuroske, J. Graham and C. A. Ryan, The regulation of synthesis and accumulation of proteinase inhibitors in leaves of wounded tomato plants in: "Mechanisms of Plant Resistance to Insects," P. Hedin, ed., ACS Monograph, (1982).

27. P. Bishop, G. Pearce, J. Bryant and C. A. Ryan, in preparation.

28. M. McNeil, A. G. Darvill, P. Albersheim, Rhamngalacturonan I, a structurally complex pectic polysaccharide in cells of suspension cultured sycamore cells. Plant Physiol. 66:1128 (1980).

29. S.-C. Lee and C. A. West, Polygalacturonase from Rhizopus stolonifer, an elicitor of casbene synthetase in castor bean (Recinus communis L.) seedlings, Plant Physiol. 67:633 (1981).

30. R. J. Bruce and C. A. West, The role of pectic fragments of the plant cell wall in elicitation by a fungal endopoly-galacturonase, Plant Physiol. 69:1181 (1982).

31. Hahn, G. M., A. G. Darvill and P. Albersheim, The endogenous elicitor, a fragment of plant cell wall polysaccharide that elicits phytoalexin accumulation in soybeans, Plant Physiol. 68:1161 (1981).

32. M. Walker-Simmons, L. Hadwiger and C. A. Ryan, in preparation.

33. C. A. West, Fungal elicitors of the phytoalexin response in higher plants, Naturewissenschaften 68:447 (1981).

34. C. A. Ryan, unpublished data.

35. W. Brown and C. A. Ryan, in preparation.

MITOCHONDRIAL GENES AND THEIR EXPRESSION IN HIGHER PLANTS

C. J. Leaver, L. K. Dixon, E. Hack, T. D. Fox[*] and
A. J. Dawson

Department of Botany, University of Edinburgh
Edinburgh, EH9 3JH, Scotland
[*]Cornell University, Ithaca, New York, 14853 USA

INTRODUCTION

Many of the major changes which occur during growth and differentiation of higher plants are associated with, or dependent upon, marked changes in mitochondrial number, structure and activity. However, very little is known about either the genes which code for mitochondrial proteins, nor the environmental, physiological and genetic factors which regulate mitochondrial biogenesis and coordinate it with development of the plant cell.

The first observations suggesting that the major energy transducing organelles of the plant cell contained their own DNA were made some 30 years ago. Since then considerable progress has been made in analysing the structure, organisation and coding function of the chloroplast genome, no doubt due to the ease of isolation of chloroplasts and their role in photosynthesis, coupled with the advent of modern cloning and sequencing techniques. Comparable studies on the plant mitochondrial genome were initiated comparatively recently, due in part to the realisation that both organellar genomes contain a previously neglected source of genetic diversity, this diversity being of potential use to the plant breeder seeking to produce higher yielding varieties of disease resistant crop plants, able to grow in a wide range of environments.

Progress in our understanding of the organisation and expression of the plant mitochondrial genome has also been stimulated by several lines of evidence which suggest that mutations in the mitochondrial DNA (mtDNA) of maize and sorghum lead to the failure of the mature plant to produce functional pollen.[1]

This maternally inherited trait is called cytoplasmic male sterility (CMS) and is used commercially in the production of hybrid seed varieties by eliminating self-fertilisation of the seed parent plant.

However, despite recent progress which has shown that the higher plant mitochondrial genome is considerably larger and more variable than comparable genomes in other organisms, our detailed understanding of mitochondrial genome organisation, information content and expression has been obtained from studies on animal and fungal mitochondria.[1,2,3] Therefore a summary of the more important features of the human and yeast mitochondrial genomes will be given, followed by a resume of the current state of knowledge of the plant mitochondrial genome and its expression (for a more detailed review see ref. 1).

ORGANISATION OF YEAST AND HUMAN MITOCHONDRIAL GENOMES

The mitochondrial DNAs of animals and fungi are covalently closed, circular molecules, which occur in many copies per mitochondrion and are autonomously replicated and transcribed within the organelle. The animal mtDNAs so far examined are about 16–17 kb in length, while in the commoner strains of yeast the genome is some five times larger at between 68–75 kb. Despite this difference in size both genomes contain essentially the same basic set of genes (Table 1) which are however organised in a strikingly different manner. These genes fall into two functionally different classes. One set codes for ribosomal and transfer RNA components of a mitochondrion specific protein synthesising system whose function is to translate the messenger RNA (mRNA) transcripts of the second set of genes. These genes code for a small number (13–20)of mitochondrial polypeptides which constitute between 5–10% of the total mitochondrial protein.[2]

Complete sequence analysis of the 16,569 bp of the human (and recently mouse and bovine) mitochondrial genomes shows a tightly packed genome with the coding capacity for 2 ribosomal RNAs, 22 transfer RNAs and 13 proteins, with very few non-coding nucleotides. Intervening as well as spacer sequences are conspicuously absent, and at each end of a coding sequence there is in almost every case a tRNA gene.[2]

The animal genome is completely and symmetrically transcribed from a single initiation site on each strand of the mtDNA. The giant transcripts are then rapidly processed by cleavage at the 5' and 3' ends of the tRNA genes to yield the individual functional RNAs, the tRNA genes apparently providing a recognition signal for the endonucleolytic processing enzyme(s). The mRNA transcripts are subsequently modified by the addition of a 3'-poly (A) tail, which in several cases generates the stop codon UAA, which is not encoded in the mtDNA, from the pre-existing 3'-terminal U or UA.[3]

In contrast to the economy of organisation shown in the animal genome, the mtDNA of yeast (Saccharomyces cerevisiae) is some five-fold larger (75-78 kb) with coding sequences organised in a completely different manner. In many cases the genes are separated by extensive stretches of non-coding AT-rich sequences and further sequence analysis has revealed that at least three genes are split and contain intervening sequences (introns).[2,4]

Table 1. Mitochondrial Genes and their Products in Animal, Yeast and Plant Mitochondria

	Animal	Yeast	Plant
MtDNA-size (kb)	16-17	75-78	250-2500
Mitochondrial Gene and/or Product			
Large ribosomal RNA	16S	21S	26S
Small ribosomal RNA	12S	15S	18S
5S ribosomal RNA	−	−	+
Transfer RNAs	22	25	'⩾30'
Cytochrome c oxidase			
Subunit I	+	+	+
Subunit II	+	+	+
Subunit III	+	+	?
Apo-cytochrome b	+	+	+
ATPase complex			
Subunit 6	+	+	?
Subunit 9	−	+	+
Ribosomal protein (Var 1)	−	+	'+'
Unassigned Reading Frames (URFs)	8	∽13	?

The large rRNA gene contains a single intron, while two protein coding genes (for apocytochrome b and subunit I of cytochrome c oxidase) contain multiple introns, some of which are optional.

In the case of the cytochrome b gene (COB), various forms of the gene, containing either 5 introns and 6 exons or 2 introns and 3 exons, have been isolated from laboratory yeast strains. Certain of these introns contain long unassigned reading frames (URFs) which are in phase with the exon immediately upstream. Apparently the long form of the COB gene, containing 5 introns, is transcribed into a precursor RNA which is ca. seven times the length required to code for the structural protein. The first small intron 1 is removed by a nuclear coded processing enzyme thus joining the first two exons. These exon sequences together with the open reading frame in intron 2 code form a hybrid protein (M_r ca. 42,000) which has been termed an 'RNA maturase'. This enzyme is involved in the excision of intron 2 which at the same time destroys its own mRNA and thus controls its own synthesis. Intron 4 of the COB gene also apparently codes for a maturase protein which is not only involved in the processing of COB gene transcripts but also affects the expression of the gene for subunit 1 of cytochrome c oxidase. At the time of writing no one has purified any of the postulated maturase proteins and the question remains as to why certain mitochondrial genes contain introns. In the absence of firm data one is forced to assume that the intricate system for RNA processing and splicing allows a more precise control over mitochondrial gene expression.[2,4,5]

The presence of only 22 tRNAs in animal and 25 tRNAs in yeast mitochondria raises the question as to how all 61 codons are read. Apparently each tRNA is specific for a codon family in the genetic code. Those tRNAs for two-codon families have G:U wobble anti-codons, while those for 4-codon families have U in the 3rd position of the anticodon so that U:N wobble is possible.[3]

Sequence analysis has also revealed that the genetic code in mitochondria differs from the previously 'universal code'.

In animals and fungi, UGA is read as tryptophan rather than 'stop'; in animals AGA, AGG are read as 'stop' rather than arginine, and AUA as methionine rather than isoleucine.[2,3]

The identification of mitochondrial translation products, coupled with the characterisation and mapping of the genes which code for them, was initially carried out in yeast. The application of rapid DNA sequencing techniques has subsequently allowed identification and mapping of homologous gene sequences in the mtDNA of several mammals and the fungus Neurospora.[6]

The major mitochondrially synthesised polypeptides in yeast are hydrophobic subunits of three oligomeric enzyme complexes which are vital for the assembly of the functional inner mitochondrial membrane. In yeast these have been identified as the three largest (I, II and III) of the seven subunits of cytochrome c oxidase, the apocytochrome b subunit of the cytochrome bc_1 complex and two subunits (6 and 9) of the ten subunit, oligomycin-sensitive ATPase complex. In addition a single polypeptide of the small ribosomal subunit (Var 1) is also coded and synthesised in yeast and Neurospora mitochondria.[2,6]

The remainder of the 300-400 mitochondrial proteins, namely those of the outer membrane, the matrix space (including the enzymes of the TCA cycle and those required for replication and transcription of mtDNA and for translation), and a large proportion of the inner membrane, are encoded in nuclear DNA, synthesised on cytoplasmic ribosomes and subsequently transported into the mitochondrion.[7]

In contrast to our extensive knowledge of the sequence, coding capacity and organisation of the mitochondrial genome, our understanding of the participation of nuclear genes coding for mitochondrial proteins and the control of their expression during mitochondrial biogenesis is very limited. In yeast and Neurospora it has been shown that many mitochondrial proteins are synthesised on free cytoplasmic polysomes with amino-terminal extensions. The apparent molecular weights of these precursors are 500-10,000 daltons higher than the corresponding mature proteins. Translocation of polypeptides from the cytosol into the mitochondrial matrix or inner mitochondrial membrane requires an electrochemical potential across the membrane and is usually accompanied by the proteolytic cleavage of the precursor by specific chelator -sensitive protease(s) in the matrix space.[7] Current research is directed towards the identification of receptor proteins on the outer membrane which provide a specific binding site for the mitochondrial protein precursors.

Thus the synthesis of functional mitochondria capable of electron transport and coupled oxidative phosphorylation requires the coordinated expression of both mitochondrial and nuclear genomes. The morphological complexity of the organelle, coupled with the fact that the synthesis of the constituent proteins and lipids occurs in two spatially separated compartments of the cell, indicates that the assembly of the mitochondrion is a highly ordered process, whose most general features remain unknown.

THE MITOCHONDRIAL GENOME OF HIGHER PLANTS

The higher plant mitochondrial genome is much larger and more variable in size than the mitochondrial genomes of fungal and animal cells.[1] Recent estimates suggest a variation in mtDNA size of 250-2500 kb between species, with a seven to eight-fold variation within a single plant family, the cucurbits.[8] Electron microscopy of mtDNA from a number of species reveals a high

proportion of linear molecules of varying size, together with
multiple size classes of circular molecules (1-100 kb).[9] In an
attempt to produce a complete physical map of maize mtDNA,
Lonsdale and his colleagues at the Plant Breeding Institute in
Cambridge have cloned a large proportion of the maize mitochondrial genome into cosmid vectors and carried out restriction
enzyme mapping. To date they have produced a restriction map some
650 kb in length, which can be organised into two large linkage
groups of ca. 200-240 kb and two small linkage groups. These
large linkage groups contain several large repeated sequences of
ca. 26, 14 and 12 kb and it is assumed that as more mapping data
becomes available a single large linkage group, corresponding to
the whole mitochondrial genome, will be obtained. (D. Lonsdale
personal communication).

     The production of a circular, physical map, together with
identification and localisation of specific coding sequences, will
eventually provide a more complete picture of the organisation of
the plant mitochondrial genome, which at present appears to differ
considerably from that described in other organisms.

Why is the Plant Mitochondrial Genome so Large

     Two important questions which must eventually be answered
are, why is the plant mitochondrial genome so large and what is
the functional significance, if any, of the wide range of genome
sizes found in different plants? Does plant mtDNA contain
additional structural genes not found in other organisms? Are
there additional 'regulatory sequences' in green plant mitochondria which are involved in 'interorganellar communication' with
chloroplast and nuclear genomes, during the coordinated changes
in cellular function which occur during development and differentiation? A partial answer to some of these questions, which
also creates further fundamental problems, is provided by the
recent findings of Stern and Lonsdale.[10] They have reported that
maize mtDNA contains a 12 kb region homologous to part of the
inverted repeat of maize chloroplast DNA. In chloroplasts this
region encodes the chloroplast 16S ribosomal RNA and tRNA[ile] and
tRNA[val]. Questions concerning the extent, origin, significance
and function of these sequences in the mitochondrial genome
provide an exciting basis for future research.

Mitochondrial Genes

     Before these questions and many others besides can be
answered it will be necessary to identify and map the genes
localised on plant mtDNA. To date four genes have so far been
positively identified on plant mtDNA; three of these are the
ribosomal RNA genes which code for the 26S, 18S and 5S

mitochondrial rRNAs, and are the subject of an article in this volume by Gray et al.[11] The 5S mitochondrial rRNA is apparently unique to plant mitoribosomes and has not been identified in mitoribosomes of other organisms.[1] The only other gene that has been positively identified as being encoded in plant mtDNA is that coding for subunit II of cytochrome c oxidase.[12] The approach used in isolating the gene has opened the way for the rapid identification of specific genes on plant mtDNA and exploits the fact that the sequences of many mitochondrial genes are evolutionarily conserved. Yeast mitochondrial gene probes, specific for the oxi-1 gene (coding for subunit II of cytochrome c oxidase), were nick-translated and hybridised under conditions of very low stringency, to restriction fragments of maize mtDNA. The single 2.4 kb Eco RI fragment of mtDNA which hybridised with the yeast probe was subsequently cloned into the bacterial plasmid pBR322 and sequenced. The DNA sequence revealed several interesting features. The first being that the plant gene, unlike the homologous yeast and animal genes, contains a single, centrally located 794 bp - long intron. The intron contains two open reading frames of 118 and 110 codons, respectively; neither of them is in phase with either exon or share any homology with URF regions in yeast or mammalian mtDNA. Thus raising the question again as to why some mitochondrial genes are split in some organisms and not in others.

The two coding regions separated by the intron share an amino acid homology of 47% with the predicted yeast sequence and 40% with the bovine sequence. The sequence data also suggests a further variation in the once universal genetic code. Unlike the fungal and mammalian mitochondrial genomes which use UGA to specify tryptophan instead of 'stop', the plant apparently uses CGG (normally arginine) in addition to the usual UGG to specify this amino acid. In contrast to the situation found in the homologous gene of other organisms there are no TGA codons (coding for tryptophan) in the translated reading frame, leaving open the question of whether this codon can be read in plant mitochondria.[12,13]

The plant genes for subunit I of cytochrome c oxidase and apocytochrome b have also been identified by this approach and are currently being sequenced.

Ideally we would like to prove that a specific mitochondrial gene is present on cloned fragments of mtDNA by using a coupled transcription-translation system from E. coli, wheat germ or reticulocyte lysate. However our efforts to date have met with failure, possibly in part due to the non-universality of the genetic code and/or the absence of specific transcription or translation recognition sites encoded by the mtDNA.

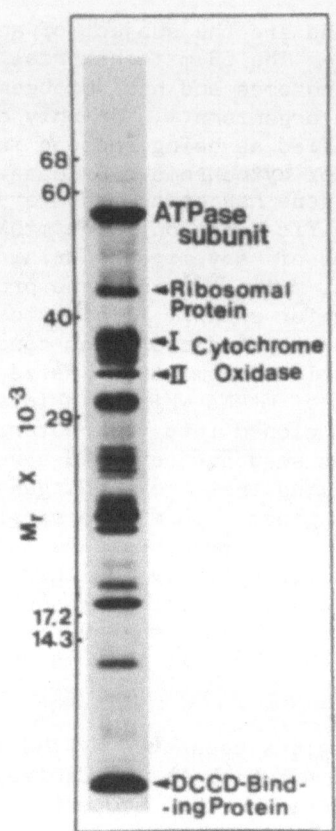

Figure 1. Polypeptides synthesised by isolated maize mitochondria
          Mitochondria were isolated from 5 day old, dark-grown
          maize seedlings and allowed to synthesise protein in
          an 'optimized' medium containing [35S]-methionine. The
          mitochondrial proteins were then solubilised in SDS,
          fractionated by electrophoresis in 15% (w/v) poly-
          acrylamide slab gels and the labelled polypeptides
          detected by autoradiography of the dried gel.

     While the approach to gene identification described in this
section will no doubt lead to the isolation of several more
genes, the ultimate limitation is the availability of homologous
gene probes from other, well characterised mitochondrial genomes.
The possibility that plant mtDNA encodes additional structural
genes requires the type of approach described in the next
section.

Mitochondrial Translation Products

     An alternative approach designed to establish the number and
identity of polypeptides synthesised within plant mitochondria and
by extrapolation encoded by mtDNA, is to analyse the proteins
synthesised by isolated mitochondria. Analysis of the radio-
actively labelled products of mitochondrial translation from a
range of plant tissues, by 1-D SDS-polyacrylamide gel electrophoresis, followed by autoradiography, reveals that an essentially
similar spectrum of some 18-20 polypeptides are synthesised (Fig.
1).[1] The higher resolution afforded by 2-D I.E.F./PAG electrophoresis suggests that in excess of 30 polypeptides are labelled,
although it is possible that certain of the labelled 'spots' are
the products of premature termination, charge modification or
proteolytic cleavage.

     The mitochondrial translation products have apparent mole-
cular weights ranging from 8,000 to 54,000. In an attempt to
localise the labelled polypeptides further we have fractionated
mitochondria into outer membrane, inter-membrane space, inner
membrane and matrix (Eilers & Leaver, unpublished observations).
As in other organisms, most of the labelled polypeptides are
associated with the inner membrane. At least two polypeptides,
however, are found in the matrix fraction; the larger has a molecular weight of ca. 54,000 and preliminary evidence suggests
that it may be the α-subunit of the F_1 component of the mitochondrial ATPase complex. The smaller labelled matrix polypeptide co-purifies with mitochondrial ribosomes and is probably
homologous to the Var-1 protein described in yeast and Neurospora.[1] (Hack & Leaver, unpublished observations). To identify
those labelled polypeptides localised in the inner membrane we
have used two approaches. The first involved immunoprecipitation
of labelled mitochondrial translation products with monospecific
antibodies prepared against purified subunits I and II of yeast
cytochrome c oxidase. This has allowed tentative identification
of the homologous plant subunits as the labelled polypeptides
with estimated molecular weights of 38,000 (subunit I) and 34,000
(subunit II) (Fig. 1).

     The second approach involves the isolation of specific
enzyme complexes from the inner mitochondrial membrane of
labelled mitochondria, followed by 1-D and 2-D gel electrophoresis of the component polypeptides. We have isolated the proton-
translocating ATPase complex by a modification of the method of
Rott and Nelson[13] and further fractionated the complex into the
hydrolytic unit - F_1, and the hydrophobic component - CF_0 which
anchors the F_1 unit to the inner membrane. Preliminary results
suggest that in maize one polypeptide of the F_1 unit and at least
one in the CF_0 component are synthesised in plant mitochondria.
The polypeptide labelled in the F_1 unit has a molecular weight of

ca. 54,000 and co-purifies with the 'α-subunit' in 2-D gels. The major labelled polypeptide in the CF_O component has a molecular weight of ca. 8,000, is soluble in butan-1-ol and specifically binds ^{14}C - dicyclohexyl-carbodiimide (DCCD) (Leaver, unpublished observations). These characteristics suggest that this polypeptide is the DCCD-binding proteolipid (ATPase subunit 9), the gene for which is located on mtDNA in yeast but on nuclear DNA in animals and <u>Neurospora</u>.

The remaining 20 or so polypeptides synthesised by, and presumably encoded within plant mitochondria, remain to be identified. The assignment of a functional role to these mitochondrially coded polypeptides is a prerequisite to further studies of both the regulation of mitochondrial differentiation and the analysis of mitochondrial mutations with important effects on the phenotype of the plant.

MITOCHONDRIAL MUTATIONS AND CYTOPLASMIC MALE STERILITY

Our understanding of mitochondrial genetics and biogenesis is mainly due to work carried out with the unicellular yeast, <u>Saccharomyces cerevisiae</u>. The unique ability of yeast to live by glycolysis alone, i.e. without functional mitochondria, has allowed the isolation and characterisation of mutations in the mitochondrial and nuclear genomes, which affect mitochondrial biogenesis. The application of a similar approach to the study of mtDNA and mitochondrial biogenesis in higher plants is almost impossible. Primarily because most of the mutations would be lethal and, unlike certain chloroplast mutations, many non-lethal mutations in plant mtDNA might go undetected.

There is however one cytoplasmically inherited trait in higher plants which is due in many cases to mutations in the mitochondrial genome. This maternally inherited trait termed cytoplasmic male sterility (CMS), prevents the formation of functional pollen and is exploited commercially in the production of F1 hybrid seed varieties in such crops as maize, sorghum, sunflower, sugar beet and onion. The majority of research on this topic has until recently been carried out with maize where the male-sterile cytoplasms have been classified into three types compared to the normal (N) fertile cytoplasm. These are designated T, C and S and can be distinguished on the basis of the specific nuclear genes (Rf genes) which restore pollen fertility. The restorer-alleles in cms-T(Rf, Rf_2) and cms-C (Rf_4)lines act at the sporophytic level, while in case of cms-S(Rf_3) restoration depends on the genotype of the pollen grains and restoration is said to be gametophytic.

In maize there are several lines of evidence supporting the contention that the genetic defects determining CMS are located in the mitochondrial genome: (a) restriction endonuclease analysis and mapping of mtDNA from fertile and male-sterile cytoplasms indicate characteristic heterogeneity in genome organisation.[1,9] This heterogeneity being a reflection of the DNA deletions and rearrangements which have occurred, (b) analysis of mitochondrial translation products reveals that characteristic variant polypeptides are synthesised by mitochondria isolated from male-sterile cytoplasms of maize, sorghum, sugar beet, wheat and field bean (see Table II),[1,14,15] (c) mitochondria (and whole plants) from the cms-T cytoplasm of maize are susceptible to low levels of a host specific toxin (T-toxin) produced by Helminthosporium maydis, race T, whereas mitochondria from N, C and S cytoplasms with similar nuclear genotypes are unaffected (see ref. 1), (d) ultrastructural studies on normal and 'male-sterile' anthers show that mitochondrial degeneration is the first indication of abnormality during pollen development (see ref. 1).

The T Cytoplasm of Maize

Mitochondria isolated from T-toxin sensitive, male sterile plants with T cytoplasm synthesise an additional 13,000 M_r polypeptide not found in other cytoplasms. When Rf alleles which restore fertility are introduced into the nuclear background of lines carrying the T cytoplasm, there is a marked and specific supression of the synthesis of the 13,000 M_r polypeptide by isolated mitochondria, coupled with a reduced sensitivity to T-toxin.[1,14] In addition, male fertile plants, resistant to T-toxin, can be regenerated from tissue cultures of maize carrying cms-T cytoplasm. Mitochondria isolated from the progeny of these regenerants are no longer sensitive to T-toxin and fail to synthesis significant levels of the characteristic 13,000 M_r polypeptide.[16] Restriction endonuclease analyses of mtDNA from these regenerants have shown that rearrangement of the mitochondrial genome occurs in the tissue culture environment or during regeneration of the plants from culture.[17,18]

Taken together these observations show that the synthesis of a specific mitochondrial polypeptide is under the control of both nuclear and cytoplasmic genes. Furthermore they provide strong evidence in support of the hypothesis that changes in mtDNA organisation result in changes in gene expression (e.g. synthesis of the 13,000 M_r polypeptide) which are causally associated with expression of the male-sterile phenotype and sensitivity to T-toxin. The inability to separate T-type cytoplasmic male sterility from disease susceptibility could be interpreted to mean that both of these agronomically important phenomena are different expressions of a single genetic defect (see ref. 1 for further speculation on the molecular basis of CMS and disease susceptibility).

Table II. Variant Mitochondrial Translation Products in Maize
and Sorghum.

Cytoplasm	Phenotype	Variant Polypeptide (M_r)	Linear 'Plasmid-Like' DNA (kb)
Maize			
N	MF	–	–
T	MS	13,000	–
C	MS	17,500	–
S	MS	42,000–85,000	5.2 & 6.2
Sorghum			
Kafir	MF	–	–
Milo[a]	MS	65,000	–
IS1112C	MS	82,000 + 12,000	5.3 & 5.7
M35-1	MS	82,000	5.3 & 5.7
9E	MS	42,000[b]	–

MF = male fertile, MS = male sterile, '-' denotes failure to detect.
a Mitochondria from 21 other cytoplasms synthesised this variant polypeptide.
b This polypeptide is an altered form of subunit I of cytochrome c oxidase and replaces the normal subunit which has an M_r of 38,000.

CMS in Sorghum

In sorghum as in maize expression of CMS is associated with variation in mitochondrial genome organisation[19] and synthesis of variant mitochondrial translation products.[15] The sorghum CMS lines can be divided into four groups on the basis of variation in mitochondrial translation products[15] (Table II). Of particular interest is the observation that mitochondria from 9E cytoplasm in any one of 14 different nuclear backgrounds, synthesise an additional 42,000 M_r polypeptide, replacing a 38,000 M_r polypeptide synthesised by 9E mitochondria from the homologous nuclear background. Immunoprecipitation of the labelled translation products confirmed that the 42,000 M_r polypeptide is in fact an altered form of subunit I of cytochrome oxidase which in its normal form has a molecular weight of 38,000. Further work is in progress to examine whether the alteration in cytochrome oxidase subunit I expression is due to mutations which affect, for example, the coding region of the gene, RNA processing, initiation or termination of translation or post-translational processing.

Linear 'Plasmid-Like' DNAs and CMS

In the last few years a number of reports have shown that
mitochondria from several higher plants contain both circular and
linear 'plasmid-like' DNA molecules. (See Leving's this volume
and ref. 1). The majority of work has concentrated on the linear
plasmid-like DNA molecules identified in the mitochondria of the
CMS-S lines of maize and the M35-1 and IS1112C cytoplasms of
sorghum.[1,15] In all cases the presence of these DNA molecules has
been found to be associated with the synthesis of a range of characteristic high molecular weight polypeptides by the isolated mitochondria.[14,15] (Table II).

Using seed provided by Dr. J. Laughnan of the University of
Illinois, we have examined whether mitochondria isolated from a
variety of S-type male-sterile plants, which have spontaneously
reverted to the fertile phenotype, synthesise the S-specific polypeptides mentioned above. In those cases in which the reversion
event has been shown genetically to be a cytoplasmic event (cytoplasmic revertants) the 'free plasmids' are no longer detectable in
the mitochondria and the S-specific polypeptides are not synthesised. In cases where the reversion to fertility have been shown to
be a nuclear event, the free plasmids are still present in the
mitochondria and the S-specific polypeptides are synthesised. In
addition, in those cases where the nuclear Rf_3 gene is present in
the nucleus, the free plasmids are present in the mitochondria and
the S-specific polypeptides are synthesised. Future work will
determine if these 'plasmid-like' DNAs are transcribed into mRNAs
which encode the characteristic high molecular weight polypeptides
and their involvement, if any, in cytoplasmic male sterility.

CONCLUSIONS AND PROSPECTS

The observations outlined in this chapter strongly suggest
that in several plants specific differences in mitochondrial
genome organisation are associated with the synthesis of additional characteristic polypeptides and the phenotypic expression of
male-sterility. Final proof for the involvement of the mitochondrial genome in CMS will require the functional identification of
the polypeptides involved and the sequencing of the mitochondrial
genes which encode them.

The results discussed also emphasise the interactions between
nucleus and cytoplasm which are involved in regulating mitochondrial gene expression. In all the cases examined when cytoplasms
are transferred from their original nuclear background (in which
the phenotype is fertile), to a foreign nuclear background (in
which the phenotype is cytoplasmic male sterile) some change in
mitochondrial gene expression results. This indicates that during
the course of evolution nuclear and cytoplasmic genes controlling

mitochondrial gene expression may have diverged so that a foreign
nuclear background cannot correctly regulate mitochondrial gene
expression. Attention must therefore eventually turn towards an
analysis of the nuclear genes encoding mitochondrial proteins and
the role of nuclear genes in regulating the expression of the
mitochondrial genome.

REFERENCES

1. C.J. Leaver and M.W. Gray, Mitochondrial genome organisation
and expression in higher plants, Ann. Rev. Plant Physiol. 33: 373
(1982).
2. P. Slonimski, P. Borst and G. Attardi (1982). "Mitochondrial
Genes", Cold Spring Harbor monograph series, 12. .
3. G. Attardi, Organisation and expression of the mammalian mitochondrial genome: a lesson in economy, Trends Biochem. Sci. 86,
100 (1981).
4. P. Borst and L.A. Grivell, One gene's intron is another gene's
exon, Nature 289: 439 (1981).
5. L.A. Grivell and P. Borst, Mitochondrial mosaics - maturases
on the move, Nature 298: 703 (1982).
6. A. Tzagoloff, G. Macino, W. Sebald, Mitochondrial genes and
translation products, Ann. Rev. Biochem. 48: 419 (1979).
7. W. Neupert and G. Schatz, How proteins are transported into
mitochondria, Trends Biochem. Sci. 6: 1 (1981).
8. B.L. Ward, R.S. Anderson and A.J. Bendich, The size of the
mitochondrial genome is large and variable in a family of plants
(Cucurbitaceae), Cell 25: 793 (1981).
9. Levings, C.S., Shah, D.M., Hu, W.W.L., Pring, D.R., Timothy,
D.H. (1979), Molecular heterogeneity among mitochondrial DNAs
from different maize cytoplasms, in:"Extrachromosomal DNA, ICN-
UCLA Symposium on Molecular and Cellular Biology", ed. D. Cumm-
ings, P. Borst, I. David, S. Weissman, C.F. Fox. Academic Press,
New York.
10. D.B. Stern and D.M. Lonsdale, Mitochondrial and chloroplast
genomes of maize have a 12 kb DNA sequence in common, Nature in
press (1982).
11. D.B. Stern, T.A. Dyer and D.M. Lonsdale, Organisation of the
mitochondrial ribosomal RNA genes in maize, Nucleic Acids Res. 11:
3333 (1982).
12. T.D. Fox and C.J. Leaver, The Zea mays mitochondrial gene
coding cytochrome oxidase subunit II has an intervening sequence,
and does not contain TGA codons, Cell 26: 315 (1981).
13. R. Rott and N. Nelson, Purification and immunological properties of proton-ATPase complexes from yeast and rat liver mitochondria, J. Biol. Chem. 256: 9224 (1981).
14. B.G. Forde and C.J. Leaver, Nuclear and cytoplasmic genes
controlling synthesis of variant mitochondrial polypeptides in
male-sterile maize, Proc. Natl. Acad. Sci. U.S.A. 77: 418 (1980).

15. L.K. Dixon and C.J. Leaver, Mitochondrial gene expression and cytoplasmic male sterility in sorghum, Plant Mol. Biol. 1: 89(1982)

16. L.K. Dixon, C.J. Leaver, R.I.S. Brettell and B.G. Gengenbach, Mitochondrial sensitivity to D. maydis T-toxin and the synthesis of a variant mitochondrial polypeptide in plants derived from maize tissue cultures with Texas male-sterile cytoplasm, Theor. Appl. Genet. 63: 75 (1982).

17. B.G. Gengenbach, J.A. Connelly, D.R. Pring and M.F. Conde, Mitochondrial DNA variation in maize plants regenerated during tissue culture selection, Theor. Appl. Genet. 59: 161 (1981).

18. R.J. Kemble, R.B. Flavell and R.I.S. Brettell, Mitochondrial DNA analyses of fertile and sterile maize plants derived from tissue culture with Texas male sterile cytoplasm, Theor. Appl. Genet. 62: 213 (1982).

19. D.R. Pring, M.F. Conde and K.F. Schertz, Organelle genome diversity in Sorghum: male sterile cytoplasms, Crop Sci. 22: 414 (1982).

RELATIONSHIPS AMONG PLASMID-LIKE DNAS OF THE MAIZE MITOCHONDRIA

C. S. Levings III, R. R. Sederoff,
W. W. L. Hu* and D. H. Timothy*

Departments of Genetics and Crop Science*
North Carolina State University
Raleigh, NC 27650

In addition to the high molecular weight DNA normally encountered in maize mitochondria, several cytoplasms contain plasmid-
like DNAs. In the S cytoplasm (cms-S), two plasmid-like DNAs are
found, S-1 and S-2, which are about 6.4 and 5.4 kilobases (kb) long,
respectively (Pring et al., 1977). Electron microscopy has shown
that these molecules have a linear configuration with defined ends.
However, these observations do not rule out the possibility that
linearity could have arisen by the breakage of native circular
molecules. Additional studies have demonstrated novel sequence ar-
rangements in that both S-1 and S-2 are terminated by inverted
repeats, which are about 0.2 kb long (Levings and Pring, 1979).
About 1.7 kb of terminally located sequence homology exist between
the S-1 and S-2 DNAs. The common sequences involve 1.5 kb, including
the inverted repeat, at one end, and at the other end, the 0.2 kb
inverted repeat.

The S-1 and S-2 DNA species are only found in the S group of
cytoplasms. Cms-S types are male steriles that are restored to
fertility by the Rf3 restorer gene. S cytoplasms are unstable; many
cases have been observed where cms-S changes from the male-sterile
to the male-fertile phenotype, (Laughnan and Gabay, 1975a; 1975b).
Two types of changes are observed, cytoplasmic changes and mutations
giving rise to new nuclear restorer genes. Most often, newly arisen
male fertiles are caused by stable cytoplasmic changes.

Studies of cytoplasmic revertant strains revealed that S-1 and
S-2 DNAs disappear when the S cytoplasm reverts to the male-fertile
phenotype (Levings et al., 1980). In addition, changes also take
place in the main mtDNAs of the revertants and importantly, these

changes most often involve sequences homologous with S-1 and/or S-2
DNAs. These findings, plus genetic studies, led to the speculation
that the plasmid-like DNAs may behave like transposable elements
by inserting S-1 and/or S-2 sequences into the main mtDNA.

Additional plasmid-like DNAs, which differ from those found in
cms-S, have recently been identified in maize (Weissinger et al.,
1982). These new species, designated R-1 and R-2, are present in
numerous South American maize accessions. The R-plasmids are isolated as linear molecules and contain terminal inverted repeats
like the S plasmids. They are distinguished from the S plasmids
by size and sequence differences (see later sections). In contrast
to the S cytoplasm, strains carrying the R plasmid-like DNAs appear
to be male fertile.

In perennial diploid teosinte (Zea diploperennis) two new
plasmid-like DNAs, designated D-1 and D-2, have been discovered
(Timothy et al., 1982). Although not yet fully characterized,
these DNA species resemble the R plasmids in structure. It also
appears that the D-1 and D-2 plasmid-like DNAs are not associated
with male sterility. These findings suggest that plasmid-like DNAs
may carry different genetic determinants.

The origin and function of the plasmid-like DNAs, S-1 and S-2,
are important because of their relationship with the S type of male
sterility and their apparent transpositional behavior. Previous
studies demonstrated that mtDNA sequences from normal (fertile)
maize share homology with both the S-1 and S-2 DNA species (Thompson
et al., 1980; Spruill et al., 1980). Restriction mapping and hybridization studies identified two regions in normal mtDNA, each
adjacent to a large 26kb duplication, which contain sequences
homologous with the S-1 and S-2 DNAs. One region contains a sequence that hybridizes to S-1 while the other region has a sequence
that hybridizes most prominently to S-2; these regions are designated the S-1 and S-2 regions, respectively (Lonsdale et al., 1982).
Five BamHI fragments,cloned into pBR322, account for most of the
S-1 and S-2 sequences of normal mtDNA (Spruill et al., 1980). The
sizes of these BamHI fragments correspond with those identified in
the S-1 and S-2 regions by Lonsdale et al. (1982). We have studied
three of the larger fragments for homology with S-1, R-1 and S-2 by
restriction mapping and heteroduplex analysis.

The insert of clone #181 is 7.0 kb long and is colinear with
approximately 66% of the S-1 molecule (Fig. 1). More precisely,
the fragment contains 4.3 kb that is homologous with an internal
segment of S-1 molecule (Fig. 2). It differs from S-1 in that it
lacks 0.6 kb at one end of S-1 and 1.5 kb at the other end. Hence,
the inverted repeats found in S-1 are absent from the fragment.
Since no BamHI cleavage sites are present in S-1, BamHI digestion
should not interrupt S-1 sequences present in this fragment.

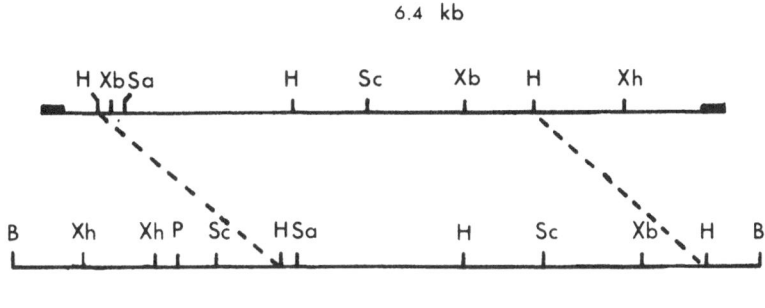

Fig. 1. Restriction maps of S-1 and clone 181. The upper line
         shows a restriction map of S-1 (Kim et al., 1982). Dark
         bars at the ends represent the inverted repeats. The
         lower line is the BamHI clone 181. The region of homology
         evident from restriction mapping is indicated between the
         dotted lines. Restriction sites are abbreviated B(BamHI),
         H(HindIII), P(PstI), Sa(SalI), Sc(SacI), Xb(XbaI),
         Xh(XhoI).

A second large BamHI fragment, isolated as clone #701, is 4.6
kb long and hybridizes prominently with S-2. Heteroduplexing
studies showed that this fragment contains a 3.7 kb internal segment which is homologous with S-2 (Fig. 3). The analysis also
indicated that 0.3 kb at one end of S-2, including the inverted
repeat, are missing from the fragment. The other end of the fragment is colinear with S-2 up to the BamHI cloning site; a BamHI
site is found in an analogous position in the S-2 molecule.
Cleavage maps show the colinearity between #701 and S-2 with respect to restriction sites (Fig. 4).

These results indicate that intact copies of S-1 and S-2 DNAs
are not present in the main mtDNAs of this particular normal maize
hybrid (NC7 x T204). It remains to be seen if intact copies of the
plasmid-like DNAs exist in the mitochondrial genomes of other normal maize cytoplasms. In the meanwhile, these findings seriously
challenge the idea that S-1 and S-2 may have arisen by whole copy
excision from the mitochondrial genome. Finally, conspicuously
absent from these large fragments are the terminal inverted repeats
which are integral parts of the plasmid-like DNAs.

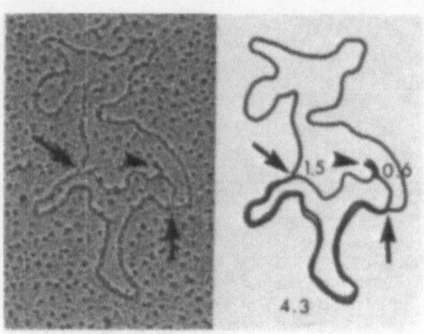 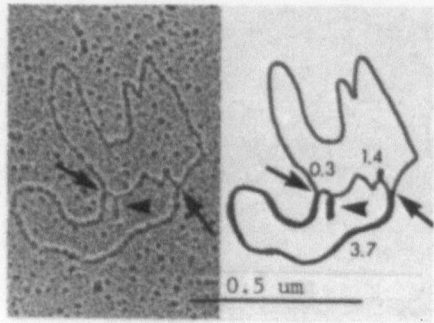

181 x S-1   701 x S-2

Fig. 2. Heteroduplex formed by   Fig. 3. Heteroduplex formed by
S-1 and BamHI clone 181.   S-2 and the BamHI clone 701.
Double stranded regions are in-   Double stranded regions are indicated by double lines; single   dicated by double lines; single
stranded by single lines. An   stranded by single lines. An
arrowhead points to the paired   arrowhead points to the paired
inverted repeats of S-1. A 4.3   inverted repeats of S-2. The 3.7
kb homologous region (double   kb homologous region (double line)
line) lies between the arrows.   lies between the arrows. The 0.3
The 0.6 and 1.5 kb segments are   and 1.4 kb segments are nonhomo-
nonhomologous (unpaired) regions   logous (unpaired) regions of S-2.
of S-1. Lengths are means of 23   Lengths are means of 24 hetero-
heteroduplexes.   duplexes.

    The occurrence of a BamHI site in #181 was unanticipated be-
cause S-1 does not have that cleavage site. However, R-1, a related
plasmid-like DNA, does contain an internal BamHI site (Weissinger
et al., 1982). Even though R-1 is only about 1 kb longer than S-1,
it contains a unique sequence of 2.6 kb, which is located in the
smaller BamHI fragment. The larger BamHI fragment of R-1 has a 4.9
kb segment that is homologous with S-1.

    Previously restriction mapping and the heteroduplexing studies
suggested that R-2 and S-2 molecules are homologous. These findings
do not, however, preclude the possibility of minor sequence differences between them.

    Heteroduplex analysis indicated that #181 contains a 4.3 kb
segment which is homologous with an internal portion of R-1 (Fig.5).
The fragment is distinguished from R-1 in that it lacks homology
with about 0.7 kb at one end of R-1. (This is the terminal end of

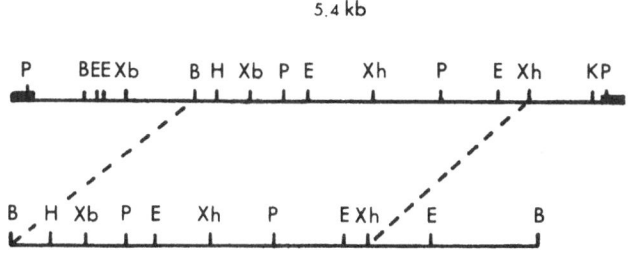

Fig. 4. Restriction maps of S-2 and clone 701. The upper line
shows a restriction map of S-2. Dark bars at the ends
represent the inverted repeats. The lower line is the
BamHI clone 701. The region of homology evident from
restriction mapping is indicated between the dotted lines.
Restriction sites are abbreviated B(BamHI), E(EcoRI),
H(HindIII), K(KpnI), P(PstI), Xb(XbaI), Xh(XhoI).

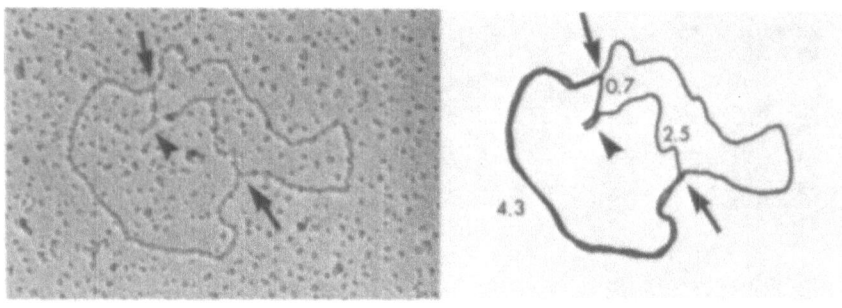

Fig. 5. Heteroduplex formed by R-1 and BamHI clone 181. Double
stranded regions are indicated by double lines; single
stranded by single lines. An arrowhead points to the
paired inverted repeats of R-1. A 4.3 kb homologous
region (double line) lies between the arrows. The 0.7
and 2.5 kb segments are nonhomologous (unpaired) regions
of R-1. Lengths are means of 16 heteroduplexes.

the large BamHI fragment of R-1). The situation at the other end
of #181 requires some explanation. R-1 has a single BamHI cleavage
site which divides the molecule into two fragments of about 5.0 and
2.4 kb. Since #181 is a BamHI fragment, homology with R-1 should
extend only to this site if R-1 and #181 are colinear. The sum of
the homologous region of R-1 and #181 and the unpaired region of
the larger BamHI fragment of R-1, is 5.0 kb (4.3 kb and 0.7 kb).
This result suggests that R-1 and #181 are colinear up to and including the BamHI site at this end of #181. Furthermore it predicts
that homology with R-1 should extend into the adjacent BamHI
fragment.

Adjacent to the 6.9 kb fragment (our clone #181) in the S-1
region is a BamHI fragment that is 3.9 kb long. This fragment has
been isolated as clone #607 and is known to hybridize weakly to
both S-1 and S-2 (Spruill et al., 1980). In contrast, hybridization
studies with labelled #607 DNA indicated a strong homology with the
smaller BamHI fragment of R-1 (not shown). Subsequent electron
microscopy studies revealed approximately 2.4 kb of homology between
#607 and R-1 (Fig. 6). Based upon this analysis, #607 appears to
contain a segment that is homologous with the entire small BamHI
fragment of R-1.

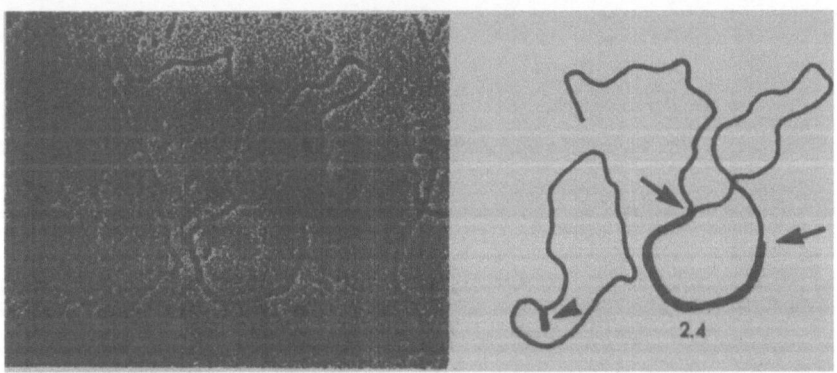

607 x R-1

Fig. 6.   Heteroduplex formed by R-1 and BamHI clone 607. Double
          stranded regions are indicated by double lines; single
          stranded by single lines. An arrowhead points to the
          paired inverted repeat of a single stranded R-1 molecule
          in a stem-loop configuration (left corner). A 2.4 kb
          homologous region (double line) of the heteroduplex
          structure lies between the arrows. The single stranded
          tail is the nonhomologous (unpaired) region of R-1.
          Lengths are means of 21 heteroduplexes.

Although hybridization studies had indicated weak homology between S-1 and #607, we have been unable to find heteroduplex structures involving these DNA species. The weak homology may be due to the inverted repeat sequence that is apparently present in #607. This argument is strengthened by the observation that S-2 and #607 also hybridize weakly with each other on Southern blots.

We estimate that clones #181 and #607 contain about 6.7 kb of sequence homology with R-1. In marked contrast, these same clones have only about 4.5 kb of homology with S-1 (Table 1). As a consequence of this substantial difference in homology, we propose that those regions of the normal mtDNA which are homologous with the plasmid-like DNAs are more closely related to R-1 and R-2 than S-1 and S-2. Interestingly, the maize strains that contain R-1 and R-2 are all male fertiles. Perhaps this is related to the fact that the plasmid-like sequences integrated into the mtDNA of normal fertile maize are similar to the R plasmids. Furthermore, it raises the possibility that some part of the unique region of R-1 is important to normal pollen development.

Collectively, our studies with the R and S plasmid-like DNAs suggest that the S-1 molecule may have arisen by a recombinational event between R-1 and R-2 (Fig. 7). The only sequence homology between R-1 and R-2 resides in the inverted repeats. Homology between R-1 and S-1 is 4.9 kb long by our most recent estimate; this places the end of homology between R-1 and S-1 very close to the BamHI site of R-1 (5.0 kb). A recombination event between R-1 and R-2 that joins 4.9 kb of R-1 with 1.5 kb of R-2 would generate a molecule like S-1. The recombinant molecule would include about 1.5 kb at one end and 0.2 kb (the inverted repeat) at the other

Table 1.   Estimated homology in kb between the plasmid-like DNAs, R-1 and S-1, and the two adjacent BamHI fragments, #181 and #607. We have estimated that #607 contains about 0.2 kb (the size of the inverted repeat) of homology with S-1 even though no homology was detected by heteroduplexing studies.

	Plasmid-Like DNAs	
Clones	R-1	S-1
#181	4.3 kb	4.3 kb
#607	2.4 kb	0.2 kb (estimated)
Total	6.7 kb	4.5 kb

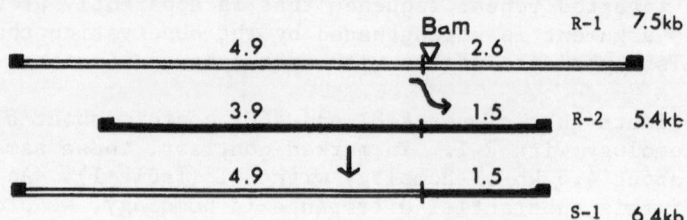

Fig. 7. Diagram of postulated recombination event between R-1 and
         R-2. R-1 (upper line) is shown with the BamHI site, the
         region homologous with S-1 (4.9 kb) and the region unique
         to R-1 (2.6 kb). R-2 is shown with 3.9 kb unique to R-2
         (or S-2) and 1.5 kb of homology shared with S-1. S-1
         shows   4.9 kb shared with R-1 and 1.5 kb shared with S-2.
         Inverted repeats are indicated as black boxes at the ends
         of the moleclues. Recombination between R-1 and R-2 at
         the indicated site (vertical line) can generate a molecule
         like S-1.

end that are common to R-2. The proposed recombinant molecule and
R-2 seem to correspond directly with the S-1 and S-2, respectively,
of the S cytoplasm. (As pointed out previously, R-2 and S-2 are
indistinguishable.) Although the recombinant event is unproven,
the organization of the plasmid-like DNAs and the main mtDNA are
consistent with this speculation.

REFERENCES

Kim, B. D., Mans, R. J., Conde, M. E., Pring, D. R., and Levings,
     C. S., III, 1982, Physical mapping of homologous segments of
     mitochondrial episomes from S male-sterile maize, Plasmid, 7:1.
Laughnan, J. R., and Gabay, S. J., 1975, Nuclear and cytoplasmic
     mutations to fertility in S male-sterile maize, In Inter-
     national Maize Symposium: Genetics and Breeding, p. 427,
     D. B. Walden, ed. New York: Wiley.
Laughnan, J. R., and Gabay, S. J., 1975, An episomal basis for in-
     stability of S male sterility in maize and some implications
     for plant breeding, In Genetics and Biogenesis of Mitochondria
     and Chloroplasts, p. 330, C. W. Birkey, P. S. Perlman, and T. J.
     Beyers, eds. Columbus: Ohio State University Press.

Levings, C. S., III, Kim, B. D., Pring, D. R., Conde, M. F., Mans, R. J., Laughnan, J. R., and Gabay-Laughnan, S. J., 1980, Cytoplasmic reversion of cms-S in maize: Association with a transpositional event, Science, 209:1021.

Levings, C. S., III, and Pring, D. R., 1979, Molecular basis of cytoplasmic male sterility of maize, In Physiological Genetics, vol. 5, p. 171, J. C. Scandalios, ed. New York: Academic Press.

Lonsdale, D. M., Thompson, R. D., and Hodge, T. P., 1981, The integrated forms of the S-1 and S-2 DNA elements of maize male sterile mitochondrial DNA are flanked by a large repeated sequence, Nucleic Acids. Res., 9:3657.

Pring, D. R., Levings, C. S., III, Hu, W. W. L., and Timothy, D. H., 1977, Unique DNA associated with mitochondria in the "S" type cytoplasm of male-sterile maize, Proc. Natl. Acad. Sci. U.S.A., 74:2904.

Spruill, W. M., Jr., Levings, C. S., III, and Sederoff, R. R., 1980, Recombinant DNA analysis indicates that the multiple chromosomes of maize mitochondria contain different sequences, Develop. Genetics, 1:363.

Thompson, R. D., Kemble, R. J., and Flavell, R. B., 1980, Variations in mitochondrial DNA organization between normal and male-sterile cytoplasms of maize, Nucleic Acid Res., 8:1999.

Timothy, D. H., Levings, C. S., III, Hu, W. W. L., and Goodman, M. M., 1982, Zea diploperennis may have plasmid-like mitochondria DNAs, Maize Genet. Coop. News Letter, 56:133.

Weissinger, A. K., Timothy, D. H., Levings, C. S., III, Hu, W. W. L., and Goodman, M. M., 1982, Unique plasmid-like mitochondrial DNAs from indigenous maize races of Latin America, Proc. Natl. Acad. Sci. U.S.A., 79:1.

ORGANIZATION AND EVOLUTION OF RIBOSOMAL RNA GENES IN WHEAT MITOCHONDRIA

Michael W. Gray, Tai Y. Huh, Murray N. Schnare,
David F. Spencer, and Denis Falconet*

Department of Biochemistry
Dalhousie University
Halifax, Nova Scotia B3H 4H7 (CANADA)

INTRODUCTION

Mitochondrial DNA (mtDNA) is known to encode the distinctive ribosomal RNA (rRNA) species found in the organelle-specific ribosomes that function in mitochondrial protein synthesis [1]. Qualitatively and quantitatively, rRNA production is a major genetic function of mtDNA, and the factors controlling mitochondrial rRNA (mt-rRNA) synthesis are therefore of great interest. Moreover, since homologous rRNA species are found in all systems (eukaryotic cytosol, prokaryotic, chloroplast, mitochondrial) having a ribosome-based translation system, comparative studies of these rRNAs and their genes are an important means of illuminating the evolutionary history of the eukaryotic cell and its organelles [2]. For these reasons, we have been investigating the organization and evolution of the rRNA genes in plant mitochondria, particularly those of wheat, Triticum aestivum.

Novel Arrangement of rRNA Genes in Plant mtDNA

T_1 Oligonucleotide fingerprinting [3] and cataloguing [4] studies and RNA sequence analysis [5-7] have shown that wheat 26S, 18S, and 5S mt-rRNAs are distinct from their cytosol counterparts, with which they share no homology detectable in rRNA-DNA hybridization experiments [8]. Identification of restriction fragments encoding the individual wheat mt-rRNAs provided the first direct demonstration of specific genes encoded by plant mtDNA [8] and led us to infer that:

---

*Present address: Laboratoire de Biologie Moléculaire Végétale, Universite de Paris-Sud, Centre d'Orsay, 91405 Orsay Cedex (FRANCE)

(1) Genes for wheat 26S and 18S mt-rRNAs must be far apart in the wheat mitochondrial genome, since they are always found on <u>different</u> fragments in a given restriction digest.

(2) Genes for wheat 5S and 18S mt-rRNAs must be closely linked in wheat mtDNA, since they are found on the <u>same</u> restriction fragments in a given digest. This localization of 5S rRNA genes differs from that in all other genomes (nuclear, prokaryotic, and chloroplast) that encode a 5S rRNA species.

(3) Since each individual rRNA probe usually hybridizes with multiple restriction fragments in each digest, there must be multiple distinct rRNA cistrons in wheat mtDNA. The 5S mt-rRNA gene (if it is colinear with the RNA sequence; [6]) should contain no internal <u>EcoRI</u> or <u>SalI</u> sites, yet 5S mt-rRNA hybridizes with at least four distinct <u>EcoRI</u> and three different <u>SalI</u> restriction fragments. ·On the other hand, the 5S rRNA hybridizes with only a single <u>XhoI</u> fragment. Taken together, these data imply that there is a basic structural unit encoding the 5S rRNA, but that sequences flanking this unit are not identical. The multiplicity of rRNA restriction fragments hybridizing with the same rRNA cannot be ascribed to incomplete endonuclease cleavage of wheat mtDNA arising from partial methylation of restriction sites, since identical restriction and rRNA hybridization patterns are observed when wheat mtDNA is digested with either <u>MspI</u> or <u>HpaII</u> [9].

More recently, we have examined other plant mtDNAs (rye, corn, broad bean, pea, cucumber) in order to determine whether this novel arrangement of mt-rRNA genes is peculiar to wheat or is more widespread. The results [10] suggest that this same pattern of rRNA gene organization (18S and 5S genes close together but remote from 26S genes) is a general (perhaps universal) feature of angiosperm mtDNA.

rRNA Genes in Cloned Fragments of Wheat mtDNA

We have collaborated with F. Quetier's group (Orsay) in examining cloned restriction fragments carrying wheat mt-rRNA genes. <u>SalI</u> fragments of wheat mtDNA were inserted into pBR322 by the Orsay group, and selected recombinant plasmids hybridizing with wheat 18S and 5S mt-rRNAs were characterized in our laboratory. Restriction maps of <u>Sal</u> fragments S21 and S19 [8] (5.5 and 6.2 kbp, respectively) are shown in FIG. 1. It can be seen that the two fragments share identical restriction sites over most of their lengths, starting at the same leftward <u>SalI</u> site (S_L) and proceeding at least as far as a common <u>ClaI</u> site 4760 bp away. The remaining lengths of S21 (740 bp) and S19 (1440 bp) bear no homology detectable by restriction analysis, and the fragments terminate at distinct rightward <u>SalI</u> sites (S_R).

Initial Southern hybridization experiments localized the coding regions for the 18S and 5S mt-rRNAs within a <u>PstI-XhoI</u> subfragment 2750 bp long and common to both <u>Sal</u> inserts. The 3'-end of the 18S

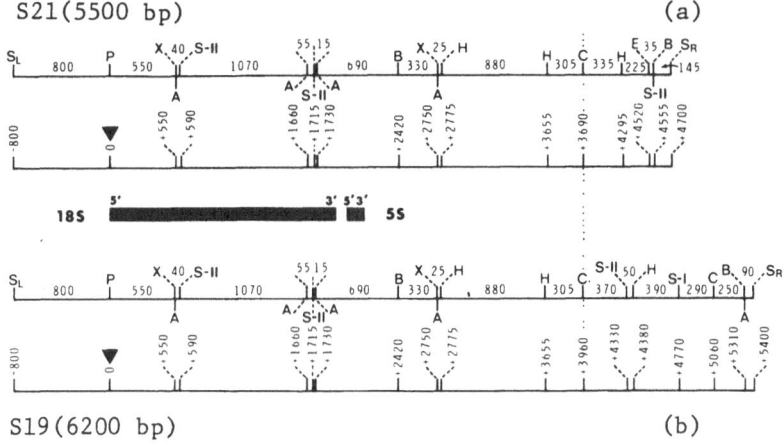

S21(5500 bp)   (a)

S19(6200 bp)   (b)

Fig. 1.   Restriction maps of fragments S21 (a) and S19 (b), cloned
           from a SalI digest of wheat mtDNA. S_L and S_R = leftward and
           rightward SalI sites, respectively; A = AvaI; B = BamHI; C =
           ClaI; E = EcoRI; H = HindIII; P = PstI; S-I = SstI; S-II =
           SstII; X = XhoI. Restriction site coordinates (in bp) are
           calculated relative to the unique PstI site (solid
           triangle). The dotted line denotes the point at which S21
           and S19 diverge in restriction sites. Solid bars mark the
           18S and 5S rRNA coding regions.

gene was placed close to the 5S gene by hybridization experiments
which employed a 3'-specific probe derived from [5'-^{32}P]pCp-labeled
wheat 18S mt-rRNA [7]. Coding boundaries have since been refined by
sequence analysis of cloned rDNA. Based on 5'- [unpublished] and 3'-
[7] nucleotide sequences directly determined from the 18S mt-rRNA, the
5' end of the 18S gene is 25 bp downstream from the unique PstI site
(which is 800 bp from S_L), while the 3'-terminus is 200 bp downstream
from the +1730 AvaI site. By comparison of the DNA sequence
determined for this region of cloned rDNA with the primary sequence of
wheat 5S mt-rRNA [6], the 5'-end of the 5S gene has been positioned
about 105 bp downstream from the 3'-end of the 18S gene, on the same
strand. This arrangement raises the possibility that the 18S and 5S
mt-rRNAs are co-transcribed from a single promoter.

Multiple Distinct Cistrons for 18S and 5S rRNA Genes in Wheat mtDNA

        In addition to bands corresponding to S21,and S19, a third band
of hybridization (>16 kbp) was evident when SalI digests of wheat
mtDNA were probed with either 18S or 5S mt-rRNAs [8]. In screening
for clones which might account for this latter hybridization, we
uncovered two additional, high-molecular-weight fragments carrying 18S
and 5S mt-rRNA genes. Detailed restriction analysis has shown that

these fragments, designated S5,6a (18.4 kbp) and S5,6b (19.1 kbp), share the same leftward SalI site, different from that in S21 and S19, and are identical over most of their lengths, diverging close to their rightward ends. We also found (somewhat unexpectedly) that in the region of divergence, each of the larger fragments is identical to one of the smaller fragments (either S21 or S19). These relationships are illustrated in FIG. 2, which shows the XhoI restriction maps of the four SalI fragments. Note that each possesses the same basic 18S-5S rRNA coding unit, largely contained within the common 2200 bp XhoI subfragment that is the main site of 18S hybridization, and exclusive site of 5S hybridization, in XhoI digests of wheat mtDNA [8].

It seems likely, although not yet definitively proven, that there is one genome equivalent of each of the rDNA fragments identified in this study. Based on analysis of densitometer tracings [8], S19 and S21 are present in amounts roughly equimolar with each other and with neighboring fragments in gels of SalI digests of wheat mtDNA. As shown in FIG. 3, this implies that the same rRNA coding sequence (R) is repeated four times in the wheat mitochondrial genome, and is flanked by different arrays of other repeated sequences (U, V, W, W'). How these SalI fragments are organized within wheat mtDNA remains to be investigated.

Assuming a stoichiometry of one for S21 in SalI digests of wheat mtDNA, and based on its known size (5.5 kbp) and the mass proportion it occupies in a SalI digest (determined from densitometer tracings of

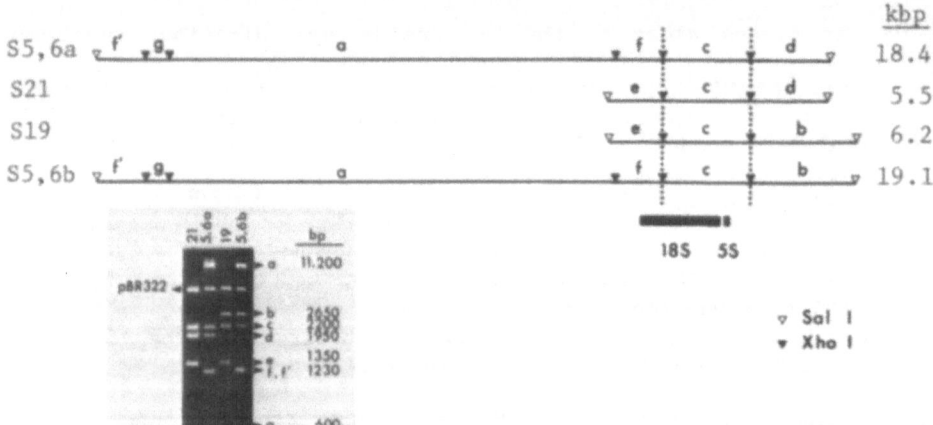

Fig. 2.   XhoI restriction maps showing the structural relationships among SalI rDNA fragments cloned from wheat mtDNA. Dotted lines delineate the common XhoI fragment (c, 2200 bp) that carries most of the 18S, and all of the 5S, gene (Fig. 1). The inset shows restriction profiles visualized after agarose gel electrophoresis of double digests (XhoI + SalI) of recombinant plasmids carrying the SalI rDNA inserts.

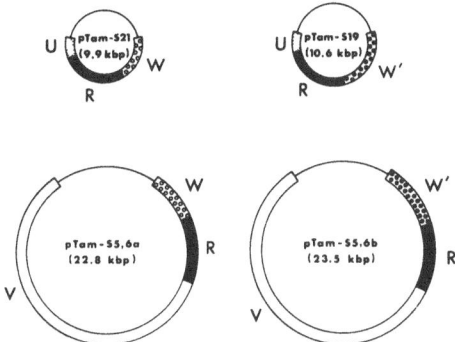

Fig. 3.   Structural relationships among recombinant plasmids carrying
wheat mt-rRNA genes. Mitochondrial DNA inserts represent
rDNA-containing SalI fragments cloned into the SalI site of
pBR322 (thin line).   R = common rRNA coding unit
corresponding to the 2.75 kbp PstI-XhoI fragment (0 to
+2750) shown in Fig. 1. The sizes (in kbp) of the flanking
regions are: U = 0.8; V = 13.7; W = 1.95; W' = 2.65. W and
W' show extensive restriction site homology (Fig. 1).

a SalI restriction pattern; see Fig. 2 of [8]), we estimate that the
physical size of wheat mtDNA is minimally about 225 kbp (150 MDal),
which would make it some 14 times as large as animal mtDNA. The four
cloned SalI fragments described here total 49 kbp, and so would
account for about 20% of the wheat mitochondrial genome, if they are
each present in unimolar amounts.

Evolutionary Origin of Plant Mitochondrial rRNAs

Ribosomal RNA sequence data have been instrumental in solidifying
the view that chloroplasts are of endosymbiotic, specifically
eubacterial, origin [2].   In contrast, conclusions about the
evolutionary origin of mitochondria, drawn from similar data, are
complicated by the pronounced diversity in primary sequence, base
composition, and size of the mitochondrial rRNAs [1,2]. This may be
due in part to a variable (and in some cases, quite rapid) rate of
evolution of mtDNA and its contained rRNA genes [1]. Plant mt-rRNAs,
however, are not "atypical" in size and base composition [11] and
strong evidence in support of an endosymbiotic, eubacterial, origin of
mitochondria has come from studies of the primary structure of plant
mt-rRNAs.

We showed a number of years ago that the T_1 oligonucleotide
catalogue of wheat 18S mt-rRNA strongly resembles T_1 oligonucleotide
catalogues of eubacterial and chloroplast 16S rRNAs, but lacks
detectable homology with the T_1 catalogue of wheat cytosol 18S rRNA

[4]. In addition, among those T_1 oligonucleotides which the 18S mt-rRNA shares with eubacterial and chloroplast 16S rRNAs, there is an especially high proportion of ones identified [12] as conserved in the evolution of eubacterial 16S but not eukaryotic cytosol 18S rRNA species [13]. More recently, direct determination of the sequences of the 3'-terminal ca. 100 nucleotides of wheat mitochondrial and cytosol 18S and E. coli 16S rRNAs [7] has demonstrated that:

(1) There is a substantially greater degree of primary sequence homology between wheat mitochondrial 18S and E. coli 16S rRNAs (72%) than between either wheat mitochondrial and cytosol 18S rRNAs (53%) or wheat cytosol 18S and E. coli 16S rRNAs (60%). In fact, except that it lacks the "Shine-Dalgarno" sequence [14] present in E. coli and chloroplast 16S rRNAs, wheat mitochondrial 18S rRNA is as homologous to E. coli 16S rRNA in this region as is maize chloroplast 16S rRNA.

(2) At a position occupied by 3-methyluridine (m^3U) in E. coli 16S rRNA, the same (or a very similar) modified nucleoside is present in wheat mitochondrial 18S rRNA but not in wheat cytosol 18S rRNA. Interestingly, m^3U is present in a "universal" T_1 oligonucleotide (U*AACAAGp of [12]) in E. coli 16S rRNA. Since two other eubacterial 16S universals, CCm^{7}GCGp and m^4CmCCGp, also appear in the wheat 18S mt-rRNA T_1 catalogue [4,13], the latter rRNA shows evidence of being highly homologous to eubacterial 16S rRNAs not only in primary sequence, but in post-trancriptional modification pattern, as well.

Extensive primary sequence homology between E. coli and wheat mitochondrial rRNAs is also indicated by the fact that the bacterial 16S and 23S rRNAs hybridize specifically to those restriction fragments containing wheat mitochondrial 18S and 26S rRNA genes, respectively [7]. The high degree of primary sequence homology found within the 3'-terminal 100 nucleotides of E. coli 16S and wheat mitochondrial 18S rRNAs has now been confirmed by DNA sequence analysis of the coding region of the latter. From the primary sequence data we have accumulated to date, overall homology to E. coli 16S rRNA appears to be 70-75%, with some impressively long stretches (in excess of 20 nucleotides) of complete identity.

Although we initially thought that the 18S mt-rRNA coding sequence was about 1750 bp long [15], precise determination of the ends of the gene now raises this estimate to about 1900 bp, making the wheat 18S mt-rRNA gene some 360 bp longer than that of E. coli 16S rRNA, and even longer than those of S. cerevisiae (1789 bp) and X. laevis (1825 bp) 18S rRNAs! We should therefore expect to find regions of non-homology between E. coli 16S and wheat mitochondrial 18S rRNA genes, corresponding to "inserts" in the mitochondrial gene sequence. One such example occurs within the 3'-terminal 200 nucleotides of the 18S mt-rRNA gene. Comparison with secondary structure models of E. coli and other small subunit rRNAs [16-18] shows that 47 nucleotides of the mitochondrial sequence have no counterpart in the bacterial sequence. The extra nucleotides in this part of wheat 18S mt-rRNA are localized within a helical region that is highly variable in size (ranging from 64-130 nucleotides) among small subunit rRNAs [18 & unpublished]. This secondary structure element is flanked by single-stranded segments (14 and 16 nucleotides long) that are absolutely conserved in E. coli and Z. mays chloroplast 16S rRNAs and wheat mitochondrial 18S rRNA.

In view of the pronounced eubacterial phylogenetic affinity of wheat 18S mt-rRNA, it has been somewhat surprising to find that wheat 5S mt-rRNA is not obviously eubacterial or eukaryotic in primary sequence or potential secondary structure, but in these parameters shows characteristics of both classes of 5S rRNA, as well as some unique features [6,19,20]. Nevertheless, the secondary structure model proposed by us for wheat 5S mt-rRNA [6] can be accommodated within a uniform model that has recently been shown to fit all known 5S rRNA sequences [21]. When scored in terms of positions within this uniform model that are diagnostic for different classes of 5S rRNA, wheat 5S mt-rRNA shares a somewhat higher number (7) of such positions with eubacterial 5S rRNA than with either eukaryotic (4 positions) or archaebacterial (2 positions) 5S rRNAs. The fact that wheat 18S mt-rRNA is obviously eubacterial in nature, whereas wheat 5S mt-rRNA is decidedly less so, may indicate that functional contraints on primary sequence divergence are more pronounced in 16S/18S rRNA than in 5S rRNA.

CONCLUDING REMARKS

Technical advances centered on recombinant DNA and nucleotide sequence analysis have confirmed a novel arrangement of rRNA genes in plant mitochondria, led to the identification of multiple rRNA cistrons in wheat mtDNA, and provided strong additional support for an endosymbiotic, specifically eubacterial, origin of plant mitochondria. Extension of these techniques should soon allow us to determine how these multiple copies of rRNA genes are organized with respect to each other and to other genes in the wheat mitochondrial genome, and the manner in which remotely located 26S and 18S genes, and closely linked 18S and 5S genes, are coordinately expressed.

ACKNOWLEDGMENTS

Continuing financial support from the Medical Research Council of Canada (grant MT-4124) is gratefully acknowledged.

REFERENCES

[1] Gray, M.W. (1982) Can. J. Biochem. 60:157-171.
[2] Gray, M.W. and Doolittle, W.F. (1982) Microbiol. Rev. 46:1-42.
[3] Cunningham, R.S., Bonen, L., Doolittle, W.F. and Gray, M.W. (1976) FEBS Lett. 69:116-122.

[4] Bonen, L., Cunningham, R.S., Gray, M.W. and Doolittle, W.F. (1977) Nucleic Acids Res. 4:663-671.

[5] MacKay, R.M., Spencer, D.F., Doolittle, W.F. and Gray, M.W. (1980) Eur. J. Biochem. 112:561-576.

[6] Spencer, D.F., Bonen, L. and Gray, M.W. (1981) Biochemistry 20:4022-4029.

[7] Schnare, M.N. and Gray, M.W. (1982) Nucleic Acids Res. 10:3921-3932

[8] Bonen, L. and Gray, M.W. (1980) Nucleic Acids Res. 8:319-335.

[9] Bonen, L., Huh, T.Y. and Gray, M.W. (1980) FEBS Lett. 111:340-346.

[10] Huh, T.Y. and Gray, M.W. (1982) Plant Mol. Biol. (in press).

[11] Leaver, C.J. and Gray, M.W. (1982) Annu. Rev. Plant Physiol. 33:373-402.

[12] Woese, C.R., Fox, G.E., Zablen, L., Uchida, T., Bonen, L., Pechman, K., Lewis, B.J. and Stahl, D. (1975) Nature 254:83-86.

[13] Cunningham, R.S., Gray, M.W., Doolittle, W.F. and Bonen, L. (1977) In Acides Nucléiques et Synthèse des Protéines Chez les Végétaux (Bogorad, L. and Weil, J.H., eds), pp. 243-248, Centre National de la Recherche Scientifique, Paris.

[14] Shine, J. and Dalgarno, L. (1974) Proc. Natl. Acad. Sci. U.S.A. 71:1342-1346.

[15] Gray, M.W., Bonen, L., Falconet, D., Huh, T.Y., Schnare, M.N. and Spencer, D.F. (1982) In Mitochondrial Genes (Slonimski, P., Borst, P. and Attardi, G., eds), pp. 483-488, Cold Spring Harbor Laboratory, Cold Spring Harbor, N.Y.

[16] Woese, C.R., Magrum, L.J., Gupta, R., Siegel, R.B., Stahl, D.A., Kop, J., Crawford, N., Brosius, J., Gutell, R., Hogan, J.J. and Noller, H.F. (1980) Nucleic Acids Res. 8:2275-2293.

[17] Stiegler, P., Carbon, P., Zuker, M., Ebel, J.-P. and Ehresmann, C. (1981) Nucleic Acids Res. 9:2153-2172.

[18] Zwieb, C., Glotz, C. and Brimacombe, R. (1981) Nucleic Acids Res. 9:3621-3640.

[19] Gray, M.W. and Spencer, D.F. (1981) Nucleic Acids Res. 9:3523-3529.

[20] MacKay, R.M., Spencer, D.F., Schnare, M.N., Doolittle, W.F. and Gray, M.W. (1982) Can. J. Biochem. 60:480-489.

[21] De Wachter, R., Chen, M.-W. and Vandenberghe, A. (1982) Biochimie 64:311-329.

DNA POLYMERASE AND DNA SYNTHESIS IN WHEAT EMBRYO MITOCHONDRIA

S. Litvak, L. Keclard-Christophe, M. Echeverria
and M. Castroviejo

Institut de Biochimie Cellulaire et Neurochimie du CNRS
1 rue Camille Saint Saëns, 33077 Bordeaux Cedex, France

INTRODUCTION

The study of mitochondria isolated from differenct sources has shown that these organelles possess a unique DNA. In the case of mitochondria from lower eucaryotes or animal cells this DNA is a double stranded circular molecule[1]. In animal cells, DNA polymerase γ, the enzyme involved in the replication of the organelle genome, has been studied in some detail[2-5]. The mitochondria of higher plants perform the same function as the organelles from other sources. However, the size of the mitochondrial DNA from plants is much bigger than its animal counterpart[6]. We have previously reported a preliminary study of the wheat mitochondrial DNA polymerase[7]. This enzyme differs in some of its properties from the animal mitochondrial DNA polymerase γ. In this communication we present further studies of the highly purified wheat mitochondrial DNA polymerase, as well as the results we have obtained with a DNA synthesizing system using whole purified wheat mitochondria.

PROPERTIES OF THE PURIFIED WHEAT MITOCHONDRIAL DNA POLYMERASE

Four DNA polymerases have been purified from wheat embryo in our laboratory[8,9]. Two of these polymerases are of the α type, one is a γ-like DNA polymerase and the last is the mitochondrial polymerase. A scheme of the purification steps leading to a highly purified mitochondrial DNA polymerase is shown in Figure 1. The enzyme has been purified 440 folds starting from purified mitochondria. The specific activity of the purified enzyme is 111 nmoles TMP incorporated into activated DNA per mg of protein per hour. The incubation mixture and conditions are described in reference 7.

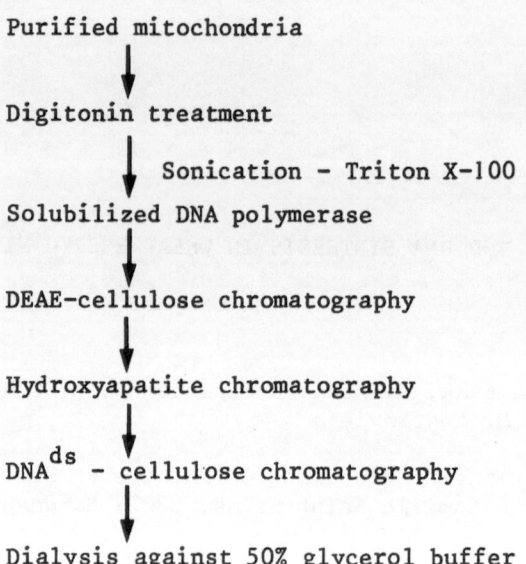

Purified mitochondria

Digitonin treatment

Sonication - Triton X-100

Solubilized DNA polymerase

DEAE-cellulose chromatography

Hydroxyapatite chromatography

DNA^{ds} - cellulose chromatography

Dialysis against 50% glycerol buffer

Fig. 1. Scheme of the purification steps leading to the wheat mitochondrial DNA polymerase.

Some properties of this polymerase are shown in Table I. The animal and plant mitochondrial DNA polymerases are inhibited, with a similar pattern, by the following reagents: N-ethyl maleimide, dideoxyTTP and ethidium bromide. Aphidicolin, a specific inhibitor of DNA polymerase α, does not affect the activities of the plant and animal mitochondrial DNA polymerases. The size of both polymerases are very similar (about 180 kd). They seem to be tetramers: α_4 in the case of the animal polymerase and $\alpha_2\beta_2$ in the case of the wheat organelle enzyme. However, template recognition is very different with both enzymes. Animal polymerase γ is very active with a poly rA-dT$_{12}$ template, while the plant polymerase recognizes this template very poorly if at all. An interesting property of the wheat mitochondrial DNA polymerase is its ability to use an RNA primer. If mitochondrial DNA replication in plants is initiated on RNA primers, like in the animal organelle, it is expected that the polymerase involved in the duplication of the mitochondrial genome be able to use a template-primer of the poly dT-oligo rA type.

DNA SYNTHESIS WITH WHOLE MITOCHONDRIA

Using purified mitochondria we have found the optimal conditions for DNA synthesis when labeled TTP is used as precursor. The incubation mixture contains: 50 mM Tris-HCl pH 7.9, 2 mM DTT, 50 μM dNTP, 40 mM KCl, 20 mM MgCl$_2$, 2 mM ATP and 100 μg/ml of bovine

Table I. General properties of the wheat mitochondrial DNA poly-
          merase.

Molecular weight (native)	180 kd
Molecular weight (SDS)	50 kd + 40 kd
Optimum $MgCl_2$	10 - 20 mM
Optimum $MnCl_2$	0.5 mM
Optimal KCl (Mg^{+2})	30 mM
Optimal KCl (Mn^{+2})	150 mM
% Inhibition by:	
N-ethyl maleimide (5 mM)	70
ddTTP (ddTTP/TTP = 20)	83
Aphidicolin (40 µg/ml)	5
Ethidium bromide (10 µM)	55
Template specificity (nmoles dNMP/mg protein/hour)	
Poly dA-dT$_{12}$ (Mg-TTP)	52
Poly dC-dG$_{12}$ (Mg-dGTP)	98
Poly rA-dT$_{12}$ (Mg-TTP)	1
Poly rA-dT$_{12}$ (Mn-TTP)	2
Activated DNA (Mg-TTP)	25
Poly dT-rA$_{12}$ (Mg-dATP)	74

serum albumin. Incubation was carried out at 37°C and gave an average value of about 150 pmoles of TMP incorporated per mg of mitochondrial protein per hour of incubation. It is interesting to point
out that Mn^{+2} cannot replace Mg^{+2} in our conditions. In the case of
DNA synthesis with isolated animal mitochondria the opposite requirement is observed, since optimal DNA synthesis is observed with
Mn^{+2}.

As shown in Table II the effect of inhibitors is almost identical when using either purified mitochondrial DNA polymerase or
whole mitochondria. These results point out to the conclusion that
the enzyme involved in the replication of the plant organelle genome and the DNA polymerase we have purified from isolated mitochondria are the same. The synthesis of mitochondrial DNA is dramatically enhanced by ATP when the activity is measured in whole
mitochondria, while ATP inhibits strongly the activity of the purified polymerase (not shown).

Table II. Effect of inhibitors on whole mitochondrial or pu-
           rified DNA polymerase.

Inhibitor	% Inhibition	
	Whole mitochondria	Purified DNA polymerase
Aphidicolin (40 µg/ml)	3	5
ddTTP (ddTTP/TTP = 20)	76	83
Ethidium bromide (10 µM)	61	55

We have studied the changes of mitochondrial DNA synthesis activity during wheat embryo germination. Our results indicate that
the level of mitochondrial DNA polymerase is already high in quies-
cent embryos and stays constant during the first 20 hours of germination, while the level of DNA synthesis with isolated whole mitochondria increased dramatically during the same period, as seen in
Table III.

Thus, DNA polymerase seems not to be the limiting factor in the
control of the onset of mitochondrial DNA replication. We are
currently studying other protein factors that may be involved in the
replication of the organelle genome.

Table III. Changes in DNA synthesis and DNA polymerase acti-
            vity in wheat mitochondria during germination.

	Ungerminated	Germinated (20 h.)
	Activity (pmoles TMP/mg protein)	
DNA polymerase	378	316
Mitochondrial DNA synthesis	64	185

The results summarized in this article indicate that the DNA
polymerase purified from wheat mitochondria cannot be considered as
a typical γ-like DNA polymerase. However, we have reported previously the presence of a DNA polymerase of the γ type in the soluble cytoplasm of wheat embryos[10]. These results can be explained
in view of the recent report that the DNA polymerase purified from
chloroplast is a γ-like polymerase showing a very high level of activity with a template poly rA-dT$_{12}$[11]. Thus, our DNA polymerase γ
from wheat could be a leakage product from the chloroplast fraction
during enzyme purification.

This work was supported by the C.N.R.S. (Action Thématique Programée: Biologie Moléculaire Végétale) and the University of Bordeaux II. We are very grateful to Dr. A. H. Todd (I.C.I. United Kingdom) for a gift of aphidicolin and to Dr. A. Berville (I.N.R.A. Dijon. France) for helpful discussion and training concerning the mitochondria isolation.

REFERENCES

1. D.A. Clayton. Cell 28: 693 (1982).
2. A. Bolden, G. Pedrali-Noy and A. Weissbach. J.Biol.Chem. 252: 3351 (1977).
3. U. Bertazzoni, A. I. Scovassi and G. Brun. Eur.J.Biochem. 81: 237 (1977).
4. A. I. Scovassi, R. Wicker and U. Bertazzoni. Eur.J.Biochem. 100: 491 (1979).
5. L. Tarrago-Litvak, O. Viratelle, D.Darriet, R. Dalibart, P.V. Graves and S. Litvak. Nucleic Acids Res. 5: 2197 (1978).
6. F. Quetier and F. Vedel. Nature 268: 365 (1977).
7. L. Christophe, L. Tarrago-Litvak, M. Castroviejo and S. Litvak. Plant Sc.Letters 21: 181 (1981).
8. M. Castroviejo, D. Tharaud, L. Tarrago-Litvak and S. Litvak. Biochem.J. 181: 193 (1979).
9. M. Castroviejo, M. Fournier, M. Gatius, J.C. Gandar, B.Labouesse and S. Litvak. Biochem.Biophys.Res.Comm.107: 294 (1982).
10. L. Tarrago-Litvak, M. Castroviejo and S. Litvak. FEBS Letters 59:125 (1975).
11. F. Sala, A. R. Amileni, B. Parisi and S. Spadari. Eur.J.Biochem. 112:211 (1980).

TRANSFORMATION OF PLANT PROTOPLASTS IN VITRO

F.A. Krens, G.J. Wullems and R.A. Schilperoort

Department of Biochemistry
State University of Leiden, Wassenaarseweg 64
2333 AL Leiden, The Netherlands

INTRODUCTION

In genetic manipulation one can distinguish between the mixing of more or less complete genomes and the more accurate introduction of well defined genes. In the first case use is being made of somatic cell fusion and the uptake of isolated chromosomes and organelles. It might particularly contribute in the transfer of complex genetic traits, like polygenic complexes, that affect yield in agricultural production. In the second case use is being made of recombinant DNA and transformation of protoplasts. By this approach only one or a small number of genes are transferred into an otherwise unaltered genetic background, which has many advantages over less accurate procedures. It is quite clear that plant genetic manipulation is at an early stage of development and that much has still to be learned. Nevertheless, it is proven that this technology can overcome restrictions on gene flow between widely different organisms. Its use will enable us to understand e.g. genomic organization and regulation of gene expression in higher plants. Unless much more is known about this subject and the molecular processes, that underly plant phenotype in general, it can not be expected that somatic and molecular genetics will significantly contribute to applications of practical use. Here, we only deal with the transformation of plant cells, which requires a procedure for introducing DNA into cells followed by its expression. The major obstacle to DNA uptake in plant cells is the cell wall, but this can be circumvented by using plant protoplasts, i.e. cells freed of their cell walls by enzymatic digestion. Using appropriate media, protoplasts regenerate a new cell wall and subsequently divide. After sustained cell divisions small cell clumps arise.

387

Strategies for plant cell transformation are based on the construction of DNA vectors that either are capable to integrate into
the host genome or show autonomous replication. DNA vectors should
meet various requirements among which are those that are needed for
their use as shuttle between bacteria and plant cells. Bacteria come
into play because they are preferentially used in recombinant-DNA
operations and in addition allow isolation of sufficient amounts of
pure DNA for transformation experiments. Plant DNA vectors, therefore,
should carry sites in which genes can be inserted stably, selectable
markers for both bacteria and plant cells, DNA sequences for replication in bacteria and either a plant replication-origin for autonomous replication or DNA sequences for integration into the plant
genome. The latter is preferred for stable maintenance and transmission into offspring and is a condition when genetically engineered
plants have to be propagated sexually. Obviously, genes inserted in
plant DNA vectors should contain all the types of regulatory sequences
that are needed for expression in plant cells.

For development of plant DNA vectors use can be made of DNA
viruses and the Ti-plasmids of Agrobacterium tumefaciens. Of the
viruses, the double-stranded DNA caulimoviruses of which cauliflower
mosaic virus (CaMV) is the best studied and the single-stranded gemini
viruses are receiving the most attention. Here, we will concentrate on
the Ti-plasmid as the most promising plant DNA vector at present. This
plasmid confers on its host the capacity to induce tumors, that are
called Crown galls, on dicotyledons. Monocotyledons are not susceptible
to A. tumefaciens. Via the bacterium, which attaches to the plant cell
but itself stays outside, a defined part of the Ti-plasmid, called
T-DNA, is introduced into the cells where it is integrated into the
nuclear DNA and is expressed into mRNA and proteins. T-DNA encodes
enzymes responsible for the synthesis of tumour specific amino acid
derivatives such as octopine or nopaline, which the bacterium, harbouring the corresponding octopine type or nopaline type Ti-plasmid, can
use as a sole source of carbon and nitrogen. T-DNA also carries genes,
on separated loci, that give rise to an auxin- and cytokinin-like
phenotype and by which the transformed cells acquire the ability to
grow in the absence of phytohormones. Auxin and cytokinin are hormones
that are usually required for growth of normal cells in tissue culture.
Thus, T-DNA carries genes for selection and identification of plant
cell transformants, while the complete Ti-plasmid replicates in a
bacterium. It, moreover, has been shown that T-DNA, present in plants
regenerated from tumour cells, is transmitted into offspring in a
mendelian fashion, proving its stable integration into chromosomes.
Ti-plasmids, therefore, possess all requirements that were posed for
a plant DNA vector. Crown gall as a model system for transformation
of plants, furthermore, offers possibilities to understand plant cell
development and regeneration by investigating the function of the
small number of genes on T-DNA, that show a phytohormone-like phenotype and cause autonomous growth.

THE CROWN GALL SYSTEM

Crown gall induction on plants

A.tumefaciens, like A.rhizogenes which causes the hairy root disease on dicotyledons, needs a wound in order to induce a tumour. Wounding appears to be essential for the development of "conditioned" cells. These are cells, at the wound site, that are susceptible to the tumour inducing stimulus during a restricted period of time, i.e. before the first cell division takes place.[1] The plant's wound sap is used by the bacteria as a source of nutrition. Only bacteria that are metabolically active have the capacity to induce tumours. Dead bacteria or metabolically inactive bacteria, e.g. multiple auxotrophs if inoculated without addition of the requirements for their growth, are unable to initiate tumours. The bacteria, moreover, seem to need a "bacterial adjustment phase" before they can accomplish tumour induction.[2] In order to transform the plant cells agrobacteria must attach to the cell wall. During attachment bacteria compete for a limited number of attachment sites.[2,3] Various types of experiments indicate that attachment occurs via the lipopolysaccharide (LPS) component of agrobacterial cell wall.[4] It seems that the polygalacturonic acid fraction in plant cell walls of dicotyledons is responsible for binding of A.tumefaciens, since pre-incubation of agrobacteria with this cell wall fraction prior to inoculation into fresh wounds prevents tumour formation. The polygalacturonic acid fraction from cell walls of monocotyledons is not inhibitory suggesting that monocotyledonous cells do not contain attachment sites. However, after this fraction is incubated with pectinesterase, which results in demethylation of the polygalacturonic acid fraction, binding of agrobacteria is observed. The polygalacturonic acid fraction from crown gall cells also seems to be methylated.[5] This could be a possible explanation for the insusceptibility of both monocots and certain plants regenerated from crown gall cells (see the cocultivation procedure). At present virtually nothing is known about the molecular process by which DNA is transferred from virulent agrobacteria into plant cells. Studies on plants have shown that this process is accomplished within about 20 h. whereafter the bacteria can be killed without affecting tumour development.[1] The process of tumour induction contains at least one step that is thermosensitive. For various plant species, tumour induction appears to be inhibited at temperatures between 28°C and 30°C, while no tumours are formed at higher temperatures.[1,6] The growth of neither agrobacteria nor plant cells is negatively influenced by this condition. For Mazzard cherry it is observed that when roots are kept at a soil temperature of 35°C for 5 days, following inoculation with A.tumefaciens, galls are more numerous and larger than on control plants kept at 25°C.[7] This suggests that temperature sensitivity of tumour induction concerns a step in the process that takes place in the host plant. Detailed information on Crown gall can be found in a number of recent review.[8,9]

T-DNA characteristics and tumour-morphology mutants

A large plasmid, ranging in size between 100-150 Mdalton, in both A.tumefaciens and A.rhizogenes is essential for the capacity of these microorganisms to cause the crown gall and hairy root disease, respectively. The plasmids in question are called tumour inducing or Ti-plasmid and root inducing or Ri-plasmid. Three classes of Ti-plasmids have been described. These are the octopine-, nopaline- and null-type or agropine Ti-plasmids. A common feature, besides tumour induction, of these plasmids is, that they are responsible for the synthesis of tumour specific amino acid derivates, having the general name of opines, in crown gall tissue. The synthesis of opines such as octopine or nopaline is coded for by Ti-plasmids that carry the corresponding name.[10,11] The various Ti- and Ri-plasmids encode degradative pathways for their respective opines, which enable virulent agrobacteria to use these compounds as a source of nitrogen, carbon or energy. For octopine and nopaline Ti-plasmids, as well as for Ri-plasmids more recently, it has been demonstrated that a defined area of the plasmid, referred to as T-region, is stably integrated in the plant genome.[12,13] This part of Ti- or Ri-plasmids in transformed cells is called transferred-DNA or T-DNA. Detailed data are only available for T-DNA of octopine and nopaline tumour tissues. Here we will mainly concentrate on octopine T-DNA to which most of our studies are related.

Biochemical studies with cell organelles and later on genetic studies with flowering plants regenerated from tumour cells have revealed that T-DNA is present in the nucleus.[14,15,16] Studies with crown gall DNA clones, harbouring T-DNA and plant/T-DNA borders from a few callus lines, have proven that T-DNA is covalently joined to the plant DNA.[17] They also show that both single copy DNA and repeated DNA are sites, used for T-DNA integration. Moreover, several copies of T-DNA per cell can be present at different sites of integration. Although these data suggest that no preferred DNA sequences are used for T-DNA integration more extensive studies are needed to establish whether the integration takes place at random indeed. Nopaline tobacco tumours can carry from one to at least four different T-DNA copies, each with a size of about 16 Mdalton. For two independent lines it is observed that the copies can be arranged in a head to tail tandem configuration. The T-DNA in octopine tumours can be composed of either one, namely T_L-DNA with a size of about 8 Mdalton, or two Ti-plasmid segments, T_R-DNA and T_L-DNA. (Fig.1) Callus tissues derived from tobacco tumours always contain T_L-DNA in one or a few copies and occasionally the additional T_R-DNA is observed. In one tumour line T_R-DNA is shown to be amplified to a high copy number. Sunflower octopine tumour tissues have been reported to contain both T_L- and T_R-DNA. It is not known yet whether the presence of T_R-DNA is determined by the plant species used or by differences in octopine Ti-plasmids. Although T_L-DNA usually has a well defined size, occasionally small extensions and deletions are observed at the ends. On the octopine Ti-plasmid map the T_R-region is located to the right of the T_L-region.

Since T_L-DNA invariably is found in tumour tissues it is likely that it carries genes for the tumourous character of the cells. However, genes on T_R-DNA could have been present at early stages of tumour initiation and lost at a later stage. In that case they might have a temporary function in tumour induction. To investigate this possibility we isolated a series of octopine Ti-plasmid deletion mutants.[18] They show that deletion of the T_R-region does not affect virulence, but that deletion of T_L- plus T_R-region or of the T_L-region alone results in loss of the tumour inducing capacity. With this result it is proven conclusively that only T_L-DNA and not T_R-DNA carries genes that are required for tumour development. A considerable part of T_L-DNA has common DNA sequences with a nopaline T-DNA segment, which indicates that they share several gene functions that apparently are essential in tumour formation and maintenance.[19] Studies on expression of T-DNA show that almost all of it is transcribed but that not all segments seem to be transcribed equally well. Transcripts are detected in both poly A^+ and poly A^- RNA fractions.[20,21] Using purified active nuclei from crown gall cells it is demonstrated that α-amanitin, at low concentrations, inhibits the transcription of T-DNA.[22] This indicates that T-DNA transcription is performed by RNA polymerase II. In total 7 transcripts appear to be made from T_L-DNA and the direction of transcription has been established. (Fig. 1) Evidence has been presented that initiation and termination of RNA synthesis takes place within T-DNA. Therefore, the prokaryotic T-region appears to carry all the required signals for the plant RNA polymerase II. One transcript (number 3) of about 1400 bases, coming from the right end of T_L-DNA, is shown by in vitro translation to code for a protein of about M_R 40.000. By immunoprecipitation it is demonstrated that this protein is the enzyme for octopine synthesis, which is called lysopine dehydrogenase or octopine synthase.[23]

Since T-DNA must play a role in the phytohormone independent growth of crown gall cells we were interested to see whether T-DNA genes could be identified with a function that directly could be correlated to well known auxin and cytokinin activities. Some physiological effects of auxin are the elongation of cells, the stimulation of root formation and inhibition of lateral shoot development (apical dominance). Auxins are produced in shoot tips; by cell-to-cell polar transport it is transported downwards. Physiological effects of cytokinins can oppose those of auxins: inhibition of root development, stimulation of lateral shoot formation. Cytokinins are produced particularly in the root system. The hormone is transported upwards in the stem and the leaves through the xylem in the vascular bundles. The addition to culture medium of balanced concentrations of both an auxin and a cytokinin results in the stimulation of undifferentiated callus growth. Relatively high concentrations of cytokinins versus auxins give rise to shoot development in normal tobacco callus, where-

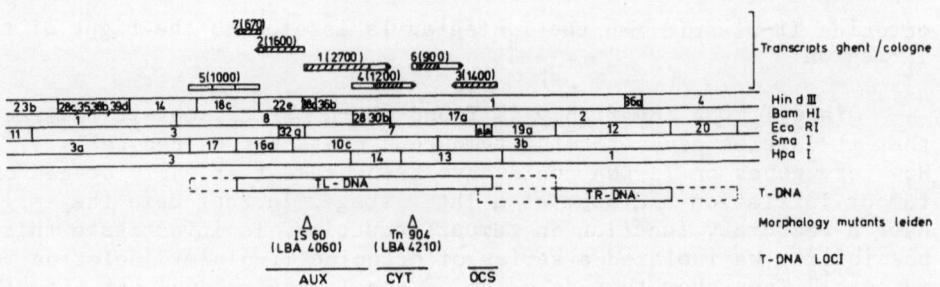

Fig.1. Map of the T-region of an octopine Ti-plasmid with indicated
       positions of transcripts, T_L- and T_R-DNA, transposon/insertion
       mutations giving rise to tumour morphology mutants, and loci
       for tumour functions. aux: auxin, cyt: cytokinin, ocs: octopine
       synthesis.

as the reverse situation results in root development. To identify
T-DNA genes that might promote auxin- and cytokinin-like activities
in tumour cells we investigated octopine Ti-plasmid mutants that were
obtained by random transposon-mutagenesis. A number of them appear to
induce tumours with an aberrant morphology and carry an insertion in
T-DNA.[24] Three mutants (LBA1501, LBA4060 and LBA4210) are hardly virulent on tomato but induce tumours of practically normal size on
Nicotiana rustica and N.debneyi. Two of these (LBA1501 and LBA4060)
carry an insertion at the left part of the T_L-region, which for T_L-
DNA is at the position of transcript 2 and 1, respectively (Fig]).
They form tumours on tobacco stems from which, in contrast to normal
octapine tumours, shoots develop and on Kalanchoë daigremontiana stems
they induce small, unorganized tumours without the adventitious roots
normally observed for tumours induced by the wild-type strain. Above
tumours on Kalanchoë, that were induced by LBA4060, the apical dominance appears to be abolished, since lateral shoots develop from buds
only above the tumours. This indicates that, contrary to what is
observed for normal tumours, a growth factor is released, which is
transported in an upwards direction and gives cause to a phenomenon
that is reminiscent to cytokinin activity. This is further supported
by the absence of adventitious roots around the tumour. On Kalanchoë
leaves LBA4060 is hardly virulent. Mutant LBA4210, which has an
insertion at the middle of the T_L-region (position of transcript 4 on
T_L-DNA) induces tumours on tobacco from which, in contrast to normal
tumours, roots develop. On Kalanchoë stems, tumours with a strongly
increased number of adventitious roots are formed. The stimulation
of root development suggests a relatively high auxin-like activity.
On leaves of Kalanchoë LBA4210 is weakly virulent. Inoculation with
a 1:1 mixture of the two types of mutants (LBA4060 and LBA4210)
results in the formation of tumours that are identical in all respects

to those induced by the wild-type on the various plants tested (tomato, tobacco, Kalanchoe stems and leaves). In order to investigate the molecular basis of the observed complementation explants of tumours, that are obtained after mixed infection with both types of mutants, are brought in tissue culture on medium without hormones.[25] Subsequently, from one tumour callus, subclones are derived via protoplasts. Six subclones, that both grow in the absence of phytohormones and produce octopine, are analyzed for their T-DNA content. All six clones appeared to contain T-DNA that originated from each of both mutants, suggesting that they are derived from doubly infected cells. Genetic complementation in the tumour cells might therefore at least partly account for the normal tumour development. Recombination, leading to a non-mutated T_L-DNA, is not observed. From all of these data, we postulated that T_L-DNA contains loci for an auxin- and cytokinin-like phenotype. Inactivation of the auxin-locus, like in LBA1501 and LBA4060, would then result in a cytokinin-like effect in plant cells, because the activity of the cytokinin-locus is not anymore counterbalanced by the activity of the auxin-locus. Likewise inactivation of the cytokinin-locus, as in LBA4210, would result in an auxin-like effect. Following this model we assumed that T-DNA introduced into plant cells via the Ri-plasmid might have an extremely active auxin-locus and lack a cytokinin-locus. Sequence homology has been detected indeed recently between part of the auxin-locus of the Ti-plasmid and the T-region of a Ri-plasmid.[26] We further tested our model by investigating the influence of auxin and cytokinin on tumour formation by both types of Ti-plasmid tumour morphology mutants. It is found that the addition of a cytokinin, in contrast to an auxin, stimulates tumour formation on tomato by the mutant LBA4060 with an insertion in the cytokinin-locus.[24] Auxin stimulates tumour formation on tobacco by the mutant LBA4210 with an insertion in the auxin-locus. Also the introduction of a Ri-plasmid into mutants with a mutation in the auxin-locus results in normal tumour formation on tomato, suggesting the possibility that Ri-plasmid derived T-DNA and mutant Ti-plasmid derived T-DNA can complement each other genetically. (Hooykaas et al., unpublished results) The Ri-plasmid then contributes an active auxin-locus. Earlier it had been observed already that A.rhizogenes, which normally induces root formation on Kalanchoë leaves, by the addition of a cytokinin during infection gives rise to tumours rather than roots.[27] Recently many more transposon-insertion mutants in the T-region of the octopine Ti-plasmid have been isolated by others. With these mutants the auxin- and cytokinin-loci, which by these authors are called tms (tumour morphology shooting) and tmr (tumour morphology rooting)-locus respectively, are mapped more accurately.[28] In addition a new locus is identified. An insertion in this locus leads to the formation of tumours of a much larger size than normal on Kalanchoë stems, but not on tobacco stems. This locus has been named tml (tumour morphology large). The tumour morphology mutants carrying inactivated T-DNA genes show that by mutation the wide host range can become more limited and that even organ specificity is expressed. This shows the importance of host's

physiology in its response to the tumour inducing stimulus and by
this also the role of T-DNA in determining, at least partly, the
host range.

THE COCULTIVATION PROCEDURE

The cocultivation procedure can be considered as being tumour
induction under artificial conditions. Virulent agrobacteria are
temporary cocultivated with protoplasts from the moment that the
protoplasts have regenerated a new cell wall.[29] Protoplasts are comparable to the earlier mentioned conditioned cells, that arise from
differentiated cells after wounding a plant. Protoplasts are isolated
from leaves of axenically grown Nicotiana tabacum SRI shoots; SRI is
a streptomycin resistant tobacco mutant. The protoplasts are suspended
at a density of $10^5 - 10^6$ protoplasts/ml in K_3 culture medium, containing a reduced level of hormones (0,1 mg NAA; 0,2 mg kinetin per
liter) compared to their use in callus cultures. Petridishes containing 10 ml of protoplast suspension are kept at $26^{\circ}C$ in the dark
for the first 24 h. and thereafter at 2000 lux for 48 h. At day 3
i.e. well before cell division takes place and when new cell wall
material has formed as indicated by calcofluor white staining, the
cells are mixed with agrobacteria in a 400:1 bacteria/protoplast
ratio. After a cocultivation period of 32 h., during which heavy
aggregation of protoplasts and bacteria occurs, free bacteria are
removed by repeated washing. The plant cells are further cultured in
K_3 medium supplemented with hormones. Carbenicillin (250 μg/ml) is
added to kill remaining bacteria. Three to four weeks later small
calli are plated at a 1:10 dilution on hormone free medium solidified
with agar. Continued selective pressure allows only calli consisting
of transformed cells to survive; habituated tissue, consisting of
cells that spontaneously have acquired hormone autotrophy, is not
obtained with the SRI protoplasts.

When virulent agrobacteria are added to freshly isolated protoplasts or to one day old protoplasts neither bacterial attachment
nor transformation is observed. The presence of newly formed cell
wall constituents, as present on 3 day old protoplasts, could be one
of the essential conditions for transformation via agrobacteria. This
assumption is supported by the use of inhibitors of cell wall formation.(coumarin, colchicin, 2,6 dichlorobenzonitril) We also found
that EDTA, a chelating agent of divalent cations, but not EGTA, an
agent that only binds Ca^{2+}, inhibits both attachment and transformation. Since a cell wall already had formed in the experiments with
these chelators, the results suggest that certain divalent cations,
like Mg^{2+} but not Ca^{2+}, are involved possibly at the level of binding
the bacteria effectively. As has been suggested for other bacterium-
plant interactions lectins, which are hydroxyproline-rich glycoproteins, might play a role. Their activity seems to depend on the
presence of divalent cations. We found that substantial amounts of
hydroxyproline is present both in cell wall material extracted from

3 day old protoplasts and in material isolated from medium in which
protoplasts are grown. If lectins, which interact with sugar groups,
play a role in the bacterial attachment indeed they perhaps could
function as a bridge in binding the polygalacturonic acid component
in the cell wall of dicotyledons on the one side and the LPS component
of the agrobacterial wall on the other side. Since agrobacteria often
show a wide host range, the function of any compound which controls
effective attachment can neither be plant species nor Agrobacterium
species specific. It might, however, have a specific function in
establishing an effective attachment only within the system of the
Agrobacterium-dicotyledonous plant interaction. In this respect it
is worth to note, that the LPS fraction of E.coli does not inhibit
tumour induction by A.tumefaciens and that E.coli does not show
attachment to 3 day old protoplasts. This, moreover, indicates that
the attachment observed for agrobacteria in vitro is not mainly an
aspecific phenomenon. Also Agrobacterium related bacteria like
Rhizobium trifolii attach to cell wall regenerating protoplasts and
earlier it is shown that when they have acquired a Ti-plasmid they
are able to induce tumours.[30] However, R.meliloti, carrying a Ti-
plasmid, does not have the capacity to induce tumours neither
attaches to protoplasts, with a regenerated cell wall. Agrobacteria
that have been cured of their Ti-plasmid, and therefore are avirulent,
still have the capacity to attach to such protoplasts. Their LPS
fraction also inhibits tumour induction by virulent agrobacteria.
Therefore it is likely that genes on the Agrobacterium chromosome
determine the bacterial attachment.

When A.tumefaciens is cocultivated with aggregates of normal
tobacco cells, that have developed from dividing protoplasts after
16 days, attachment is observed, but no transformants are found. In
this case either the Ti-plasmid (or T-DNA) transfer-mechanism does
not function completely or plasmid DNA is transferred, but tobacco
cells in culture are not or much less "competent" or "conditioned"
for stable transformation. This observation is in agreement with
results obtained from tumour induction on plants. These already had
lead to the conclusion that cells at the wound site are "conditioned"
during a period before cell division takes place, whereafter no
transformation occurs. Whether this is generally true for all plant
species has still to be established. Crown gall cells are different
from normal cells in that they do not show attachment of
A.tumefaciens. We observed, however, that 3 day old protoplasts,
that are isolated from tobacco crown gall cells or from leaves of
T-DNA containing transformed plants, do attach A.tumefaciens. This
capacity appears to be lost again when protoplasts have divided and
cell aggregates are tested. This indicates that a componenet, probably in the cell wall, required for attachment is synthesized at
the protoplast stage but modified, masked or even absent at the
cellular stage.

Via the cocultivation procedure we have isolated hormone autotrophic calli using agrobacteria of the octopine- and the nopaline-type and also with agrobacteria harbouring a cointegrate plasmid consisting of an octopine and nopaline Ti-plasmid[31] In the octopine Ti::nopaline Ti-plasmids studied sofar the cointegration invariably occurred in the common sequence of their T-DNAs. This results in two well separated composite T-DNAs. The one carries one part of the octopine T-DNA linked to one part of the nopaline T-DNA, whereas in the other the remaining parts of both types of T-DNA are linked[32] Tumourous tissues are obtained with a frequency of 1 to 0,1% of the starting population of protoplasts. The characterization of presumed transformants is based on expression of the crown gall specific markers: hormone autotrophy (Aut) and opine synthesis (Ocs or Nos). In table 1 the various phenotypes that are found are summarized. The results clearly demonstrate a segregation of tumour markers among these in vitro transformants, indicating that somehow the final result of the transformation is not always perfect i.e. that not all markers are invariably expressed. Such a situation is not observed for crown galls on plants, nor for calli derived from them. The difference between in vivo and in vitro tumours probably lies in the fact, that we observed, that protoplasts derived subclones of an in vitro tumour are all identical with respect to T-DNA structure and organization while this is not true for an in vivo tumour[33] In vitro transformation, thus, gives rise to calli with a homogeneous composition while in vivo tumour induction leads to calli consisting of a mixed population of tumour cells. Segregation of tumour markers will not be detected if in the mixed population only a small number of cells show this phenomenon. The homogenicity of in vitro tumours also is demonstrated by subcloning of a transformant line derived from cocultivation with a strain harbouring an octopine Ti::nopaline Ti cointegrate plasmid. The primary callus produces both octopine and nopaline. More than 100 subclones, obtained without selection, all show Ocs^+ and Nos^+ phenotype. A number of them are analysed for T-DNA and the presence of the two composite T-DNAs is demonstrated[32] The architecture of T-DNA in amorphous octopine type transformants obtained in vitro is not significantly different from that of T-DNA found in calli derived from tumours on plants. None of the in vitro obtained transformants analysed contain T_R-DNA; T_L-DNA of a fairly fixed size is present. Whether the observed phenotypic variation is due to deviations from normal T_L-DNA or to bad expression of T-DNA genes has still to be established.

Another interesting feature of the cocultivation method is that it often gives rise to octopine type transformants with a high shooting capacity. Regeneration of shoots has neither been observed for octopine tumours on plants nor for callus tissues derived from them. The percentage of shoot development from nopaline type trans-formants is even higher but also on plants this type of tumours develop shoots or teratomata. In the few cases that have been studied sofar e.g. $SRI-4013-3^+$ in fig. 2, we observed that shooting tissue contains T_L-DNA which lacks part of the left side of normal T_L-DNA.

The deletions concerned affect at least part of the auxin-locus and this could well explain the spontaneous shooting capacity of the calli. One of the characteristics of the shoots, and after they have been grafted on decapitated tobacco plants also of the flowering transformed plants, is that they do not develop roots. In analogy with the tumour-morphology mutants, carrying an affected auxin-locus, this property might be due to the activity of the cytokinin-locus that is still present. Non-rooting flowering plants also are obtained from nopaline type calli. The one of them that has been studied in detail also contains a left-side T-DNA deletion affecting the auxin-locus but not the cytokinin-locus.

Table 1. Phenotypic variation observed for transformed tissues obtained after cocultivation of tobacco protoplasts with different A.tumefaciens strains.

type of bacteria	phenotype	frequency (%)
octopine	Aut^+, Ocs^+	69
	Aut^+, Ocs^-	30
	Aut^-, Ocs^+	1
nopaline	Aut^+, Nos^+	77
	Aut^+, Nos^-	33
oc-nop cointegrate	Aut^+, Ocs^+, Nos^+	13
	Aut^+, Ocs^+, Nos^-	33
	Aut^+, Ocs^-, Nos^+	33
	Aut^+, Ocs^-, Nos^-	17
	Aut^-, Ocs^+, Nos^-	4

Aut: phytohormone autotrophy
Ocs: octopine synthesis
Nos: nopaline synthesis

Transformed plants of octopine and nopaline type, carrying a substantial segment of T-DNA, still have other newly acquired properties: abnormal flowers and insusceptibility towards infection with A.tumefaciens.[34] All their flowers show a remarkable outgrowth of the pistil (heterostyly), which to that extent is not observed for grafted control plants, derived from normal SRI callus tissue or SRI seeds. Whilst flowers on control plants form seedbulbs as a result of self-fertilization, the flowers of the transformants fall off without

seed formation. Crosses are performed by applying normal pollen on
the stamen of transformants and vice versa. Only in the first way
seeds are obtained, indicating that these transformed plants are male
sterile. When transformant derived seeds are germinated on culture
medium, initially all seedlings develop a root tip. But about two
weeks later approximately half of them show a normal development,
while the others develop a transformed phenotype: thick, sprouting
shoots and a lack of root development i.e. the root tips form callus.
The group of transformed seedlings give rise to plants with identical
characteristics, including T-DNA, as the parental regenerants. These
results clearly demonstrate that T-DNA is transmitted as a single
Mendelian trait. Like normal seedlings octopine type transformed
seedlings derived from SRI-4013-3^{+} contain 48 chromosomes, which to
our surprise is different from the number found in cells derived from
buds of the parental regenerant. Here we observe a variation in chromosome number between 48 and more than 100 per cell. Less than 10%
of the cells contain 48 chromosomes. The difference, in this respect,
between parental plant and its transformed seedlings suggests to us
that the meiotic division might have acted as a selective barrier
for those cells having an aneuploid chromosome number.

Although both transformed plants and transformed F1 progeny are
not susceptible to A.tumefaciens we found that with A.rhizogenes an
enormous swelling occurs of internodes having one infected wound.
No local tumours develop. Since all available evidence indicate a
similar mechanism for transformation by A.tumefaciens and A.rhizogenes
we assume that no T-DNA transfer takes place, but that the observed
swelling is a response to some growth factor with a pronounced
auxin-like activity, that is excreted by A.rhizogenes. This activity
together with a presumed high cytokinin-like activity in cells of
the transformed tobacco plants, might also trigger cells more outside the wound site to divide. The presumed involvement of a high
cytokinin-like activity in development and in some of the phenotypic
traits of our transformed tobacco plants is tested by repeatedly
spraying normal tobacco plants with kinetin. We found that such a
treatment results in thickening of stems and sprouting of lateral
buds, giving these plants quite a transformed plant appearance. These
plants turned out to be not susceptible to A.tumefaciens either. If
transformed plants are not susceptible to A.tumefaciens because of
an abnormal plant cell wall, by which the agrobacteria can not attach
themselves, then we might postulate that some activity of the
cytokinin-locus determines the alteration in tumour cell walls.

DNA TRANSFORMATION OF PLANT PROTOPLASTS

General transformation procedures

Recipient cells that are used for DNA transformation experiments
vary from bacteria to eukaryotic cells derived from animals or plants.

Each system requires its own particular conditions for the uptake of DNA, but some basic features are similar in several methods. In bacteria, like E.coli, it is important first to make the bacteria competent by a $CaCl_2$ treatment or to use a bacterial species from which competent cells can be isolated directly as with Bacillus subtilis. DNA uptake is often achieved by a heat shock treatment[35] or bacterial protoplasts are used which, after the addition of DNA, are mixed with a polyethyleneglycol (PEG) solution (final concentration 30% w/v).[36] The exposure to PEG lasts for a few minutes after which the solution is diluted. The protoplasts are then washed and plated onto selective medium containing an osmotic stabilizer to allow cell wall regeneration. For organisms that possess a cell wall it is usual to first prepare protoplasts or spheroplasts, which is done by enzymatic digestion of the cell wall. Yeast is transformed by using protoplasts that are incubated with DNA in the presence of 10mM $CaCl_2$ and PEG (20-40% w/v).[37,38] The combination of $CaCl_2$ and PEG is characteristic for many procedures of DNA transformation applied to different organisms.

PEG is also well known for its capacity to fuse cells. Fusion of bacterial protoplasts with rat cells has been used to introduce and to express genes of polyoma and SV40.[39] The bacteria contained recombinant plasmids carrying viral genes. In another procedure, red blood cells, via fusion, are used as injection vehicles.[40] They take up macromolecules during hypotonic hemolysis and after they have resealed the blood cells are fused to counterparts by the use of sendai virus. This method, however, does not work well with nucleic acids or proteins larger than 300 Kdalton. Also use has been made of pinocytic vesicles that are formed by cultured mouse cells when they are exposed to a medium containing 0,5 M sucrose, 10% (w/v) PEG 1000 and the macromolecule that has to be introduced.[41] The cells are subsequently placed in hypotonic culture medium, in order to induce breakage of the pinocytic vesicles as a result of an increased internal osmotic pressure. The macromolecules are thus delivered into the cytosol. Via this method certain enzymes, dextran 70.000 and antibodies have successfully been introduced. Whether it can be applied also for the introduction and stable integration of nucleic acids is still unknown. Extensive studies have been performed by another type of vesicles namely liposomes. Liposomes can be easily prepared by evaporating an ether solution, containing phospholipids, to dryness, by which a lipid film on the inside of a glass tube is formed. After addition of an aqueous solution, lipid vesicles are obtained through vortexing or sonication. Most of the vesicles formed in this way consist of multiple layers of lipid and are therefore called multilamellar vesicles (MLVs) . However, the enclosed volume is rather small and this makes them less suitable for DNA transformation experiments. Therefore, several methods have been developed for the preparation of large unilamellar vesicles (LUVs). The principle procedures are the ether vaporization method, the cochleate

cylinder method and the reverse phase evaporation (REVs) method.[42]
Dependent on the type of phospholipids, the liposomes can have a
positive, negative or neutral net charge. The charge is important
in the liposome-cell interaction. The stability of the vesicles also
depends on the type of lipids used and it has been found that
inclusion of cholesterol greatly enhances the maintenacne of stability and reduces cell-induced leakage. Chloreterol, furthermore,
increases the amount of encapsulated material which is delivered
intracellularly. This can further be stimulated by pretreatment of
target cells with PEG.[43,44] Fusion of the liposomes with recipient
cells via PEG has also been used to introduce the content of the
liposomes into cells. It is found that nucleic acids remain physically intact upon encapsulation within liposomes and are protected
against nuclease degradation. To demonstrate the biological activity
of nucleic acids after liposome mediated transfer to cells SV40 DNA
is used.[45] Sensitive plaque and fluorescence assays exist to monitor
the expression of viral antigens in the monkey cells to which SV40
DNA is delivered. It is shown that transformation via liposomes is
as efficient as the "calciumphosphate-DNA coprecipitate" method.
This method was initially developed to transform human cells with
human adenovirus 5 DNA.[46] A modification of this procedure is used
in further experiments with other cell types and DNAs.[47] The basic
principle of this method is that a fine calciumphosphate precipitate
is allowed to form in the presence of DNA. Cell monolayers are then
incubated with the DNA-calciumphosphate precipitate and postincubated
in a medium containing a high concentration of Ca^{2+}. This procedure
is at present a well established way for the transformation of
mammalian cells.

The last method to be mentioned here is microinjection. In
general micropipettes are made with the aid of a mechanical puller.
Micromanipulators are used to guide the pipette through which the
injection solution is delivered into the cell by aid of pressure
from a syringe.[48] This method was initially applied to systems consisting of cells of sufficient size, e.g. oocytes, and at present
also for mammalian tissue culture cells that are well immobilized
in a monolayer. The frequency of transformation must be high to
overcome the relatively small number of cells which can be manipulated.

Uptake of nucleic acids by plant protoplasts

Plant protoplasts excrete nucleases which obviously will have
a negative effect on the uptake of nucleic acids. Endo- and/or
exonuclease activity has been shown to be secreted into the medium
by tobacco and Datura protoplasts as well as to be associated with
them.[49,50] Therefore, $ZnCl_2$, which inhibits plant ribonuclease
activity or high pH (pH 10) are often used in the experiments.
Nucleic acids can also be made inaccessible to nucleases by encapsulation in liposomes. Much research is carried out on determining

optimal conditions for DNA encapsulation in and DNA transfer from
liposomes to plant protoplasts. Since liposomes can be toxic to
protoplasts, one carefully has to look for the appropriate liposomes,
protoplasts ratio. A biological assay is necessary to demonstrate
true uptake of DNA or RNA. In the case of RNA such an assay is
provided by tobacco mosaic virus (TMV) against which antibodies are
raised. Virus production in tobacco protoplasts is demonstrated for
TMV RNA that has been encapsulated in liposomes containing cholesterol. Polyethyleneglycol (PEG) and polyvinylalcohol (PVA) are found
to enhance nucleic acid transfer.[51,52] Many procedures not involving
liposomes have been tried as well. In order to achieve RNA-uptake
by protoplasts, incubation mixtures with polycations, like poly-
L-ornithine (PLO), or PEG and high Ca^{2+} concentration (to accomplish
RNA uptake) are used. RNA uptake is also forced by osmotic shock.
Various concentrations and combinations of the additives are tested
with variable success. The only procedure that has been reported
to give reproducible results for different viruses and plant species
made use of protoplasts and RNA in the presence of approximately
40% (w/v) PEG and 3 mM $CaCl_2$ for 10 to 30 seconds, followed by
dilution of the PEG with growth medium containing $CaCl_2$ prior to
washing.[53] It thus appears to be possible to introduce RNA into
protoplasts either via liposomes or by PEG/Ca^{2+} treatment.

More recently studies on DNA uptake by plant cells, including
algae, have been reported. Transformation has been demonstrated for
cell wall-deficient, arginine-requiring Chlamydomonas reinhardii
cells which are treated with a recombinant plasmid consisting of
pBR322, the yeast arg 4 locus and a yeast replication-origin.[54]
Uptake of plasmid and carrier DNA is accomplished in the presence
of either poly-L-ornithine and $ZnSO_4$ for 30 min. or with PEG(approx.
30% w/v) and $CaCl_2$ for 15 min. Arg^+ cells examined by Southern blot
hybridization are shown to contain fragments of yeast DNA. For the
introduction of octopine T-DNA, bacterial protoplasts of A.tumefaciens
are fused with Vinca protoplasts by using PEG and $CaCl_2$.[55] Hormone
autotrophic transformants are obtained among which only a small
number that synthesized octopine. The transformed nature of the
transformants has still to be confirmed by demonstrating the presence
of T-DNA. The more general applicability and the reproducibility of
this procedure is still unknown. In order to achieve uptake of
Ti-plasmid DNA by Petunia protoplasts a few methods have been
published.[56] Protoplasts are incubated with either PLO and DNA or
with $CaCl_2$ and DNA for 15 sec. at $25^{\circ}C$ followed by addition of PEG/
Ca^{2+} and incubation for 2 min. at $34^{\circ}C$. The reported results are
somewhat ambiguous. Transformants are found to be unstable and although by Southern blot hybridization one small fragment is observed
with DNA-sequence homology to the T-region of the Ti-plasmid, the
main internal restriction fragments of T-DNA are not detected and
therefore genetic information that is essential for the tumourous
character of crown gall cells seems to be absent. Another peculiar
point is that the same fragment having homology to T-DNA is found

in every transformant. In our laboratory a method is developed which
is proven to be reproducible and which results in stable transformants carrying large, but variable stretches of T-DNA.

TRANSFORMATION WITH TI-PLASMID DNA

Many of the mentioned general transformation procedures, in
various combinations, have been tried at our laboratory in order to
achieve stable transformation of tobacco protoplasts with octopine
Ti-plasmid DNA. We were only successful with one procedure that is
based on the use of PEG/Ca^{2+}. In this procedure 1 ml of a suspension
of tobacco SR1 leaf protoplasts (5.10^5 protoplasts/ml in K3 medium
with phytohormones) is mixed with 0.5 ml F medium (among other salts
containing 125 mM CaCl$_2$) supplemented with 40% (w/v) PEG 6000. The
final concentrations of Ca^{2+} and PEG are thus approximately 40 mM
and 13%, respectively.[60] During the preparation of F-medium a fine
calcium phosphate precipitate is formed, which is not removed. To
the mixture is added 10 μg Ti-plasmid DNA and 50 μg calf thymus DNA
as a carrier. After incubation for 30 min. at 26°C, the PEG is decreased and the Ca^{2+} concentration is increased stepwise with F-
medium during a postincubation period, which in total lasts about
20 min. Higher concentrations of PEG result in more cell death and
appearance of fusion bodies. No transformants were obtained at lower
concentrations of Ti-plasmid DNA or when carrier DNA was omitted.
Lower concentrations of Ca^{2+} during postincubation or an one-step
addition of F-medium followed by 20 min. postincubation also gave
negative results.

After selection on phytohormone free medium, as a final step,
tissue lines are obtained showing again different phenotypes with
regard to regeneration capacity, LpDH activity and even hormone-
autotrophy. By Southern blot hybridization the T-DNA structure and
organization has been studied using T-region clones. All transformants contain T-DNA. A small number of them, coming from one experiment, show the same banding pattern, suggesting that they might
have originated from one transformant the tissue of which is
disrupted at an early stage. The others show banding patterns that
are different among themselves, which makes it likely that they
have originated from independent transformation events within one
experiment. The PEG/Ca^{2+} procedure is fairly reproducible since
stable transformants are obtained in repeated experiments. As can
be seen in Fig.2, representing some of the most remarkable results,
the T-DNA in DNA transformants differs largely from that found in
tumour tissue obtained via A.tumefaciens in vivo or in vitro. DNA
transformants are found that carry a continuous stretch of T-DNA
extending more to the left as well as to the right of T$_L$-DNA. Some
contain T$_R$-DNA present in a considerable higher copy number than
T$_L$-DNA in the same transformant. Also transformants are isolated
showing a very complex banding pattern in which all or most of the
known internal T-DNA restriction fragments are lacking. In this case

various rearrangements in T-DNA as well as integration of parts of
T-DNA at different sites in the plant genome might have occurred.

It has been reported that the octopine and nopaline T-region
at its ends has nucleotide sequences that are preferred for T-DNA
integration in plant DNA.[57,17] Such border sequences, determining a
well defined fragment of DNA, seem much less used when Ti-plasmid
DNA instead of A.tumefaciens, carrying the same Ti-plasmid, is used
in transformation experiments. This might indicate that these border
sequences play a role in a mechanism, functioning in the bacterium,
by which a more fixed piece of T-DNA is integrated in tumour cells
via A.tumefaciens. It has been shown that virulence genes exist far
outside the T-region on the left half of the Ti-plasmid. Genetic
complementation studies recently have indicated that these genes act
in trans and, therefore, most likely have to be expressed in the
bacterium for virulence.[58,59] It can be envisaged that this set of
genes is involved in determining the fixed size of T-DNA, through
the recognition of border sequences, as well as its transfer into
plant cells.

CONCLUDING REMARKS

If an optimal result has to be reached with transformation
experiments, the DNA of interest must be incubated with a large
population of target cells, in order to obtain a few cells that have
stably incorporated the desired gene. In this respect, the methods
described here, based on single plant protoplasts as target cells,
are similar to those used in bacterial, yeast and mammalian cell
genetics. Millions of single plant cells can be exposed to the
transforming bacteria or Ti-plasmid DNA from which transformants
can be selected.

The advantage of the use of Agrobacterium itself, instead of
naked DNA, as a microinjector for the introduction of genes into
plant cells, lies in the relatively high frequency of transformation
observed (0.1 - 1% of the initial protoplast number) and the non-
scrambled, distinct size of transferred DNA. Both aspects make the
use of A.tumefaciens more reliable than DNA transformation. The
present knowledge about the architecture of T-DNA, its expression
into RNA and proteins and its inheritability justifies the view
that transformation systems based on the Ti-plasmid of Agrobacterium
can be used to transfer foreign genes at will into plants. Plant
DNA vectors, therefore, will be constructed that can replicate and
maintain themselves in Agrobacterium and, furthermore, only contain
from T-DNA the genetic information that is essential for transfer,
and subsequent accurate integration and expression of genes, in the
plant cell. If selection of transformants is still required, suitable
marker genes will replace in T-DNA the genes for tumourous, phytohormone independent growth.

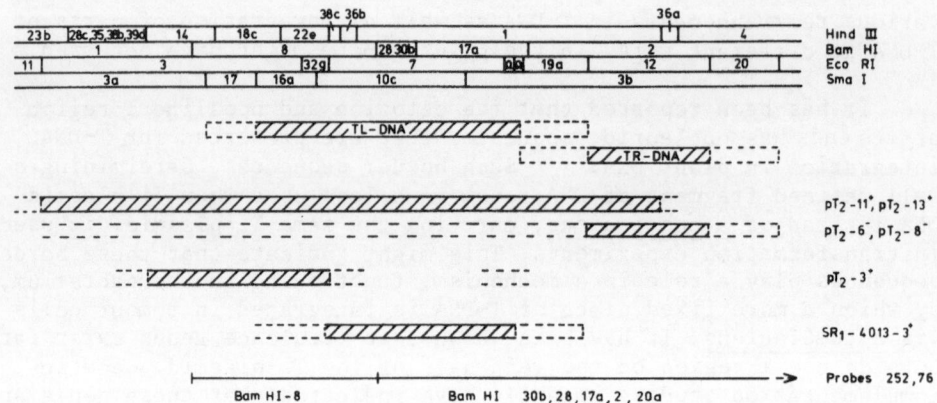

Fig.2. Aberrant T-DNA structure in tumourous tissues derived from
       DNA transformation and cocultivation. Interrupted lines
       indicate areas in which homology with T-DNA clones is demon-
       strated, but for which the precise position of borders is
       not yet known. pT: DNA transformant; +: Ocs.

    DNA transformation, on the other hand, presumably is the most
promising method for monocotyledons, since these are not susceptible
to A.tumefaciens infection. Also in this case genetic information
from T-DNA, that is important for integration and expression of
foreign DNA in plant cells, might successfully be used.

REFERENCES

1. J.Lipetz, Crown gall tumorigenesis II. Relations between wound
     healing and the tumorigenic response, Cancer Res. 26:1597
     (1966).
2. R.A.Schilperoort, Investigations on plant tumors. Crown Gall. On
     the biochemistry of tumor induction by Agrobacterium
     tumefaciens, thesis, Univ. Leiden (1969).
3. B.B.Lippincott and J.A.Lippincott, Bacterial attachment to a
     specific wound site as an essential stage in tumor initiation
     by Agrobacterium tumefaciens, J.Bacteriol. 97:620 (1969).
4. M.H.Whatley, J.S.Bodwin, B.B.Lippincott and J.A.Lippincott, Role
     for Agrobacterium cell envelope lipopolysaccharide in infection
     site attachment, Infect.Immun. 13:1080 (1976).
5. J.A.Lippincott and B.B.Lippincott, Microbial adherence in plants,
     in Bacterial adherence (Receptors and Recognition, Series B,
     volume 6), E.H.Beachey, e.d., Chapman and Hall, Londen (1980).
6. A.C.Braun, Thermal inactivation studies on the tumor-inducing
     principle in crown gall, Phytopathology 40:3 (1950).
7. I.W.Deep and H.Hussin, Effect of postinoculation temperature

on crown gall development on cherry, Phytopathology 52:360
(1962).

8. A.C.Braun ed., Plant tumor research, in Progress in Experimental
    Tumor Research, vol.15, S.Karger, Basel (1972).

9. G.Kahl and J.Schell,eds., Molecular Biology of Plant Tumors,
    Academic Press, New York (1982).

10. G.Bomhoff, P.M.Klapwijk, H.C.M.Kester, R.A.Schilperoort, J.P.
    Hernalsteens and J.Schell, Octopine and nopaline synthesis and
    breakdown genetically controlled by a plasmid of Agrobacterium
    tumefaciens, Mol.Gen.Genet. 145:177 (1976).

11. A.L.Montoya, M.-D.Chilton, M.P.Gordon, D.Sciaky and E.W.Nester,
    Octopine and nopaline metabolism in Agrobacterium tumefaciens
    and crown gall cells:role of plasmid genes, J.Bacteriol.129:
    101 (1977).

12. M.-D.Chilton, M.H.Drummond, D.J.Merlo, D.Sciaky, A.L.Montoya,
    M.P.Gordon and E.W.Nester, Stable incorporation of plasmid
    DNA into higher plant cells: the molecular basis of crown
    gall tumorigenesis, Cell 11:263 (1977).

13. M.-D.Chilton, D.A.Tepfer, A.Petit, C.David, F.Casse-Delbart and
    J.Tempé, Agrobacterium rhizogenes inserts T-DNA into the
    genomes of the host plant root cells, Nature 295:432 (1982).

14. L.Willmitzer, M.De Beuckeleer, M.Lemmers, M.Van Montagu and J.
    Schell ,DNA from Ti-plasmid present in nucleus and absent from
    plastids of crown gall plant cells, Nature 287:359 (1980).

15. M.-D.Chilton, R.K.Saiki, N.Yadav, M.P.Gordon and F.Quetier,
    T-DNA from Agrobacterium Ti-plasmid is in the nuclear DNA
    fraction of crown gall tumor cells, Proc.Natl.Acad.Sci. USA
    77:4060 (1980).

16. L.Otten, H.de Greve, J.P.Hernalsteens, M.Van Montagu, O.Schieder,
    J.Straub and J.Schell,Mendelian transmission of genes intro-
    duced into plants by the Ti-plasmids of Agrobacterium
    tumefaciens, Mol.Gen.Genet. 183:209 (1981).

17. P.Zambryski, M.Holsters, K.Kruger, A.Depicker,J.Schell, M.Van
    Montagu and H.M.Goodman, Tumor DNA structure in plant cells
    transformed by A.tumefaciens, Science 209:1385 (1980).

18. G.Ooms, P.J.J.Hooykaas, R.J.M.van Veen, P.van Beelen, T.J.G.
    Regensburg-Tuink and R.A.Schilperoort, Octopine Ti-plasmid
    deletion mutants of Agrobacterium tumefaciens with emphasis
    on the right side of the T-region, Plasmid 7:15 (1982).

19. G.Engler, A.Depicker, R.Maenhaut, R.Villaroel, M.Van Montagu
    and J.Schell,Physical mapping of DNA base sequences homologous
    between an octopine and nopaline Ti-plasmid of Agrobacterium
    tumefaciens, J.Mol.Biol. 152:183 (1981).

20. L.Willmitzer, G.Simons and J.Schell, The T_L-DNA in octopine crown-
    gall tumours codes for seven well-defined polyadenylated
    transcripts, EMBO Journal 1:139 (1982).

21. S.B.Gelvin, M.F.Thomashow, J.C.McPherson, M.P.Gordon and E.W.
    Nester, Sizes and map positions of several plasmid-DNA-encoded
    transcripts in octopine-type crown gall tumors, Proc.Natl.

Acad.Sci. USA 79:76 (1982).

22. L.Willmitzer, W.Schmalenbach and J.Schell, Transcription of T-DNA
    in octopine and nopaline crown gall tumours is inhibited by
    low concentrations of α-amanitin, Nucl.Acids Res. 9:4801 (1981).
23. J.Schröder, G.Schröder, H.Huisman, R.A.Schilperoort and J.Schell,
    The mRNA for lysopine dehydrogenase in plant tumor cells is
    complementary to a Ti-plasmid fragment, FEBS Lett.129:166
    (1981).
24. G.Ooms, P.J.J.Hooykaas, G.Moolenaar and R.A.Schilperoort, Crown
    gall plant tumours of abnormal morphology, induced by Agro-
    bacterium tumefaciens carrying mutated octopine Ti-plasmids;
    analysis of T-DNA functions, Gene 14:33 (1981).
25. G.Ooms, L.Molendijk and R.A.Schilperoort, Double infection of
    tobacco plants by two complementing octopine T-region mutants
    of Agrobacterium tumefaciens, Plant Mol.Biol. 3 in press (1982).
26. L.Willmitzer, J.Sanchez-Serrano, E.Buschfeld and J.Schell, DNA
    from Agrobacterium rhizogenes is transferred to and expressed
    in axenic hairy root plant tissues, Mol.Gen.Genet. 186:16(1982).
27. R.Beiderbeck, Wurzelinduktion an Blättern von Kalanchoë daigre-
    montiana durch Agrobacterium rhizogenes und der Einfluss von
    Kinetin auf diesen Prozess, Z.Pflanzenphysiol. 68:460 (1973).
28. D.J.Garfinkel, R.B.Simpson, L.W.Ream, F.F.White, M.P.Gordon and
    E.W.Nester, Genetic analysis of crown gall: Fine structure
    map of the T-DNA by site directed mutagenesis, Cell 27:143
    (1981).
29. L.Márton, G.J.Wullems, L.Molendijk and R.A.Schilperoort, In vitro
    transformation of cultured cells from Nicotiana tabacum by
    Agrobacterium tumefaciens, Nature 277:129 (1979).
30. P.J.J.Hooykaas, P.M.Klapwijk, M.P.Nuti, R.A.Schilperoort and
    A.Rörsch, Transfer of the Agrobacterium tumefaciens Ti-plasmid
    to avirulent agrobacteria and to rhizobium ex planta, J.Gen.
    Microbiol. 98:477 (1977).
31. P.J.J.Hooykaas, H.den Dulk-Ras, G.Ooms and R.A.Schilperoort,
    Interactions between octopine and nopaline plasmids in
    Agrobacterium tumefaciens, J.Bacteriol. 143:1295 (1980).
32. G.Ooms, T.J.G.Regensburg-Tuink, M.H.Hofker, A.Hoekema, P.J.J.
    Hooykaas and R.A.Schilperoort, Studies on the structure of
    cointegrates between octopine and nopaline Ti-plasmids and
    their tumour-inducing properties, Plant Mol.Biol., in press
33. G.Ooms, A.Bakker, L.Molendijk, G.J.Wullems, M.P.Gordon, E.W.
    Nester and R.A.Schilperoort, T-DNA organization in homogeneous
    and heterogeneous octopine-type crown gall tissues of Nicotianum
    tabacum, Cell, in press.
34. G.J.Wullems, L.Molendijk, G.Ooms and R.A.Schilperoort, Retention
    of tumor markers in F1 progeny plants from in vitro induced
    octopine and nopaline tumor tissues, Cell 24:719 (1981).
35. S.N.Cohen, A.Y.C.Chang and L.Hsu, Non chromosomal antibiotic
    resistance in bacteria: genetic transformation of Escherichia
    coli by R-factor DNA, Proc.Natl.Acad.Sci. USA 69:2110 (1972).

36. S.Chang and S.N.Cohen, High frequency transformation of Bacillus subtilis protoplasts by plasmid DNA, Mol.Gen.Genet. 168:111 (1979).

37. A.Hinnen, J.B.Hicks and G.R.Fink, Transformation of yeast, Proc. Natl.Acad.Sci. USA 75:1929 (1978).

38. J.D.Beggs, Transformation of yeast by a replicating hybrid plasmid, Nature 275:104 (1978).

39. M.Rassoulzadegan, B.Binetruy and F.Cuzin, High frequency of gene transfer after fusion between bacteria and eukaryotic cells, Nature 295:257 (1982).

40. R.A.Schlegel and M.Rechsteiner, Microinjection of thymidine kinase and bovine serum albumin into mammalian cells by fusion with red blood cells, Cell 5:371 (1975).

41. C.Y.Okada and M.Rechsteiner, Introduction of macromolecules into cultured mammalian cells by osmotic lysis of pinocytic vesicles, Cell 29:33 (1982).

42. R.Fraley and D.Papahadjopoulos, New generation liposomes: the engineering of an efficient vehicle for intracellular delivery of nucleic acids, TIBS March (1981).

43. C.Kirby, J.Clarke and G.Gregoriadis, Effect of cholesterol content of small unilamellar liposomes on their stability in vivo and in vitro, Biochem.Journ.186:591 (1980).

44. R.Fraley, R.M.Straubinger, G.Rule, E.L.Springer and D.Papahadjopoulos, Liposome-mediated delivery of deoxyribonucleic acid to cells: enhanced efficiency of delivery related to lipid composition and incubation conditions, Biochemistry 20:6978 (1981).

45. R.Fraley, S.Subramani, P.Berg and D.Papahadjopoulos, Introduction of liposome-encapsulated SV40 DNA into cells, J.Biol.Chem. 255: 10431 (1980).

46. F.L.Graham and A.J.van der Eb, A new technique for the assay of infectivity of human adenovirus 5 DNA, Virology 52:456 (1973).

47. M.Wigler, A.Pellicer, S.Silverstein, R.Axel, G.Urlaub and L. Chasin, DNA-mediated transfer of the adenine phosphoribosyl transferase locus into mammalian cells, Proc.Natl.Acad.Sci USA 76:1373 (1979).

48. E.G.Diacumakos, Methods for micromanipulation of human somatic cells in culture, in "Methods in cell biology", D.M.Prescott, ed., Academic, New York (1973).

49. A.E. Oleson, A.M.Janski and E.T.Clark, An extracellular nuclease from suspension cultures of tobacco, Biochim.Biophys.Acta 366:89 (1974).

50. A.Schaefer, K.Ohyama and O.L.Gamborg, Detection by agarose gel electrophoresis of nucleases associated with cells and protoplasts from plant suspension cultures using Agrobacterium tumefaciens Ti-plasmid, Agric.Biol.Chem. 45:1441 (1981).

51. T.Nagata, K.Okada, I.Takebe and C.Matsui, Delivery of tobacco mosaic virus RNA into plant protoplasts mediated by reverse-phase evaporation vesicles (liposomes), Mol.Gen.Genet. 184:161 (1981).

52. R.T.Fraley, S.L.Dellaporta and D.Papahadjopoulos, Liposome-
    mediated delivery of tobacco mosaic virus RNA into tobacco
    protoplasts: a sensitive assay for monitoring liposome-
    protoplast interactions, Proc.Natl.Acad.Sci USA 79:1859 (1982).
53. A.J.Maule, M.I.Boulton, C.Edmunds and K.R.Wood, Polyethylene
    Glycol-mediated infection of cucumber protoplasts by cucumber
    mosaic virus and virus RNA, J.Gen.Virol. 47:199 (1980).
54. J.-D.Rochaix and J.van Dillewijn, Transformation of the green
    alga Chlamydomonas reinhardii with yeast DNA, Nature 296:70
    (1982).
55. S.Hasezawa, T.Nagata and K.Syono, Transformation of Vinca proto-
    plasts mediated by Agrobacterium spheroplasts, Mol.Gen.Genet.
    182:206 (1981).
56. J.Draper, M.R.Davey, J.P.Freeman, E.C.Cocking and B.J.Cox,
    Ti-plasmid homologous sequences present in tissues from
    Agrobacterium plasmid-transformed Petunia protoplasts, Plant
    & Cell Physiol. 23:451 (1982).
57. R.B.Simpson, P.J.O'Hara, W.Kwok, A.L.Montoya, C.Lichtenstein,
    M.P.Gordon and E.W.Nester, DNA from the A6S/2 crown gall tumor
    contains scrambled Ti-plasmid sequences near its junctions with
    plant DNA, Cell 29:1005 (1982).
58. J.Hille, I.Klasen and R.A.Schilperoort, Construction and appli-
    cation of R prime plasmids, carrying different segments of an
    octopine Ti-plasmid from Agrobacterium tumefaciens, for comple-
    mentation of vir genes, Plasmid 7:107 (1982).
59. H.J.Klee, M.P.Gordon and E.W.Nester, Complementation analysis of
    Agrobacterium tumefaciens Ti-plasmid mutations affecting onco-
    genicity, J.Bacteriol. 150:327 (1982).
60. F.A.Krens, L.Molendijk, G.J.Wullems and R.A.Schilperoort, In vitro
    transformation of plant protoplasts with Ti-plasmid DNA, Nature 29
    72 (1982).

T-DNA OF THE AGROBACTERIUM TI AND RI PLASMIDS AS VECTORS

Mary-Dell Chilton[*], Annick De Framond[*], Michael Byrne[*],
Rob Fraley[+], W. Scott Chilton[@], Lucille Fenning[*], Kenneth
A. Barton[*], Andrew N. Binns[*], Antonius J. M. Matzke[*],
Michael Bevan[*], Jane Koplow[*], George Jen[*], Chantal David[#]
and Jacques Tempé[#]

[*]Department of Biology, Washington University
St. Louis, Missouri 63130, U.S.A.

[+]Monsanto Company, 800 N. Lindbergh Boulevard
St. Louis, Missouri 63167, U.S.A.

[@]Department of Biology, University of Pennsylvania
Philadelphia, Pennsylvania 19104, U.S.A.

[#]Institut de Microbiologie, Faculté de Science d'Orsay
F91405 Orsay, France

INTRODUCTION

Crown gall and hairy root disease are incited by <u>Agrobacterium
tumefaciens</u> strains carrying large virulence plasmids (Zaenen et al.,
1974; Van Larebeke et al., 1974, 1975; Watson et al., 1975; White &
Nester, 1980a). These are groups of related plasmids and have been
designated Ti (tumor-inducing) and Ri (root-inducing) plasmids
(Sciaky et al., 1978; Chilton et al., 1982), based on morphology of
the infected plant tissue. The pathogenic bacteria genetically
transform the host plant cells by an unknown mechanism that results
in incorporation of a specific part of the virulence plasmid into
the host plant genome (Chilton et al., 1977, 1982; White et al.,
1982). This foreign DNA element, called T-DNA (transferred DNA),
is covalently joined to host plant nuclear DNA (Chilton et al.,
1980; Willmitzer et al., 1980; Yadav et al., 1980; Zambryski et al.,
1980). T-DNA contains genes that function in the transformed plant

cells, producing polyadenylated transcripts (Drummond et al., 1977;
Gelvin et al., 1981, 1982; Gurley et al., 1979; Willmitzer et al.,
1981, 1982; Bevan and Chilton, 1982). The morphology of tumor cells
is affected when specific transcripts are inactivated by transposon
insertion mutagenesis (Ooms et al., 1981; Garfinkel et al., 1981;
Leemans et al., 1982). The auxin and cytokinin autotrophy of
tobacco crown gall tumor cells can be eliminated individually by
specific T-DNA mutations (Barton et al., 1982; Binns et al., 1982).
An additional genetic function encoded by T-DNA is the synthesis by
tumor tissue of novel metabolites, called opines, catalyzed by
enzymes encoded by mapped T-DNA genes (Holsters et al., 1980;
Garfinkel et al., 1981; Murai and Kemp, 1982; Schröder et al., 1981).
Because the opines serve as specific catabolic substrates for the
inciting Agrobacterium strain (Petit et al., 1970; Tepfer and Tempé,
1981), the transformation of thehost plant cells can be rationalized
as an example of genetic engineering by a prokaryotic organism.

The ability of T-DNA to insert into the host plant genome can
be exploited to introduce novel DNA into plant cells: a transposon
inserted into the T-DNA portion of a Ti plasmid is incorporated
into tumor cells together with the flanking T-DNA (Hernalsteens et
al., 1980). Development of techniques for site-directed mutagenesis
of the Ti plasmid (Leemans et al., 1981; Matzke and Chilton, 1981)
has made it feasible to introduce desired foreign genetic information
into predetermined sites within T-DNA (Barton et al., 1982). These
techniques can clearly be employed for isolation of crown gall tumor
lines of normal or aberrant morphology (Ooms et al., 1981; Garfinkel
et al., 1981) that contain desired novel genes, in order to test
for their expression in plant cells. Detailed study of expression
of such foreign genes in intact plants requires regeneration of
plants and/or organs from transformed plant cells.

Carrot cells transformed by A. rhizogenes or A. tumefaciens
strains carrying Ri plasmids develop into rapidly growing roots
that can be propagated as organ cultures and cloned from individual
growing root tips (Tepfer and Tempé, 1981; Chilton et al., 1982).
Such transformed roots contain T-DNA (Chilton et al., 1982), and
if engineered by available procedures such roots would afford a
convenient means of testing foreign genes for ability to express
in carrot roots. Tobacco cells transformed by nopaline-type Ti
plasmids grow as teratomata and after single-cell cloning, continue
to produce shoots of abnormal morphology (Binns et al., 1981). Such
shoots, upon grafting to decapitated tobacco plants, regenerate into
more or less normal-appearing shoots in which the tumorous phenotype
has been suppressed (Binns et al., 1981) although full length T-DNA
remains (Yang et al., 1980; Lemmers et al., 1980). Such suppressed
leaves could be produced from engineered nopaline teratomata to
test foreign genes for expression in tobacco leaves, stems or
apices. Such a strategy would clearly be inferior to the use of
whole plants for gene expression studies.

REGENERATION OF WHOLE PLANTS FROM TRANSFORMED PLANT CELLS

The ultimate goal of a T-DNA vector for crop plant genetic engineering will require techniques for regenerating whole plants from transformed plant cells. Regenerants from cloned crown gall tumors have fallen into two categories: A. those with the characteristics of suppressed shoots described above, which are unable to form roots and which usually contain opines (Binns et al., 1981; Wullems et al., 1981a, 1981b); and B. those with physiologically normal characteristics that have large deletions in T-DNA (Yang and Simpson, 1981; Otten et al., 1981; J. Schell, personal communication). Because selection for normal plant phenotype affords plants that have deletions in the central region of T-DNA, it appears that one or more gene products encoded by that region must be incompatible with regeneration and normal plant morphology.

In contrast with crown gall tumor cells, carrot roots transformed by Ri plasmid T-DNA can produce intact plants with roots (Chilton et al., 1982) that contain T-DNA (David et al., in preparation). A single transformed root tip was cultured first as a root organ culture, then on phytohormone-supplemented agar as a callus, and finally as a suspension in liquid medium with no hormones. In the latter phase, carrot cells underwent spontaneous embryogenesis to form plantlets, which eventually grew into healthy intact plants. The presence of the diagnostic opine (mannopine) in 100% of the regenerated plants, and T-DNA hybridization studies of DNA from their cultured roots, show that these plants are still transformed (Chilton et al., 1982; David et al., in preparation). These results indicate that the genes in T-DNA of the Ri plasmid are not deleterious and do not prevent regeneration. It seems clear that the hormonal balance resulting from insertion of Ri T-DNA is quite different from that in octopine or nopaline tumors containing Ti T-DNA.

A class of insertion mutants in pTi T37 exhibiting the "rooty" phenotype (Garfinkel et al., 1981; Ooms et al., 1981) has recently been observed to produce transformed tobacco cells capable of facile regeneration of hundreds of whole plants with roots (Barton et al., 1982). The cloned transformed plant cells were found to require cytokinin for rapid growth; thus the "rooty" locus is responsible for the cytokinin autotrophy of crown gall tumors (Barton et al., 1982). This experiment demonstrates that a single mutation can disarm T-DNA, at least with respect to tobacco host plants.

IS THE RI PLASMID A "ROOTY" MUTANT OF THE TI PLASMID?

Inoculation of bacteria containing "rooty" mutants of pTi T37 onto carrot discs produces outgrowths of roots resembling those incited by strains containing Ri plasmids. We have found that such roots can be excised and grown as root organ cultures, and that

such cultures synthesize nopaline, indicative that the roots are
indeed transformed. These observations suggest that the "rooty"
mutation in nopaline T-DNA converts it to a form functionally
similar to the T-DNA of the Ri plasmid. As pointed out above,
that mutation is the one that inactivates a gene conferring cytokinin autotrophy.

DNA homology studies show, however, that the Ri plasmid is
not simply a defective or mutant form of Ti plasmid, for T-DNA
of the Ti plasmid hybridizes with Ri plasmid DNA only at extremely
low stringency. For example, pRi 15834 labeled probe DNA fails
to hybridize to Southern blots containing cloned T-DNA fragments
from the octopine Ti plasmid unless the temperature is dropped to
41° below Tm (White and Nester, 1980b). Using the reverse approach,
we have found that four cloned T-DNA probes from pTi T37 fail to
hybridize to the plasmid of virulent A. rhizogenes strain A4, while
they hybridize strongly to homologous control DNA, pTi T37 fragments on the same Southern blot (Figure 1). Taken together, these
results show that the Ri plasmids of strains A4 and 15834, which
are very closely related to one another (White and Nester, 1980b),
do not hybridize well to the T-DNAs of two wide host range Ti
plasmids. The Ri plasmids appear to represent a distinct evolutionary line.

OTHER DISARMED VECTORS DERIVED FROM TI AND RI PLASMIDS

Although "rooty" Ti plasmid mutants and wild type Ri plasmids
appear sufficiently disarmed for certain types of host plants, it
may in other cases be essential to delete additional T-DNA genes
(for example those conferring auxin autotrophy). The ultimate disarmed vector would be a Ti (De Framond et al., in preparation) or
Ri plasmid containing the border signal repeats (Yadav et al.,
1982; Simpson et al., 1982; Zambryski et al., 1982) and a solitary
opine gene, for example that encoding nopaline synthase. No genes
mapping within T-DNA have been found essential for T-DNA transfer
to plant cells (Garfinkel et al., 1981); thus there is every reason
to suppose that such a disarmed vector will genetically transform
plant cells and produce no tumorous phenotype. A technical problem
will be that of finding the transformant cell lines, which could
not be selected on hormone-free medium. For octopine-synthase-
containing lines, homoarginine (a toxic amino acid analogue accepted
as substrate by octopine synthase) has been found to confer a selective advantage (Van Slogteren et al., 1982). A more general
approach that has been used successfully is "brute force" screening
of candidate clones for nopaline synthase activity (Barton et al.,
1982; R. Fraley, unpublished data).

CONCLUSIONS

Progress on the design of disarmed Ti and Ri plasmid vectors

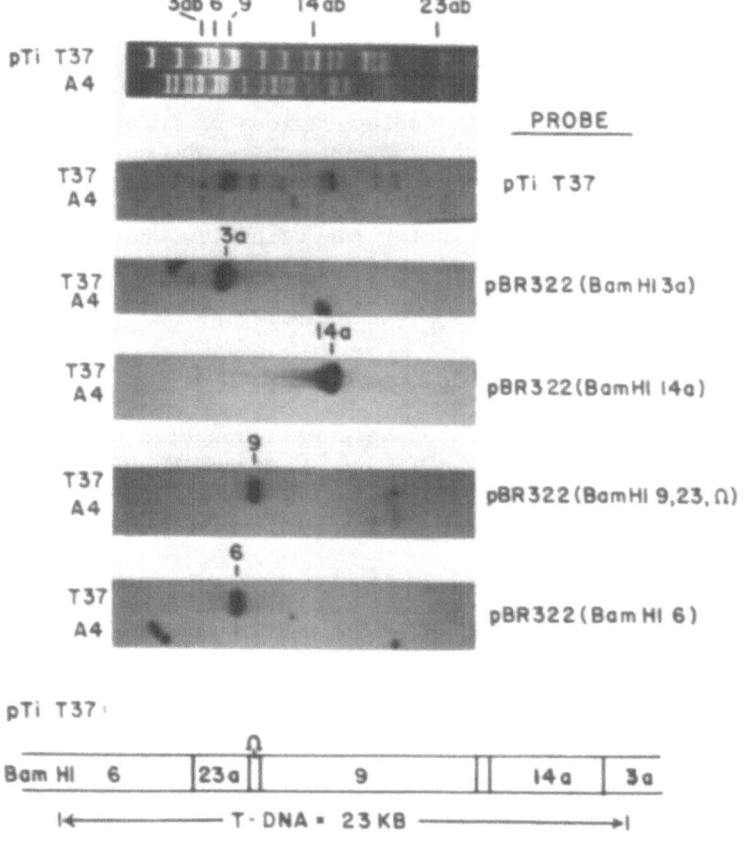

Figure 1. pTi T37 T-DNA probe hybridization to pTi T37 DNA vs.
A. rhizogenes A4 plasmid DNA. Plasmid DNA was isolated
from A. tumefaciens strain A208 (containing pTi T37)
and from A. rhizogenes strain A4 by the method of
Currier and Nester (1976). Plasmid DNAs were digested
to completion with Bam HI (Biolabs) and 2 ug per track
(five replicates) fractionated by horizontal agarose
gel electrophoresis (Sciaky et al., 1978). The top
track shows the fragment pattern visualized by ethidium
bromide staining and UV illumination. Relevant bands
of the pTi T37 digest are numbered. Southern blots of
five tracks, prepared as described (Chilton et al.,
1978), were hybridized with the indicated plasmid DNAs,
labelled by nick translation. Hybridization and wash
conditions were those of Thomashow et al., (1980): 68°,
3 x SSC. Bands of hybridization were visualized by
autoradiography on Kodak X-ray film for 3-18 hours.
The location of the four probe fragments on pTi T37
T-DNA is shown on the fragment map at the bottom of
the figure.

has confirmed the feasibility of the approach. The remaining
unsolved problem is that of bringing about expression of foreign
genes introduced into plants by such vectors. At present no such
expression has been reported; chimeric gene constructions with
T-DNA promoters attached to coding regions of foreign genes are
under construction and testing at present. The development of
dominant markers selectable in planta will provide a superior
solution to the problem of finding transformed plant cells. Perhaps
the most intriguing question for the future is whether T-DNA will
possess important biological advantages as a vector, or whether
small plasmids can be constructed and in vitro transformation
procedures devised to achieve the same end at comparable efficiency.

ACKNOWLEDGMENTS

Unpublished research discussed here was supported by American
Cancer Society grant NP194, D. O. E. Contract ERa0889 and U. S. D.
A. grant 59-2294-1-1-640-0 to M. D. C.; N. S. F. grant PCM-8104064
to A. N. B.; and C. N. R. S. grants ATP and AI 032750 to J. T.

K. L. B., A. J. M. M. and M. W. B. were supported by postdoctoral
fellowships from Monsanto Company; A. D. F. was supported by a
predoctoral fellowship from C. N. R. A. (France).

REFERENCES

Barton, K. A., Binns, A. N., Matzke, A. J. M. and Chilton, M.-D.,
    Regeneration of complete tobacco plants containing genetically
    engineered T-DNA from pTi T37. Submitted (1982).
Bevan, M. W. and Chilton, M.-D., Nopaline T-DNA encodes 13 transcripts
    in BT37 tumor tissue. Submitted (1982).
Binns, A. N., Sciaky, D. and Wood, H. N., Variation in hormone
    autonomy and regenerative potential of cells transformed by
    strain A66 of Agrobacterium tumefaciens is due to a mutation
    in T-DNA. Submitted (1982).
Binns, A. N., Wood, H. N. and Braun, A. C., 1981, Suppression of the
    tumorous state in crown gall teratomas of tobacco: a clonal
    analysis, Differentiation, 19:97.
Chilton, M.-D., Drummond, M. H., Merlo, D. J., Sciaky, D., Montoya,
    A. L., Gordon, M. P. and Nester, E. W., 1977, Stable incorpora-
    tion of plasmid DNA into higher plant cells: the molecular
    basis of crown gall tumorigenesis, Cell, 11:263.
Chilton, M.-D., Montoya, A. L., Merlo, D. J., Drummond, M. H.,
    Nutter, R. C., Gordon, M. P. and Nester, E. W., 1978, Restric-
    tion endonuclease mapping of a plasmid that confers oncogenicity
    upon Agrobacterium tumefaciens strain B6-806, Plasmid, 1:254.
Chilton, M.-D., Saiki, R. K., Yadav, N., Gordon, M. P. and Quétier,
    F., 1980, T-DNA from Agrobacterium Ti plasmid is in the nuclear
    fraction of crown gall tumor cells, Proc. Natl. Acad. Sci. USA,
    77:2693.

Chilton, M.-D., Tepfer, D. A., Petit, A., David, C., Casse-Delbart,
    F. and Tempé, J., 1982, Agrobacterium rhizogenes inserts T-DNA
    into the genomes of the host plant root cells. Nature (Lond.),
    295:432.
Currier, T. C. and Nester, E. W., 1976, Isolation of covalently
    closed circular DNA of high molecular weight from bacteria,
    Anal. Biochem., 66:431.
Drummond, M. H., Gordon, M. P., Nester, E. W. and Chilton, M.-D.,
    1977, Foreign DNA of bacterial plasmid origin is transcribed
    in crown gall tumors, Nature (Lond.), 269:535.
Garfinkel, D. J., Simpson, R. B., Ream, L. W., White, F. F., Gordon,
    M. P. and Nester, E. W., 1981, Genetic analysis of crown gall:
    fine structure map of the T-DNA by site-directed mutagenesis,
    Cell, 27:143.
Gelvin, S. B., Gordon, M. P., Nester, E. W. and Aronson, A. A.,
    1981, Transcription of the Agrobacterium Ti plasmid in the
    bacterium and in crown gall tumors, Plasmid, 6:17.
Gelvin, S., Thomashow, M. F., McPherson, J. C., Gordon, M. P.
    and Nester, E. W., 1982, Sizes and map positions of several
    plasmid DNA encoded transcripts in octopine-type crown gall
    tumors. Proc. Natl. Acad. Sci. USA, 79:76.
Gurley, W. B., Kemp, J. D., Albert, M. J., Sutton, D. W. and Callis,
    J., 1979, Transcription of Ti plasmid-derived sequences in
    three octopine-type tumor lines, Proc. Natl. Acad. Sci. USA,
    76:2828.
Hernalsteens, J. P., Van Vliet, F., De Beuckeleer, M., Depicker, A.,
    Engler, G., Lemmers, M., Holsters, M., Van Montagu, M. and
    Schell, J., 1980, The Agrobacterium tumefaciens Ti plasmid
    as a host vector system introducing foreign DNA in plant cells,
    Nature (Lond.), 287:654.
Holsters, M., Silva, B., Van Vliet, F., Genetello, C., De Block, M.,
    Dhaese, P., Depicker, A., Inze, D., Engler, G., Villarroel,
    R., Van Montagu, M. and Schell, J., 1980, The functional
    organization of the nopaline A. tumefaciens plasmid pTi C58,
    Plasmid, 3:212.
Leemans, J., Deblaere, R., Willmitzer, L., De Greve, H., Hernalsteens,
    J. P., Van Montagu, M. and Schell, J., 1982, Genetic identi-
    fication of functions of T_L-DNA transcripts in octopine crown
    galls, The EMBO Journal, 1:147.
Leemans, J., Shaw, C., Deblaere, R., De Greve, H., Hernalsteens,
    J. P., Maes, M., Van Montagu, M. and Schell, J., 1981, Site
    specific mutagenesis of Agrobacterium Ti plasmids and transfer
    of genes to plant cells, J. Mol. Appl. Genet., 1:149.
Lemmers, M., De Beuckeleer, M., Holsters, M., Zambryski, P.,
    Hernalsteens, J. P., Van Montagu, M. and Schell, J., 1980,
    Internal organization, boundaries and integration of Ti
    plasmid DNA in nopaline crown gall tumors, J. Mol. Biol.,
    144:353.
Matzke, A. J. M. and Chilton, M.-D., 1981, Site specific insertion
    of genes into T-DNA of the Agrobacterium Ti plasmid: an

approach to genetic engineering of higher plant cells, J. Mol. Appl. Genet., 1:39.

Murai, N. and Kemp, J. D., 1982, Octopine synthase mRNA isolated from sunflower crown gall callus is homologous to the Ti plasmid of Agrobacterium tumefaciens, Proc. Natl. Acad. Sci. USA, 79:86.

Ooms, G., Hooykaas, P. J. J., Moolenaar, G., and Schilperoort, R. A., 1981, Crown gall plant tumors of abnormal morphology induced by Agrobacterium tumefaciens carrying mutated octopine Ti plasmids: analysis of T-DNA functions, Gene, 14:33.

Otten, L., De Greve, H., Hernalsteens, J. P., Van Montague, M., Scheider, O., Straub, J. and Schell, J., 1981, Mendelian transmission of genes introduced into plants by the Ti plasmids of Agrobacterium tumefaciens, Mol. Gen. Genet., 183:209.

Petit, A., Delhaye, S., Tempe, J. and Morel, G., 1970, Recherches sur les guanidines des tissues de crown gall. Mise en évidence d'une relation biochimique spécifique entre les souches d'Agrobacterium tumefaciens et les tumeurs qu'elles induisent, Physiol. Vég., 8:205.

Schröder, J., Schröder, G., Huisman, H., Schilperoort, R. A. and Schell, J., 1981, The mRNA for lysopine dehydrogenase in plant tumor cells is complementary to a Ti plasmid fragment, FEBS Lett., 129:166.

Sciaky, D., Montoya, A. L. and Chilton, M.-D., 1978, Fingerprints of Agrobacterium Ti plasmids, Plasmid, 1:238.

Simpson, R., O'Hara, P., Lichtenstein, C., Montoya, A. L., Kwok, W., Gordon, M. P. and Nester, E. W., 1982, The DNA from A6S/2 tumor contains scrambled Ti plasmid sequence near its junction with plant DNA, Cell, 29:1005.

Tepfer, D. A. and Tempé, J., 1981, Production d'agropine par des racine formées sous l'action d'Agrobacterium rhizogenes souche A4, C. R. Acad. Sci. Paris, 292:153.

Thomashow, M. F., Nutter, R., Montoya, A. L., Gordon, M. P. and Nester, E. W., 1980, Integration and organization of Ti plasmid sequences in crown gall tumors, Cell 19:729.

Van Larebeke, N., Engler, G., Holsters, M., Van den Elsacker, S., Zaenen, I., Schilperoort, R. A. and Schell, J., 1974, Large plasmid in Agrobacterium tumefaciens essential for crown gall inducing ability, Nature (Lond.), 252:169.

Van Larebeke, N., Genetello, C., Schell, J., Schilperoort, R. A., Hermans, A. K., Hernalsteens, J. P. and Van Montagu, M., 1975, Acquisition of tumor inducing ability by non-oncogenic agrobacteria as a result of plasmid transfer, Nature (Lond.), 255:742.

Van Slogteren, G. M. S., Hooykaas, P. J. J., Planqué, K. and de Groot, B., 1982, The lysopinedehydrogenase gene used as a marker for the selection of octopine crown gall cells, Plant Molec. Biol., 1:133.

Watson, B., Currier, T. C., Gordon, M. P., Chilton, M.-D. and

Nester, E. W., 1975, Plasmid required for virulence of
    Agrobacterium tumefaciens, J. Bacteriol. 123:255.

White, F. F., Ghidossi, G., Gordon, M. P. and Nester, E. W., 1982,
    Tumor induction by Agrobacterium rhizogenes involves the
    transfer of plasmid DNA to the plant genome, Proc. Natl.
    Acad. Sci. USA, 79:3193.

White, F. F. and Nester, E. W., 1980a, Hairy root: plasmid encodes
    virulence traits in Agrobacterium rhizogenes, J. Bacteriol.,
    141:1134.

White, F. F. and Nester, E. W., 1980b, Relationship of plasmids
    responsible for hairy root and crown gall tumorigenicity,
    J. Bacteriol., 144:710.

Willmitzer, L., De Beuckeleer, M., Lemmers, M., Van Montagu, M.
    and Schell, J., 1980, DNA from Ti plasmid present in nucleus
    and absent from plastids of crown gall plant cells, Nature
    (Lond.), 287:359.

Willmitzer, L., Otten, L., Simons, G., Schmalenbach, W., Schröder,
    J., Schröder, G., Van Montagu, M., de Vos, G. and Schell, J.,
    1981, Nuclear and polysomal transcripts of T-DNA in octopine
    crown gall suspension and callus cultures, Mol. Gen. Genet.,
    182:255.

Willmitzer, L., Simons, G. and Schell, J., 1982, The T_L-DNA in
    octopine crown gall tumors codes for seven well-defined
    polyadenylated transcripts, The EMBO Journal, 1:139.

Wullems, G. J., Molendijk, L., Ooms, G., and Schilperoort, R. A.,
    1981a, Differential expression of crown gall tumor markers
    in transformants obtained after in vitro Agrobacterium tume-
    faciens induced transformation of cell wall regenerating
    protoplasts derived from Nicotiana tabacum, Proc. Natl.
    Acad. Sci. USA, 78:4344.

Wullems, G. J., Molendijk, L., Ooms, G. and Schilperoort, R. A.,
    1981b, Retention of tumor markers in F1 progeny plants from
    in vitro induced octopine and nopaline tumor tissue, Cell,
    24:719.

Yadav, N. S., Postle, K., Saiki, R. K., Thomashow, M. F. and
    Chilton, M.-D., 1980, T-DNA of a crown gall teratoma is
    covalently joined to host plant DNA, Nature (Lond.),
    287:458.

Yadav, N. S., Vanderleyden, J., Bennet, D., Barnes, W. M. and
    Chilton, M.-D., 1982, Short direct repeats flank the T-DNA
    on a nopaline Ti plasmid, Proc. Natl. Acad. Sci. USA,
    in press.

Yang, F. M., Montoya, A. L., Merlo, D. J., Drummond, M. H.,
    Chilton, M.-D., Nester, E. W. and Gordon, M. P., 1980,
    Foreign DNA sequences in crown gall teratomas and their
    fate during the loss of the tumorous traits, Mol. Gen.
    Genet., 177:704.

Yang, F. M. and Simpson, R. B., 1981, Revertant seedlings from
    crown gall tumors retain a portion of the bacterial Ti
    plasmid sequences, Proc. Natl. Acad. Sci. USA, 78:4151.

Zaenen, I., Van Larebeke, N., Teuchy, H., Van Montagu, M. and
    Schell, J., 1974, Supercoiled circular DNA in crown gall
    inducing Agrobacterium strains, J. Mol. Biol., 86:109.
Zambryski, P., Depicker, A., Kruger, K. and Goodman, H. M., 1982,
    Tumor induction by Agrobacterium tumefaciens: analysis of
    the boundaries of T-DNA, J. Molec. Appl. Genet., 1:361.
Zambryski, P., Holsters, M., Kruger, K., Depicker, A., Schell,
    J., Van Montagu, M. and Goodman, H., 1980, Tumor DNA
    structure in plant cells transformed by A. tumefaciens,
    Science, 209:1385.

THE CAULIFLOWER MOSAIC VIRUS MINICHROMOSOME

Tom Guilfoyle, Neil Olszewski, and Gretchen Hagen

Department of Botany
University of Minnesota
St. Paul, Minnesota 55108

INTRODUCTION

Plant viruses which contain DNA genomes have recently gained popularity as potential vehicles for introducing foreign DNA into plants (reviewed by Howell, 1982; Hohn et al., 1982). The most intensively studied of these DNA viruses is cauliflower mosaic virus (CaMV) which contains a double-stranded DNA genome of about 8 kilobases. The infective DNA purified from virus particles is circular, but not covalently closed (i.e., generally two to three site-specific discontinuities occur in the genome; Hull and Howell, 1978; Volovitch et al., 1978). One of the discontinuities occurs in the α-strand of CaMV DNA and is generally considered as map position 0/1 on the circular genome. The complementary or β-strand of CaMV DNA usually contains two discontinuities at map positions 0.20 and 0.53. In one case, however, the CM4-184 isolate of CaMV contains a deletion of about 421 base pairs in and around map position 0.20 which eliminates one of the discontinuities in the α-strand. In the virus particle, the DNA is surrounded by a protein capsid shell (reviewed by Hohn et al., 1982), but additional proteins such as histones or other chromosomal proteins are not associated with the encapsidated DNA.

Transcription of CaMV DNA occurs in a clockwise direction on the circular genome and appears to be asymmetric since stable RNA transcripts are exclusively coded by the α-strand of CaMV DNA (Hull et al., 1979; Howell and Hull, 1978). Two major transcripts of CaMV DNA have been identified and characterized (Odell et al., 1981; Covey et al., 1981; Howell, 1981; Dudley et al., 1982). One of these transcripts is full genome in length (approximately 8 kilobases), and the 5'-end of this transcript is located just counterclockwise

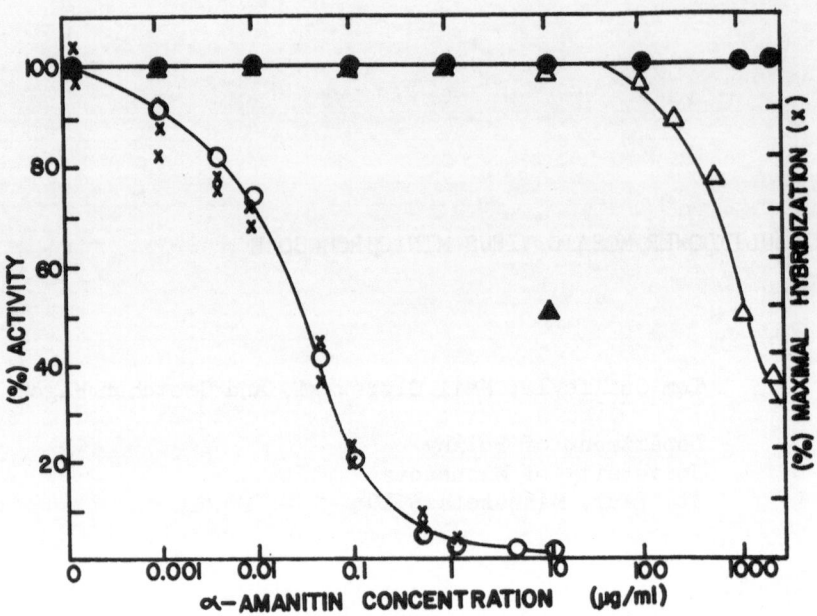

Fig. 1.   Inhibition of RNA polymerase II activity and viral-specific
transcription by α-amanitin. In vitro transcription was
carried out as described by Guilfoyle (1980) with nuclei
purified from CaMV-infected turnip leaves (Olszewski et al.,
1982) or with purified RNA polymerases. Inhibition curves
are displayed for purified turnip RNA polymeras I (●——●)
and II (○——○) and cauliflower RNA polymerase III (△——△).
The point of 50% inhibition of a more α-amanitin sensitive
plant class III enzyme (e.g., wheat germ) is shown (▲).
Hybridization (% maximal at 0 µg/ml α-amanitin) of ^{32}P-
labeled in vitro RNA transcripts to CaMV DNA immobilized
on nitrocellulose (x).

to the discontinuity in the α-strand of CaMV DNA. The function of
this large transcript is unknown, but it may be possible that this
RNA is processed into smaller mRNAs that code for the viral coat
protein and other unidentified viral-coded polypeptides. The second
major transcript is initiated at around map position 0.7 and has the
same 3'-end as the larger transcript. This smaller transcript codes
for a polypeptide called P66 which is associated with viral inclusion
bodies (Odell and Howell, 1980).

We have initiated studies to determine the intracellular localization, the cellular machinery, and the nature of the CaMV genome
during transcription and replication of the viral DNA.

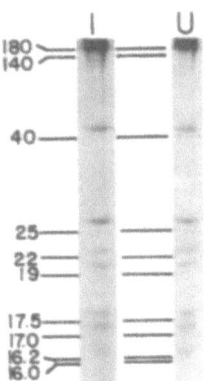

Fig. 2. Subunit structures of turnip nuclear RNA polymerase II
purified from uninfected and CaMV-infected turnip leaves.
Enzymes were purified by the methods described by Jendrisak
and Guilfoyle (1978) with the addition of heparin-Sepharose
chromatography as a final purification procedure. Subunit
molecular weights are given in kilodaltons next to the
stained gels (15% polyacrylamide containing dodecyl sulfate;
Laemmli, 1970). I: CaMV-infected; U: Uninfected.

RESULTS AND DISCUSSION

     Nuclei purified from CaMV-infected, but not uninfected, turnip
leaves synthesize RNA transcripts in vitro which hybridize to CaMV
DNA restriction fragments encompassing the entire viral genome, but
to only the α-strand of CaMV DNA (Guilfoyle, 1980). Viral-specific
transcription in isolated nuclei is inhibited by low concentrations
of α-amanitin (Guilfoyle, 1980), and the progressive decrease in
viral-specific in vitro RNA synthesis in isolated nuclei parallels
the inhibitory action of the fungal toxin on purified turnip nuclear
RNA polymerase II activity (Fig. 1). These results indicate that
host RNA polymerase II is largely, if not entirely, responsible for
transcription of the viral genome. Viral infection results in no
readily observable alteration in host RNA polymerase II; the subunit
structures of RNA polymerase II purified from uninfected and CaMV-
infected turnip leaves are identical (Fig. 2). The salt optimum for
the production of viral-specific in vitro RNA transcripts in isolated
nuclei is identical to that of chromatin-associated RNA polymerase
II (Guilfoyle, 1980), and this observation suggests that the transcriptionally active form of CaMV DNA may possess a chromatin
structure.

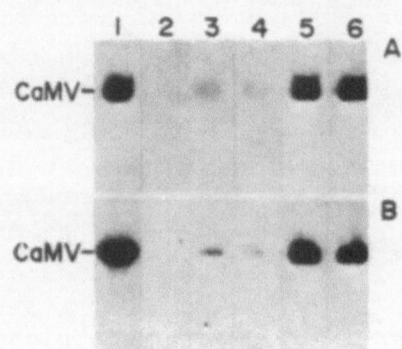

Fig. 3. Effect of inhibitors on viral-specific in vitro tran-
         scription in isolated nuclei (A) and purified CaMV tran-
         scription complexes (B). In vitro transcription was
         carried out, and the RNA was purified and hybridized to
         CaMV DNA immobilized on nitrocellulose filters (Guilfoyle,
         1980). Transcription conditions were: (1) no inhibitors;
         (2) 1 µg/ml α-amanitin; (3) 50 µg/ml Actinomycin D; (4) 200
         µg/ml Actinomycin D; (5) 10 µg/ml heparin; and (6) 0.1%
         Sarkosyl.

        To further investigate the nature of the transcriptionally
active viral DNA template, we prepared a turnip nuclear lysate
enriched for viral transcription complexes (Olszewski et al., 1982).
The purified CaMV DNA complexes produced a typical nucleosome pattern
when digested with micrococcal nuclease, suggesting that the CaMV
DNA in the complexes is associated with host chromosomal proteins
(i.e., histones). In vitro transcription with purified CaMV DNA
complexes has characteristics identical with that observed for
viral-specific transcription in isolated nuclei from infected
turnip leaves. In both systems, in vitro transcription is asymmetric (Guilfoyle, 1980; Olszewski et al., 1982), inhibited by low
concentrations of α-amanitin and Actinomycin D, and refractory to
inhibition by the transcription initiation inhibitors, heparin and
Sarkosyl (Fig. 3). These results indicate that with both isolated
nuclei and purified CaMV transcription complexes, in vitro transcription is catalyzed by turnip nuclear RNA polymerase II, is
DNA-dependent, and represents propagation of RNA transcripts that
were most likely initiated in vivo prior to cellular disruption.

        To determine the structure of CaMV DNA in these transcription
complexes, the purified complexes were deproteinized and the CaMV
DNA was analyzed. In contrast to virus encapsidated CaMV DNA which
possesses characteristic site-specific discontinuities, the CaMV
DNA purified from these transcription complexes is, largely, covalently closed circles. The covalently closed, supercoiled nature

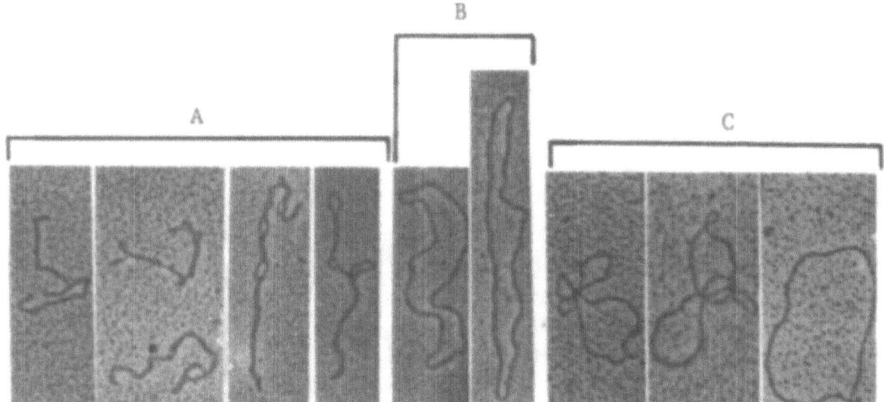

Fig. 4.   Electron micrographs of supercoiled and open circular CaMV
           DNAs.   Molecules were prepared for electron microscopy by
           the aqueous spreading technique of Davis et al., 1971.
           Grids were stained with uranyl acetate, shadowed with
           platinum-palladium and photographed in a Zeiss electron
           microscope.   A: supercoiled CaMV DNA purified from mini-
           chromosomes; B: relaxed circular CaMV DNA purified from
           minichromosomes; and C: "knotted" and relaxed circular
           CaMV DNA purified from virus particles.

of the CaMV DNA circles associated with transcription complexes is
supported by a wide range of experimental evidence including:
(1) increased mobility of this DNA on agarose gels compared to open
circular and linear forms of CaMV DNA; (2) resistance of this DNA
to heat denaturation (i.e., the double-stranded DNA does not denature
into single-strands); (3) greater density of this DNA on cesium
chloride density gradients containing ethidium bromide; (4) relax-
ation of this DNA by wheat germ topoisomerase (Olszewski et al.,
1982), and (5) appearance of supercoiled CaMV DNA molecules in
electron micrographs (Fig. 4).   From the above results, we conclude
that CaMV DNA present in transcription complexes is a covalently
closed circular genome associated with host nucleosomal proteins
and host nuclear RNA polymerase II.   This complex can appropriately
be referred to as a minichromosome.

     The CaMV minichromosome offers a model system to study tran-
scription and possibly replication in higher plants.   The isolation
of transcriptionally active CaMV minichromosomes provides a system
where a defined plant DNA sequence that is extrachromosomal and
present in multiple copies per cell can be studied in its native
chromatin structure.   This system may allow identification of
components associated with RNA polymerase II transcription complexes
and of factors required for faithful transcription in vitro on a
native chromatin template.

ACKNOWLEDGMENTS

This work was funded by NIH and USDA/SEA Competitive Research
Grants. N. O. is an NIH predoctoral trainee. G. H. is an NIH
postdoctoral fellow.

REFERENCES

Covey, S. N., Lomonossoff, G. P., and Hull, R., 1981, Characterization
        of cauliflower mosaic virus DNA sequences which encode major
        polyadenylated transcripts, Nucl. Acids Res., 9:6735.
Davis, R. W., Simon, M., and Davidson, N., 1971, Electron microscope
        heteroduplex methods for mapping regions of base sequence
        homology in nucleic acids, Methods in Enzymology, 21D:413.
Dudley, R. K., Odell, J. T., and Howell, S. H., 1982, Structure and
        5'-termini of the large and 19S RNA transcripts encoded by
        the cauliflower mosaic virus genome, Virology, 117:19.
Guilfoyle, T. J., 1980, Transcription of cauliflower mosaic virus
        genome in isolated nuclei from turnip leaves, Virology, 107:
        71.
Hohn, T., Richards, K., and Lebeurier, G., 1982, Cauliflower mosaic
        virus on its way to becoming a useful plant vector, Current
        Topics in Microbiology and Immunology, 96:193.
Howell, S. H., 1981, Ultraviolet mapping of RNA transcripts encoded
        by the cauliflower mosaic virus genome, Virology, 112:488.
Howell, S. H., 1982, Plant molecular vehicles: potential vectors for
        introducing foreign DNA into plants, Ann. Rev. Plant Physiol.,
        33:609.
Howell, S. H. and Hull, R., 1978, Replication of cauliflower mosaic
        virus and transcription of its genome in turnip leaf proto-
        plasts, Virology, 86:468.
Hull, R., Covey, S. N., Stanley, J., and Davies, J. W., 1979, The
        polarity of the cauliflower mosaic virus genome, Nucl. Acids
        Res., 7:669.
Hull, R. and Howell, S. H., 1978, Structure of the cauliflower mosaic
        virus genome. II. Variation in DNA structure and sequence
        between isolates, Virology, 86:482.
Jendrisak, J. J. and Guilfoyle, T. J., 1978, Eukaryotic RNA polymer-
        ases: comparative subunit structures, immunological propert-
        ies, and α-amanitin sensitivities of the class II enzymes
        from higher plants, Biochemistry, 17:1322.
Laemmli, U. K., 1970, Cleavage of structural proteins during assembly
        of the head of bacteriophage T4, Nature, 227:680.
Odell, J. T., Dudley, R. K., and Howell, S. H., 1981, Structure of
        the 19S RNA transcript encoded by the cauliflower mosaic
        virus genome, Virology, 111:377.
Odell, J. T. and Howell, S. H., 1980, The identification, mapping
        and characterization of mRNA for P66, a cauliflower mosaic
        virus-coded protein, Virology, 102:349.

Olszewski, N., Hagen, G., and Guilfoyle, T. J., 1982, A transcript-
        ionally active, covalently closed minichromosome of cauli-
        flower mosaic virus DNA isolated from infected turnip leaves,
        Cell, 29:395.
Volovitch, M., Drugeon, G., and Yot, P., 1978, Studies on the single-
        stranded discontinuities of the cauliflower mosaic virus
        genome, Nucl. Acids Res., 5:2913.

THE POTENTIAL OF CAULIFLOWER MOSAIC VIRUS AS A GENE VECTOR

R. Hull and S. N. Covey

John Innes Institute
Norwich, England

INTRODUCTION

Cauliflower mosaic virus (CaMV) is the type member of the
caulimoviruses, a group of plant viruses which have genomes of
double-stranded DNA. CaMV is the most studied member of the group
as it can be purified most easily. The encapsidated viral DNA is a
circular molecule of 8Kbp which has two unusual features. Many of
the molecules have a twisted conformation (Hull et al., 1976; Hull,
1981; Hohn et al., 1982) which is not due to them being covalently
closed. The DNA of all CaMV isolates has site specific
discontinuities (Hull & Howell 1978; Volovitch et al., 1978) which
have been shown by sequencing to be overlaps (Franck et al., 1980;
Richards et al., 1981). Most CaMV isolates have three
discontinuities (gaps), one [G1] in one strand (the α strand) (Fig
1) and two [G2 and G3] in the other, giving the β and γ strands.
One isolate (CM4-184) which has a deletion in the region of one
discontinuity [G3] thus has only two discontinuities, one in each
strand (Hull & Howell, 1978). The DNAs of other caulimoviruses also
have discontinuities, all with one in one strand, some with two in
the complementary strand, others with three (Hull and Donson, 1982).

The DNA of two isolates of CaMV has been sequenced (Franck et al.,
1980; Gardner et al., 1981). Only the α strand appears to be
transcribed (Howell and Hull, 1978) and the sequence shows six (or
possibly eight) closely spaced and even overlapping open reading
frames in this strand. There are two non-coding regions, one small
(about 100bp) [IR2] between open reading frames V and VI and one
large (about 1000bp)[IR1] (Fig.1) which traverses the discontinuity.

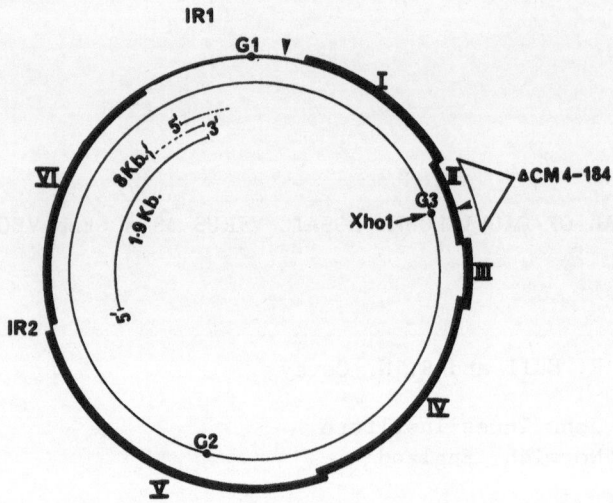

Fig. 1. Features of the CaMV genome described in the text. The
         outer ring represents the α strand with the single dis-
         continuity [G1], the 6 open reading frames (I-VI) and
         the two intergenic regions [IR1 and IR2]. Also shown
         are the two sites [▼] where insertions have been made
         and the region deleted in CM4-184. The next ring rep-
         resents the complementary strand and shows the positions
         of the other two discontinuities [G2,G3]. Within this
         are shown the cutting site of <u>Xho</u> I and the 3'- and
         5'-ends of the 8Kb and 1.9Kb transcripts.

CaMV DNA (and that of other caulimoviruses) has been suggested as
a possible candidate for carrying 'foreign' DNA into and
expressing in plant cells (see Szeto et al., 1977; Hull, 1978;
Howell, 1982). Among the advantages of the CaMV system are that it
replicates in most cells of susceptible plants, it reaches a high
copy number (estimated as about 50,000 per cell) and it is
expressed efficiently. Some of the disadvantages will be
discussed later.

We have two main approaches to developing a higher plant gene
vector from CaMV DNA. In the first, attempts are being made to
find sites in the full-length or nearly full-length CaMV genome
into which foreign DNA can be inserted without impairing the
ability for replication and expression. In the second, the
transcriptional and replication strategies of the virus are being
studied and the DNA sequences which control these functions
identified.

Inserting Foreign DNA

The effect of mutagenising CaMV DNA by either insertion or deletion is usually the loss of infectivity. However, two sites have been found at which inserting DNA does not result in the loss of infectivity. In the large intergenic region, IRl,(Fig.1) an 8bp Eco Rl linker has been ligated into an Alu l site (Howell et al., 1981)and the DNA was still infectious. Various bacterial DNA fragments have been inserted into the unique Xho I site in open reading frame II (Shepherd et al., 1981; Gronenborn et al., 1981). When 60bp and 250bp fragments were inserted, CaMV DNA was infectious and the fragments retained, at least for a few transfers. Larger insertions of 500bp and 1200bp resulted in loss of infectivity. This limit to the size of "foreign" DNA is thought to reflect limits on encapsidation which, in turn, may be needed for cell to cell spread.

As noted above, CaMV isolate CM4-184 is a natural deletion variant. The deletion of 421bp (Howarth et al., 1981) is around the Xho I site (Fig.1) at which insertions can be made in non-deleted strains. J.R. Penswick in our laboratory has constructed deletions of 126bp and 402bp flanked by Xho I sticky ends in a previously non-deleted isolate. Both these deleted molecules are infectious and the larger is being used for inserting DNA the size of small genes

CaMV Transcripts

Two species of poly[A]+ RNA, about 8Kb and 1.9Kb long, are the most abundant CaMV-specific RNAs 18-22 days after inoculation (Covey and Hull, 1981; Odell et al., 1981). The 1.9Kb RNA is transcribed from the region of CaMV DNA which includes open reading frame VI (Fig.1 (Odell and Howell, 1980; Covey and Hull, 1981; Odell et al., 1981), predicted to encode a protein of 61,000 MW (Franck et al., 1980). This RNA has been translated in vitro to produce a protein of 62,000-66,000 MW (Al Ani et al., 1980; Odell and Howell, 1980; Covey and Hull, 1981). Covey and Hull (1981) showed, by peptide fingerprint analysis, that the 62,000 MW polypeptide synthesised in vitro using hybrid-selected CaMV-specific RNA was very similar to a major protein, of the same size, associated with virus inclusion bodies isolated from infected leaves. The 8Kb RNA is a full-length transcript of the DNA α strand (Covey and Hull, 1981).

More precise mapping of these RNAs using the SI nuclease protection procedure revealed that their termini were located in the intergenic regions IR1 and IR2 (Fig.1.) (Covey et al., 1981; Dudley et al., 1982). We (Covey et al.,1981) have sequenced the 5'-end of the 1.9Kb inclusion body protein mRNA by primer extension in the presence of dideoxy nucleoside triphosphates (Fig.2a). The

```
              Open reading frame VI
              ATAGTTTTCCGATGACGGATAAATTTGTGTAGAGACCTCTGACTCTTTT-
5' -ACTTGTGGCTGATATCAAAAGGCTACTGCCTATTTAAACACATCTCTGGAGACTGAGAAAA-
              •
              5713


     5'        fmet^glu_asn^ile_glu_lys        protein
       GACCUCCAAGCAUGGAGAACAUAGAAAAACU- 3' messenger RNA

  -AGTCTGGAGGTTCGTACCTCTTGTATCTTTTTGA- 5' DNA coding strand
  -TCAGACCTCCAAGCATGGAGAACATAGAAAAACT- 3' DNA non-coding strand
     •              •
     5765          5776
```

(b)

```
 orf VI
 TTTCGTTCACCTAACT
-AAAGCAAGTGGATTGATGTGATATCTCCACTGACGTAAGGGATGACGCACAATCCCACTATCCTT-

                        ...............5'-end 8kb RNA
-CGCAAGACCCTTCCTCTATATAAGGAAGTTCATTTCATTTGGAGAGGACACGCTGAAATCACCAG-


-TCTCTCTCTACAAATCTATCTCTCTCTATAATAATGTGTGAGTAGTTCCCAGATAAGGGAATTAG-


-GGTTCTTATAGGGTTTCGCTCATGTGTTGAGCATATAAGAAACCCTTAGTATGTATTTGTATTTG-

                                        ..............
-TAAAATACTTCTATCAATAAAATTTCTAATTCCTAAAACCAAAATCCAGTACTAAAATCCAGATC-

 ...3'-end 8kb & 1.9kb RNAs
-TCCTAAAGTCCCTATAGATCTTTG-
                  •
                  7672
```

(a)

Fig. 2. Nucleotide sequences around the termini of the two major
         transcripts. (a) The 5'-terminal sequence of the 1.9Kb
         inclusion body protein mRNA is aligned above the DNA
         strand encoding it with the AT-rich region (underlined)
         situated about 30 nucleotides upstream. (b) Part of the
         DNA sequence of IR1 showing the positions of the 8Kb 5'-
         and 3'-termini and the 3'-terminus of the 1.9Kb mRNA.
         Putative CAT and TATA boxes and the poly(A) signal se-
         quence are underlined. Nucleotides are numbered accor-
         ding to Franck et al., [1980].

1.9Kb mRNA has a leader of eleven nucleotides which exhibits some
complementarity with a consensus sequence at the 3'-end of 18S
rRNA. About 30 nucleotides upstream of the putative cap-site is an
AT-rich sequence similar to the TATA box found in the promotor
region of many eucaryotic genes. This might indicate, as suggested
by Howell (1981), that transcription of this messenger is promoted
from within IR2.

The 3'-end of the 1.9Kb RNA maps within IR1 and is co-terminal with
that of the 8Kb RNA and close to a putative terminator-associated
poly(A) signal sequence AATAAA. However, the 5'-end of the 8Kb RNA
is located about 200 nucleotides upstream of its 3'-end (Covey et
al., 1981); it is therefore longer than the DNA α strand from which
it is transcribed and has a terminal repeat of about 200
nucleotides. Within IR1 and upstream of the 8Kb RNA 5'-terminus are
DNA sequences with strong positional and sequence homology with
characterised encaryotic promoter regions (Fig.2b).

The mechanism of transcription of the 8Kb CaMV RNA apparently has to
overcome two obstacles. Firstly the polymerase has to pass the
polyadenylation signal before continuing around the rest of the
DNA. Having gone round the DNA, the polymerase then has to
terminate the second time it passes the polyadenylation signal; thus
the sequences around the overlap region effect transcriptional
control by means not yet understood. The second obstacle is that the
transcript apparently has to traverse the discontinuity in the
strand. This has led to the search for covalently-closed CaMV DNA
molecules among the non-encapsidated DNA.

CaMV Non-Encapsidated DNAs

There are at least eight different molecular species of CaMV DNA
present in total DNA extracted from infected leaves (Covey & Hull,
in preparation). The DNA isolation methods do not release
significant amounts of encapsidated DNA and very little of the DNA
forms found in CaMV particles appear to be free in the cell. Most
of CaMV DNA species are linear molecules delineated to a greater or
lesser extent by the discontinuities. In fact, all of the species
expected from the three discontinuities have been found, but two,
one from G1 to G2 in a counter clockwise direction (see Fig.1) and
the other from G1 to G3 in the same direction, preponderate.
As well as these forms, CaMV DNA exists as covalently closed
circular molecule within the nucleus (Menissier et al., 1982;
Olszewski et al.,1982). Olszewski et al., (1982) have shown that the
covalently closed CaMVDNA can exist as a minichromosome which is
transcriptionally active thus explaining how the 8Kb transcript
apparently passes G1.

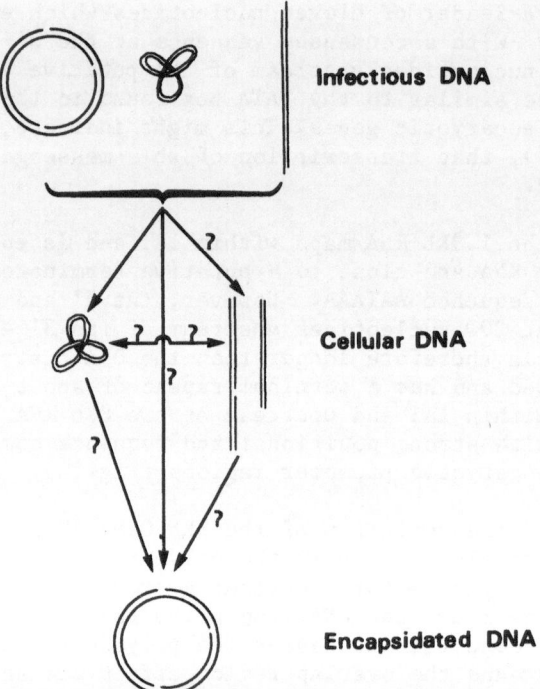

Fig. 3.   Replication of CaMV DNA. The infectious DNA is either
           the gapped circular form or linear and religated cir-
           cular molecules from cloned DNA. Supercoiled and
           various linear forms are found within the cell but
           only gapped circular molecules are encapsidated. The
           arrows indicate possible replication pathways; that
           without is the only one to be demonstrated.

CaMV DNA Replication

Little is known yet about the mechanism of CaMV DNA replication.
Shepherd et al. (1981) quote unpublished data suggesting that CaMV
replication takes place in the nucleus. From the observations
above and the fact that as well as virion DNA, cloned CaMV DNA is
infectious (Howell et al., 1980; Lebeurier et al., 1980) we can
draw up the scheme shown in Fig.3. This scheme raises the
question of why only the circular DNA with discontinuities is
encapsidated. It is possible that the discontinuities might prime
or control encapsidation and that only the full sized molecule
with discontinuities can form stable capsids. However, this
raises the question of the role of the unencapsidated linear
molecules. Among the various possibilities are that they might

be intermediates or premature terminations of DNA replication or be templates for some transcriptional events. If they are the former, it is interesting to note their association with discontinuities and to speculate that these regions might be associated with DNA replication.

The Future

We have briefly reviewed some of the observations pertinent to the development of CaMV DNA as a plant vector. Some of the disadvantages that a relatively unmodified CaMV DNA has as a vector have been mentioned above viz. the possible limitation on the size of inserts and the concomitant likely need for encapsidation for cell to cell spread. This problem might be overcome by the use of protoplasts. Other disadvantages include relatively limited host range and the production of symptoms (though this at present provides a good marker). The availability of various CaMV isolates with different symptom expression and of other caulimoviruses with different host ranges coupled with the use of recombitant DNA technology should enable us to identify which virus functions determine symptom expression and host range. This, together with knowledge of DNA sequences which control replication and transcription, should lead us to develop a broader host range, symptomless, non-integrating vector system.

REFERENCES

Al Ani, R., Pfeiffer, P., Whitechurch, O., Lesot, A., Lebeurier, G. & Hirth, L. 1980. A virus specified protein produced upon infection by cauliflower mosaic virus. Ann Virol (Institut Pasteur) 131E:33.

Covey, S.N. & Hull, R. 1981. Transcription of cauliflower mosaic virus DNA. Detection of transcripts, properties and location of the gene encoding the virus inclusion body protein. Virology 111:463.

Covey, S.N., Lomonossoff, G.P. & Hull, R. 1981. Characterisation of cauliflower mosaic virus DNA sequences which encode major polyadenylated transcripts. Nucl. Acids Res. 9:6735.

Dudley, R.K., Odell, J.T. and Howell, S.H. 1982. Structure and 5' termini of the large and 19S RNA transcripts encoded by the cauliflower mosaic virus genome. Virology 117:19.

Franck, A., Jonard, G., Richards, K., Hirth, L., & Guilley, H. 1980. Nucleotide sequence of cauliflower mosaic virus DNA. Cell 21:285.

Gardner, R.C., Howarth, A.J., Brown-Luedi, M., Shepherd, R.J. & Messing, J. 1981. The complete nucleotide sequence of an infectious clone of cauliflower mosaic virus by M13mp^7 shotgun sequencing. Nucl. Acids Res. 9:2871.

Gronenborn, B.,, Gardner, R.C., Schaefer, S., & Shepherd, R.J. 1981. Propagation of foreign DNA in plants using cauliflower mosaic virus as vector. Nature, London 294:773.

Hohn, T., Richards, K. and Lebeurier, G. 1982. Cauliflower mosaic virus on its way to becoming a useful plant vector. Current Topics in Microbiol & Immunol. 96:193.

Howarth, A.J., Gardner, R.C., Messing, J. & Shepherd, R.J. 1981. Nucleotide sequence of naturally occurring deletion mutants of cauliflower mosaic virus. Virology 112:678.

Howell, S.H. 1981. Ultraviolet mapping of RNA transcripts encoded by the cauliflower mosaic virus genome. Virology. 112:488.

Howell, S.H. 1982. Plant molecular vehicles: potential vectors for introducing foreign DNA into plants. Ann. Rev. Plant Physiol., 33:609.

Howell, S.H. & Hull, R. 1978. Replication of cauliflower mosaic virus and transcription of its genome in turnip leaf protoplasts. Virology 86:468.

Howell, S.H., Walker, L.L. & Dudley, R.K. 1980. Cloned cauliflower mosaic virus DNA infects turnips Brassica rapa. Science 208:1265.

Howell, S.H., Walker, L.L. & Walden, R.M. 1981. Rescue of in vitro generated mutants of cloned cauliflower mosaic virus genome in infected plants. Nature, Lond. 293: 483.

Hull, R. 1978. The possible use of plant viral DNAs in genetic manipulation in plants. Trends in Biochem. Sci.3:254.

Hull, R. 1981. Cauliflower mosaic virus DNA as a possible gene vector for higher plants. In Genetic Engineering in the Plant Sciences, ed. N.J. Panopoulos, pp 99-109, Praeger Scientific.

Hull, R. & Donson, J. 1982. Physical mapping of the DNAs of carnation etched ring and figwort mosaic viruses. J.Gen.Virol. 60:125.

Hull, R. & Howell, S.H. 1978. Structure of the cauliflower mosaic
    virus genome. II. Variation in DNA structure and sequence
    between isolates. Virology 86:482.

Hull, R., Shepherd, R.J. & Harvey, R.D. 1976. Cauliflower mosaic
    virus: an improved purification procedure and some properties
    of the virus particles. J.Gen.Virol. 31:93.

Lebeurier, G., Hirth, L., Hohn, T. & Hohn, B. 1980. Infectivities
    of native and cloned DNA of cauliflower mosaic virus. Gene
    12:139.

Menissier, J., Lebeurier, G. and Hirth, L. 1982. Free cauliflower
    mosaic virus supercoiled DNA in infected plants. Virology
    117:322.

Odell, J.T., Dudley, K & Howell, S.H. 1981. Structure of the 19S RNA
    transcript encoded by the cauliflower mosaic virus genome.
    Virology 111: 377.

Odell, J.T. & Howell, S.H. 1980.The identification, mapping and
    characterisation of messenger RNA for P66, a cauliflower mosaic
    virus coded protein. Virology 102:349.

Olszewski, N., Hagen, G. and Guilfoyle, T.J. 1982. A
    transcriptionally active, covalently closed minichromosome of
    cauliflower mosaic virus DNA isolated from infected turnip
    leaves. Cell, 29: 395.

Richards, K.F., Guilley, H. and Jonard, G. 1981. Further
    characterisation of the discontinuities in cauliflower mosaic
    virus DNA. FEBS. Lett. 134:67.

Shepherd, R.J., Gronenborn, B., Gardner, R. & Daubert, S.D.
    1981. Molecular cloning of foreign DNA in plants using
    cauliflower mosaic virus as a recombitant vector. In Genetic
    Engineering in the Plant Sciences, ed. N.J. Panapoulos, pp.
    255-257. Praeger Scientific.

Szeto, W.W., Hamer, D.H., Carlson, P.S. & Thomas, C.A. 1977.
    Cloning of cauliflower mosaic virus DNA in Escherichia
    coli.Science 196:210.

Volovitch, M., Drugeon, G. & Yot, P. 1978. Studies on the
    single-stranded discontinuities of the cauliflower mosaic
    virus genome. Nucl. Acids. Res. 5:2913.

STRUCTURE AND FUNCTION OF PLANT VIRUS GENOMES

Lous van Vloten-Doting, John F. Bol, Annette Nassuth,
Jan Roosien and Alberto N. Sarachu

Department of Biochemistry, State University of Leiden
P.O. Box 9505, 2300 RA Leiden, The Netherlands

STRUCTURE AND ORGANISATION OF PLANT VIRUS GENOMES

When the presently classified viruses are grouped according
to their genetic material (DNA, RNA, double-stranded, single-
stranded, plus - or minus-type) we see (Table 1) that the majority
of plant viruses has a genome consisting of single-stranded RNA of
the plus polarity (virion RNA has the same polarity as mRNA). Within this group both the structural features (number of genome parts,
structure present at the 5' or the 3' termini of the RNA) as well
as the strategy of expression are extremely diverse (Table 2)[2,3]
(and references therein).

Table 1. Genetic material of classified groups
of viruses[a]

	Plants	Animals	Bacteria
ds DNA	1	6	6
ss DNA	1	1	2
ds RNA	3	2	1
- ss RNA	1	5	0
+ ss RNA	22	6[b]	1

[a]Based on the fourth report of the international
committee on taxonomy of viruses[1].
[b]Includes also the retroviridae (DNA step in replication cycle).

437

Table 2.   Translation strategy and structural features of plant
           viruses with single-stranded plus type RNA genomes[a]

Number of genomic RNAs	Group[b]	Translation strategy[c]	Structure at 5'[d]	3'[e]
	tobamo	sub/read	cap	tRNA
	tymo	sub/read/cleav	cap	tRNA
	potex	sub/read	cap	X_{OH}
1	TCV	sub/read	?	?
	CarMV	polycistronic?	?	X_{OH}
	TNV	polycistronic?	(p)ppX	X_{OH}
	sobema	sub/read	VPg	X_{OH}
	poty	sub/read/cleav	VPg	polyA
	como	cleav	VPg	polyA
2	nepo	cleav	VPg	polyA
	tobra	sub/read	cap	X_{OH}
2 or 3	hordei	sub	cap	tRNA
	bromo	sub	cap	tRNA
3	cucumo	sub	cap	tRNA
	ilar[f]	sub/read	cap	X_{OH}

[a]For references see 2 and 3.
[b]Classified as in [1], TCV, CarMV and TNV are ungrouped viruses.
[c]sub: subgenomic mRNA; read: stop and/or readthrough; cleav: cleavage of protein, observed *in vitro*, for comoviruses also *in
vivo*.
[d]VPg: RNA linked protein.
[e]tRNA: virion RNA can be charged with amino acid.
[f]Includes also alfalfa mosaic virus (AMV)[4].

      For several multipartite viruses it has been found that the
information for structural protein(s) is separated from the information for the proteins involved in RNA replication. The latter
information is located on the large RNA of the viruses with a bipartite genome[5,6] or on the combination of the two largest RNAs of
the viruses with a tripartite genome[7,8]. The capsid of plant
viruses is built of one type of proteins. To date the only exception known are the comoviruses (bipartite genome). The capsids of
these viruses consist of an equal number of large and small subunits, which are derived from a common precursor. The information
for the structural protein(s) is mostly located close to the 3'
terminus of the genomic RNA (monopartite viruses) or on the smal-

lest genome part (bi- and tripartite viruses)[2,3].
It is remarkable that among the viruses with a multipartite genome, there is no virus with a genome part carrying exclusively the information for the capsid protein(s). When the information is expressed via subgenomic mRNA(s) the additional cistron(s) are nearly always located proximal to the 5' terminus of that genome part[2,3]. This organisation might be required for the regulation of the expression of the capsid protein(s), alternatively it could be required to prevent the loss of the information for the capsid protein.

To date the only virus coded proteins with known function(s) are the capsid protein and the genome linked protein of the poty-, como- and nepoviruses. For the other virus coded proteins we can only offer indications (and speculations), which are mainly based on genetic experiments. The fact that mutants are often thermosensitive in one host and not in other hosts[9] (and references therein) points to a tight interplay between virus coded and host coded proteins. Since plant viruses contain only a limited amount of information several virus coded proteins may be involved in more than one process.

FUNCTION(S) OF CAPSID PROTEIN

The most obvious function of capsid protein is to associate with virion RNA and to protect the RNA against nucleases. The association between the nucleic acid and the capsid protein should be (i) *stable*, both in the plant cell and during transmission of the virus by the vector (aphids, nematodes etc.); (ii) *not too rigid*, since upon entrance of a virus particle in a new host cell the RNA has to be (nearly) completely uncoated; (iii) *highly specific*, to avoid packaging of host cell RNAs. For several viruses it has been shown that the N-terminal part of the protein, which is rich in basic amino acids, is involved in the binding of the protein to the RNA[10] (and references therein). For two viruses it has been shown that there is a particular part of the RNA with a very high affinity for the coat protein. For tobacco mosaic virus (TMV, tobamogroup) it has been shown that this part is located about 1,000 nucleotides from the 3' terminus. The assembly of the virions starts at this position and than proceeds bidirectionally[11]. This method of assembly seems to be typical for TMV, and does not hold for other helical viruses[12]. For alfalfa mosaic virus (AMV, ilarvirusgroup) an RNA sequence showing a high affinity for coat protein is located at the 3' terminus of all three genomic RNAs[13] (since the subgenomic mRNA represents the 3' half of the corresponding genomic RNA, it does also contain this coat protein binding site). On the largest AMV RNA (RNA 1) there is besides the coat protein binding site discussed above, an additional coat pro-

tein binding site about halfway the RNA molecule (Zuidema *et
al.*, to be published). Since all RNAs are separately encapsidated
each RNA species should have an initiation site for assembly, this
might be the 3' terminal coat protein binding site. However, we
have to realise that the coat protein of AMV (as well as that of
other ilarviruses) fulfils an additional role early in the infection cycle.

For infectivity the genomic RNAs of the ilarviruses have to
be supplemented with coat protein or the subgenomic mRNA for coat
protein. The functional equivalence between coat protein and its
messenger rules out the possibility that coat protein is required
for penetration of the host cell. It is remarkable that although
there is no chemical or serological relationship between the coat
proteins of the different ilarviruses, nor any base sequence homology (detectable by hybridization techniques) between the RNAs of
the different viruses, the coat protein of most ilarviruses is
able to activate the genome of other ilarviruses[14].

A number of AMV mutants with *ts* defects in the early function
of the coat protein has been isolated[9]. Plants infected with mixtures of one RNA species complexed with mutant coat protein and
two RNA species complexed with wild type coat protein produced at
the non-permissive temperature hardly any virus[15]. Apparently all
three genomic RNAs have to be complexed (presumably at the 3' terminus of the RNA) with active coat protein to be infectious. This
supports the hypothesis[16] that the coat protein of the ilarviruses
is involved in the template recognition by the replicase. It is
possible that the 3' terminal coat protein binding site plays, depending on the concentration of coat protein, a role in the RNA
replication or in the virion assembly.

VIRUS CODED FUNCTIONS INVOLVED IN RNA REPLICATION

It has been disputed a long time whether plant viruses code
for a replicase (subunit) or depend completely on the RNA replicating enzyme coded for by the host. At present genetical as well as
biochemical evidence that virus coded functions are involved in
RNA replication is accumulating. As yet there is no conclusive
evidence that virus coded proteins are really (part of) the RNA
replicating enzyme.

For tobacco mosaic virus (TMV, tobamogroup) there is evidence
that at least one virus coded function is involved in the synthesis
of double-stranded RNA[17] and one in the synthesis of single-stranded RNA[18]. These functions can operate in the absence of coat protein since a TMV mutant has been described[19] which does not induce
the synthesis of coat protein.

In the viruses with a bipartite genome the information for
virus replication is located on the large RNA (tobra-[20], como-[5]
and nepogroup[6]). For como-[21] and nepoviruses this could only be

demonstrated in *in vitro* infected protoplasts, suggesting that the process is confined to the primary infected cells. The 5' terminus of the como- and nepovirus RNAs is linked to a small virus coded protein (VPg)[2,3]. In analogy to the picornaviruses it is assumed that this protein originates from the replicase. The immidiate precursor of VPg of cowpea mosaic virus (CPMV, comovirus) is a 60K protein[18] which was shown to be exclusively present in the membrane fraction, containing the viral replicase activity[22].

For some viruses with a tripartite genome the situation may be more complex. For brome mosaic virus (BVM, bromovirus) the information present in one or both of the two largest genomic RNAs (RNA 1 and/or RNA 2) is sufficient for virus RNA replication in protoplasts[7]. Moreover, a protein identical (based on comparison of tryptic digests) to the protein directed by RNA 1 *in vitro* was found to be present in a template-dependent and template-specific RNA polymerase preparation extracted from BMV infected barley[23]. These results are in contrast with the finding that *ts* mutations located on RNA 3 of cowpea chlorotic mottle virus (CCMV, another bromovirus) resulted in the loss of virus RNA synthesis at the non-permissive temperature[24]. For AMV (ilarvirus) it could be shown that a combination of the two largest nucleo-protein components (containing RNA 1 and RNA 2) did induce RNA synthesis in protoplasts[8]. However, these protoplasts contained only a small amount of plus type progeny RNA, and much more minus type RNA than protoplasts infected with the complete genome[25]. Apparently information present in the smallest genomic RNA (RNA 3) is involved in (the regulation of) plus strand RNA synthesis.

Analysis of RNA synthesized in protoplasts infected with two AMV *ts* mutants at the non-permissive temperature showed that mutations in each of the two largest RNAs resulted in a strongly reduced synthesis of minus strand RNA. It is remarkable that in both mutants mainly the minus strand RNA synthesis is affected. In all cases where minus strand RNA was detectable plus type RNA was abundantly present (Sarachu *et al.*, to be published). These results could indicate that only coat protein (together with host proteins) is responsible for transcription of minus RNA, or more likely that the products directed by both RNA 1 and RNA 2 have several functions which can be mutated independently. This is in accordance with genetic studies[9,26], which showed that the mutants located on RNA 1 as well as those located on RNA 2 fall into two complementation groups. Combinations of RNA 2 mutants belonging to the same complementation group often showed interference. This result might indicate that the RNA 2 product has two functional domains and is active in a multimeric form[26].

Our present knowledge about AMV replication has led to the model presented in Figure 1[25]. AMV nucleoproteins (represented by a single particle) are uncoated to give biological active entities of viral RNA complexed with a few coat protein subunits at the 3' termini (step 1). Proteins P1 and P2 translated from RNA 1 and

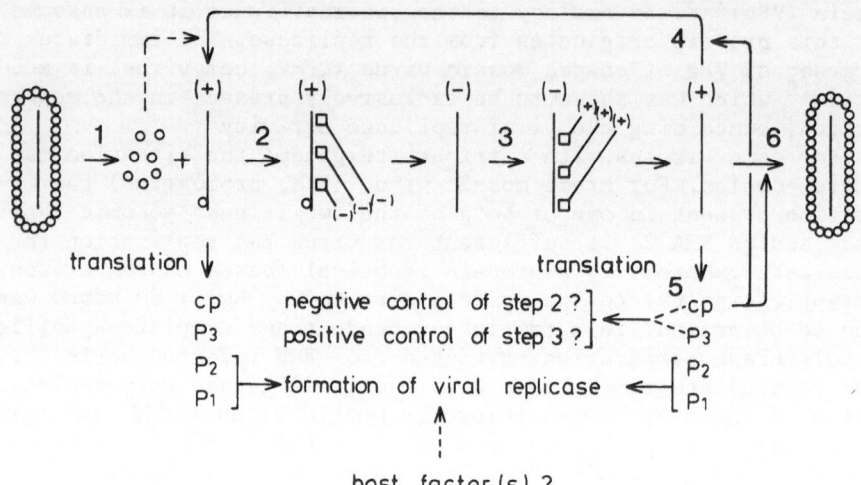

Fig. 1.   Schematic representation of the replication cycle of AMV.
          The tri-partite genome is represented by a single bar.
          Small circles and squares denote the viral coat protein
          (CP) and RNA polymerase(s), respectively. P1, P2 and P3
          are the translation products of RNAs 1, 2 and 3, respec-
          tively. The numbers 1 to 6 refer to steps in the replica-
          tion cycle discussed in the text.

RNA 2, respectively, are involved in the formation of an RNA polymerase activity ("replicase") that is able to synthesize viral
minus strand RNA (step 2) and plus strand RNA (step 3) with equal
efficiency. Probably, recognition of minus strand RNA by the enzyme does not require the binding of coat protein to the template.
Plus strand progeny RNA can enter three different routes. After
binding of a few coat protein subunits it may serve as a template
for new rounds of RNA synthesis (step 4). Translation of progeny
RNA (step 5) will yield additional replicase; a protein encoded by
RNA 3 (the coat protein?) makes the RNA synthesizing machinery
switch from the symmetric production of plus and minus strand RNA
to an asymmetric production of plus strand RNA. Later in infection
encapsidation of progeny RNA will be the major route (step 6).
Ultimately, at least 80% of the newly synthesized genomic RNA is
found in virions.

VIRUS CODED FUNCTIONS INVOLVED IN TRANSPORT THROUGH THE HOST

Transport of virus through the host is apparently a complex event in which both virus coded functions as well as host coded functions (host defense!) play a role[27]. We will distinguish cell to cell movement, which is relatively slow (6-13 μm/hr) from the more rapid transport through the vascular tissue (1.5-8 cm/hr).

Cell to Cell Movement

The finding that for several multipartite viruses part of the genome can induce detectable RNA synthesis in protoplasts but not in plants (see above), suggests that some factor required for transport of the newly synthesized RNA from the initially infected cell to the neighbouring cells is located on the missing part of the genome. Since several virus isolates lacking (functional) coat proteins are able to spread from cell to cell it is less likely that this transport factor is the coat protein itself. By this reasoning one could deduce that for the viruses with a tripartite genome the 35K protein (the only non-structural protein coded for by RNA 3) could be involved in cell to cell transport of virus.

Studies with a *ts* mutant of TMV[28] suggest that for this virus a 30K protein[29] is involved in cell to cell movement. On the genetic map this 30K protein is located at the lefthand side of the coat protein (as is the 35K protein of the viruses with a tripartite genome).

There are indications that plasmodesmata are involved in cell to cell spread of viruses. Recently it has been reported that tissue infected with the TMV *ts* mutant mentioned above and incubated at the non-permissive temperature showed much less plasmodesmata than the mutant infected tissue incubated at the permissive temperature[30]. There was no significant difference in number of plasmodesmata of mock infected or wild type TMV infected tissue incubated at the two different temperatures. This results would indicate that the mutated non-functional virus protein (30K protein?) is responsible for the disappearance of plasmodesmata.

Long Distance Movement

For a number of viruses isolates are known which can infect plants systemically as well as isolates in which the newly synthesized virus is confined to a local lesion (of several hundred cells) in the inoculated leaf. We do not know whether the confinement is due to triggering of a host response (blocking virus transport), or to the loss of a virus coded function actively involved in virus transport. The fact that from an AMV strain which could infect french beans systemically isolates inducing only local lesions were frequently observed, while the reverse (from local lesion isolate to systemic infection) has only been observed once[26], argues in favour of the latter explanation. By constructing pseudo-recombinants between an AMV strain which could move systemically and one which induced only local infections, it could be demonstrated that the information present on RNA 2 is involved in the confinement in this host[31]. This is in accordance with the results obtained with the mutants described above, which are mapped on RNA 2[26].

For other virus/host combinations similar types of experiments have been performed. The results show that the information for movement or confinement in a particular host can be located on one RNA species, while for some other host information on two or even three RNAs may act in concert[14,27,32].

VIRUS CODED FUNCTIONS INVOLVED IN TRANSPORT BY VECTORS

In the field plant viruses are mainly spread by vectors (nematodes and arthropods). Some viruses can also multiply in these vectors and should be regarded as both plant and animal viruses. Even with viruses which do not multiply in their vector the relationship with the vector is often more than just passive transport of the virus[27].

It has been shown that wounding of a plant, growing in virus containing soil, by a nematode does not result in infection. Apparently the wounding itself is not sufficient. Between nematodes and viruses there is considerable virus-vector specificity, which for nepoviruses is located on the small genome part, suggesting that the coat protein may be the vector specificity determinant[33].

Aphids can transmit virus in two different ways: non-persistent (also called stylet born), when virus survives only for a short period in the vector and is always lost following a molt, persistent (also called circulative), when virus is ingested by the insect (sometimes multiplies) and is transported to the salivary glands. Some aphids will only transmit one particular virus (mostly persistent) while some others can transmit up to 70 viruses (in a non-persistent way).

Several virus isolates of the cucumo- and ilarviruses have been kept on plants for over 20 years by mechanical inoculation. There are no reports about loss of genome parts. Apparently, the virus coded factors involved in vector transmission is (coupled to a factor) essential for virus replication in plants.

The specificity of aphid-cucumber mosaic virus (CMV, cucumovirus) relationship may be determined by coat protein, since the genome part coding for the capsid protein (and one other protein) determines the aphid transmissibility[34].

Sometimes the situation may be more complex, since in plants infected with potyviruses and caulimoviruses (a ds DNA virus) an additional factor is formed which is essential for virus transmission[27]. This so-called "helper" component, which is group specific, has in the case of the potyviruses been identified as a protein (MW 100-200 x 10^3) serologically unrelated to coat protein or inclusion protein. It is possible that this helper protein (which may be virus coded or virus induced host coded) is required for the attachment of the virus to the vector. A similar role can sometimes be played by a "helper" virus[27].

Wound tumor virus (WTV, reovirus; ds RNA) can be transmitted by and multiplied in leaf-hoppers. When virus isolates are maintained for a long time in plants some isolates loose their ability to be multiplied in leaf-hoppers. Analysis of these isolates showed that 2 (out of the 12) genome segments are missing[35]. Since these isolates replicated normally in sweet clover and had a full capacity to induce the characteristic tumours, the missing genome parts are only essential for transmission by and multiplication in leaf-hoppers, but not for replication in the plant.

VIRUS CODED FUNCTIONS INVOLVED IN MODIFICATION OF HOST CHARACTERS.

Modification of the Phenotype of the Host

The phenotype of plants may be changed drastically due to virus infection. Well known examples are the colour breaking in tulip flowers due to tulip breaking virus, and the beautiful leaf variegation of Abutilon plants due to abutilon mosaic virus. Furthermore, viruses can induce severe wilting, reduction of growth or fruit, as well as malformation of leaves etc.[27,36]. Only for very few cases we do have indications which virus coded products are involved.
Tobacco streak virus (TSV, ilarvirus) induces in tobacco a peculiar symptom, namely toothing of the leaves. The information for this characteristic is probably located on one of the two largest RNAs[37].
Severe necrosis of tomato plants was induced upon infection of plants with CMV isolates containing a satellite RNA. It could be shown that not CMV but the satellite RNA was responsible for induction of necrosis[38]. It is unknown whether a protein is involved or that it is due to the satellite RNA itself.

On the microscopic level a large number of modifications can be distinguished[27]. Virus coded proteins will certainly play a role in the induction of these modifications; however, at present very little is known. In virus infected plants inclusion bodies are often observed, sometimes they consist of semi-crystalline arrays of (empty) virus particles. However, in some cases they consist of protein not related to capsid protein. For the potyviruses it has been shown that the three types of inclusion bodies are all chemically different and virus coded[39]. The function of these inclusion bodies is unknown, they could represent aggregates

of redundant virus coded proteins. Recently[21], it was shown that the
large RNA of CPMV alone can induce cytopathic structures in cowpea
protoplasts. Apparently the development of these cytopathic structures is not linked to the accumulation of virus particles but to
the replication and expression of the large viral RNA.

Modification of the Genotype of the Host

Genetic changes are mainly caused by DNA viruses or by RNA
viruses which have a DNA step in their replication cycle. This
latter type of virus has not yet been found in plants. However, a
genetic abnormality of maize induced by barley stripe mosaic virus
(BSMV, hordeivirus) has been described. Originally it was thought
that the virus was responsible for the induction of mutations as
well as for the phenomenon called Aberrant Ratio (AR)[40]. Recently
it was shown that the latter phenomenon was due to the presence of
hitherto undetected recessive alleles[41]. In plants carrying mutations induced by infection with BSMV no viral sequences could be
detected by hybridisation assays[42], nor by "Northern blotting"
(Wienand *et al.*, to be published), suggesting that the mutations
are due to some indirect interaction between the virus and the
host genome.

PROSPECTS

In the near future we expect an accumulation of data on the
sequences of plant virus RNAs. These data may give insight in the
mechanism of virus protein expression. DNA recombinant techniques
may give the possibility to construct mutants in the test tube.
Analysis of the phenotype of these well defined mutants may give
information about virus genome expression as well as insight in
the interaction between viruses and their hosts.

REFERENCES

1. R.E.F. Matthews, Classification and nomenclature of viruses,
      Fourth report of the international committee on taxonomy
      of viruses, Intervirology 17: 1 (1982).
2. L. van Vloten-Doting, and L. Neeleman, Translation of plant
      virus RNAs, in: "Encycl. Plant. Phys." 14B, D. Boulter and
      B. Parthier, eds., Springer Verlag, Berlin, Heidelberg,
      New York, pp. 297 (1982).
3. J.W. Davies, and R. Hull, Genome expression of positive strand
      RNA viruses, J. Gen. Virol. 61: 1 (1982).
4. L. van Vloten-Doting, R.I.B. Francki, R.W. Fulton, J.M. Kaper,
      and L.C. Lane, Tricornaviridae- a proposed family of plant
      viruses with tripartite, single-stranded RNA genomes,
      Intervirology 15: 198 (1981).

5. R. Goldbach, G. Rezelman, and A. van Kammen, Independent replication and expression of B-component RNA of cowpea mosaic virus, Nature 286: 297 (1980).

6. D.J. Robinson, H. Barker, B.D. Harrison, and M.A. Mayo, Replication of RNA 1 of tomato black ring virus independently of RNA 2, J. Gen. Virol. 51: 317 (1980).

7. P. Kiberstis, L.S. Loesch-Fries, and T.C. Hall, Viral protein synthesis in barley protoplasts infected with native and fractionated brome mosaic virus RNA, Virology 112: 804 (1981).

8. A. Nassuth, F. Alblas, and J.F. Bol, Localization of genetic information involved in the replication of alfalfa mosaic virus, J. Gen. Virol. 53: 207 (1981).

9. L. van Vloten-Doting, J.A. Hasrat, E. Oosterwijk, P. van 't Sant, M.A. Schoen, and J. Roosien, Description and complementation analysis of 13 temperature sensitive mutants of alfalfa mosaic virus, J. Gen. Virol. 46: 415 (1980).

10. J.F. Bol, B. Kraal, and F.Th. Brederode, Limited proteolysis of alfalfa mosaic virus: Influence on the structural and biological function of the coat protein. Virology 58: 101 (1974).

11. G. Lebeurier, A. Nicolaeiff, and K.E. Richards, Inside-out model for self-assembly of tobacco mosaic virus, Proc. Natl. Acad. Sci. USA 74: 149 (1977).

12. M. Abou Haidar, Polar assembly of clover yellow mosaic virus, J. Gen. Virol. 57: 199 (1981).

13. E.C. Koper-Zwarthoff, F.Th. Brederode, P. Walstra, and J.F. Bol, Nucleotide sequence of the 3'-noncoding region of alfalfa mosaic virus RNA 4 and its homology with the genomic RNAs, Nucleic Acids Res. 7: 1887 (1979).

14. L. van Vloten-Doting, and E.M.J. Jaspars, Plant covirus systems: Three-component systems, in: "Comprehensive Virology" Vol. 11, H. Fraenkel-Conrat and R.R. Wagner, eds., Plenum Press, New York, London, pp. 1 (1977).

15. C.H. Smit, J. Roosien, L. van Vloten-Doting, and E.M.J. Jaspars, Evidence that alfalfa mosaic virus infection starts with three RNA-protein complexes, Virology 112: 169 (1981).

16. C.J. Houwing, and E.M.J. Jaspars, Coat protein binds to the 3'-terminal part of RNA 4 of alfalfa mosaic virus. Biochemistry 17: 2927 (1978).

17. W.O. Dawson, and J.L. White, A temperature-sensitive mutant of tobacco mosaic virus deficient in synthesis of single-stranded RNA, Virology, 93: 104 (1979).

18. W.O. Dawson, and J.L. White, Characterisation of a temperature-sensitive mutant of tobacco mosaic virus deficient in synthesis of all RNA species, Virology 90: 209 (1978).

19. S. Sarkar, and P. Smitamana, A truly coat protein-free mutant of tobacco mosaic virus, Naturwissenschaften 68: 145 (1981).

20. R.M. Lister, Functional relationships between virus-specific products of infection by viruses of the tobacco rattle type, J. Gen. Virol. 2: 43 (1968).

21. G. Rezelman, H.J. Franssen, R.W. Goldbach, T.S. Ie, and A. van Kammen, Limits to the independence of bottom component RNA of cowpea mosaic virus. J. Gen. Virol. 60: 335 (1982).

22. P. Zabel, M. Moerman, F. van Straaten, R. Goldbach, and A. van Kammen, Antibodies against the genome-linked protein VPg of cowpea mosaic virus recognize a 60,000-dalton precursor polypeptide. J. of Virology 41: 1083 (1982).

23. J.J. Bujarski, S.F. Hardy, W.A. Miller, and T.C. Hall, Use of dodecyl-β-D-maltoside in the purification and stabilization of RNA polymerase from brome mosaic virus-infected barley. Virology 119: 465 (1982).

24. W.O. Dawson, Effect of temperature-sensitive, replication-defective mutations on RNA synthesis of cowpea chlorotic mottle virus. Virology 115: 130 (1981).

25. A. Nassuth, and J.F. Bol, Altered balance of the synthesis of plus- and minus-strand RNAs induced by RNA 1 and RNA 2 of alfalfa mosaic virus in the absence of RNA 3. Virology, in press.

26. J. Roosien, J., and L. van Vloten-Doting, Complementation and interference of UV induced M ts mutants of alfalfa mosaic virus. J. Gen. Virol., in press.

27. R.E.F. Matthews, "Plant Virology", 2nd edition, Academic Press, New York, London, Toronto, Sydney, San Francisco (1981).

28. M. Nishiguchi, F. Motoyoshi, and N. Oshima, Behaviour of a temperature sensitive strain of tobacco mosaic virus in tomato leaves and protoplasts, J. Gen. Virol. 39: 53 (1978).

29. D.A. Leonard, and M. Zaitlin, A temperature-sensitive strain of tobacco mosaic virus defective in cell to cell movement generates an altered viral-coded protein, Virology 117: 416 (1982).

30. T.A. Shalla, L.J. Petersen, and M. Zaitlin, Restricted movement of a temperature-sensitive virus in tobacco leaves is associated with a reduction in numbers of plasmodesmata, J. Gen. Virol. 60: 355 (1982).

31. A. Dingjan-Versteegh, L. van Vloten-Doting, and E.M.J. Jaspars, Alfalfa mosaic virus hybrids constructed by exchanging nucleoprotein components, Virology 49: 716 (1972).

32. A.L.N. Rao, and R.I.B. Francki, Distribution of determinants for symptom production and host range on the three RNA components of cucumber mosaic virus. J. Gen. Virol. 61: 197 (1982).

33. B.D. Harrison, A.F. Murant, M.A. Mayo, and J.M. Roberts, Distribution of determinants for symptom production, host range and nematode transmissibility between the two RNA components of raspberry ringspot virus. J. Gen. Virol. 22: 233 (1974).

34. D.W. Mossop, and R.I.B. Francki, Association of RNA 3 with aphid transmission of cucumber mosaic virus. Virology 81: 177 (1977).

35. D.V.R. Reddy, and L.M. Black, Isolation and replication of mutant populations of wound tumor virions lacking certain genome segments, Virology 80: 336 (1977).
36. L. Bos, "Symptoms of Virus Diseases in Plants", 3rd edition, Pudoc, Wageningen (1978).
37. R.W. Fulton, Inheritance and recombination of strain-specific characters in tobacco streak virus, Virology 50: 810 (1972).
38. J.M. Kaper, and H.E. Waterworth, Cucumber mosaic virus associated RNA 5: Causal agent for tomato necrosis, Science 196: 429 (1977).
39. W.G. Dougherty, and E. Hiebert, Translation of potyvirus RNA in a rabbit reticulocyte lysate: Identification of nuclear inclusion proteins as products of tobacco etch virus RNA translation and cylindrical inclusion protein as a product of the poty virus genome, Virology 104: 174 (1980).
40. G.F. Sprague, and H.M. McKinney, Further evidence on the genetic behavior of AR in maize, Genetics 67: 533 (1971).
41. K.M. Brakke, R.G. Samson, and W.A. Compton, Specific Aberrant Ratio is due to recessive alleles, Genetics 99: 481 (1981).
42. D.R. Pring, Barley stripe mosaic virus infection of corn and the "aberrant ratio" genetic effect, Phytopathology 64: 64 (1974).

STRUCTURE AND EXPRESSION OF THE CAULIFLOWER MOSAIC VIRUS GENOME

H. Guilley, R.K. Dudley[*], G. Jonard, E. Balazs and
K. Richards
Laboratoire de Virologie
Institut de Biologie Moléculaire et Cellulaire
15 rue Descartes, 67000 Strasbourg, France

INTRODUCTION

Cauliflower mosaic virus (CaMV) is the type member of the caulimoviruses, the only plant viruses known to possess a double-stranded DNA genome (Shepherd, 1979). The genome of CaMV is circular and about 8000 bp in length. Two topologically distinct forms of CaMV DNA have been recognized. One such form is virion DNA, which contains three single-strand discontinuities, two in one strand and one in the other, at well defined sites on the circular DNA molecule (Hull and Howell, 1978 ; Volovitch et al., 1978). (Preparations of virion DNA also contain linear molecules but most of these are thought to arise from the circular form by adventitious breakage). The discontinuities in the circular virion DNA are not nicks or gaps but, rather, regions of sequence overlap where the 5' and 3' ends of the interrupted DNA strand overlap by 8 to 20 nucleotides (Richards et al., 1981). Consequently the DNA in the vicinity of each overlap is triple-stranded with one of the broken ends being displaced from its complementary strand by the other.

The other form of CaMV DNA (Ménissier et al., 1982 ; Olszewski et al., 1982) is supercoiled, hence lacking the inter-ruptions characteristic of virion DNA, and may be found associated with histones in a minichromosome structure in infected cells (Olszewski et al., 1982). The supercoiled form of viral DNA is undoubtedly the template for most viral RNA transcription although we will show below that the discontinuous (virion) form of DNA is probably transcribed as well.

---

[*]Present address : Chester Beatty Research Institute, London.

The complete nucleotide sequence of three strains of CaMV has been determined with about 5 % sequence difference between strains (Franck et al., 1980 ; Gardner et al., 1981 ; Balázs et al., 1982). The sequence corresponding to the β-strand, the strand possessing two discontinuities, contains six long open reading frames (ORFs) which together cover about 85 % of the genome (Figure 1). No long

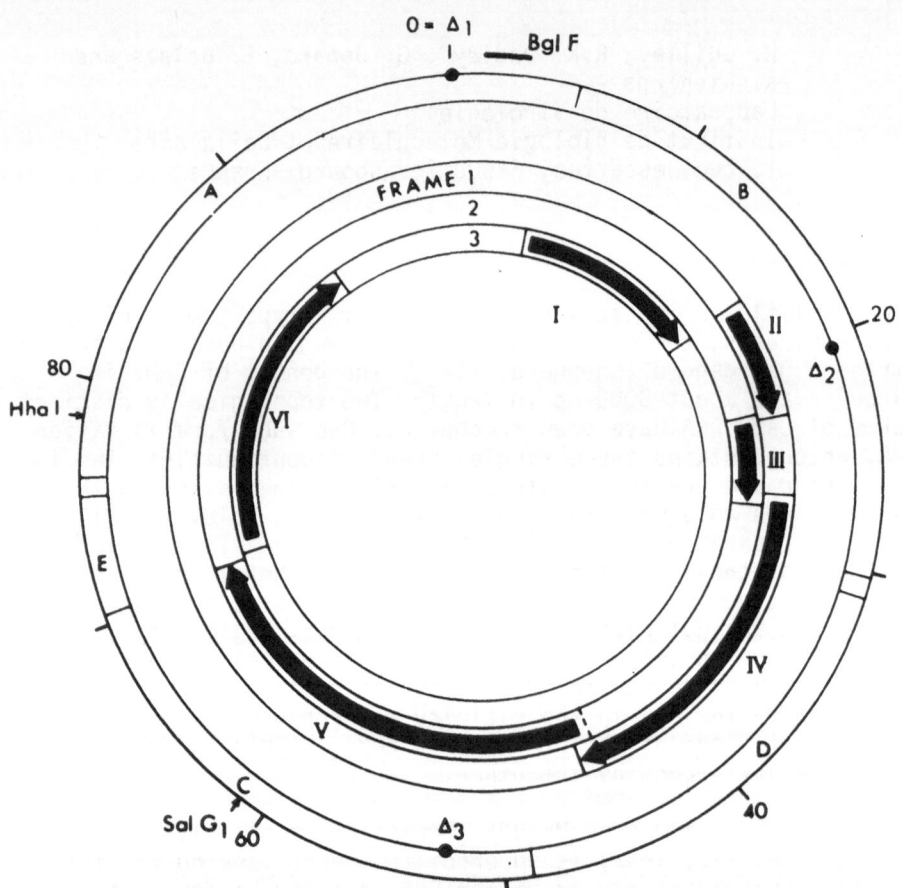

Fig. 1.   Coding regions on CaMV DNA. Inner circles give the position on the DNA α-strand of the six long open reading frames described in the text. The outer circle gives the position of Eco RI fragments A-E and the three discontinuities (Δ) in virion DNA. The position of Bgl II fragment F (see text) is indicated by a small bar alongside the outer circle.

open reading frames are present in the complementary α-strand. With two exceptions, the successive open reading frames in the coding sequence follow one another very closely, with little if any intervening noncoding sequence. The two exceptions are the short intergenic region (104 base pairs) between ORF's V and VI and the long intergenic region (1050 base pairs) separating ORF's VI and I (Figure 1). As will be seen below these two intergenic regions contain signals governing initiation and termination of CaMV transcription.

At present only two of the six ORF's detected in the DNA sequence have been assigned to known viral polypeptides. Poly-adenylated RNA isolated from CaMV-infected but not from healthy leaves directs the in vitro synthesis of a ≃ 62 kd polypeptide in the reticulocyte lysate system (Odell and Howell, 1980 ; Al Ani et al., 1980 ; Covey and Hull, 1981). A serologically cross-reacting polypeptide of similar size is the major structural protein of CaMV-induced inclusion bodies, large electron-dense structures of irregular shape (often harboring virus particles) found in the cytoplasm of virus-infected cells. Hybrid-arrested translation experiments (Odell and Howell, 1980) and N-terminal sequence analysis (Xiong et al., 1982) have shown that the in vitro 62 kd translation product is encoded by ORF VI. The mRNA directing its synthesis, termed 19 S RNA, is readily detected in the polyadenylated RNA fraction from infected tissue (see below). The viral coat protein is known to be encoded by ORF IV upon the basis of its amino acid composition (Franck et al., 1980) and the capacity of recombinant plasmids containing this coding region to direct synthesis of coat protein in bacteria (see Hahn and Shepherd, 1982). Efforts to obtain synthesis of coat protein (or translation products corresponding to the other four ORF's) in the reticulocyte lysate primed with polyadenylated or total RNA from infected tissue have been unsuccessful, suggesting that the mRNA's encoding these species are present in very low abundance or do not lend themselves to translation in the in vitro system.

CaMV transcripts

Synthesis of CaMV RNA's is assymmetric with only the α-strand being transcribed (Howell and Hull, 1978 ; Hull et al., 1979 ; Al Ani et al., 1980). Polyadenylated RNA isolated from CaMV infected leaves may be denatured by glyoxylation and electrophoresed through an agarose gel. After transfer to diazobenzyloxymethyl paper, viral RNAs are detected by hybridization with nick-translated viral DNA. Three major viral specific species, termed 35 S, 19 S and 8 S RNAs, are visible in such experiments (Figure 2). After separation from one another by sucrose gradient centrifugation the extremities of the various viral transcripts have been localized by S1 nuclease mapping and primer extension techniques (Covey et al., 1981 ; Dudley et al., 1982 ; Guilley et al., 1982). We have

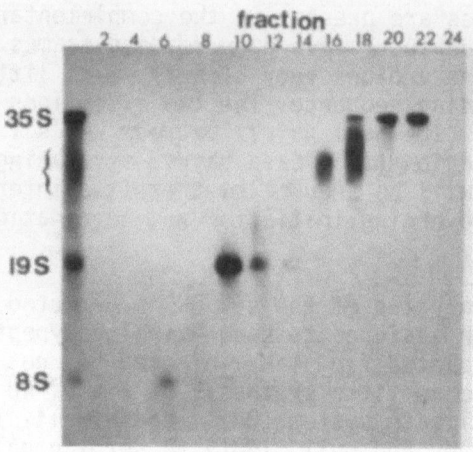

Fig. 2.   Identification of CaMV-specified polyadenylated RNAs by
           Northern hybridization and separation of the 8 S, 19 S
           and 35 S transcripts from one another by sucrose
           gradient centrifugation. Brackets indicate uncharacterized
           heterogenous RNA thought to be degradation products of
           35 S transcript.

used the S1 nuclease mapping method of Weaver and Weissmann (1979)
to show that the 35 S RNA fraction contains two transcripts. In
this technique the α-strand of a restriction fragment, 5'32p-
labelled, is hybridized with the gradient purified 35 S RNA and
nonhybridized nucleic acid is eliminated by S1 nuclease digestion.
The length of the shortened nuclease resistant radioactive DNA
fragment, as determined by polyacrylamide gel electrophoresis
under denaturing conditions, provides a measure of the distance
separating the restriction site from the 5' extremity of the
transcript. A similar procedure using 3' end labelled restriction
fragments permits the localization of 3' extremities. In preliminary experiments we found that the end-labelled α-strands of
cloned Eco RI fragments B, C, D and E were totally protected from
S1 nuclease by hybridization with gradient-purified 35 S RNA,
indicating that no RNA extremities lie within these fragments.
In the case of 5'-labelled Eco RI fragment A, the S1 nuclease
mapping procedure revealed two shortened nuclease resistant
bands (Figure 3) one major band and one minor band, corresponding
to 5' extremities at nt 7435 and Δ1, respectively. (The precise
coordinates of the extremities were established by high resolution
S1 nuclease mapping with shorter end-labelled restriction fragments).

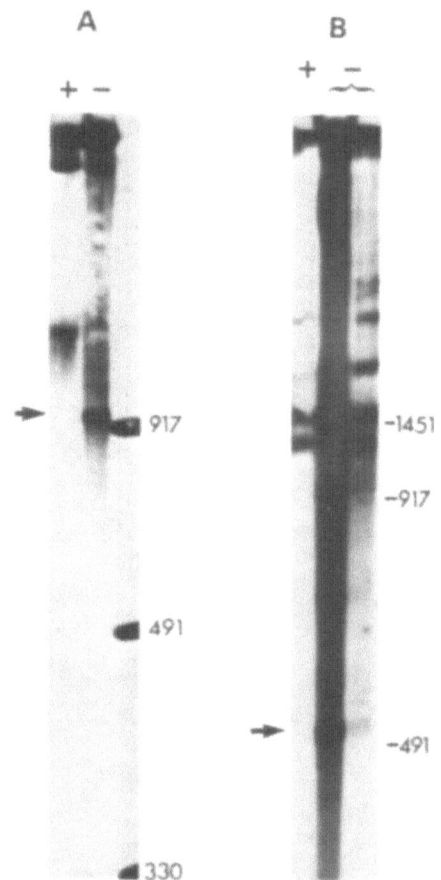

Fig. 3.   S1 nuclease mapping of 35 S RNA with 5' end-labelled (A)
           and 3' end-labelled (B) Eco RI fragment A (α-strand).
           Electrophoresis was in a denaturing 5 % polyacrylamide
           gel. Lane 1 : no S1 nuclease ; lane 2 : 300 units S1
           nuclease ; lane 3 : 600 units ; lane 4 : 3000 units.
           MAJ and MIN are the bands corresponding to the extremities
           of the 35 S maj and 35 S min species. Length markers were
           single-stranded CaMV DNA restriction fragments.

The 3' extremities of the major and minor species, termed 35 S maj
and 35 S min, respectively, were mapped with 3' end labelled Eco RI
A α-strand, to nts 7615 (35 S maj) and Δ1 (35 S min). The coordinates
of these two transcripts are indicated schematically in Figure 4.

    A noteworthy feature of the S1 mapping experiments shown in
Figure 3 is that a sizable proportion of the end-labelled restriction
fragment is totally protected by hybridization with the 35 S RNA.
This observation could signal the existence of 35 S transcripts

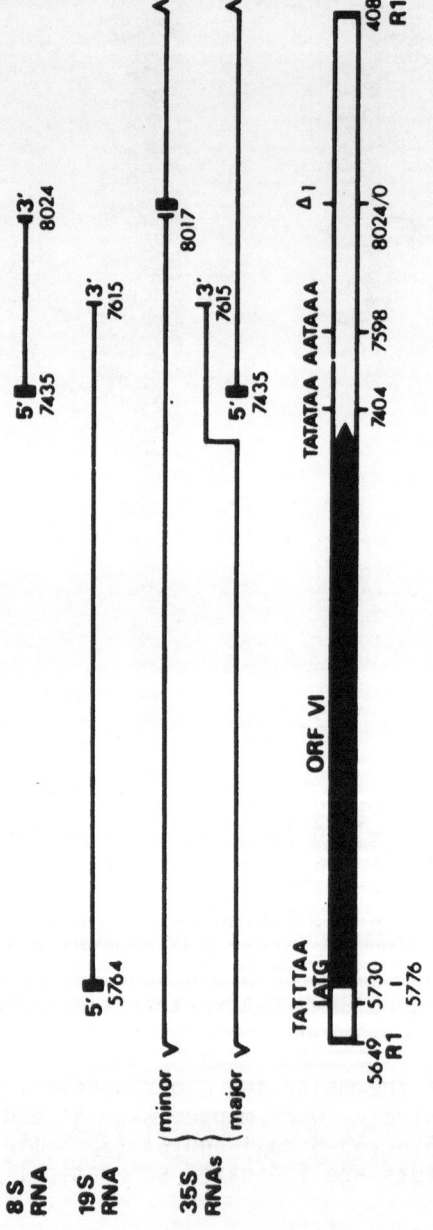

Fig. 4.   Coordinates of the four viral transcripts described in the text.

with extremities outside of Eco RI fragment A or with no extremities at all, i.e. circular molecules. To test this possibility, reverse transcriptase was used to synthesize DNA copies of 35 S RNA in the region encompassed by Eco RI fragment A. The α-strand of Bgl II fragment F (see Figure 1), 5'^{32}P-labelled, was used as primer. After annealing to 35 S RNA, the primer was extended with reverse transcriptase in the presence of actinomycin D and the cDNA products were analyzed by polyacrylamide gel electrophoresis. Two major cDNA bands migrating more slowly than the unextended primer of 129 nucleotides were visible in the gel : a major species of about 800 nucleotides and a minor species of 230 nucleotides (Figure 5). The lengths of these cDNAs correspond closely to expectation for reverse transcription terminating by run-off at nt 7435 and Δ1,

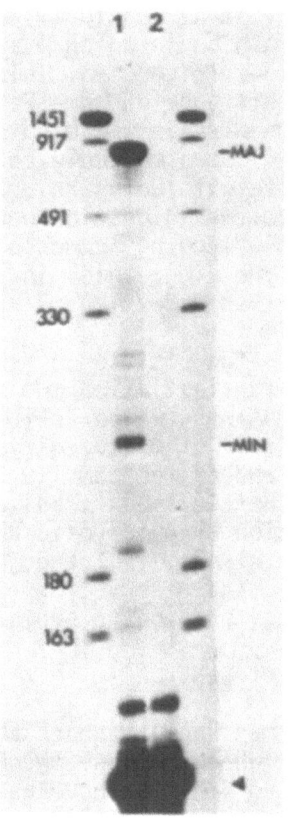

Fig. 5.   Mapping the 5' termini of 35 S RNAs by primer extension. The primer was 5'^{32}P-labelled α-strand of Bgl II F (see Figure 1). Position of unextended primer indicated by black triangle. cDNA's were synthesized with 35 S RNA fraction from CaMV infected (lane 1) and healthy (lane 2) plants. Outer lanes contain length markers.

respectively, thus substantiating our hypothesis that 35 S RNA
possesses 5' termini at these two points. Furthermore, no cDNA
longer than 800 nucleotides can be detected, arguing against the
existence of long transcripts with 5' termini outside of Eco RI
fragment A. We conclude that the protection of full-length Eco RI
fragment A by 35 S RNA is artifactual, resulting from the overlap
between the 3' and 5' terminal sequences of the 35 S maj transcript
(see below).

The Weaver and Weissmann S1 nuclease mapping technique was
also used to localize the 5' and 3' extremities of the 19 S and
8 S transcripts. The results are summarized in Figure 4. The 19 S
transcript has its 5' extremity at nucleotide 5764 in the short
intergenomic region and is 3' coterminal with 35 S maj at nt 7615
The 8 S transcript is 5' coterminal with 35 S maj RNA at nt 7435
and has its 3' extremity at Δ1. A significant feature of the 35 S
maj transcript is the fashion in which its 5' and 3' extremities
overlap by 180 nucleotides (Figure 4). This overlap is presumably
responsible for the persistance of some S1 nuclease resistant
full-length Eco RI fragment A in the mapping experiments shown
in Figure 2. A single 35 S maj molecule could sometimes loop back
upon itself and hybridize with both the 3' and 5' portions of
the DNA fragment. S1 nuclease digestion would eliminate the RNA
tail displaced by the overlapping sequence but the resulting
RNA-DNA duplex with only a single nick in the RNA chain would be
rather resistant to further digestion.

Figure 4 also shows the position of several sequence motifs
which may be important for initiation and termination of transcription. The sequence AATAAA, which is found about 20 nucleotides
upstream of the poly A tail of most eucaryotic mRNAs, occurs 18
nucleotides before the end of the CaMV 19 S and 35 S maj transcripts.
A sequence resembling the "TATA box", believed to be important for
promotion of transcription by eucaryotic RNA polymerase II
(Breathnach and Chambon, 1981), is found just upstream of the 19 S
and 35 S maj 5' termini. The observations described below suggest
that these sequences can function to promote CaMV transcription.

In vitro Transcription of CaMV DNA

The 19 S and 35 S maj RNAs are both abundant in CaMV-infected
cells leading us to ask whether these two RNAs have promotors at
their 5' termini. To study this we have used the in vitro transcription system of Manley et al. (1980) prepared from lysed HeLa
cells. Fragments of the viral genome encompassing the 5' end of
each RNA were cloned into pBR 322 and plasmid DNA prepared. The
inserted DNA was excised with the appropriate enzyme and purified
by sucrose gradient centrifugation. When purified Eco RI fragment

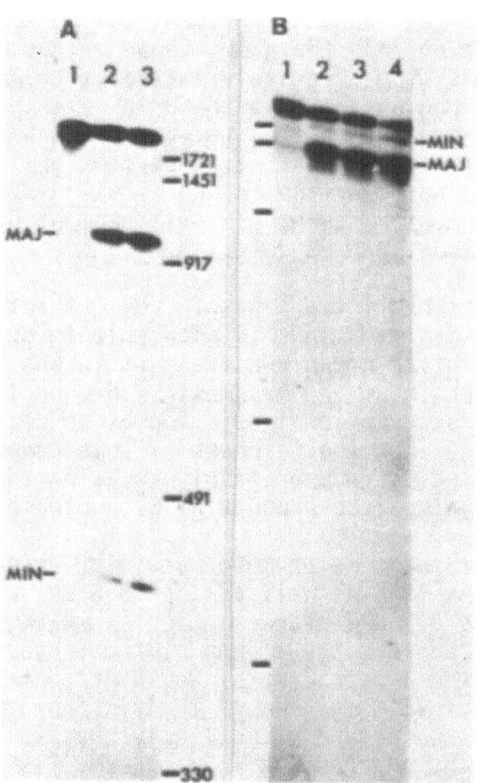

Fig. 6.   In vitro transcription of restriction fragments from
          cloned CaMV DNA containing the 35 S and 19 S promotors.
          (A) Transcription of Eco RI fragment A in the
          presence (+) or absence (-) of α-amanitin. DNA
          concentration : 80 µg/ml.
          (B) Transcription of small Sal I-Hha I fragment (see
              Figure 1) in the presence (+) or absence (-) of
              α-amanitin. DNA concentration : 80 µg/ml (lane 1)
              and 120 µg/ml (lane 2). Arrows denote run-off
              transcripts described in text.

A (Figure 1) was added to the in vitro transcription system a
transcript of approximately one kilobase was synthesized (Figure 6).
In an identical reaction containing α-amanitin (1 μg/ml) this band
was not synthesized, demonstrating that it is a product of RNA
polymerase II transcription. Presuming this band to represent a
true run-off transcript its 5' terminus must lie at about nt 7440.
The 5' end of the in vitro transcript was mapped exactly by the S1
nuclease technique and found to be identical to that of the 35 S
maj transcript, at nt 7435 (data not shown). Thus our results show
that the in vitro system accurately initiates transcription on
viral DNA in this region and that the HeLa cell RNA polymerase II
can recognize the sequence acting to promote 35 S maj RNA synthesis.
By way of contrast, the transcription start signal for 35 S min
RNA synthesis does not function in the in vitro system using
cloned Eco RI fragment A, as no run-off fragment of the predicted
size, 415 nucleotides, can be detected.

     A cloned Sal I-Hha I fragment of CaMV DNA (nts 4857-6283)
containing the 19 S 5' terminus is also able to promote α-amanitin
sensitive transcription of an RNA fragment in the in vitro system
(Figure 6). The length of the fragment, ≈ 520 nucleotides, is
consistent with transcription initiation at or near the authentic
19 S RNA 5' terminus but the weakness of this promotor in vitro
has so far prevented us from precisely locating the 5' terminus
of the in vitro synthesized product by S1 nuclease mapping.

     The fact that there is promotor activity associated with the
5' extremity of the 19 S as well as the 35 S maj transcript tends
to rule out models of CaMV transcription in which the smaller
species is processed from the 3' end of the larger RNA. The
discontinuity in the α-strand at Δ1 would present an obstacle
to transcription of 35 S maj RNA if the virion form of DNA was
the template. Thus we regard it as likely that 35 S maj RNA is
transcribed from the supercoiled form of CaMV. 19 S RNA may be
transcribed from the supercoiled DNA as well. The 8 S transcript
is 5' coterminal with 35 S maj RNA and its synthesis is presumably
controlled by the same promotor. The template for transcription,
however, is probably the interrupted virion form of DNA with
termination of synthesis occurring by run-off at the Δ1
discontinuity.

     There is no TATA box sequence near Δ1 and we have failed to
detect promotor activity associated with this region of the
uninterrupted cloned DNA used in in vitro transcription experiments.
This need not preclude transcription initiation of minor 35 S RNA
at the Δ1 discontinuity of the virion form of DNA, however, as
RNA polymerase II can bind specifically to DNA and start RNA
synthesis at a discontinuity (Lewis and Burgess, 1980 ; Cooke
et al., 1981).

An unusual characteristic of the 35 S maj transcript is the 180 nucleotide sequence overlap between its 5' and 3' extremities (Figure 4). The significance of this overlap is unknown. Likewise unknown is the mechanism by which the polymerase II molecule, during synthesis of 35 S maj RNA, passes a termination signal at the position of the 3' end of the transcript on its first circuit of transcription but stops at the same signal the second time around. One possibility is that the termination signal is leaky, in which case one would expect to find transcripts longer than 35 S, corresponding to two full circuits around the genome, as well as an RNA of 180 nucleotides, corresponding to a stop on the first passage. Leaky termination of 19 S transcript should also occur. None of these forms has been detected. A second possibility is that the signal governing transcription termination involves sequence or secondary structure on a part of the nascent transcript lying upstream of the 35 S maj 5' terminus. In these circumstances termination can occur only after the upstream region has been transcribed. A similar suggestion has been put forth to explain readthrough of the termination signal in the left-hand long terminal repeat of integrated retrovirus DNA (Benz et al., 1980).

Only one of the four transcripts described above can be readily assigned a function : the 19 S transcript, which directs synthesis of the inclusion body structural protein. The great majority of eucaryotic mRNAs are monocistronic or, if they contain several adjacent cistrons as in many plant viral RNAs, only the 5' terminal one is expressed (Kozak, 1978). Nevertheless, in view of the large amount of 35 S maj RNA which accumulates in infected cells and of our failure to detect mRNAs corresponding to the other ORF's of the CaMV genome it is reasonable to speculate that the 35 S maj transcript is responsible for synthesis of the other proteins. In this regard it is noteworthy that efforts to isolate polysomes containing 35 S maj transcript from infected plants have failed ; the 35 S transcript, as well as the 19 S transcript, is associated with the 10,000xg pellet when the cells are broken open by conventional polysome purification techniques (authors' personal observations). Perhaps the 35 S maj transcript is bound to specialized structures (the viral inclusion bodies ?) in which its internal cistrons are made accessible to proteosynthetic machinery.

In so far as the 8 S and 35 S min RNAs arise by transcription of the interrupted rather than the supercoiled form of CaMV DNA it is possible that they are without function, resulting from adventitious fixation of polymerase to the pool of interrupted virion form of DNA existing free in the infected cell (Ménissier et al., 1981). Nevertheless, we feel that an alternate hypothesis also merits consideration : that the 8 S and 35 S min transcripts, as well as the 19 S and 35 S maj species, all function in the viral infectivity cycle and that generation of the single-strand discontinuity at Δ1 represents a mechanism for switching from one class of transcript to the other.

ACKNOWLEDGEMENTS

The authors would like to thank Prof. Hirth and their other colleagues for sharing ideas and discussions and C. Kédinger for advice on in vitro transcription. This work was supported by ATP 4255 of Centre National de la Recherche Scientifique. R.K.D. was a recipient of a Royal Society Fellowship.

REFERENCES

Al Ani, R., Pfeiffer, P., Whitechurch, O., Lesot, A., Lebeurier, G., and Hirth, L., 1980, Ann. Virol. (Inst. Pasteur), 131E:33.

Balăzs, E., Guilley, H., Jonard, G., and Richards, K. E., 1982, Gene, in press.

Benz, E. W., Wydro, R. M., Nadal-Ginard, B., and Dina, D., 1980, Nature, 288:665.

Breathnach, R., and Chambon, P., 1981, Ann. Rev. Biochem., 50:349.

Cooke, R., Durand, R., Teissere, M., Penon, P., and Ricard, J., 1981, Biochem. Biophys. Res. Comm., 98:36.

Covey, S., and Hull, R., 1981, Virology, 1111:463.

Covey, S. N., Lomonossoff, G. P., and Hull, R., 1981, Nucleic Acids Res., 24:6735.

Dudley, R. K., Odell, J. T., and Howell, S. H., 1982, Virology, 117:19.

Franck, A., Guilley, H., Jonard, G., Richards, K. E., and Hirth, L., 1980, Cell, 21:285.

Gardner, R. C., Howarth, A. J., Hahn, P., Brown-Luedi, M., Shepherd, R. J., and Messing, J. C., 1981, Nucleic Acids Res., 9:2871.

Guilley, H., Dudley, R. K., Jonard, G., Balăzs, E., and Richards, K. E., 1982, Cell, in press.

Hahn, P., and Shepherd, R. J., 1982, Virology, 116:480.

Hull, R., and Howell, S. H., 1978, Virology, 86:482.

Hull, R., Covey, S. N., Stanley, J., and Davies, J. W., 1979, Nucleic Acids Res., 7:669.

Kozak, M., 1980, Cell, 22:7.

Lewis, M. K., and Burgess, R. R., 1980, J. Biol. Chem., 255:4928.

Manley, J. L., Fire, A., Cano, A., Sharp, P. A., and Gefler, M. L., 1980, Proc. Natl. Acad. Sci. USA, 77:3855.

Ménissier, J., Lebeurier, G., and Hirth, L., 1982, Virology, 117:322.

Odell, J. T., and Howell, S. H., 1980, Virology, 102:349.

Olszewski, N., Hagen, G., and Guilfoyle, T. J., 1982, Cell, 29:395.

Richards, K. E., Guilley, H., and Jonard, G., 1981, FEBS Lett., 134:67.

Shepherd, R. J., 1979, Ann. Rev. Plant Physiol., 30:405.

Volovitch, M., Drugeon, G., and Yot, P., 1978, Nucleic Acids Res., 5:2913.

Weaver, R. F., and Weissmann, C., 1979, Nucleic Acids Res., 7:1175.

Xiong, C., Muller, S., Lebeurier, G., and Hirth, L., 1982, EMBO J., in press.

HYDROXYPROLINE-RICH GLYCOPROTEINS EXTRACTED FROM THE CELL WALLS OF AERATED CARROT ROOT SLICES

J.E. Varner and J.B. Cooper

Department of Biology
Washington University
St. Louis, MO 63130, U.S.A.

Hydroxyproline containing proteins were discovered in plants in F.C. Steward's laboratory in the 1950s (reviewed in Lamport, 1965). In 1960 Dougall and Shimbayashi and Lamport and Northcote independently reported that the bulk of the bound hydroxyproline released on acid hydrolysis was present in the cell wall (reviewed in Lamport, 1965). Since then work from several laboratories has made it clear that hydroxyproline occurs in at least three kinds of proteins —all glycoproteins. These are: 1) the cell wall proteins, 2) the arabinogalactan proteins and 3) certain lectins. These are easily separated from one another and distinguished from one another by virtue of their isoelectric points, amino acid compositions and carbohydrate compositions (reviewed in Lamport, 1981). We shall briefly review the work that has brought us to our present understanding of hydroxyproline-rich glycoproteins and present work from our laboratory on the characterization of a cell wall protein that accumulates in aerated carrot slices.

Hydroxyproline constitutes one to seven percent of the total cellular amino acids of the various tissues of lupin seedlings (Steward et al. 1954), and five to 21 mole percent of the amino acids of walls isolated from various dicotolydenouss species in tissue culture (Lamport, 1965). In monocot species the levels of hydroxyproline are lower by a factor of 10 to 20 (Table I). As shown in Table II, it was evident early on that the level of peptidylhydroxyproline is developmentally regulated. Further evidence for this is shown in Table I and in Tables III through VII and in Figs. 1 through 3.

Table I. Hydroxyproline Distribution in Various Plant Parts

	percentage dry weight		
		hydroxyproline	
		Whole	Cell
Species	Part	tissue	walls
Pisum sativum	Root	n.d.	1.1
	Epicotyl	n.d.	0.58
	Cotyledon	0.2	n.d.
	Cotyledon callus	0.8	n.d.
Phaseolus vulgaris	Hypocotyl	0.36	0.88
Eruca sativa	Hypocotyl	0.08	0.17
Acer pseudoplatanus	Cambial tissues	0.05	n.d.
Citrus paradisi	pericarp	0.03	0.14
Helianthus annus	Hypocotyl	0.02	0.1
Festuca sp.	Leaf	0.02	0.05
Avena sativa	Coleoptile	0.03	0.05
Zea mais	Coleoptile and leaf	0.02	0.05
Pyrus communis	Pericarp	0.01	0.04

Adapted from LAMPORT, 1965

Table II. Peptidylhydroxyproline level is developmentally
            regulated.

	Potato tuber		Kalanchoe		
	Original	Tissue	Normal	Tumor-	Leaf
	explant	culture	leaves	bearing leaves	tumors
Hydroxyproline*	0.0	4.8	0.0	0.0	1.06

*Hydroxyproline nitrogen as % of total protein nitrogen

Adapted from STEWARD et al., 1958.

Table III.   Hydroxyproline Distribution in Tissue Cultures

Species	Percentage dry weight hydroxyproline Whole tissue	Cell Walls
Phaseolus vulgaris	0.42	2.7
Solanum tuberosum (2n)	1.42	2.4
Galega officinalis	0.97	1.6
Apium graveolens	0.74	1.5
Acer pseudoplatanus	0.5	1.2*
Daucus carota	0.5	1.1
Ginkgo biloba (2n)	0.6	1.1
Lepidium sativum	0.56	0.95
Oryza sativa	n.d.	0.2
Ginkgo biloba (n)	n.d.	0.07

*This figure has decreased very slightly since the original isolation of the culture in 1958. No significant difference has been found in the hydroxyproline content of walls isolated from cells in log phase or stationary phase, plasmolysed or unplasmolysed.

Adapted from LAMPORT, 1965

Table IV.   Amino Acid Composition of Wall Protein of Marked
Segments of Etiolated Pea Stems

The segments were isolated at the indicated times after marking.

Amino Acid	Time after Marking (h)					
	0	12	24	48	72	96
	n moles/mg wall		% of initial concn			
Hyp	19.6	149	325	371	444	424
Asp	17.7	98	141	163	141	153
Thr	12.3	99	146	170	141	179
Ser	18.0	123	186	219	213	227
Glu	14.9	88	133	153	103	134
Pro	23.6	89	124	138	125	164
Gly	18.1	102	130	165	142	159
Ala	11.8	102	132	156	136	136
Val	12.4	113	172	194	176	185
Met	1.1	91	164	209	145	191
Ile	7.3	101	149	158	134	153
Leu	13.9	94	125	142	112	123
Tyr	5.8	148	226	240	222	248
Phe	5.6	112	146	178	146	155
Lys	11.1	124	209	250	224	255
His	4.8	148	240	264	252	233
Arg	6.9	90	123	129	103	109

Adapted from KLIS, 1976.

Table V. Amino acid composition of cell wall protein from
          different parts of dark-grown bean hypocotyls.

Amino acids	Residues per 1000 in hypocotyl segments				
	Hook	0 to 10 mm	10 to 20 mm	20 to 30 mm	60 to 70 mm
Hyp	16	20	38	69	70
Asx	101	102	101	93	89
Thr	47	51	44	39	38
Ser	68	65	69	84	94
Glx	132	129	123	106	106
Pro	53	57	57	63	42
Gly	86	88	96	114	93
Ala	84	86	83	72	77
Val	54	47	53	45	48
Met	11	12	12	11	7
Ile	36	38	36	27	28
Leu	88	88	83	70	70
Tyr	27	28	26	30	30
Phe	36	37	33	27	31
His	49	36	40	48	61
Lys	66	67	72	77	90
Arg	46	39	34	25	26

Adapted from Van HOLST et al., 1980

Table VI. Protein-bound hydroxyproline (Hyp) content of the cell
           walls of successive segments (2 mm) cut basipetally
           from the root tip of Pisum sativum

Distance from root tip (mm)	Hyp (µg/ ten segments)	Hyp content (µg of Hyp/mg of cell-wall	Hyp (pg of Hyp/cell)
0–2	8.4	29.0	5.5
2–4	10.1	42.1	9.2
4–6	10.6	55.8	21.6
6–8	13.1	87.3	59.5
8–10	15.5	100.0	86.1
10–12	16.0	114.3	100.0

Adapted from VAUGHAN and CUSENS, 1974.

Table VII.   Effect of light on in situ elongation and hydroxy-
             proline content.

A 1-cm region was marked on the third internode of intact plants.
Light treatments (5 min) were given and the plants returned to
darkness for the indicated period.   The region between the marks
was measured with a vernier caliper and then excised for
hydroxyproline determination.   Each datum is the average of at
least 2 separate analyses; there were at least 15 plants in each
treatment group in each analysis.

Time h	Treatment	Final Length cm	Hydroxyproline Content (μg/g fresh wt
1	Dark		54
	Red		58
	Far red		53
	Red + Far red		54
3	Dark	1.16	54
	Red	1.08	61
	Far red	1.15	52
	Red + Far red	1.14	48
6	Dark	1.32	64
	Red	1.14	88
	Far red	1.29	68
	Red + Far red	1.28	72
12	Dark	1.39	72
	Red	1.11	86
	Far red	1.43	73
	Red + Far red	1.34	79

Adapted from PIKE, 1979

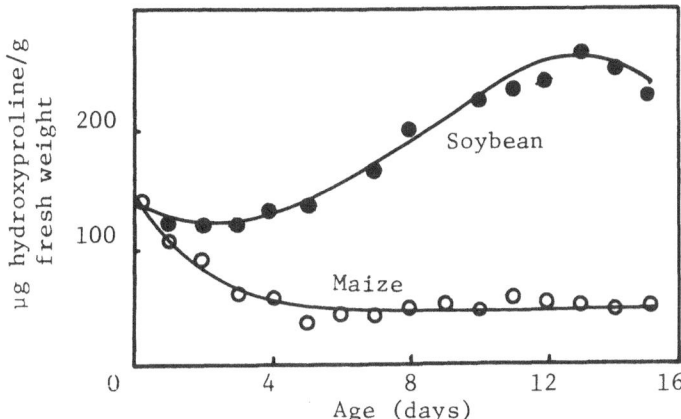

Fig. 1.   The hydroxyproline content of etiolated soybean and maize
seedlings during germination and growth (E.R. STout and G.J. Fritz
personal communication).   The hydroxyproline content was measured
in seedlings minus endosperm and seed coat.

Adapted from LAMPORT, 1965

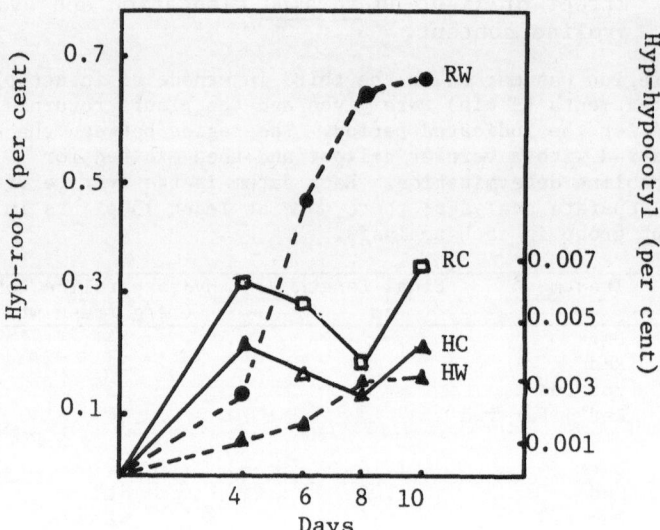

Fig. 2. Summary of alterations in hydroxyproline levels for root
wall (RW) and cytoplasm (RC) as well as hypocotyl wall (HW) and
cytoplasm (HC) from light-grown soya-bean seedlings; values are
expressed on a total root or hypocotyl dry-weight basis rather
than on a wall or cytoplasmic fraction basis.

Adapted from CHAO and DASHEK, 1973

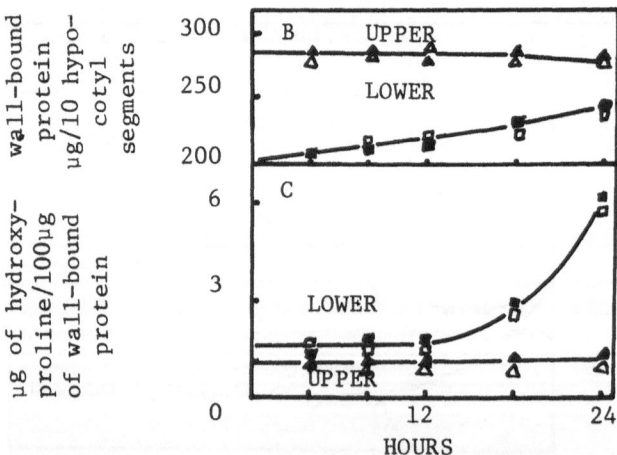

Fig. 3. Accumulation of wall dry weight, wall bound protein and
protein-bound hydroxyproline in the upper and lower halves of
intact radish hypocotyls during 24 h of growth. Open symbols =
light; filled-in symbols = dark.

Adapted from LANG, 1976

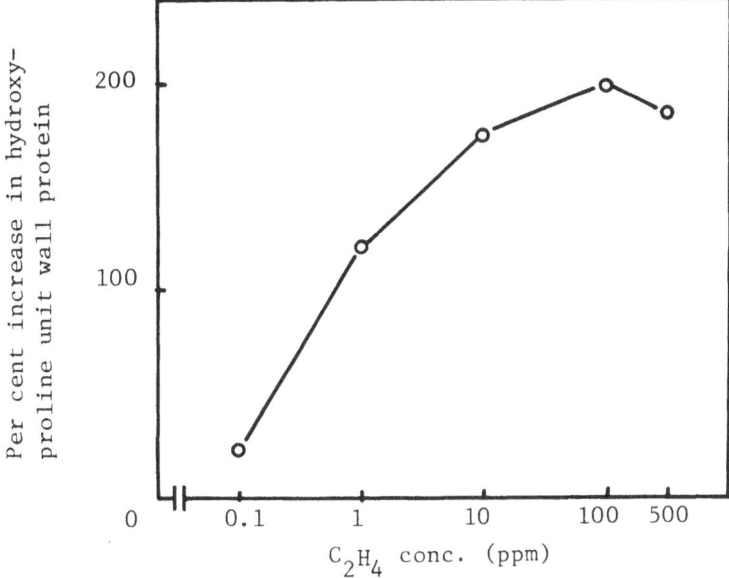

Fig. 4. Increases in wall hydroxyproline in apical tissue after 3 days in ethylene (0.1-500 ppm). Initial level of hydroxyproline at day 0 = 5.33 μg, 100 mg wall protein.

Adapted from RIDGE and OSBORNE

Also the level of peptidylhydroxyproline is regulated by the level of ethylene (Fig. 4; Toppan et al. 1982).

A developmentally regulated protein(s) of unusual composition located in the cell wall is of course of great interest with respect to a possible role in determining the form and function of a plant cell.

The initial characterization of the hydroxyproline-rich proteins of plant cell walls was accomplished by examining the peptides and glycopeptides obtained by partial hydrolysis of isolated cell walls. The amino acid sequence −ser (hyp)$_4$− occurs repetitively (Table VIII). Alkaline hydrolysis of the cell walls releases hydroxyproline arabinosides containing from one to four arabinose residues. The hydroxyproline arabinoside profile is species specific (Table IX), and developmentally modulated (Table X). The alkaline hydrolysates of the hydroxyproline-rich potato lectin has the Hyp-ara profile shown in Table XI. The hydroxy- proline glycosides obtained by alkaline hydrolysis of Chlamydomonas cell wall proteins (Table XII) and bean arabano- galactan proteins (Table XIII) are quite different from those obtained from potato lectin and from the cell wall protein.

Table VIII.   Sequences found in peptides released by wall
              hydrolysis.

- SER - (HYP)$_4$ - SER - HYP - SER (HYP)$_4$ - "TYR" - TYR - LYS
- SER - (HYP)$_4$ - SER - HYP - LYS
- SER - (HYP)$_4$ - THR - HYP - VAL - TYR - LYS
- SER - (HYP)$_4$ - LYS
- SER - (HYP)$_4$ - VAL - "TYR" - LYS - LYS

Adapted from LAMPORT, 1977

Table IX.   Hydroxyproline Arabinosides Released by Alkaline
            Hydrolysis of Cell Walls of Different Plants

Group	Species	Hydroxyproline Arabinosides				Unsubstituted Hydroxyproline
		Hyp ara$_4$[1]	Hyp ara$_3$	Hyp ara$_2$	Hyp ara	
		%				
Algae	C. vulgaris	0	4	16	6	74
Liverworts	Sphaerocarpos	1	30	26	3	40
Mosses	Funaria hygrometrica	3	8	18	8	63
Ferns	Onoclea sensibilis (leaves)	21	32	6	8	33
Horsetails	Equisetum sp. (sporophyte)	19	19	5	5	52
Gymnosperms	Ginko biloba (culture)	33	44	6	4	13
	Cupressus sp. (culture)	26	34	8	6	26
	Ephedra sp. (culture)	27	37	4	6	26
Monocotyledons	Zea mays (pericarp)	4	13	2	15	66
	Avena sativa (coleoptile)	6	11	3	5	75
	Iris kaempferi (pericarp)	10	11	3	5	71
	Allium porrum (pericarp)	6	13	3	5	73
Dicotyledons	A. pseudoplatanus (culture)	75	17	3	2	3
	Lycopersicon esulentum (culture)	52	28	4	6	10
	Convolvulus arvensis (culture)	63	22	6	4	5
	Vicia tetrasperma (culture)	52	31	5	4	8
	Pisum sativuum (root)	33	41	7	6	13

[1]Hyp ara$_4$ is hydroxyproline tetra-arabinoside.

Adapted from LAMPORT and MILLER, 1971

Table X. Hydroxyproline (Hyp) content of cell wall protein and
          arabinosylation patterns of wall-bound Hyp from
          different parts of dark-grown bean hypocotyls.

Segment of hypocotyl	Hydroxyproline wall protein %	Hydroxyproline arabinosylation (% of total wall-bound Hyp)				
		Hyp	Hyp Ara_1	Hyp Ara_2	Hyp Ara_3	Hyp Ara_4
Hook	1.6	28	2	1	22	47
10-20 mm	3.8	24	3	2	20	51
30-40 mm	6.9	18	3	3	18	58
60-70 mm	7.0	16	3	3	19	59

Adapted from VAN HOLST et al., 1980

Table XI. Hyp oligosaccharides from potato lectin

Hyp Ara	15.5%
Hyp $(Ara)_2$	23.5%
Hyp $(Ara)_3$	34.5%
Hyp $(Ara)_4$	37.3%

Adapted from ASHFORD et al., 1982

Table XII. Tentative Sequence of Hyp Oligosaccharides
            in Chlamydomonas cell wall protein

HYP-ARA-GLC-ARA-GAL-ARA
HYP-ARA-GLC-ARA-GAL
HYP-ARA-ARA-GAL-ARA
HYP-ARA-GLC-ARA
HYP-ARA-GLC
HYP-ARA

Adapted from MILLER et al. 1972

Table XIII. Hydroxyproline glycosides in bean hypocotyl
             arabinogalactan protein.

Hyp-$(Ara_{14},Gal_{22},Glc,Rha)$
Hyp-(Ara,Gal_4)
Hyp-(Ara_2,Gal),Hyp-(Ara_2,Glc)
Hyp-Ara_2
Hyp-Ara,Hyp-Gal,Hyp-Glc

Adapted from VAN HOLST and KLIS, 1981

The structures of the hydroxyproline tri- and tetra-arabinosides of potato lectin (Ashford et al. 1982) and of cell wall protein (Akiyama et al. 1980) are identical and are as follows:

$$\beta ARAf1 \to 2\beta ARAf1 \to 2\beta ARAf1 \to HYP$$
$$\alpha\text{-}ARAf1 \to 3\beta ARAf1 \to 2\beta ARAf1 \to 2\beta ARAf1 \to HYP$$

The amino acid composition of the potato lectin (Table XIV) and of Chlamydomonas cell wall protein (Table XIV) have been available for some time. The recent purification of a cell wall protein from aerated carrot slices (Stuart and Varner, 1980) and of an arabinogalactan protein from bean (Van Holst et al. 1981) allows us to compare the amino acid compositions of these hydroxy-proline-rich proteins (Table XIV). These proteins presumably have some sequences in common because of their richness in hydroxyproline and serine. Clearly each also has unique sequences

Table XIV. Amino Acid Analysis of several hydroxyproline-rich glycoproteins

	Potato Lectin[a]	Datura Lectin[b]	Carrot CWP[c]	Bean AGP[d]	Chlamydomonas CWP (2BII)[e]
HYP	16.5	14.1	50.8	26.0	15.0
ASX	4.6	7.1	0.4	3.9	10.2
THR	6.0	5.9	1.1	7.1	7.0
SER	12.9	13.5	12.8	18.2	7.8
GLX	7.4	7.1	0.4	4.5	6.0
PRO	7.4	6.5	1.1	2.6	7.1
GLY	12.9	13.5	0.7	6.5	6.9
ALA	4.6	4.1	0.6	16.2	9.0
CYS	11.5	12.9	0.0	0.6	–
VAL	0.5	5.9	3.0	3.2	6.7
MET	0.5	0.6	0.0	0.6	1.1
ILE	1.8	1.2	0.3	1.2	3.3
LEU	1.3	1.8	0.3	3.2	6.5
TYR	3.2	2.3	10.1	0.6	3.6
PHE	0.0	1.2	0.0	0.6	3.9
HIS	0.5	0.6	11.4	0.6	–
ORN	0.5	0.0	0.0	0.6	–
LYS	4.1	1.8	6.9	2.6	2.6
ARG	0.5	2.9	0.2	0.6	3.0
TRP	3.7	1.8	N.D	N.D	–

A bacterial agglutinin isolated from potatoes (Leach, 1981) has an amino acid and carbohydrate composition similar to that of the carrot cell wall protein. The carrot cell wall protein has an agglutination titer equal to that of the potato lectin.

a.   Allen et al., 1978.   d.   Van Holst, et al., 1981.
b.   Ashford et al., 1982.   e.   Roberts, 1974.
c.   Stuart and Varner, 1980.

because of the great differences in cysteine, histidine, and alanine content. Both the potato lectin (Allen et al. 1978) and the Chlamydomonas cell wall protein (Roberts, 1979) have the bulk (perhaps all) of their hydroxyproline in hydroxyproline-rich domains. In the case of the Chlamydomonas cell wall protein these domains have the conformation of a polyproline II helix (Homer and Roberts, 1979). For the carrot cell wall protein the entire molecule seems to have the polyproline II structure (Fig. 5).

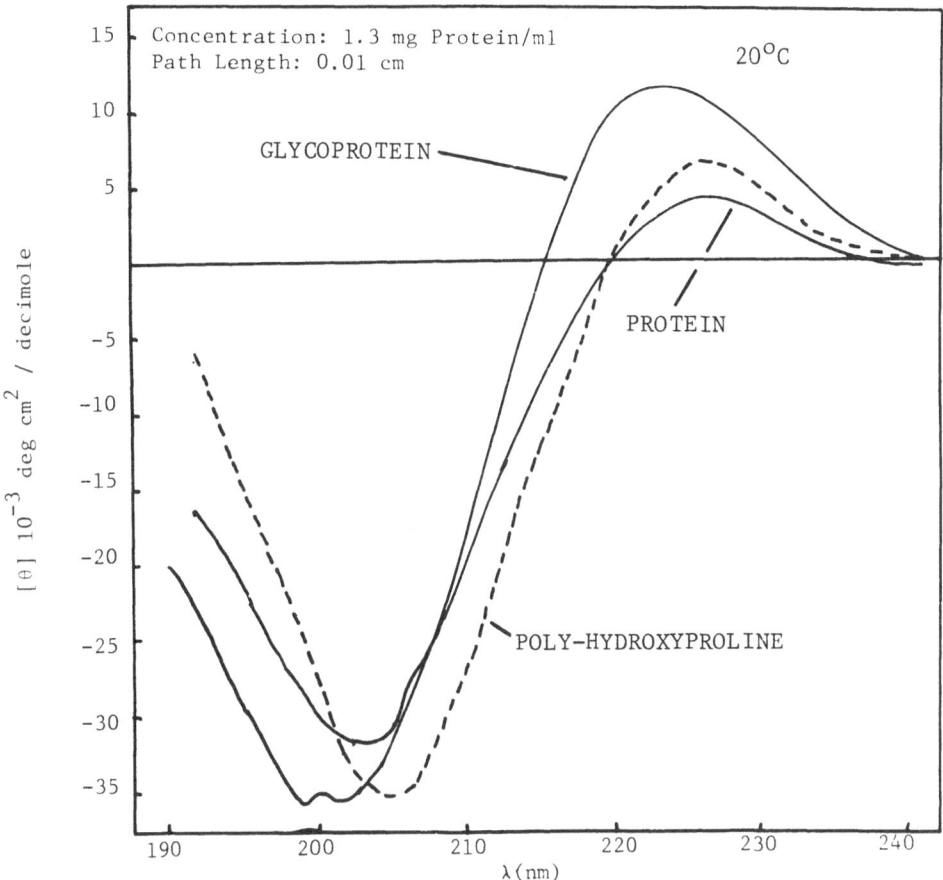

Figure 5. Circular Dichroism spectra of Carrot Cell Wall Glyco-protein, Deglycosylated Protein and Poly-hydroxyproline.

VAN HOLST, unpublished

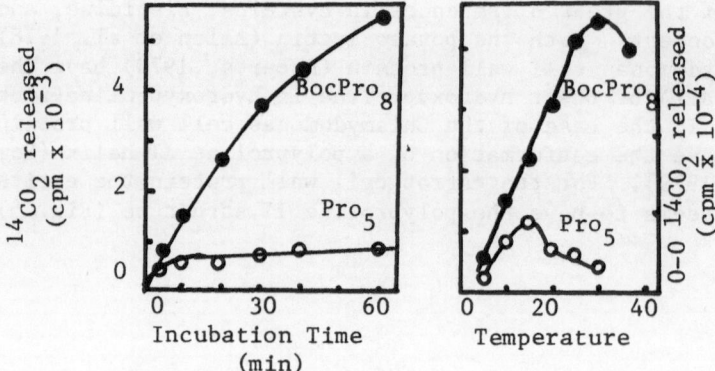

Fig. 6. Time course of prolylhydroxylase toward Pro_5 and $Boc-Pro_8$ at preincubation temperature of 0°C.

Optimum temperatures of prolyl hydroxylase toward Pro_5 and $Boc-Pro_8$. The enzyme and bovine serum albumin were preincubated with Pro_5 or $Boc-Pro_8$ at a temperature illustrated on the abscissa, and then the separately preincubated mixture containing cofactors and co-substrate was added at the same temperature.

Adapted from TANAKA et al., 1981

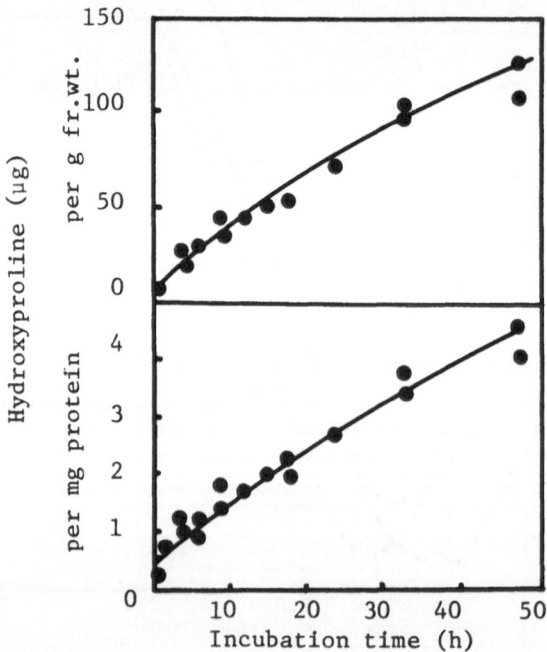

Fig. 7. Hydroxyproline accumulation during ageing in carrot disks. Tissues (2 g) aged for various periods and analysed for hydroxyproline content.

Adapted from SADAVA and CHRISPEELS, 1978

Because the plant prolylhydroxylase appears to recognize proline only when it is in the polyproline II conformation (Fig. 6) it may be that hydroxyproline residues occur only in the polyproline II conformation.

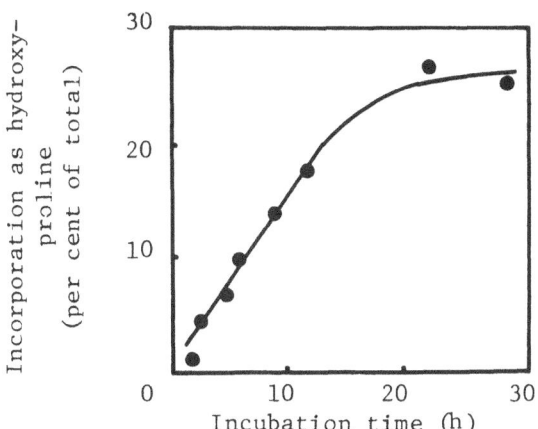

Fig. 8. Tissue (1 g) incubated and labelled with 1 μCi of [^{14}C]-proline and 100 nmol of carrier proline for 1 h. Radioactivity in peptidyl-proline and peptidyl-hydroxyproline was determined on an aliquot of the total homogenate.

Adapted from CHRISPEELS, et al., 1974

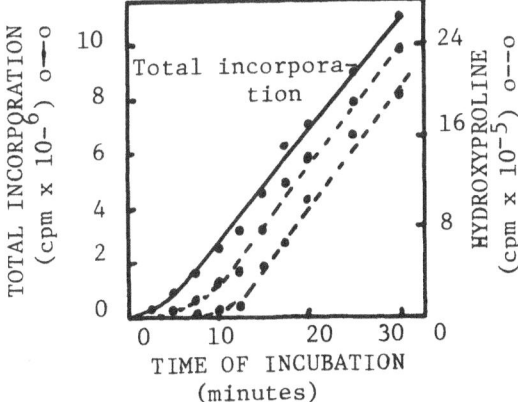

Fig. 9. Kinetics of glycosylation of peptidylhydroxyproline. Aged carrot disks were labeled with [^{14}C]proline for the times indicated and then homogenized. Aliquots of the homogenate were used to determine total incorporation, radioactivity in peptidylhydroxyproline (after acid hydrolysis of the proteins), radioactivity in peptidylhydroxyproline arabinoside (after alkaline hydrolysis of the proteins).

Adapted from CHRISPEELS and SADAVA, 1974

The aerated carrot slice is a convenient source of hydroxyproline-rich cell wall protein. Its capacity to synthesize this
protein increases during aeration (Fig. 7), and the cell wall
protein is quantitatively an important protein (Fig. 8).
Synthesis of the peptide, hydroxylation of the proline residues,
and glycosylation occur sequentially in the endoplasmic reticulum
and in the Golgi (Fig. 9). After the protein is secreted into the
cell wall space it becomes increasingly insolubilized with time.
Free radical scrubbers and antioxidants can prevent this
insolubilization (Table XV). Such insolubilization appears to be
due, at least in part, to the formation of isodityrosine (Fig. 10)
crosslinks (Fry 1982; Cooper, 1982). We presume that the "tyr" of
Table VIII is one of these crosslinks.

Table XV. Inhibitors of Cell Wall Glycoprotein Insolubilization,
          in vivo.

Compound	Concentration	% Insolubilization
Buffer Controls		100%
Mannitol	0.1 M	98
Phlorglucinol	15 μM	81
Glycine Ethyl Ester	0.25 M	78
Potassium Cyanide	2 mM	32
n-Propyl Gallate	2 mM	21
Butylated Hydroxy Anisole	1 mM	40
Butylated Hydroxy Toluene	1 mM	50
3,4,5-Trichlorophenol	0.2 mM	45
L-Ascorbate	4 mM	7

Adapted from COOPER, 1982

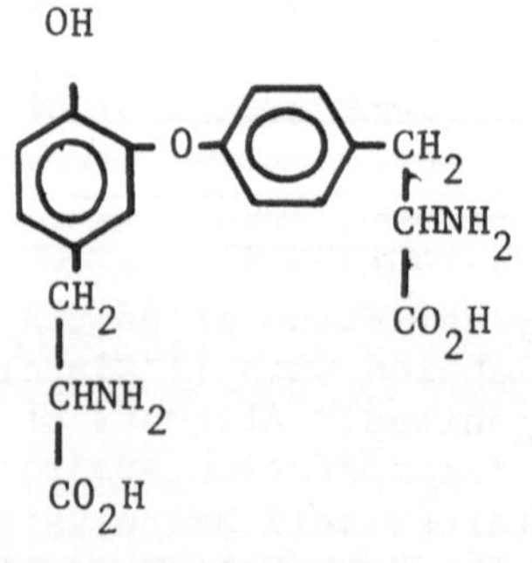

Isodityrosine

Fig. 10. Adapted from FRY, 1982.

The codons for proline are CCU, CCC, CCA, and CCG. Thus the mRNA for the proline-rich precursor of cell wall protein should have C-rich regions. Fractionation of the poly(A) RNA from aerated carrot slices on an oligo(dG) column yielded a fraction whose translation product co-migrated with the in vivo labeled proline-rich fraction (Fig. 11) and was proline-rich (Table XVI). Cloning of cDNA made from the mRNA should yield a probe of great usefulness for 1) determining the relatedness of the various hydroxyproline-rich proteins and 2) studying the control of the expression of the genes of such proteins.

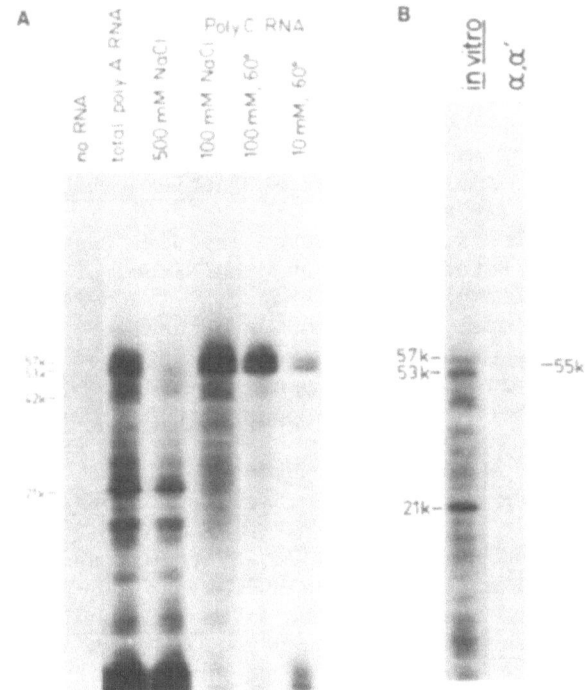

Fig. 11. In vitro translation products of poly (A) RNA from carrots analyzed by SDS-polyacrylamide gel electrophoresis. Translation was done in the presence of 3 μCi [^{3}H]-Pro. A. Translates of mRNA fractionated on oligo(dG) cellulose. B. Comparison of the mobility of in vitro translation products of poly (A) RNA (in vitro) and in vivo labeled precursor to HRGP extracted from cell walls of tissue labeled with [^{3}H]-Pro in the presence of 0.1 mM α,α'dipyridyl (α,α').

Adapted from STUART et al., 1982

Table XVI. The ^{14}C to ^{3}H ratio of trichloroacetic acid
precipitable cpm from in vitro translation products
labeled in the presence of 3 µCi ^{3}H-Glu and 0.3 µCi
^{14}C-Pro.

RNA added to reaction	^{14}C/^{3}H
No RNA (endogenous activity)	0.121
Poly A^{+} RNA	0.242
C-rich mRNA eluted at:	
100 mM NaCl, 23 C	0.471
100 mM NaCl, 60 C	0.588

Adapted from STUART et al., 1982

REFERENCES

Akiyama, Y., M. Mori and K. Kato, 1980, ^{13}C-NMR Analysis of
    Hydroxyproline Arabinosides from Nicotina tabacum. Agric.
    Biol. Chem. 44:2487-2489.
Allen, A.K., N.M. Desai, A. Neuberger and J.M. Creeth, 1978,
    Properties of Potato Lectin and the Nature of its
    Glycoprotein Linkages. Biochem. J. 171:665-674.
Ashford, D., N.N. Desai, A.K. Allen, A. Neuberger, M.A. O'Neill
    and R.R. Selvendran, 1982, Structural Studies of the
    Carbohydrate Moieties of Lectins from Potato (Solanum
    tuberosum) Tubers and Thorn-apple (Datura stramonium) Seeds.
    Biochem. J. 201:199-208.
Chao, H-Y. and W.V. Dashek, 1973, Hydroxyproline Metabolism
    during Mungbean and Soya-bean Seedling Growth. Ann. Bot.
    37:95-105.
Chrispeels, M.J. and D. Sadava, 1974, Synthesis and Secretion of
    Proteins in Plant Cells: The Hydroxyproline-rich
    Glycoprotein of the Cell Wall. In Macromolecules Regulating
    Growth and Development, E.D. Hay, T.J. King and J.
    Papaconstantinon, eds. (Academic Press, New York and London)
    pp. 131-152.
Chrispeels, M.T., D. Sadava and Y.P. Cho, 1974, Enhancement of
    Extensin Biosynthesis in Ageing Disks of Carrot Storage
    Tissue. J. Exp. Bot. 25:1157-1166.
Cooper, J.B., 1982, Techniques for studying the role of
    hydroxyproline-rich cell wall protein. Ph.D. Thesis.
    Washington University, St. Louis.
Desai, N.N., A.K. Allen and A. Neuberger, 1981, Some Properties
    of the Lectin from Datura stromonium (Thorn-apple) and the
    Nature of its Glycoprotein Linkages. Biochem. J.
    197:345-353.

Dougali, D.K. and K. Shimbayashi, 1960, Factor Affecting Growth
    of Tobacco Callus Tissue and its Incorporation of Tyrosine.
    Plant Physiol. 35:396-404.
Fry, S.C., 1982, Isodityrosine, a New Crosslinking Amino Acid
    from Plant Cell-Wall Glycoprotein. Biochem. J. 204:449-455.
Homer, R.B. and K. Roberts, 1979, Glycoprotein Conformation in
    Plant cell Walls. Planta 146:217-222.
Klis, F.M., 1976, Glycosylated Seryl Residues in Wall Protein of
    Elongating Pea Stems. Plant Physiol. 57:274-226.
Lamport, D.T.A. and D.H. Northcote, 1960, Hydroxyproline in
    Primary Cell Walls of Higher Plants. Nature 188:665-666.
Lamport, D.T.A., 1965, The Protein Component of Primary Cell
    Walls. In Advances in Botanical Research, R.D. Preston, ed.
    (Academic Press, London and New York), pp. 151-218.
Lamport, D.T.A. and D.H. Miller, 1971, Hydroxyproline
    Arabinosides in the Plant Kingdom. Plant Physiol.
    48:454-456.
Lamport, D.T.A., 1977, Structure, Biosynthesis and Significance
    of Cell Wall Glycoproteins. In Recent Advances in
    Phytochemistry, Vol. II, F.A. Loewus and V.C. Runeckles, eds.
    (Plenum Press, New York) pp. 79-115.
Lamport, D.T.A. and J.W. Catt, 1981, Glycoproteins and Enzymes
    of the Cell Wall. In Plant Carbohydrates II, Encyclopedia of
    Plant Physiology, New Series 13B, W.A. Tanner and F.A.
    Loewus, eds. (Springer-Verlag, Berlin, Heidelberg, New York)
    pp. 133-165.
Lang, W., 1976, Biosynthesis of Extensin During Normal and
    Light-Inhibited Elongation in Radish Hypocotyls. Z.
    Pflanzenphysiol. 78:228-235.
Leach, J.E., 1981, Localization, characterization, and
    quantification of a bacterial agglutinin from potatoes.
    Ph.D. Thesis. University of Wisconsin, Madison.
Miller, D.H., D.T.A. Lamport, and M. Miller, 1972, Hydroxyproline
    Heterooligosaccharides in Chlamydomonas. Science
    176:918-920.
Pike, C.S., H. Un, J.C. Lystash, and A.M. Showalter, 1979,
    Phytochrome Control of Cell Wall-bound Hydroxyproline Content
    in Etiolated Pea Epicotyls. Plant Physiol. 63:444-449.
Ridge, I., and D.J. Osborne, 1970, Hydroxyproline and
    Peroxidases in Cell Walls of Pisum sativum: Regulation by
    Ethylene. J. Exp. Bot. 21:843-856.
Roberts, K., 1974, Crystalline Glycoprotein Cell Walls of Algae:
    Their Structure, Composition and Assembly. Phil. Trans. R.
    Soc. Lond. B 268:129-146.
Roberts, K., 1979, Hydroxyproline--It's Assymetric Distribution
    in a Cell Wall glycoprotein. Planta 146:275-280.
Sadava, D., and M.J. Chrispeels, 1978, Synthesis and Secretion
    of Cell Wall Glycoprotein in Carrot Root Discs. In
    Biochemistry in Wounded Plant Tissues. G. Kahl, ed. (Walter
    de Grupter, Berlin, New York) pp. 85-102.

Steward, F.C., R.H. Wetmore, J.F. Thompson and J.P. Nitsch, 1954,
    A Quantitative Chromatographic Study of Nitrogenous
    Components of Shoot Apices. Am. J. Bot. 41:123-134.
Steward, F.C., J.F. Thompson, and J.K. Pollard, 1958, Contrasts
    in the nitrogenous Composition of Rapidly Growing and
    Non-growing Plant Tissues. J. Exp. Bot. 25:1-10.
Stuart, D.A. and J.E. Varner, 1980, Purification and
    Characterization of a Salt-extractable Hydroxyproline-Rich
    Glycoprotein from Aerated Carrot Discs. Plant Physiol.
    66:787-792.
Stuart, D.A., T.J. Mozer and J.E. Varner, 1982, Cytosine-Rich
    Messenger RNA from Carrot Root Discs. Biochem. Biophys. Res.
    Comm. 105:582-588.
Tanaka, M., K. Sato, and T. Uchida, 1981, Plant Prolyl
    Hydroxylase Recognizes Poly(L-proline)II Helix. J. Biol.
    Chem. 256:11397-11400.
Toppan, A., D. Roby and M-T Esquerre-Tugaye, 1982, Cell Surfaces
    in Plant-Microorganism Interactions. III. In Vivo Effect of
    Ethylene on Hydroxyproline-Rich Glycoprotein Accumulation in
    the Cell Wall of Diseased Plants. Plant Physiol. 70:82-86.
VanHolst, G.J., F.M. Klis, F. Bouman and D. Stegwee, 1980,
    Changing Cell-Wall Compositions in Hypocotyls of Dark-grown
    Bean Seedlings. Planta 149:209-212.
VanHolst, G.J., F.M. Klis, P.J.M. deWildt, C.A.M. Hazenberg, J.
    Buijs and D. Stegwee, 1981, Arabinogalactan Protein from a
    Crude Cell Organelle Fraction of Phaseolus vulgaris L. Plant
    Physiol. 68:910-913.
VanHolst, G.J. and F.M. Klis, 1981, Hydroxyproline Glycosides in
    Secretory Arabinogalactan-Protein of Phaseolus vulgaris L.
    Plant Physiol. 68:979-980.
Vaughan, D., and E. Cusens, 1974, Protein-Bound Hydroxyproline
    and Root Extension Growth. Biochem. Soc. Trans. 2:124-126.

TOBACCO REVISITED: A FOOD FROM TOBACCO FRACTION 1 PROTEIN PLUS A SAFER SMOKING MATERIAL

S.G. Wildman*

Leaf Proteins, Inc.
P.O. Box 28023
Raleigh, North Carolina

A little more than a decade ago, Fraction 1 protein was crystallized for the first time. The discovery was made by Nobumaro Kawashima (1), working in my laboratory at UCLA while on study leave from the Japan Tobacco Monopoly Corporation. The first crystals were obtained from tobacco leaves by a complicated, laborious, and not always successful procedure. Gradually, as often happens following a significant scientific discovery, a simpler and more reliable method evolved. Today, Fraction 1 protein is crystallized from tobacco plants by a process which may be the ultimate in simplicity for obtaining any crystalline protein in high yield. Moreover, the process of crystallizing Fraction 1 protein from tobacco leaves a residue which can be converted into a relatively safe smoking tobacco. With the costs of its production at least partially covered by the economic value of the smoking tobacco, crystalline Fraction 1 protein may be an economical as well as a highly nutritious human food. In the ensuing paragraphs, I will attempt to trace the events which have brought crystalline Fraction 1 protein from its beginning as a laboratory curiosity to its present position as a potential agricultural commodity of major economic and humanitarian importance.

Laboratory Studies of Tobacco Fraction 1 Protein

An immediate consequence of the crystallization of Fraction 1 protein by Kawashima was the opportunity to study

*Permanent address: 1024 Centinela Ave., Santa Monica, CA 90403.

new facets of the physico-chemical and enzymatic properties of
this, the world's most abundant enzyme. At that time, skepti-
cism still lingered as to whether ribulose-1-5-bisphosphate
carboxylase (rubisco) and the 0.5 million dalton Fraction 1
protein were identical macromolecules.   Using the crystalline
product, we were able to demonstrate that the rubisco activity
was inseparable from the Fraction 1 protein.

In the time-honored tradition of enzymology, the first
method of crystallizing Fraction 1 protein used elaborate pre-
cautions to keep extracts and solutions cold at all times.
Chlorophyll-bearing particulate matter was removed from a green
juice extracted from tobacco leaves and the now yellow juice
passed through a G-25 Sephadex column to remove phenols, the
protein   in   the   eluate   concentrated   with $(NH_4)_2SO_4$,   and
the Fraction 1 protein separated from other proteins by G-200
Sephadex chromatography followed by DEAE-cellulose chromatography.   Crystallization of Fraction 1 protein would often, but
not always, occur after the highly purified protein was dialyzed
using a collodion bag.

Subsequent work by Kawashima and Shalini Singh (2) showed
that the rubisco activity withstood heating to $50^{o}C$ for some
minutes and was stable at ambient temperature for prolonged
periods.   Less than two years after the original discovery,
Singh, Pak-hoo Chan, and Katsuhiro Sakano (3) were able to
dispense entirely with the Sephadex G-200 and DEAE-cellulose
chromatography steps as well as the need to work in a cold room.
Fraction 1 protein crystallized after the soluble proteins of
tobacco leaves were passed through the G-25 Sephadex column at
room temperature, followed by threefold concentration of the
eluted proteins by pressurized membrane filtration and dialysis
with collodion bags.

What astonished me was the quantity of crystalline protein
obtained with the greatly simplified procedure.   A mg of
Fraction 1 protein was regularly obtained from each gm of fresh
tobacco leaves.   Previous estimation by analytical centrifugation had placed the amount of Fraction 1 protein in tobacco
leaves at about 10 mg per gm of leaf tissue. Thus it appeared
that about 10 percent of the Fraction 1 protein was being
recovered as crystals.

Our high recovery rate of Fraction 1 protein led me to
estimate what these yields would be under field conditions. We
had been growing rather large quantities of tobacco plants in a
greenhouse under conditions which partially simulated those in
the field with regard to biomass yields. Extrapolating from our
experience as greenhouse tobacco farmers, we concluded that as
much as 125 kg of crystalline Fraction 1 protein could be

obtained per ha of tobacco plants in one growing season. Protein production of such magnitude is comparable to that obtained from soybean crops. With this information in hand, it appeared worthwhile to pursue the potential of tobacco Fraction 1 protein as a food.

Fraction 1 Protein as Food. During the second World War, N.W. Pirie of the Rothamstead Experiment Station in England commenced work on the use of concentrated leaf proteins as a possible means of alleviating protein scarcities caused by the war. With the conclusion of hostilities, his work expanded because of its promise of enriching, at low cost, protein-deficient diets which are the norm in the Third World. His proteins were basically the coagulated product obtained by heating a green extract of leaves. Different kinds of plants were used as a source of green juice, one favorite being alfalfa. While the proteins so prepared were comparable in nutritional quality to animal proteins, their texture, odor, color and taste rendered them unacceptable as food. It is an irony of human nature that tradition of how a food should appear, taste, feel or smell can be much more decisive than nutritional quality in determining our willingness to eat the food.

Using our simplified laboratory process, we were able to make enough crystalline protein at óne time to demonstrate that Fraction 1 protein, either as crystals or after drying the crystals by lyophilization, had no taste and no odor. Thus, crystalline Fraction 1 protein might overcome the organoleptic problems that previously had negated acceptance of leaf proteins as human food. I tried to bring this idea to the attention of the scientific community by submitting a manuscript for publication in an American journal, to no avail. One reviewer, who kept confusing wet and dry weights, reported to the editor that my projections seemed more like the product of Hollywood than of nearby Westwood where UCLA is located. Undaunted, I submitted another manucript to an English journal, this one hopefully clarified with regard to wet and dry weights. Again it was rejected, this time because the reviewer warned: "I don't feel the idea is feasible or sensible....There is no reason to think that plain, green leaf protein made in simple equipment won't do."

Thanks to sympathetic friends, I had the opportunity to present the idea of tobacco for food before small groups of scientists. One of these scientists, Dr. Richard Lowe, then at the University of Kentucky, developed a further simplification of the process for obtaining crystalline Fraction 1 protein (4). Lowe found that when tobacco leaves were homogenized in their own internal liquid to produce a concentrated green

juice, passage of the soluble proteins through the G-25
Sephadex column substituted for dialysis. Crystallization of
Fraction 1 protein frequently occurred even before all of the
proteins had been eluted from the void space of the column.

With Lowe's simplification, we were able to increase our
production of crystalline Fraction 1 protein to as much as 10 g
per day. This opened up a new opportunity, that of demonstrating the nutritional quality of the protein by animal feeding
tests. My friend and authority on nutrition at UCLA, Prof.
Rosalind Alfin-Slater, advised me that a minimum of one pound
of protein would be needed for even the most elementary test
using rats. The National Science Foundation provided funding
for the production of the protein, thanks in large part to the
enthusiasm of the Program Director, Dr. H. T. Huang. Dr.
Prachuab Kwanyuen organized a system for growing tobacco plants
in our greenhouse and obtaining crystalline Fraction 1 protein
from them at a rate sufficient to produce the required pound of
protein in about four months. Dr. Alfin-Slater, who was on
sabbatical leave, arranged to have the feeding tests performed
by another eminent nutritionist, Dr. B. H. Ershoff, in his
private Institute for Nutritional Studies. As shown in Table 1,
tobacco Fraction 1 protein proved to be slightly superior in
nutritional quality to casein, which is the standard for
judging other proteins.

In his long experience, Ershoff had not encountered
another plant protein with such excellent nutritional
properties that was also tasteless and odorless. It was 1979
and I had reached the age of mandatory retirement at UCLA.
Ershoff persuaded me to join him and a few others in forming
Leaf Proteins, Inc. to exploit the commercial possibility of
using tobacco Fraction 1 protein for human food.

Leaf Proteins, Inc. was able to obtain the services of
Kwanyuen, who proceeded to discover what is probably the
ultimate simplification of the process for obtaining
crystalline Fraction 1 protein. He found that when tobacco
plants were homogenized in their own juice, the residue
separated from the green juice and the chlorophyll-bearing
particulate matter removed from the latter, crystals of
Fraction 1 protein appear in the solution after it has been
allowed to stand a few hours.

Smoking Tobacco Product. In contemplating crystallization
of Fraction 1 protein on a commercial scale, it became evident
that the largest part of the tobacco plants was going to end up
as a residue of questionable value. Prof. Shuh-Ji Sheen of the
University of Kentucky came up with the idea and a technique

for turning this residue into a smoking material. He extracted
the green pigments and water from the residue with an organic
solvent, leaving a white, fibrous material. After the proteins
had been removed from the green juice, he concentrated the
remaining water-soluble, low molecular weight compounds and,
after some further treatment, added the concentrated material
to the fibers to give them the appearance, odor and flavor of
cigarette tobacco.

The possibility of obtaining a smoking material as a
byproduct of Fraction 1 protein production greatly improved the
prospects of Leaf Proteins, Inc. World demand for smoking
tobacco is enormous. Last year, about four trillion (4 x
10^{12}) cigarettes were manufactured worldwide. In the United
States alone, nearly one million metric tons of tobacco were
consumed, requiring almost one million acres of land to grow
the tobacco plants. While concern for health has caused a per
capita reduction in cigarette consumption, total production of
cigarettes continues to increase as world population increases.
The probable trend in the foreseeable future is not a decrease
in world tobacco production, but rather an increase in efforts
to make cigarette smoking less harmful. The Leaf Proteins
smoking product would be a beneficiary of this trend.

Table 2 compares the protein, nicotine and tar composition
of two kinds of conventional tobacco, making up about 90 percent
of American cigarettes, to the composition of cigarette tobacco
prepared from the residue of Fraction 1 protein production by
the Sheen method. Proteins, which have been implicated as a
significant source of hazardous volatile compounds in cigarette
smoke, are lower in the residue than in conventional tobacco.
Lipoidal materials, which contribute to tar in cigarette smoke,
are removed from the residue by organic solvent extraction.
Nicotine in the residue is reduced because the plants used for
Fraction 1 protein manufacture are harvested when still young,
before they have had time to accumulate much alkaloid. Thus
the components of tobacco known or suspected to have adverse
effects on cigarette smokers are considerably reduced in the
Leaf Proteins smoking tobacco.

Pilot Plant Production of Fraction 1 Protein

To summarize our laboratory studies, two lines of
development occurred during the decade following Kawashima's
discovery of crystalline Fraction 1 protein. First, a series
of simplifications was introduced into the process for obtaining crystalline Fraction 1 protein from tobacco, culminating in
the elimination of costly Sephadex columns and making it
possible to produce Fraction 1 protein on a large scale at

reasonable cost. Second, a series of tests was done to
establish that both crystalline Fraction 1 protein and the
smoking material made from the residue of the tobacco plant
were of potential economic value. The next step, taken by Leaf
Proteins Inc. in 1980, was to scale up the laboratory procedure
to the size necessary for commercial evaluation of the products.
This was accomplished by designing and building a pilot plant
in Lucama, North Carolina, in the heart of the tobacco-growing
country.

Transformation of a laboratory procedure into a pilot
plant process is not without its traumas, as we soon learned.
Two exasperating years went by before the pilot plant worked
properly. Perfection of the process was attributable in large
part to the imagination and first-hand attention of John Becker,
General Manager of Leaf Proteins, Inc. Although trained as a
lawyer and public accountant, he has a remarkable flair for
engineering.

Pilot Plant Process. Recently harvested, aerial portions
of tobacco plants are conveyed at about 30 kg per min to a
disintegrator, which reduces them to a fine pulp. A solution
of sodium metabisulfite in water is sprayed on the plants as
they drop into the disintegrator. The pulp is pumped to a
rotary press where a very fine screen retains a residue of cell
walls but allows escape of a concentrated green juice at a rate
of about 4 liters per min. The residue is continually
discharged at one end of the press. The green juice is pumped
through an exchanger where it is heated momentarily to 50°C
and cooled to ambient temperature before passing through a
centrifuge which removes all of the starch and about 80 percent
of the chlorophyll-bearing particular matter, discharging them
as a green sludge. The remaining chlorophyll-bearing particles
are removed by vacuum filtration of the juice, utilizing a
rotary drum type filter whose surface is covered with a thick
layer of diatomaceous earth. The filtered brown juice is sent
to a storage tank where crystallization of Fraction 1 protein
occurs. Some hours later, the Fraction 1 protein crystals are
collected. The mother liquor is then acidified to precipitate
Fraction 2 proteins. After the Fraction 2 proteins are
collected, the low molecular weight solids in the deproteinized
liquid are concentrated by evaporation of the water.

Pilot Plant Yields. Several different cultivars of tobacco
at different stages of growth have given the consistent yield
of products shown in Table 2. Our latest method results in
quantitative recovery of Fraction 1 protein as crystals and
provides Fraction 2 proteins free from Fraction 1 protein.

Prof. R. C. Long of North Carolina State University has been studying ways to maximize the biomass of tobacco during the rather short (five month) growing season in North Carolina. Table 4 shows Prof. Long's yields for different cultivars growing under conditions of close spacing. Combining the data in Tables 3 and 4, we see that annual production in North Carolina would be in the range of 400 kg of dry crystalline Fraction 1 protein per ha accompanied by 200 kg of dry Fraction 2 proteins, about 600 kg of insoluble proteins, and about 5 metric tons of dry residue.

The yields of total protein from various crops are compared with the yield from tobacco in Table 5. It is evident that tobacco, processed by the Leaf Proteins, Inc. process, is an oustandingly efficient source of protein wherever space to grow crops is limited.

Uses for Products. Crystalline Fraction 1 protein from tobacco has properties which make it useful as a source of protein for patients with various medical problems as well as for the general population. When washed free of sodium and potassium, the crystals can be used in patients with kidney failure to meet their amino acid requirement without taxing the kidney's inability to eliminate cations. Crystalline Fraction 1 protein can also be used to meet the entire protein requirement of patients with acute gastrointestinal problems or patients recovering from surgery of the alimentary canal.

Because they are odorless and tasteless, crystals of Fraction 1 protein can be added to food without altering its organoleptic qualities. As a dry, almost white powder, it can be mixed with cereal grains to improve their protein content. It can be used as a milk replacer in countries which lack a dairy industry. In its soluble form, tobacco Fraction 1 protein can be added to soft drinks, removing them from the junk food category.

Crystals of Fraction 1 protein contain about 80 percent water in their structure. The protein in crystals exposed to cations at neutral pH will dissolve to form solutions containing more than 10 percent protein, about the same as the concentration of albumin in the white of eggs. Like albumin, Fraction 1 protein irreversibly gels when heated above 80°C. It therefore has functional properties, such as "heat set," similar to egg albumin or casein which are widely used throughout the packaged food industry. We frequently demonstrate the nutritional use of our Fraction 1 protein by preparing a whipped topping from the powder which tastes and looks like a whipped cream.

Fraction 2 proteins have an essential amino acid composition that qualifies them, like Fraction 1 protein, for use as supplements to improve the nutritional quality of other foods.

The insoluble proteins from tobacco are similar in essential amino acid composition to the protein in soybean after extraction of the oil. Insoluble soybean protein has been modified to permit its widespread use in the food industry; presumably the insoluble proteins of tobacco could follow the same course of development.

The deproteinized residue may be converted by the Sheen method to a cigarette tobacco low in tar and nicotine. This smoking product can be used alone or combined with conventional tobacco to provide a safer cigarette.

Prospects for Commercialization. In the United States, where land to grow crops is plentiful and there is a surplus of food, the commercialization of tobacco as a combined source of food and of safer smoking tobacco rests entirely on economic considerations. Tobacco Fraction 1 protein must compete in the marketplace with casein and albumin, which currently sell for about $4 per kg. Similarly, the smoking tobacco made from the residue must compete with conventional tobacco, also currently selling for about $4 per kg. The success of the pilot plant operation is making it possible to obtain realistic estimates of the costs of producing Fraction 1 protein and its byproduct smoking tobacco. Further investment will depend on how these costs compare with those of the competing products.

In countries such as China where population is dense and space to grow crops is at a premium, commercialization of tobacco as a food crop may be accelerated as an efficient use of land. China now grows 0.5 million ha of tobacco with a yield of about 2 metric tons of dried smoking material per ha. Using close-grown tobacco and the Sheen processing method, China could produce the same amount of cigarette tobacco on around 200,000 ha, releasing 300,000 ha for vital food crops. In addition to a less harmful smoking tobacco, Fraction 1 protein amounting to 80,000 metric tons would be obtained -- enough to meet the total annual protein requirement for nearly 5 million inhabitants. Added to this would be substantial amounts of Fraction 2 and insoluble protein of nutritional value.

REFERENCES

1.   N. Kawashima and S. G. Wildman, Studies on Fraction 1
            protein . I. Effects of crystallization of Fraction
            1 protein from tobacco on ribulose diphosphate

Table 1. Comparative Effects of Casein and Crystalline Fraction 1 Protein from Tobacco. (a) Average Weight Increment and (b) Protein Efficiency Ratio (PER) in 10 Rats. Adapted from ref. (5).

Days of Feeding	(a) Weight Increment				(b) Protein Efficiency Ratio			
Days of Feeding	7	14	21	28	7	14	21	28
ANRC Casein	18.1	51.5	80.8	114.4	2.73	3.07	2.88	2.82
Tobacco Fr1	25.7	65.2	100.6	139.1	3.40	3.44	3.10	3.01

Table 2. Protein, Nicotine and Tar Content (in Percentage of
Dry Weight) of Deproteinized Tobacco and Conventional Cigarette
Tobacco.

	Protein	Nicotine	Tar*
Conventional flue-cured tobacco, variety NC 95	2.25	2.0	6.77
Deproteinized NC 95	1.84	0.6	0.70
Conventional burley tobacco, variety KY 14	4.15	3.0	6.07
Deproteinized KY 14	3.00	0.7	0.82

*Estimated from amount of solids extracted by petroleum ether.

Table 3. Dry Weight of Products Obtained from Tobacco (in kg.
per metric ton of Fresh Biomass).

Product	Yield
Crystalline Fr. 1 protein	4
Fraction 2 Proteins	2
Insoluble Proteins + Starch	19*
Residue	46

* Weight of starch fluctuates

Table 4.   Annual Fresh Biomass Yield of Various Cultivars of Tobacco in North Carolina in 1981.

Cultivar	Yield metric ton per ha
TI 174	146
MD 609	139
TI 560	139
C 347	130
TI 1112	130
LA 53	129
G 28	116
TI 785	113

Table 5.   Dry Weight of Harvest and Total Protein Yield (in metric tons/ha) for Various Crops.

Crop	Harvest	Total Protein
Tobacco	10	1.2
Alfalfa*	6.5	0.71
Soybeans*	1.8	0.64
Corn*	5.1	0.46
Wheat*	2.3	0.27

*Data from ref. (6).

carboxylase activity, Biochim. Biophys. Acta. 229: 240 (1971).

2. N. Kawashima, S. Singh, and S. G. Wildman, Reversible cold inactivation and heat reactivation of RuDP carboxylase activity of crystalline tobacco Fraction 1 protein, Biochem. Biophys. Res. Comm. 42: 664 (1971).

3. P. H. Chan, K. Sakano, S. Singh, and S. G. Wildman, Crystalline Fraction 1 protein: preparation in large yield, Science 276: 1145 (1972).

4. R. Lowe, Large scale crystallization of Fraction 1 protein from tobacco by a simplified procedure, FEBS Letters 78:98 (1977).

5. B. H. Ershoff, S. G. Wildman and P. Kwanyuen, Biological evalution of crystalline Fraction 1 protein from tobacco, Proc. Soc. Exper. Biol. Med. 157:626 (1978).

6. D. Pimentel, W. Dritschilo, J. Krummel, and J. Kutzman, Energy and land constraints in food protein production, Science 190:754 (1975).

493